Touch & Movement
Palpation *and*
Kinesiology *for*
Massage Therapists

Julie Goodwin

CENGAGE
Learning™

Australia • Brazil • Japan • Korea • Mexico • Singapore • Spain • United Kingdom • United States

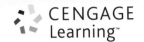

Touch & Movement: Palpation and Kinesiology for Massage Therapists
Julie Goodwin

President, Milady: Dawn Gerrain

Director of Content and Business Development:
Sandra Bruce

Acquisitions Editor: Martine Edwards

Associate Acquisitions Editor: Philip Mandl

Product Manager: Maria Moffre-Barnes

Editorial Assistant: Sarah Prediletto

Director of Marketing and Training:
Gerard McAvey

Senior Production Director: Wendy A. Troeger

Production Manager: Sherondra Thedford

Senior Content Project Manager:
Nina Tucciarelli

Technology Director: Sandy Charette

Senior Art Director: Benjamin Gleeksman

For product information and technology assistance, contact us at
Professional & Career Group Customer Support, 1-800-648-7450

For permission to use material from this text or product,
submit all requests online at **cengage.com/permissions**
Further permissions questions can be emailed to
permissionrequest@cengage.com

Library of Congress Control Number: 2011937627

ISBN-13: 978-1-4390-5657-8

ISBN-10: 1-4390-5657-9

Milady
5 Maxwell Drive
Clifton Park, NY 12065-2919
USA

Cengage Learning products are represented in Canada by Nelson Education, Ltd.

For your lifelong learning solutions, visit **milady.cengage.com**

Visit our corporate website at **cengage.com**

Printed in the United States of America
1 2 3 4 5 XX 15 14 13 12 11

BRIEF CONTENTS

CONTENTS

CHAPTER 2   Posture Assessment   55

CHAPTER 3   Gait Assessment   101

CHAPTER 4   Deconstructing Complex Movements   129

CHAPTER 5   The Science of Palpation   161

CHAPTER 6   The Art of Palpation   187

CHAPTER 8   Palpating Superficial Muscles on the Axial Skeleton   303

CHAPTER 9   Palpating Superficial Muscles on the Extremities   337

CHAPTER 10 Palpating Deeper Muscles and Muscle Groups 397

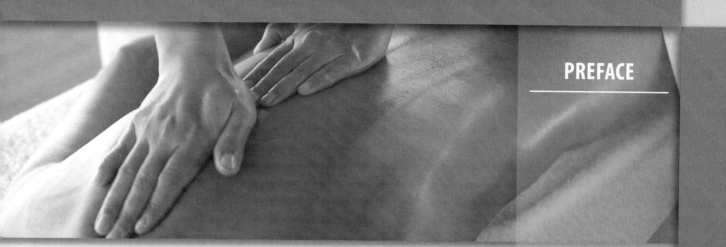

Welcome to *Touch & Movement: Palpation and Kinesiology for Massage Therapists,* and congratulations on your decision to pursue a career in the healing arts. This book is designed for massage therapy students enrolled in 500- to 1,200-hour training programs and for bodywork professionals who want to enhance both their palpation skills and their understanding of the elements of movement. *Touch & Movement: Palpation and Kinesiology for Massage Therapists* arises from the belief that effective therapeutic massage treatment begins with assessment of a client's structures and movements—posture, gait, and palpation—and that massage therapy students, their instructors, and massage professionals will benefit from a textbook dedicated to these techniques.

How Touch & Movement: Palpation and Kinesiology for Massage Therapists *differs from other textbooks*

This book stands apart from other palpation and kinesiology textbooks in the following ways:

- It is conceived and written by a massage therapist with several decades of experience in private practice and more than a decade as an instructor in hands-on classrooms, bringing a depth of experience that is reflected on every page.
- The way it is organized takes the reader through the client assessment process step-by-step: comprehensive assessments of posture and gait are performed, and complex movements are deconstructed to reveal patterns of strain or injury. Using the results of those assessments, structures are targeted for palpation and a treatment plan is created.
- The assessments examine the structure and movement of the body from the core toward the extremities. This focus acknowledges that movement is initiated within the core and is expressed by the extremities. Immediate application of hands-on techniques is emphasized through experiential exercises tied to each new skill. Information about potential dysfunctions and pathologies assures safe and effective assessment of client postures and gait.

- The reader learns to systematically deconstruct common complex movements to assess patterns of strain and injury efficiently and effectively and practices deconstructing complex movements, choosing from more than 30 illustrated examples, in a monitored classroom setting.
- A layered approach to palpation of the body's structures is presented, beginning with palpation of deeper structures, specific bony landmarks, and important connective tissue structures, before muscles are palpated for assessment. This focus acknowledges the dynamic interaction of somatic structures and that effective palpation includes palpation of all structures that are safely palpable.
- The Four-Step Palpation Protocol provides the reader with a template for palpating any body structure safely, comfortably, and effectively, while also learning how to utilize assessment results for treatment planning. The extensive instruction in palpation technique, including focus on endangerment zones, cautions, and contraindications, and an array of palpation practice exercises encourage true mastery of palpation for assessment.

Organization of Touch & Movement: Palpation and Kinesiology for Massage Therapists

This book is organized to mirror the sequence in which a massage therapist performs assessments:

- Chapter 1, Introduction to Palpation and Kinesiology, grounds the reader in the fundamentals of joint and muscle anatomy and physiology for application in assessments of structures and movements.
- Chapter 2, Posture Assessment, describes the anatomical and physiological bases of posture and gait and potential dysfunctions and pathologies and provides techniques for posture and gait assessment.
- Chapter 3, Gait Assessment, outlines the components of common complex movements, describes movement dysfunctions that may produce injuries, and presents techniques for deconstructing complex movements.
- Chapter 4, Deconstructing Complex Movements, applies techniques learned in Chapter 3 to the deconstruction of more than 30 complex movements that may produce patterns of strain or injuries commonly experienced among massage therapy clients.
- Chapter 5, The Science of Palpation, introduces the reader to the fundamentals of the anatomy and physiology of palpation, describes pathologies that may interfere with palpation, and links the concepts presented to the experience of palpation.
- Chapter 6, The Art of Palpation, presents the fundamentals of palpation technique and teaches the reader how to apply them to palpation of body structures.

- Chapter 7, Palpating Bony Landmarks and Fascial Structures, orients the reader to the bony landmarks and fascial structures in the human body and presents techniques for palpating these structures.
- Chapter 8, Palpating Superficial Muscles on the Axial Skeleton, describes the attachments and actions of the superficial muscles of the axial skeleton and applies the palpation techniques learned in prior chapters to systematic palpation of each muscle.
- Chapter 9, Palpating Superficial Muscles of the Extremities, describes the attachments and actions of the superficial muscles of the extremities and applies the palpation techniques learned in prior chapters to systematic palpation of each muscle.
- Chapter 10, Palpating Deeper Muscles and Muscle Groups, describes the attachments and actions of deeper muscles and applies the palpation techniques learned in prior chapters to systematic palpation of these muscles and muscle groups.

Learning Strategies included in Touch & Movement: Palpation and Kinesiology for Massage Therapists

Touching anatomical structures as we learn their names and functions enhances our understanding of them. We also benefit from moving our bodies to apply new techniques and we reinforce learning by working in groups. *Touch & Movement: Palpation and Kinesiology for Massage Therapists* addresses the needs of tactile, kinesthetic learners, who value interactive exercises:

- *Learning enhancement activities* encourage readers to take concepts and techniques outside the classroom and into their daily lives, reinforcing that learning opportunities abound for the massage therapist in any setting, at any time.
- *In the Treatment Room* sections bring real-life experiences to the reader for discussion and application in practice sessions.
- *Here's a Tip* and *Did You Know?* boxes scattered throughout chapters introduce readers to extra material that adds to the chapter's basic information and helps it to come alive.
- *Lab activities* at the end of each chapter allow readers to immediately use touch and movement as they experience the concepts described and apply the techniques outlined in the preceding text.
- *Case profiles* at the end of each chapter encourage group discussion of the assessment and treatment issues contained within each case.

Touch & Movement: Palpation and Kinesiology for Massage Therapists also offers features for traditional and visual learners that provide for easy organization of study time:

- *Learning objectives* at the beginning of each chapter alert the reader to the organization of the chapter's material.

- *Chapter introductions* prepare the reader for each chapter's contents.
- *Chapter summaries* reinforce each chapter's major concepts and alert the reader to upcoming topics and tasks.
- *A running glossary* throughout each chapter defines new terms as they are introduced, to allow the reader to easily review the terms within the body of the chapter.
- *Pronunciation keys and word derivations* for terms as they are introduced allow the reader to understand new terms and organize them for review, as well as enabling the massage therapist to use the terms as appropriate in speech.
- *Study questions* at the end of each chapter prepare the reader to be tested on the chapter's material and encourage critical thinking and application of the chapter's concepts.
- *Full color photos, illustrations, and tables* help the reader with visual representations of concepts and technique to reinforce them for classroom application.
- *Appendices* provide topics both for review of information and for reference.

Touch & Movement: Palpation and Kinesiology for Massage Therapists is presented in a classroom-friendly form that allows the reader to easily apply its instructions in the hands-on classroom and to consult its contents in the treatment room, for years to come.

ABOUT THE AUTHOR

Julie Goodwin, BA, LMT, graduated from Kent State University and the Desert Institute of the Healing Arts. Her career as a massage therapist and bodywork instructor has spanned more than 20 years. Ms. Goodwin has been an instructor in academic and technique classes at Desert Institute of the Healing Arts, Providence Institute, Cortiva Institute-Tucson, and the Arizona School of Acupuncture and Oriental Medicine.

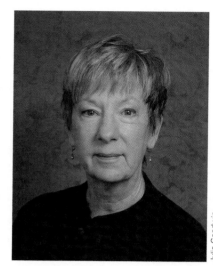

Julie Goodwin

ACKNOWLEDGEMENTS

The creation of any textbook requires collaboration, and I have been blessed with help and support throughout the process of bringing *Touch & Movement: Palpation and Kinesiology for Massage Therapists* to life. I am forever grateful to Philip Mandl, for his gentle and informed guidance, and also to Maria Moffre-Lynch; to Martine Edwards, for her creativity and energy; and to Maria Hebert, whose belief in this project from the start was an inspiration. The input from reviewers who invested their time and expertise has been invaluable and is greatly appreciated.

As a massage therapist and bodywork instructor, I have depended on the support of mentors and colleagues: Margaret Avery Moon has been a mentor, role model, and friend, whose contributions to the profession have benefitted thousands and without whom my own accomplishments would not have been possible. Deanna Sylvester has provided me with a "teaching home" and with unqualified support. My students and teaching colleagues at Desert Institute of the Healing Arts, Cortiva Institute-Tucson, The Providence Institute, and Arizona School of Acupuncture and Oriental Medicine have shared their knowledge and experience and have provided me with much motivation and material.

Finally, I thank my daughter, Jennifer Baldwin, LMT, and my grandchildren, Katt, Nick, Naomi, and Gabriel, for their never ending encouragement and patience and for making sure I maintain balance in my life.

REVIEWERS

Thank you to the many reviewers, for their assistance, comments, and expertise in reviewing the developing text.

Lurana S. Bain, LMT
Elgin Community College, Elgin, IL

Monique Blaize , LMT
Cooper City, FL

Sheila DeCora, DC, LMT
Los Angeles, CA

Jonathan Drummy, LMT
Saco, ME

Kathleen Hunt, LMT
Methuen, MA

Monica Roseberry, MA, CMT
Clayton, CA

EXTENSIVE TEACHING AND LEARNING PACKAGE

Several ancillary materials accompany *Touch & Movement: Palpation and Kinesiology for Massage Therapists,* 1st Edition. These materials are designed to support student learning and to provide massage instructors with everything they need to teach the concepts in the core textbook successfully.

Touch & Movement: Palpation and Kinesiology for Massage Therapists, 1st Edition, COURSE MANAGEMENT GUIDE cd-ROM

Theory and Practice of Therapeutic Massage Course Management Guide CD-ROM is an innovative instructor resource to support customized instruction. This CD-ROM for instructors contains excellent tools, including

- A detailed lesson plan for each chapter in the book.
- Learning-reinforcement ideas or activities that can be implemented in the massage therapy classroom.
- The answers to the review questions for the *Theory and Practice of Therapeutic Massage Workbook.*
- A *Computerized Test Bank* of over 1,100 questions in multiple-choice, matching, and short-answer format, as well as the accompanying answers, organized by chapter, which can be used to generate quizzes and tests.
- A searchable *Image Library* containing all of the color drawings and figures from *Theory and Practice of Therapeutic Massage,* 5th Edition, to incorporate into lectures, electronic presentations, assignments, testing, and handouts.
- *Student Skills Proficiency Checklists* in both ready-to-use PDF and customizable MS Word formats.
- A *Customizable Syllabus* that instructors can tailor to meet individual teaching styles and course objectives, complete with course schedules, assignments, grading options, paper topics, and more.

The Course Management Guide CD-ROM is a powerful resource that instructors can customize to fit their individual instructional goals.

Touch & Movement: Palpation and Kinesiology for Massage Therapists, 1st Edition, Instructor-Support Slides

(Microsoft® PowerPoint® Presentation)

The MS PowerPoint® presentation created to accompany the CD-ROM makes lesson plans simple, yet effective. Complete with *Touch & Movement: Palpation and Kinesiology for Massage Therapists,* 1st Edition, with photos and art, this CD-ROM has ready-to-use, chapter-by-chapter presentations that will help to engage students' attention and keep their interest through its varied color schemes and styles. Instructors can use it as is or adapt it to their own classrooms by, for example, importing photos they have taken, changing the graphics, or adding more slides.

Touch & Movement: Palpation and Kinesiology for Massage Therapists, 1st Edition, CourseMate:

Touch & Movement: Palpation and Kinesiology for Massage Therapists, 1st Edition, *CourseMate* is a unique tool for both students and instructors.

- Students and instructors benefit from easy access to interactive teaching and learning tools: quizzes, flashcards, videos, and more.
- Students also benefit from an integrated eBook, complete with highlighting and notetaking capabilities and an interactive glossary, which can be used to complement or substitute for the textbook.
- Instructors have access to the Engagement Tracker, which monitors student preparation and engagement in the text and allows instructors to easily plan intervention for students at risk of failing the course.

Introduction to Palpation and Kinesiology

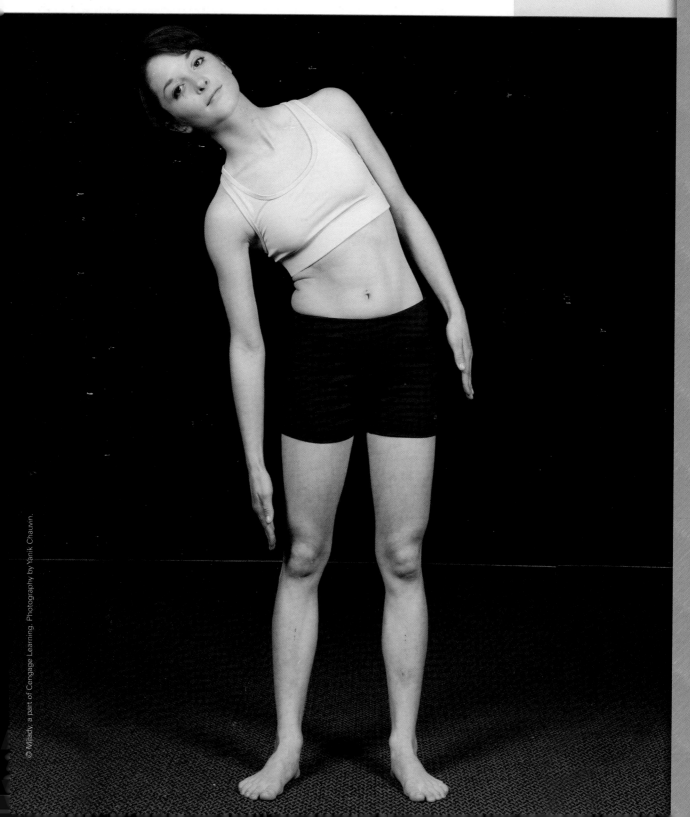

CHAPTER OUTLINE

- TOUCH AND MOVEMENT IN CLIENT ASSESSMENT
- JOINT STRUCTURE AND FUNCTION
- JOINT ACTIONS
- MUSCLE STRUCTURE AND FUNCTION
- TYPES OF MUSCLE CONTRACTION
- ROLES MUSCLES CAN PLAY
- MUSCLE NAMES

LEARNING OBJECTIVES

- Understand the role of posture and gait analysis and palpation in client assessment.
- Describe the structures and functions of the types of joints in the human body.
- Describe joint actions and movements through the planes of the body.
- Compare gross and microscopic muscle anatomy, and describe the role of the neuromuscular junction, neurotransmitters, and motor units in skeletal muscle contraction.
- Describe the types of skeletal muscle contraction and the roles skeletal muscles play in human movement by action, function, shape, and fiber type.
- Understand how the names of muscles divulge their shapes, locations, and actions.

INTRODUCTION

Assessment is the first service you perform for your client. The value of your subsequent treatment depends on the effectiveness of your initial assessments. Effective assessment is rooted in your thorough understanding of anatomy and physiology and the application of these principles, along with your ability to transfer this understanding to your client's structures. Chapter 1, Introduction to Palpation and Kinesiology, describes the importance of assessment in treatment planning and prepares you to apply the principles of joint and muscle actions to assessments of posture and gait and to palpation of body structures.

TOUCH AND MOVEMENT IN CLIENT ASSESSMENT

Palpation (palpare=to touch)

the application of purposeful, focused touch for therapeutic assessment of somatic structures.

Assessing your client's structure and movements, as shown in Figure 1–1, is a critical aspect of treatment planning. Complete assessment of the form and condition of your client's bones, joints and muscles of her body, and how she stands, walks, and moves her body, utilizes the concepts of palpation and kinesiology. **Palpation** [pal-PAY-shun] is the application of purposeful, focused touch for therapeutic assessment of somatic structures. **Kinesiology** [kih-nee-see-AHL-uh-jee] is the study of the anatomy and mechanics of human movements, including how an individual stands, sits, and walks. Your skills in visual observation and touch, along with evaluation of the results of your assessments, create an information bank for treatment planning.

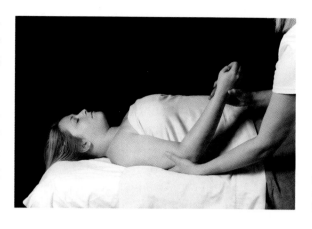

FIGURE 1–1 Assessing your client's structures and movement is crucial in treatment planning.

© Milady, a part of Cengage Learning. Photography by Yanik Chauvin.

Massage therapists use assessment tools in treatment planning for many reasons:

- To enrich our understanding of the body. A thorough foundation in human anatomy is fundamental to massage therapy education. It is essential, moreover, to be able to transfer the knowledge from textbooks about the human body to an actual client on your treatment table. No two bodies are alike, and no body in the real world looks exactly like the skeleton that hangs in most classrooms. Most of us have 24 vertebrae, but the vertebrae of a client who is 6 feet (183 cm) tall only loosely resemble those of the client who is 5 feet (152 cm) tall. Only by actively palpating individual structures, bony landmarks, muscles, and other soft tissue on as many bodies as possible can you begin to comprehend human anatomy.
- To compare contralateral structures—those on the other side of the body. While it may be interesting to compare Sophie's Rhomboid to Sam's Rhomboid, it is usually more useful for treatment planning to compare Sophie's right rhomboid to Sophie's left one. Assessing structures *on both sides of the body* is strongly recommended.
- To identify **endangerment sites**, which are discrete, specific areas on the body that indicate potential injury to the client because of their location near or over major nerves, blood vessels, or vital organs. Because each human body is unique, the anterior triangle of one client's neck may be smaller or more lateral than that of another's. Visual assessment and gentle, exploratory palpation can ensure that you are working in safe territory.
- To direct your choice of treatment modality. Assessment findings are a roadmap for the selection of the appropriate treatment modality: Is your client's skin healthy enough for myofascial work? Are her joints stable enough for complete passive or assisted range of motion? Is a temperature variance in her extremities a signal to avoid circulatory work on that area of the body?

Assessment begins with observing and measuring your client's body at rest—her posture—and in motion—her gait.

Kinesiology (kinesis-=movement)

the study of the anatomy and mechanics of human movements, large and small.

Endangerment site

a discrete, specific area on the body that may cause potential injury to the client because of its location near or over major nerves, blood vessels or vital organs.

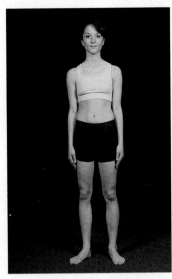

FIGURE 1–2 Posture reflects both structure and function: how your client's body is formed and how she uses it.

Posture

the arrangement of the body and limbs while standing, sitting, or reclining.

Tone

the small degree of contraction remaining in the skeletal muscles of the trunk even during relaxation which helps to maintain posture.

HERE'S A TIP

Posture assessment is repeated throughout the duration of treatment, because each assessment is a reflection of your client's posture at that moment in time. Posture is fluid and responsive to outside forces, including massage treatment.

Lab Activity 1–1 on page 48 is designed to help you develop preliminary posture-assessment skills.

Why We Assess Posture

Posture is the arrangement of the body and limbs while standing, sitting, or reclining. Posture, as shown in Figure 1–2, is created and maintained by many factors:

- Skeleton: the shape and length of your bones and their spatial relationship to one another at the joints.
- Muscles: the small amount of contraction, called **tone**, that remains in the muscles of the trunk even during relaxation.
- Connective tissues: the strength, elasticity, and tension of tendons, ligaments, and other supporting structures.
- Work and play habits: how you use your body affects—and is affected by—your posture. Posture and movement may be hampered by restrictions in skeletal formation, chronically contracted muscle fibers, and rigid tendons or ligaments.

Postural assessment gives you a wealth of information about the condition of your client's skeleton, muscles, and connective tissues, and about how she uses her body. The results of postural assessment provide you with a guide to further explore specific muscles and muscle groups to palpate and to examine your client's work and play habits.

Posture is assessed through visual measurement, touch, and comparison—comparing one aspect of your client's body to its counterpart, and comparing aspects of her body to those of others or those within the normal range of expectation.

Your client's standing posture

Assessing your client's standing posture provides you with head-to-toe information. Looking at the posture in Figure 1–2, for example, answer these questions:

- Is her head centered over her spine?
- Are her shoulders level?
- Are her elbows and hands turned inward?
- Are her hips level?
- Are her knees pointed forward?
- Are her feet pointed forward?

Your client's seated posture

Your client's seated posture also reveals a great deal of information. Compare the seated postures of the massage therapist and the client shown in Figure 1–3, answering these questions for each:

- Is her head straight or habitually tilted to one side?
- Is her spine erect or does her torso collapse into itself?
- Is her pelvis firm against the back of her chair or does it slouch toward the front edge?
- Are her legs crossed at the knee? At the ankle?
- Does she fold one leg beneath her opposite thigh as she sits?

Assessing standing and seated postures is an art that requires practice and patience. Complete postural assessment is described in Chapter 2, Posture Assessment.

Why We Assess Gait

Gait [GAYT] is one's manner or style of walking. Your gait is as individual as your fingerprints. Unlike your fingerprints, however, gait is easily altered. You constantly alter the pace, speed, length of stride, and arm swing of your gait,

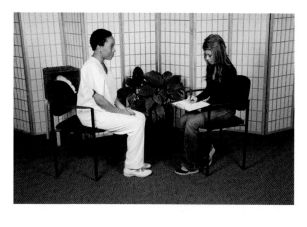

FIGURE 1–3 Your client's seated posture provides information about how she uses her body.

depending on structural conditions—perhaps one of your legs is slightly shorter than the other—and functional conditions—perhaps you're rushing to get to class on time.

| **Gait** |
| one's manner or style of walking. |

Your client's usual gait

Assessing your client's usual gait provides you with head-to-toe information:

- Does she "lead" with her head or with her hips, with her arms or with her feet? Which part of her body enters the room first?
- Is her spine straight as she walks, or is it "torqued" to one side?
- Does she swing her arms equally or does one arm swing out wide?
- Are her hips level or does one hip swing noticeably forward?
- Do her feet point forward, inward, or outward?

> ### IN THE TREATMENT ROOM
>
> Try to observe your client as she walks some distance without the awareness of being observed, such as to your clinic door from the parking lot. As you direct your client toward the treatment room, shown in Figure 1–4, allow her to walk ahead, so that you can casually observe her gait from behind. Most people alter their gait when they know they're being observed, especially when they're in a small space, such as your treatment room.

FIGURE 1–4 Casual observation of your client's gait may point you toward a more extensive assessment of her gait.

Your client's altered gait

Normal gait may be altered for a wide variety of structural or functional reasons. Assessing and recording your observations of your client's usual gait allows you to notice and assess her altered gait:

- How has the position of her head, hips, arms, and feet changed?
- How has the position of her spine changed?
- How has her arm swing changed?
- Do her feet leave the ground at the same angle and the same point during her step?

    Assessment of gait is essential in treatment planning and is described in detail in Chapter 3, Gait Assessment.

Lab Activity 1–2 on page 48 is designed to help you develop preliminary gait assessment skills.

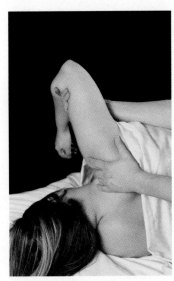

FIGURE 1–5 Even a brief, initial palpation reveals lots of information about a client's tissues.

HERE'S A TIP

Clues to your client's overall condition are given to you wherever you effectively palpate his tissues.

HERE'S A TIP

Keep in mind that gentle palpation may be the first therapeutic touch experienced by your client.

Pressure

touch that displaces tissue.

Arthrosis (arthr=joint)

another term for a joint.

DID YOU KNOW?

The term **arthritis** literally means joint inflammation: arthr=joint; -itis=inflammation.

Why We Palpate

Why do we take the time to manually explore individual structures on a client's body, rather than simply proceed with treatment? The short answer is that *palpation is more than assessment; it is part of treatment.* Palpation is not merely an academic exercise, nor is it an end in itself; it creates a more complete and effective client experience.

Your client's tissues

Palpation introduces you to the temperature, tone, and texture of your client's tissues—his bones, joints, connective tissues, and muscles. Palpation can reveal a great deal about the health of a client's tissues, as shown in Figure 1–5. Do the bony prominences seem larger than expected when compared to surrounding tissue? Do the joints feel stable or loose when palpated? Is the skin warm and intact or dry, papery, and fragile? Are muscles flaccid in any one area or throughout the body, or, for example, only on the nondominant side? Is one extremity noticeably cooler to the touch?

Palpation of your client's tissues has other significant benefits:

- To identify tissue that should not be treated: as a follow-up to interview information and visual assessment, palpation is an important tool for identifying tissue that should not be treated. If gentle palpation produces immediate, acute pain or reveals evidence of local inflammation, the acutely painful or inflamed tissue should not be treated.
- To introduce the client to your touch: palpation offers safe, nonthreatening touch to a client who is new to therapeutic massage or to your practice. An initial palpation, especially if the client has not yet disrobed, provides the opportunity for you and your client to discuss level of **pressure**, touch that displaces tissue, and areas of the body to be addressed during treatment, before she experiences the potential vulnerability of lying on a table, covered only by a sheet.
- To locate trigger points: the specific location of a trigger point can be elusive and sometimes frustrating. Accurate palpation skills contribute to successful trigger point work by increasing your touch sensitivity and your ability to anticipate trigger point location.

Effective assessment of your client's posture, gait, and tissues demands a thorough knowledge of joint and muscle anatomy and physiology. In the following sections, the structures and functions of joints and muscles are described.

JOINT STRUCTURE AND FUNCTION

A joint is also called an **arthrosis** [ar-THROH-sus]: the points where bone ends meet are called *articulations*. Joints vary in structure and in function. Some joints are structurally simple and allow little movement, while others are structurally more complex and allow a full range of multiple movements.

Types and Functions of Joints

The joints of the body are classified by structure and by the type and degree of movement they allow:

Structural classifications

Joint structure is classified by the presence or absence of a **synovial** [suh-NOH-vee-uhl] **cavity**, a binding structure that stabilizes joints that allow full range of movement.

- **Fibrous joints** have no synovial cavity. The articulating bones are held together by fibrous connective tissue. The sutures of the skull are fibrous joints.
- **Cartilaginous** [kar-tuh-la-JIN-us] **joints** also have no synovial cavity. The articulating bones are held together by hyaline cartilage or fibrocartilage. The joints between the vertebrae and between the pubic bones are cartilaginous.
- **Synovial joints** have a synovial cavity. The articulating bones are surrounded by a connective tissue capsule and other connective tissue structures. The joints between moveable parts of the skeleton, such as at the shoulder and the hip, are synovial.

Functional classifications

Joint function is classified by the degree of movement allowed:

- **Synarthrotic** [sin-ahr-THRAH-tik] **joints** are described by most sources as allowing little to no movement. Synarthrotic joints have no synovial cavity. The sutures of the skull are classified as synarthrotic.
- **Amphiarthrotic** [am-fee-arth-RAH-tik] **joints** allow slight movement. Amphiarthrotic joints have no synovial cavity. The joints between the bodies of vertebrae are amphiarthrotic.
- **Diarthrotic** [dy-ar-THRAH-tik] **joints** allow full range of movement. Diarthrotic joints have a synovial cavity and move the skeleton, such as the joints at the shoulder and the hip.

Most of the synarthrotic and amphiarthrotic joints, which allow little movement, are found in the **axial skeleton**, so-called because its structures connect to a central structure, the spine. The axial skeleton includes the skull, the hyoid bone, the thorax, the spine, and the sacrum. Synovial, diarthrotic joints—the freely moveable joints—are mostly found in the **appendicular skeleton**, so-called because its structures connect to, or append, the axial skeleton. The appendicular skeleton includes the clavicle, the scapula and the upper extremity, and the pelvis and the lower extremity.

Synovial Joint Structure

Synovial joint structure, Figure 1–6, is characterized by a surrounding fibrous capsule and an inner membrane-lined cavity that is filled with fluid. Such a structure allows the function of the joint to be diarthrotic,

---

Synovial

joint structure is characterized by a surrounding fibrous capsule and an inner, membrane-lined cavity filled with fluid; a freely moveable joint.

DID YOU KNOW?

The viewpoint of many anatomists that the sutures of the skull are immovable is disputed by practitioners of craniosacral therapy, who report that their focused palpation reveals a significant degree of movement between the bones of the skull.

Synarthrotic joints (syn=without)

a joint which does not allow palpable movement.

Amphiarthrotic joints (amphi=both or partial)

a joint which allows only slight movement.

Diarthrotic (di=twice, or double)

a freely moving joint.

Axial skeleton

the portion of the skeleton that includes the skull, the hyoid bone, the thorax, the spine, and the sacrum.

Appendicular skeleton

the portion of the skeleton that includes the clavicle, the scapula, and the upper extremity, and the pelvis and the lower extremity.

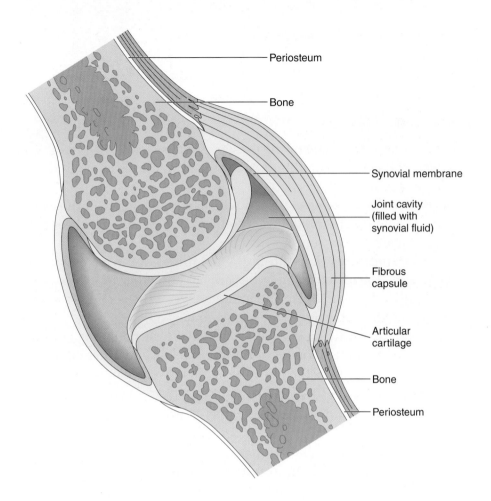

- Periosteum
- Bone
- Synovial membrane
- Joint cavity (filled with synovial fluid)
- Fibrous capsule
- Articular cartilage
- Bone
- Periosteum

FIGURE 1-6 The structure of a synovial (moveable) joint, which is surrounded by the articular capsule.

© Delmar, Cengage Learning.

or freely moving. The function of synovial joints is to allow free movement of the skeleton, in a range of types of movements and in different planes and directions.

The articular capsule

The **articular capsule**, visible in Figure 1–6, is a fibrous capsule that surrounds a synovial joint and contains the synovial cavity. The articular capsule extends from the periosteum, the outer covering, of one articulating bone to the periosteum of the other articulating bone. Contained within this fibrous capsule is the **synovial membrane**, which lines the fibrous capsule and the synovial cavity. Protection of the moving parts at synovial joints is provided by:

| **Articulation** |
| the joint itself or the site where the bones in a joint connect. |

- **Synovial fluid**, an extracellular fluid that circulates within the synovial cavity to lubricate it, to absorb shock, and to reduce friction at the joint.
- **Articular cartilage**, hyaline cartilage that lines the ends of articulating bones, reducing friction.

Associated structures at synovial joints

Connective tissue structures found at various synovial joints also provide protection and ensure the free movement required of that particular joint.

■ **Ligaments** are bands of dense, fibrous connective tissue that connect bone to bone and support the positions of the articulating bones during movement. The number and arrangement of ligaments at a joint supports the type and range of motions possible at the joint.

DID YOU KNOW?

The length and relative tension of ligaments creates the "fit" of a joint; longer, looser ligaments are one factor allowing greater range of motion. Ligaments that are too loose or overstretched, however, may fail to provide adequate support to the joint during movement. Such a joint may result in **hypermobility**, too great a range of motion that may increase the risk of injury.

■ **Meniscus** [muh-NISS-kus]: a meniscus is a plate of cartilage found at synovial joints that allows bones of different shapes to articulate and stabilize them during movement. Menisci are found at the wrist and the knee, where bones of different shapes must articulate freely.

■ **Bursa** [BUR-sah]: a bursa is a sac filled with synovial fluid that reduces friction and cushion joint parts. Bursae are found wherever friction may develop during movement by facilitating gliding: between skin and bone, tendon and bone, and ligament and bone.

■ **Tendon sheaths** are tube-like bursae that wrap around tendons traveling through areas of great friction, such as at the wrist and at the ankle.

Synovial Joint Function

Actions allowed by types of synovial joints

Six types of synovial joints create the wide variety of joint actions possible in the human body.

The structure of each type of synovial joint, shown in Figure 1–7, creates the type of action allowed at that joint.

1. At a **hinge joint**, the convex end of one bone fits into the concave end of another bone, allowing an action like that of the hinge of a door opening and closing.
2. At a **pivot joint**, a pointed end of one bone rotates around a ring-like part of another bone, allowing a rotational action.
3. At a **condyloid** [KAHN-duh-loyd] **joint**, the convex projection of one bone fits into the depression of another bone, allowing both side-to-side and up-and-down actions.
4. At a **ball-and-socket joint**, the ball-shaped end of one bone fits into the socket-shaped depression of another bone. Ball-and-socket joints allow many types of actions.
5. At a **saddle joint**, the articulating bone ends fit together as a rider does into a saddle, allowing the same types of actions found at condyloid joints.

Ligament

a band of dense, fibrous connective tissue that connect bone to bone.

Hypermobility

an excess of range of motion at a joint.

Meniscus (plural: menisci)

a plate of a cartilage plate found at synovial joints that which allows bones of different shapes to articulate and stabilizes them during movement.

Bursa (plural: bursae)

a sac filled with synovial fluid that reduces friction and cushions joint parts.

Tendon sheath

a tube-like bursa that wraps around tendons traveling through areas of great friction, such as at the wrist and the ankle.

Hinge

a joint at which a convex bone end fits into a concave bone end.

Pivot

a type of joint at which a bony process rotates around an axis.

Condyloid

a joint at which an oval-shaped condyle of a bone fits into a basin-shaped bone.

Ball-and-socket

a joint at which a ball-shaped bone end fits into the deep socket of another bone, such as at the shoulder and the hip.

Saddle

a type of joint at which the shape of one bone's articular surface looks like a saddle, while its joint partner is shaped to sit in it, as a rider would sit in a saddle.

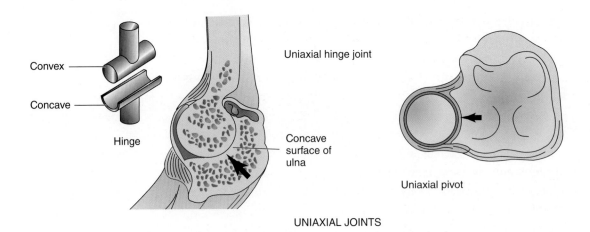

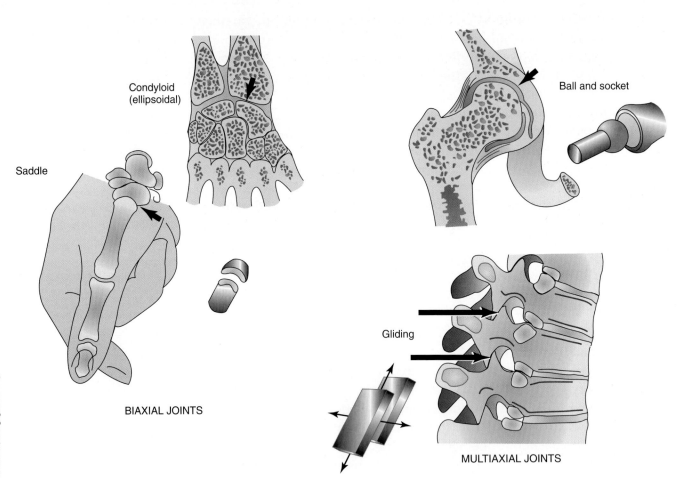

FIGURE 1-7 Types of synovial (moveable) joints.

Planar

a type of joint at which flat or slightly curved bones glide against one another.

6. At a **planar** [PLAY-nur] or **gliding joint**, the articulating bone ends are slightly curved or even flat. The actions allowed at planar joints are slight, gliding movements, either back and forth or side to side.

TABLE 1–1

TYPES OF SYNOVIAL JOINTS AND THEIR ACTIONS		
TYPE OF SYNOVIAL JOINT	ACTIONS	EXAMPLE
Hinge	Flexion and extension	The knee or the elbow.
Pivot	Rotation	The joint between the first two cervical vertebrae that allows you to shake your head "no."
Condyloid	Flexion and extension; abduction and adduction	The wrist.
Ball-and-socket	Flexion and extension; abduction and adduction; medial and lateral rotation; circumduction	The shoulder and the hip.
Saddle	Flexion and extension; abduction and adduction; opposition	The joint between the thumb and the hand.
Planar (gliding)	Gliding	The joints between the sternum and clavicle, or between the sternum and the ribs.

Table 1–1 summarizes the types of synovial joints and the actions they allow.

Table 1–2 lists the joints of the skeleton, shown in Figures 1–8 to 1–18, the articulating structures and the actions each joint allows. *From this point forward, joints will be designated by these anatomically correct names. The shoulder joint, for example, will be the glenohumeral joint.*

TABLE 1–2

JOINTS OF THE SKELETON AND THEIR ARTICULATIONS AND ACTIONS		
JOINT NAME	ARTICULATIONS	ACTIONS
Sutures of the skull (Figure 1–8)	Between the bones of the skull.	Little; slight gliding
Temporomandibular (TMJ) [TEM-puh-roh-man-dib-yuh-lur]: the jaw (Figure 1–8)	Between the mandibular fossa and tubercle of the temporal bone and the condylar process of the mandible.	Depression and elevation; protraction and retraction; deviation of the jaw
Acromioclavicular [uh-KROH-mee-oh-kluh-vik-yuh-lur]: the joint between the scapula and the clavicle (Figure 1–8)	Between the acromion of the scapula and the acromial end of the clavicle.	Slight gliding
Atlanto-axial [at-LAN-toh-AK-see-ul]: the joint between C1 and C2 (Figure 1–9)	Between the superior projection or dens on the axis, C2, and the atlas, C1.	Rotation
Intervertebral [in-tur-VUR-tuh-brul]: the joints between vertebrae (Figures 1–9)	Between the arches and bodies of adjacent vertebrae.	Flexion and extension; lateral flexion; rotation
Scapulocostal: (not pictured)	The slight articulation between the posterior scapula and thoracic ribs; not true synovial joints.	Protraction and retraction; lateral, medial, anterior and posterior tilt
Sternocostal [stur-noh-KAHS-tul]: the joints between the sternum and the ribs (Figure 1–9)	Between the sternum and pairs of ribs, one through seven.	Slight gliding
Sternoclavicular [stur-noh-kluh-VIK-yuh-lur]: the joint between the sternum and the clavicle (Figure 1–9)	Between the manubrium of the sternum and the sternal end of the clavicle.	Slight gliding
Atlanto-occipital [at-LAN-toh-ahk-SIP-it-ul]: the joint between the occiput and C1 (Figure 1–10)	Between superior facets of the atlas and the condyles of the occiput.	Flexion and extension; slight lateral flexion
Vertebrocostal [vur-tuh-broh-KAHS-tul]: the joints between the vertebrae and the ribs (Figure 1–10)	Two articulations: between the heads of ribs and bodies of vertebrae and between the tubercles of ribs and transverse processes of vertebrae.	Slight gliding

(continued)

TABLE 1-2   *(continued)*

JOINTS OF THE SKELETON AND THEIR ARTICULATIONS AND ACTIONS		
JOINT NAME	**ARTICULATIONS**	**ACTIONS**
Humeroulnar [hyoo-muh-roh-UL-nur]: the elbow joint (Figure 1–11)	Between the trochlea of the humerus, the trochlear notch of the ulna, and the head of the radius.	Flexion and extension
Glenohumeral [glee-noh-HYOO-mur-ul]: the shoulder joint (Figures 1–11 and 1–12)	Between the glenoid fossa of the scapula and the head of the humerus.	Flexion and extension; abduction and adduction; medial and lateral rotation; circumduction
Proximal and distal radioulnar [RAY-dee-oh-ul-nur]: the joints between the radius and the ulna (Figures 1–12, 1–13, and 1–14)	Proximal: between the head of the radius and the radial notch of the ulna. Distal: between the head of the ulna and the ulnar notch of the radius.	Pronation and supination
Radiocarpal [RAY-dee-oh-kar-pul]: the wrist joint (Figures 1–13 and 1–14)	Between the distal end of the radius and three carpal bones: the scaphoid, lunate, and triquetrum.	Flexion and extension; abduction and adduction
Intercarpal [in-tur-KAR-pul]: the joints between the carpal bones (Figure 1–14)	Between the proximal and distal rows of carpals.	Gliding; flexion and abduction between the rows of carpals
Carpometacarpal (CMC) [KAR-poh-met-uh-kar-pul]: the joints between the wrist and the hand (Figure 1–14)	First CMC: between the base of the thumb and the trapezium of the carpals. Second through fifth CMCs: between carpals and the bases of metacarpals.	Gliding; flexion and extension, abduction and adduction, opposition and circumduction at the thumb
Metacarpophalangeal (MCP) [MET-uh-kar-poh-fuh-lan-jee-ul]: the joints between the hand and the fingers (Figure 1–14)	Between the heads of metacarpals and the bases of proximal phalanges.	Flexion and extension; abduction and adduction; circumduction
Interphalangeal (IP) [in-tur-fuh-LAN-jee-ul]: the joints of the fingers and the toes (Figure 1–14)	Between the heads of phalanges and the bases of more distal phalanges.	Flexion and extension
Lumbosacral [lum-boh-SAY-krul]: the joint between the fifth lumbar vertebra and the sacrum (Figures 1–10, 1–15 and 1–16)	Two articulations: between the body of L5 and the base of the sacrum and between the inferior facets of L5 and the superior facets of the sacrum.	Flexion and extension; lateral flexion; rotation
Sacroiliac: the joint between the sacrum and the pelvis (Figures 1–15 and 1–16)	Between lateral surfaces of the sacrum and the ilia of the pelvis.	Slight gliding
Acetabulofemoral [as-uh-TAB-yuh-loh-fem-ur-uhl]: the hip joint (Figures 1–15 and 1–16)	Between the acetabulum of the pelvis and the head of the femur.	Flexion and extension; abduction and adduction; medial and lateral rotation; circumduction
Pubic symphysis [PYOO-bik SIM-fuh-sis] (Figure 1–16)	Between the anterior surfaces of the pubic bones.	Slight; more during pregnancy and childbirth
Tibiofemoral [tih-bee-oh-FEM-ur-uhl]: the knee joint (Figures 1–17 and 1–18)	Between the condyles of the tibia and the condyles of the femur.	Flexion and extension
Talocrural [TAY-loh-krur-ul]: the ankle joint (Figure 1–18)	Two articulations: between the medial malleolus of the tibia and the talus of the carpals and between the lateral malleolus of the fibula and the talus.	Dorsiflexion and plantarflexion
Intertarsal [in-tur-TAR-sul]: the joints between the tarsal bones (Figure 1–18)	Between tarsal bones.	Inversion and eversion
Tarsometatarsal [tar-soh-met-uh-TAR-sul]: the joints between the tarsal bones and the foot (Figure 1–18)	Between the three cuneiforms of the tarsals and the bases of the metatarsals.	Slight gliding
Metatarsophalangeal (MTP) [met-uh-TAR-soh-fay-lan-jee-ul]: the joints between the foot and the toes (Figure 1–18)	Between the heads of metatarsals and the bases of proximal phalanges.	Flexion and extension; abduction and adduction; circumduction

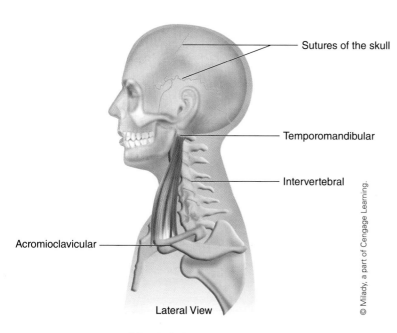

© Milady, a part of Cengage Learning.

FIGURE 1-8 Sutures of the skull; the temporomandibular joint; intervertebral joints; and the acromioclavicular joint.

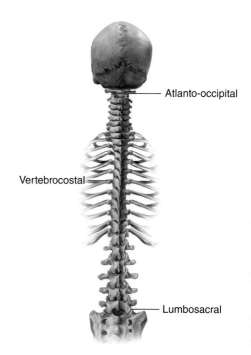

© Milady, a part of Cengage Learning.

FIGURE 1-10 The atlanto-occipital, vertebrocostal, and lumbosacral joints.

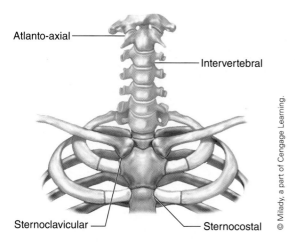

© Milady, a part of Cengage Learning.

FIGURE 1-9 The atlanto-axial joint; intervertebral joints; sternoclavicular and sternocostal joints.

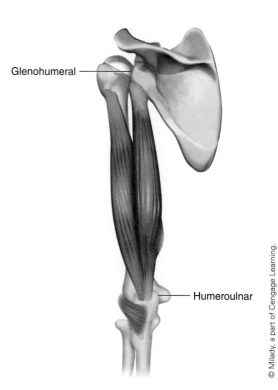

© Milady, a part of Cengage Learning.

FIGURE 1-11 The glenohumeral and humeroulnar joints.

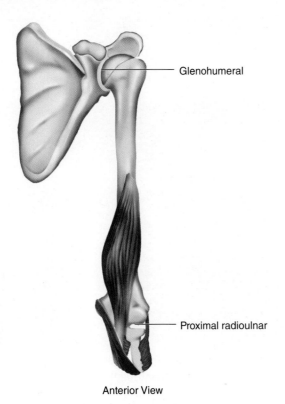

Anterior View

FIGURE 1-12 The glenohumeral and proximal radioulnar joints.

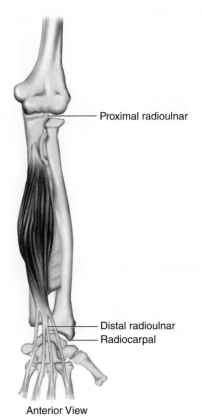

Anterior View

FIGURE 1-13 The proximal and distal radioulnar joints and the radiocarpal joint.

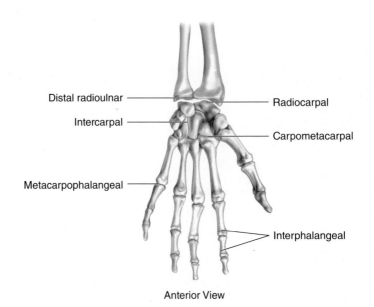

FIGURE 1-14 The distal radioulnar, radiocarpal, carpometacarpal, metacarpophalangeal, and interphalangeal joints.

Anterior View

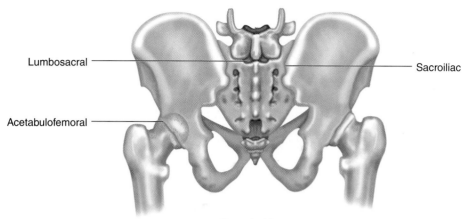

Lumbosacral

Acetabulofemoral

Sacroiliac

Posterior View

FIGURE 1-15 The lumbosacral, sacroiliac, and acetabulofemoral joints.

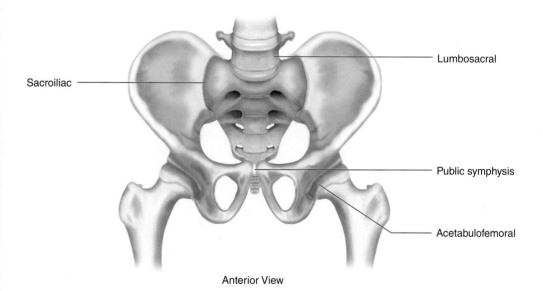

Sacroiliac

Lumbosacral

Public symphysis

Acetabulofemoral

Anterior View

FIGURE 1-16 The lumbosacral, sacroiliac, and acetabulofemoral joints and the pubic symphysis.

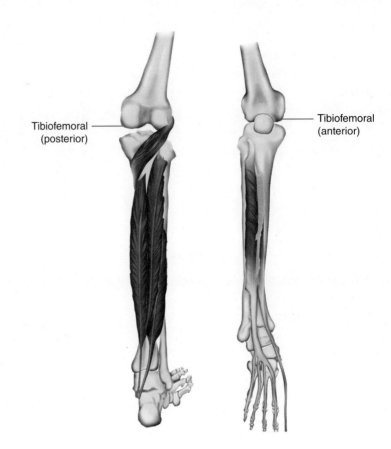

FIGURE 1-17 Anterior and posterior views of the tibiofemoral joint.

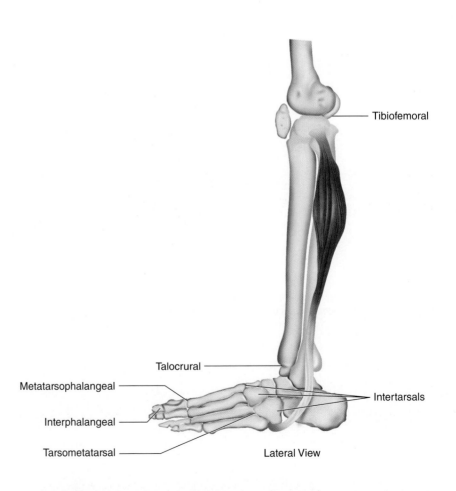

FIGURE 1-18 The tibiofemoral, talocrural, tarsometatarsal, metatarsophalangeal, intertarsal, and interphalangeal joints.

JOINT ACTIONS

Many types of actions are made possible by the body's freely moveable joints, allowing us a stunning array of choices for physical expression through movement.

Joint actions are described by naming the movement, the body part being moved, and the joint where the movement occurs. For example, lifting your arm to catch someone's attention is described as flexion, which describes the movement of the arm, the body part which is being moved at the glenohumeral joint, the joint where the movement occurs. Although there are other movements that accompany flexion of the arm at the glenohumeral joint in the action of lifting the arm, to catch someone's attention, for example, flexion of the forearm at the humeroulnar joint, hyperextension, and radial and ulnar deviation of the hand at the radiocarpal joint, the movement at the large, proximal joint—the glenohumeral joint—is described first.

Joint actions are described by their movement of a structure in relation to **anatomical position,** shown in Figure 1–19:

- The body is erect.
- The head faces forward.
- The palms of the hands face forward.
- The feet are flat and point forward.

Anatomical position

the position in which body is erect, the head faces forward, the palms of the hands face forward, and the feet are flat and face forward.

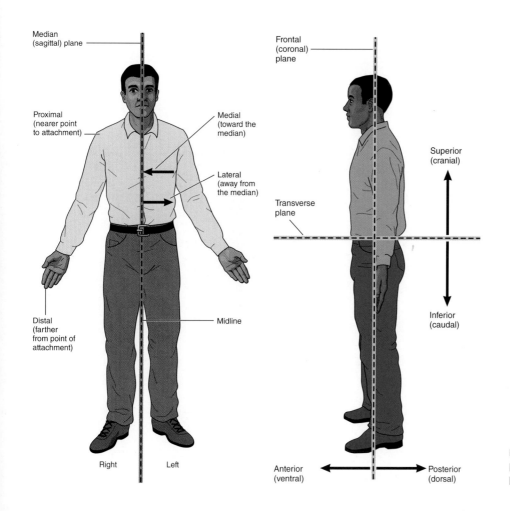

FIGURE 1-19 Anatomical position of the body showing the planes of movement.

© Milady, a part of Cengage Learning.

HERE'S A TIP

When describing joint and muscle actions, note the following:

- ■ "Arm" refers to the upper extremity, from the glenohumeral joint to the humeroulnar joint.
- ■ "Forearm" refers to the upper extremity, from the humeroulnar joint to the radiocarpal joint.
- ■ "Thigh" refers to the lower extremity, from the acetabulofemoral joint to the tibiofemoral joint.
- ■ "Leg" refers to the lower extremity, from the tibiofemoral joint to the talocrural joint.

Frontal

a plane that divides the body into anterior and posterior.

Sagittal

a plane which divides the body into left and right sections.

Transverse

a plane which divides the body into superior and inferior sections; also called the horizontal plane.

Movement through the Planes of the Body

The planes of the body are imaginary surfaces that divide the body into sections, shown in Figure 1–20:

- ■ The **frontal** plane divides the body into anterior and posterior.
- ■ The **sagittal** [SAJ-ut-ul] plane divides the body into left and right halves.
- ■ The **transverse** or **horizontal** plane divides the body into upper and lower—superior and inferior—sections.

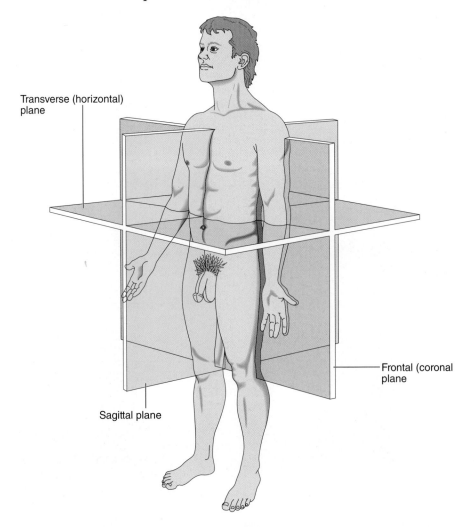

Transverse (horizontal) plane

Frontal (coronal plane

Sagittal plane

FIGURE 1–20 The planes of the body.

- An **oblique** [oh-BLEEK] plane divides the body or a section of the body at an angle.

The planes of the body are used as a reference point to describe the direction of movement *through one of the planes*:

- Adduction of the arm at the glenohumeral joint can occur by moving it through the frontal plane: from the anatomical position, the arm is lifted straight out from the side.
- Abduction of the arm at the glenohumeral joint can also occur by moving it through the horizontal plane: starting with your arm at 90° of flexion in the frontal plane, the arm is moved straight away from the midline.

Oblique

a plane that divides the body or a section of the body at an angle.

DID YOU KNOW?

The planes of the body are also used to describe the location and direction of surgical incisions.

Gliding Actions

The action of **gliding** is created when relatively flat bones move back and forth and side to side over one another, with no significant change in the relative angle between the bones. Gliding occurs mostly in the joints of the axial skeleton, or the trunk. During respiration, for example, the ribs glide slightly at their articulations with the sternum and the vertebrae to allow the chest cavity to expand and contract.

Gliding

movement during which relatively flat bones move back-and-forth and side-to-side over one another, with no significant change in the relative angle between the bones.

Angular Actions

Angular actions are so-called because they result in an increase or a decrease in the *angle* between the articulating bones, not because they may be angular in appearance.

Angular

joint actions that result in an increase or a decrease in the angle between the articulating bones.

HERE'S A TIP

Angular actions are described in their relation to the body in anatomical position: when the arm is flexed at the shoulder, for example, the angle between the articulating bones decreases as the arm leaves anatomical position.

Flexion and extension

Flexion decreases the angle between the articulating bones, and usually occurs in the sagittal plane. Examples of flexion include:

- Bowing your head toward your chest, as shown in Figure 1–21.
- Raising your arm at the shoulder, as when you're reaching for a book on a shelf.
- Curling your fingers toward the palm of your hand, as when closing your hand.
- Lifting your thigh at the hip, as when stepping onto a curb.

Flexion

movement which decreases the angle between articulating bones.

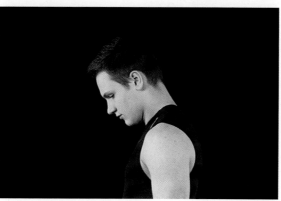

FIGURE 1–21 Flexion of the head at the spinal joints.

© Milady, a part of Cengage Learning. Photography by Yanik Chauvin.

Extension

Extension
movement which increases the angle between articulating bones.

Extension increases the angle between the articulating bones, or returns a flexed bone to anatomical position. As with flexion, extension usually occurs in the sagittal plane. Examples of extension include:

- Bringing your head back up to anatomical position, as shown in Figure 1–22.

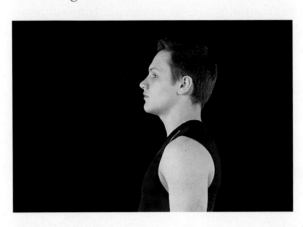

FIGURE 1-22 Extension of the head at the spinal joints.

- Bringing your arm back down to your side after you've taken a book off a shelf.
- Straightening your fingers away from the palm of your hand, as when opening your hand.
- Lowering your thigh at the hip, after you've stepped up onto the curb.

Hyperextension

Hyperextension
extension of a body part beyond anatomical position.

Hyperextension occurs when a body part extends beyond anatomical position. Hyperextension is also sometimes defined as extension beyond the normal range of motion at a joint. Examples of hyperextension include:

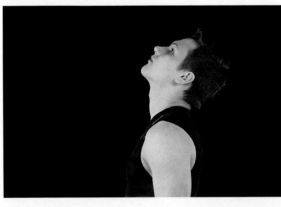

FIGURE 1-23 Hyperextension of the head at the spinal joints.

- Bending your head backward, as shown in Figure 1–23, to look at a comet streaking across the night sky.
- Reaching your arm into the backseat of your car to pick up the water bottle you dropped.
- Bending your wrist backward to stretch your forearm flexor muscles.

> ### DID YOU KNOW?
>
> Hyperextension at hinge joints, such as at the humeroulnar or tibiofemoral joint, is prevented, under normal circumstances, by the structure of the joint itself and by the tension of ligaments.

Lateral flexion

Lateral flexion
movement which bends the head or trunk to one side, in the frontal plane.

Lateral flexion is sideways bending of the head or of the trunk, as shown in Figure 1–24. Lateral flexion occurs in the frontal plane. Examples of lateral flexion include:

- Bending your head to one side to read the labels on the DVDs at the library.
- Bending your torso to one side to pick up the book beside your chair.

Abduction and adduction

Abduction and adduction occur in relation to the midline or to action on a structure, such as the hand or the foot, and usually take place in the frontal plane. **Abduction** is movement of a bone away from the midline of the body or the midline on a structure, as shown in Figure 1–25. The arm and the thigh can both be abducted: each can be moved away from the midline of the body. The fingers, thumbs, and toes can also be abducted: they can be moved away from the midline of the hand or the foot.

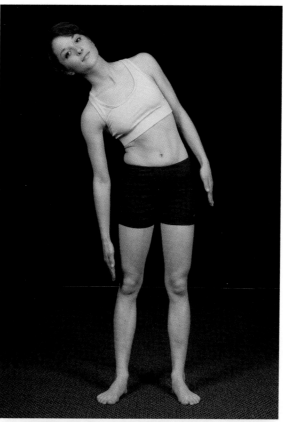

FIGURE 1–24 Lateral flexion of the trunk at the spinal joints.

© Milady, a part of Cengage Learning. Photography by Yanik Chauvin.

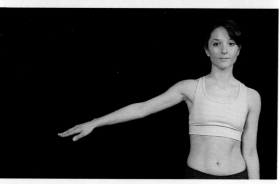

FIGURE 1–25 Abduction of the arm at the shoulder joint.

© Milady, a part of Cengage Learning. Photography by Yanik Chauvin.

HERE'S A TIP

Think of abduction as abducting or taking something away from something else—for example, you are taking away your arm from your side. When you adduct, however, you are bringing the arm back to your side—you're adding something instead of taking something away.

Abduction

movement of a limb or a structure away from the midline of the body.

Examples of abduction in the frontal plane include:
- Lifting your arms out to your sides, to say, "Here I am!"
- Sticking your leg out to one side before kicking a soccer ball.

Adduction is bringing an abducted bone back toward the midline, or even crossing the midline following abduction. Examples of adduction in the frontal plane include:
- Bringing your arms back to your sides after saying "Here I am!"
- Swinging your leg back across the midline to kick the soccer ball.

Adduction

movement of a limb or a structure toward the midline of the body.

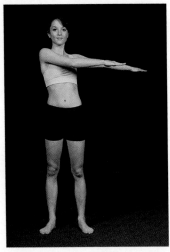

FIGURE 1–26 Abduction of the left arm and adduction of the right arm at the shoulder joints, in the horizontal plane.

Horizontal abduction

movement of a flexed limb away from the midline of the body, in the horizontal or transverse plane.

Horizontal adduction

movement of a flexed limb toward the midline of the body, in the horizontal or transverse plane.

FIGURE 1–27 Circumduction of the arm at the shoulder joint.

Circumduction

circular movement of the distal part of a limb as the proximal part of the limb remains stationary.

Joint fit

the overall structure of an articulation; the manner in which its bony parts, ligaments, and other connective tissue components fit together.

Horizontal abduction and adduction

Abduction of the arm at the shoulder or the thigh at the hip is also possible in the horizontal plane, after either limb has first been flexed to 90°. Examples of horizontal abduction include:

- Moving your flexed arms out to your sides to open a curtain.
- While seated, swinging your thigh to the side to reach down between your legs to pick up the pencil you dropped.

Adduction of the arm at the shoulder or the thigh at the hip is also possible in the horizontal plane, after the limb has first been flexed and abducted to 90°. Examples of horizontal adduction include:

- Bringing your flexed arms together to close a curtain.
- While seated, bringing your thigh back toward your seat after picking up the pencil you dropped.

Figure 1–26 demonstrates abduction of one arm and adduction of the other arm.

Circumduction

Circumduction [sur-kum-DUCK-shun] is circular movement of the distal part of a limb while the proximal part of the limb remains stationary. True circumduction occurs at the ball-and-socket joints at the glenohumeral joint, shown in Figure 1–27, and the acetabulofemoral joint. Circumduction

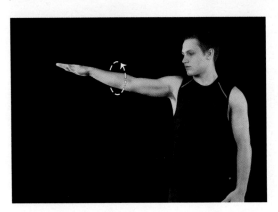

can be a very small movement or quite large. Circumduction at the glenohumeral joint or at the acetabulofemoral joint can occur in the frontal or sagittal plane. Examples of circumduction include:

- Swimming, using the backstroke.
- Drawing circles on a chalkboard.

DID YOU KNOW?

Though most sources describe circumduction as only occurring at the ball-and-socket joints, a type of circumduction occurs at the wrist or the ankle, by using the gliding movement between the carpals or the tarsals. At the metacarpophalangeal joints, too, the phalanges or fingers may seem to "twirl," though most anatomists do not describe this action as circumduction.

Joint fit and joint actions

Joint fit is the overall structure of a joint, the bones, the ligaments, and other accessory structures, and how these parts fit together. Comparing

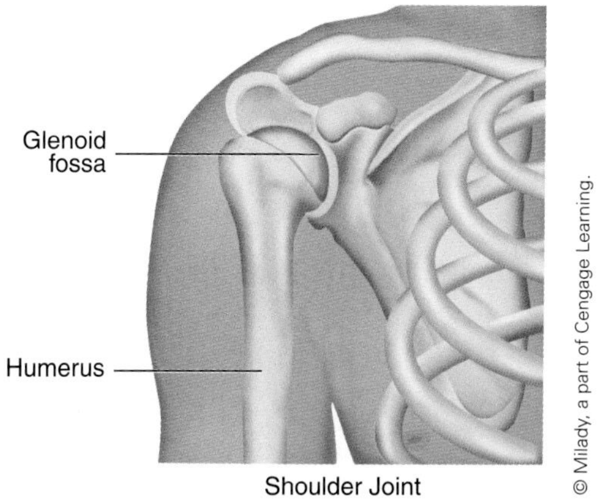

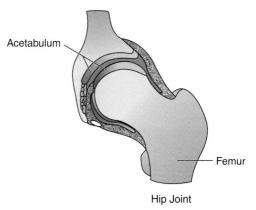

Glenoid
fossa

Humerus

Shoulder Joint

© Milady, a part of Cengage Learning.

FIGURE 1–28 The head of the humerus articulates with the shallow glenoid fossa of the scapula at the shoulder joint.

Acetabulum

Femur

Hip Joint

© Milady, a part of Cengage Learning.

FIGURE 1–29 The head of the femur articulates into the deep acetabulum of the pelvis at the hip joint.

the glenohumeral joint at the shoulder and the acetabulofemoral joint at the hip demonstrates the concept of joint fit.

The shoulder and hip joint are both ball-and-socket joints, in which the ball-shaped head of a long bone fits into the socket-shaped fossa of another bone. The difference in joint fit, their structure, creates their varying range of motion, their function:

- Comparing Figures 1–28 and 1–29, you can see that the head of the femur is much larger, relative to the size of its shaft, than the head of the humerus is in relation to its shaft, and that a longer "neck" connects the head of the femur to its shaft.
- The acetabulum of the pelvis is relatively far larger and deeper than the glenoid fossa of the scapula.
- The head of the femur is seated more deeply into the acetabulum than the head of the humerus is into the glenoid fossa.

The muscles and ligaments surrounding the acetabulofemoral joint are angled more to provide support its weight bearing function than to allow a full range of motion. The muscles and ligaments surrounding the glenohumeral joint are angled more to support a full range of motion of the head of the humerus in the absence of weight bearing of the body.

Joint fit impacts range of motion at a joint. Although both the glenohumeral joint and glenohumeral joints allow the same joint actions, the *range* of these motions is more limited in the acetabulofemoral joint. This difference in range of motion is due to the weight-bearing function at the hip: the weight of the head, the torso, and the upper extremities is transferred through the acetabulofemoral joint to the tibia. Stability, more than flexibility, is needed at the acetabulofemoral joint. By contrast, flexibility, not weight-bearing capacity, is needed in the upper extremity. The structure of the glenohumeral joint allows greater range of motion, but less stability.

Range of motion

the degree of movement, measured in a circle, allowed at a synovial joint.

Lab Activity 1–3 on page 49 is designed to help you learn how to demonstrate and identify angular joint actions.

Rotation

revolution of a bone around a single longitudinal axis.

Axis

a stationary pivot around which another structure may rotate.

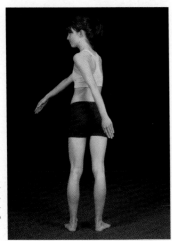

FIGURE 1–30 Rotation of the trunk at spinal joints.

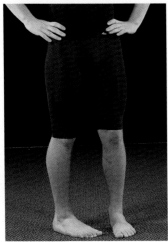

FIGURE 1–31 Medial rotation of the right thigh at the hip joint.

Medial rotation

anterior surface of a long bone rotates toward the midline of the body. Sometimes called internal rotation.

Lateral rotation

movement during which the anterior surface of a long bone rotates away from the midline of the body. Sometimes called external rotation.

Assessing range of motion at a joint is described in Chapter 2, Posture Assessment.

Rotational Movements

In **rotation**, a bone revolves around a single longitudinal **axis**, or stationary pivot, through the transverse plane. Rotations can occur at ball-and-socket and pivot joints. Rotation at pivot joints at the midline of the body rotates the head or the trunk at the spine. Rotation at ball-and-socket joints may be medial or lateral, and it moves the limb toward or away from the midline of the body.

Rotation at the midline

When rotation at the midline rotates the head to one side or the other, the action occurs at the joints between the vertebrae. Examples of midline rotation include:

- Shaking your head "no."
- Twisting your torso around in your seat to see who's behind you.

Rotation of the trunk at the spinal joints is shown in Figure 1–30.

Medial rotation

In medial rotation, the head of the humerus or the head of the femur rotates the anterior shaft of the long bone toward the midline of the body. Examples of medial rotation include:

- Turning your hip inward to look at the heel of your shoe, as in Figure 1–31.
- Reaching your hand across your body to scratch your opposite shoulder.

DID YOU KNOW?

Medial rotation is sometimes called internal or inward rotation.

Lateral rotation

In lateral rotation, the head of the humerus or the femur rotates the anterior shaft of the bone away from the midline of the body. Examples of lateral rotation include:

- Turning your hip outward to look at the sole of your foot, as in Figure 1–32.
- Reaching your arm to the side and back, to scratch someone else's shoulder.

DID YOU KNOW?

Lateral rotation is sometimes called external or outward rotation.

FIGURE 1-32 Lateral rotation of the right thigh at the hip joint.

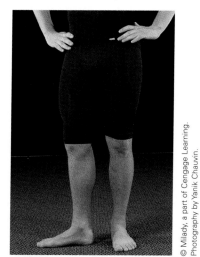

> ### HERE'S A TIP
>
> A minimal degree of medial or lateral rotation is also possible at the knee, but is accomplished by a slight gliding action, not by true rotation.

Additional Actions

These actions occur only at specific joints, and they may be variations of actions at other joints of the body although carrying a different name that sometimes acknowledges the location of the action.

Elevation and depression

Elevation is the upward movement of a body part, away from anatomical position, while **depression** is the downward movement of that body part, back into anatomical position. Elevation and depression occur at the temporomandibular joints, where depression must occur before elevation, and at the scapulocostal joints, Figures 1–33 and 1–34, where elevation must occur before depression. The pelvis may also be elevated and slightly depressed, unilaterally. Examples of elevation and depression include:

- Elevation: shrugging your shoulders in puzzlement at the world, as in Figure 1–33.
- Depression: "getting over it," as in Figure 1–34.
- Depression: opening your mouth to speak.
- Elevation: deciding to keep your mouth shut instead.

Protraction and retraction

Protraction moves a part of the body forward or to the anterior in the transverse plane. **Retraction** moves that body part back or to the posterior into anatomical position. These movements, too, occur only at the temporomandibular and scapulocostal joints, as shown in Figures 1–35 and 1–36. Examples of protraction and retraction include:

- Protraction: sticking your jaw forward to show the world you're the boss.
- Retraction: pulling it back in again when the world decides that a jaw stuck that far forward just might be a target.

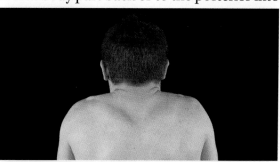

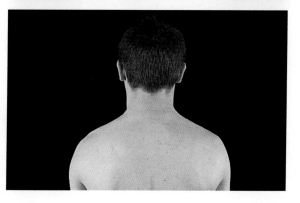

Lab Activity 1–4 on page 49 is designed to help you learn how to demonstrate and identify rotational joint actions.

> **Elevation**
> movement of a body part upward, toward the head.

> **Depression**
> movement of a body part downward, away from the head.

> **Protraction**
> movement of the shoulder or the jaw forward, toward the anterior.

FIGURE 1-33 Elevation of the shoulders at the scapulocostal joints.

FIGURE 1-34 Depression of the shoulders at the scapulocostal joints.

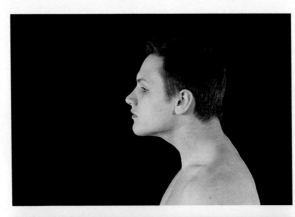

FIGURE 1-35 Protraction of the jaw at the temporomandibular joints.

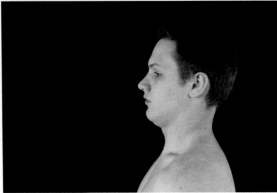

FIGURE 1-36 Retraction of the law at the temporomandibular joints.

Inversion and eversion

Inversion and **eversion** [in-VUR-zhun, ee-VUR-zhun] describe movements of the soles of the feet, the plantar aspect. As the sole of the foot is inverted, it is turned toward the midline: the soles of the feet face each other when both are inverted. As the sole of the foot is everted, it is turned away from the midline: the soles face away from each other when both are everted. Inversion and eversion occur at the intertarsal joints, between the tarsal bones of the foot. Inversion, eversion, and anatomical position of the foot are shown in Figure 1–37. Examples of inversion and eversion include:

- Inversion: turning the bottom of your foot inward so you can see what you just stepped in.
- Eversion: turning the bottom of your foot away to scrape it on the side of the curb.

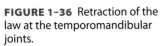

Retraction

movement of the shoulder or the jaw backward, toward the posterior.

Inversion

movement of the plantar aspect of the foot, the sole, inward or toward the midline of the body.

Eversion

movement of the plantar aspect of the foot, the sole, outward, away from the midline of the body.

DID YOU KNOW?

Inversion is sometimes called supination of the foot, and eversion is sometimes called pronation of the foot.

FIGURE 1-37 Inversion, eversion, and anatomical position of the foot.

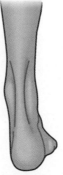 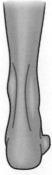 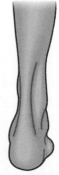

Inversion of the foot at the ankle

The foot in neutral

Eversion of the foot at the ankle

Dorsiflexion and plantarflexion

Dorsiflexion and plantarflexion are also movements of the foot: **dorsiflexion** [dor-suh-FLEK-shun] is flexion of the dorsal, or upper, aspect of the foot. Dorsiflexion points the toes toward the head in anatomical position. **Plantarflexion** [plant-ur-FLEK-shun] flexes the plantar, or bottom, aspect of the foot. Plantarflexion points the toes away from the head in anatomical position. Dorsiflexion and plantarflexion occur at the talocrural joints, the articulation of the tibia, the fibula, and the talus, as shown in Figures 1–38 and 1–39. Examples of dorsiflexion and plantarflexion include:

- Walking: when you begin to take a step, you dorsiflex your foot. When you have completed the step, you plantarflex your foot.
- Dancing: if you are performing with a Russian dance troupe, you squat and dorsiflex your foot as you throw that leg forward, with your arms crossed. If you are a ballerina, you plantarflex your foot as you rise onto the tips of your toes. During the hokey-pokey, you do both.

Pronation and supination take place at the proximal and distal radioulnar joints of the forearm and are a form of specialized rotation. During **pronation** [proh-NAY-shun], shown in Figure 1–40, the radius rotates over the ulna, turning the palm of the hand downward or to the posterior, so that it is no longer visible in anatomical position. **Supination** [SOO-puh-NAY-shun], shown in Figure 1–41, returns the palm of the hand upward or to the anterior, so that it can be seen in anatomical

Dorsiflexion

flexion of the dorsal aspect of the foot, pointing the toes toward the head.

Plantarflexion

flexion of the plantar aspect of the foot, pointing the toes away from the head.

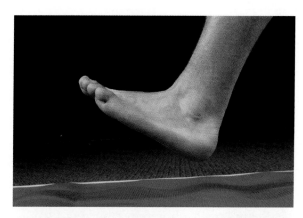

FIGURE 1–38 Dorsiflexion of the foot at the talocrural joint.

© Milady, a part of Cengage Learning. Photography by Yanik Chauvin.

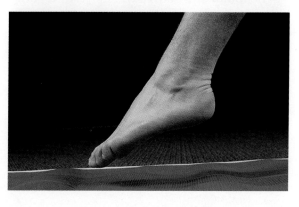

FIGURE 1–39 Plantarflexion of the foot at the talocrural joint.

© Milady, a part of Cengage Learning. Photography by Yanik Chauvin.

Pronation

a movement during which the radius revolves around the ulna, turning the palm of the hand downward.

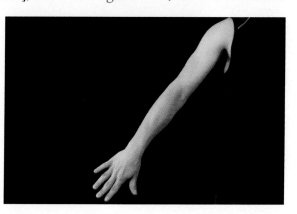

FIGURE 1–40 Pronation of the forearm at the proximal and distal radioulnar joints.

© Milady, a part of Cengage Learning. Photography by Yanik Chauvin.

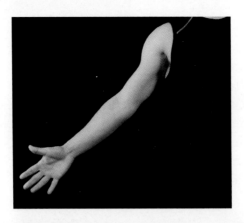

position. In both actions, the ulna remains stationary as the radius revolves around it. Examples of pronation and supination include:

- Pronation: turning your completed exam paper face down.
- Supination: turning your exam paper face up again because you forgot to write your name on it.

FIGURE 1–41 Supination of the forearm at the proximal radioulnar joint.

HERE'S A TIP

In anatomical position, the hand is supinated: the palm is visible and faces upward.

Supination

a movement during which the radius revolves around the ulna, turning the palm of the hand upward.

Tilt

the slight movement of one aspect of a structure away from anatomical position.

Tilt actions at the scapula and the pelvis

The range of movements at the scapula and the pelvis accommodate the weight-bearing function of the pelvis, though they share the action of **tilt**: the slight movement of one aspect of a structure away from anatomical position. Tilt actions of the scapula occur at its articulations with the thoracic ribs, the scapulocostal joints—not true synovial joints.

Scapular tilt, shown in Figure 1–42, may be bilateral or unilateral:

- Lateral tilt of the scapula moves the inferior angle laterally at its articulation with the ribs. Medial tilt returns it to anatomical position.
- For example, reaching one arm over the top of your head to scratch the ear on the opposite side.
- The scapula may also tilt toward the anterior or posterior at its articulation with the ribs.

DID YOU KNOW?

Scapular tilt is sometimes called rotation of the scapula.

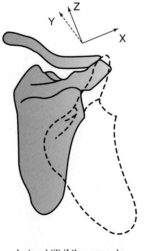

Lateral tilt if the scapula

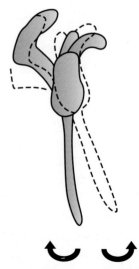

Anterior   Posterior
Anterior/Posterior tilt of the scapula

FIGURE 1–42 Lateral and anterior/posterior tilt of the scapula at scapulocostal joints.

- For example, lifting one arm to scratch an itch on the same side of your upper back.

At the pelvis, tilt is bilateral and takes place at the lumbosacral joint:

- Posterior tilt angles the pubis to the superior.
- Anterior tilt angles the pubis to the inferior.
- For example: belly dancing!

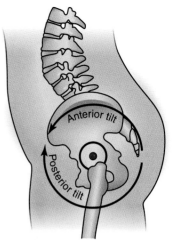

HERE'S A TIP

To visualize pelvic tilt, imagine the pelvic vault, the large opening created by the shape of the pelvic bones, as a basin: During anterior tilt, water can pour out of the basin. During posterior tilt, water cannot pour out. Figure 1–43 illustrates pelvic tilt.

FIGURE 1–43 Anterior and posterior tilt of the pelvis at the spinal joints.

Deviations at the mandible and the wrist

Additional joint movements are possible at the mandible and the wrist, sometimes called **deviations**, another term for movement of structures away from anatomical position.

Lateral or medial deviation of the mandible at the temporomandibular joint:

- In a unilateral movement, the mandible can be moved laterally, for example, while chewing.

Radial or ulnar deviation of the hand at the radiocarpal joint, shown in Figure 1–44, is also called abduction or adduction of the wrist:

- During **radial deviation** or abduction of the wrist, the thumb or radial side of the hand moves away from the midline of the body when in anatomical position, or toward the radius when in any other position.
- During **ulnar deviation** or adduction of the wrist, the little finger or ulnar side of the hand moves toward the midline of the body when in anatomical position or toward the ulna when in any other position. For example, waving hello or brushing crumbs off the table.

DID YOU KNOW?

The range of radial and ulnar deviation is limited by the styloid processes at the distal ends of the radius and the ulna.

Deviation

a term for certain movements of structures away from anatomical position.

Radial deviation

abduction of the hand at the wrist, moving it away from the midline of the body.

Ulnar deviation

adduction of the hand at the wrist, moving it toward the midline of the body

Opposition

a diagonal movement of the thumb across the hand, making contact with the other digits.

Striated

the appearance of skeletal or cardiac muscle tissue that, when viewed under a microscope, has alternating light and dark bands.

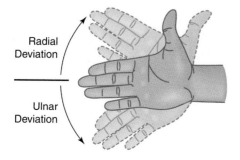

Radial Deviation

Ulnar Deviation

FIGURE 1–44 Radial and ulnar deviation of the hand at the wrist.

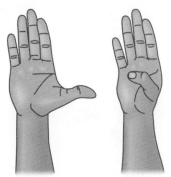

Extension of the
thumb

Flexion of the
thumb

FIGURE 1–45 Flexion and
extension of the thumb at the
first carpometacarpal joint.

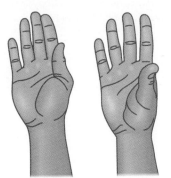

Adduction
of the thumb

Abduction
of the thumb

FIGURE 1–46 Abduction and
adduction of the thumb at the
first carpometacarpal joint.

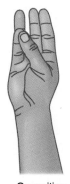

Opposition

FIGURE 1–47 Opposition
of the thumb at the first
carpometacarpal joint.

Lab Activity 1–5 on
page 50 is designed to
help you learn how to
demonstrate and identify
additional joint actions.

© Milady, a part of Cengage Learning.

Actions of the thumb

Actions of the thumb differ from actions of the other digits of the hand.
The unique saddle formation of the joint between the hand and the
thumb, the first carpometacarpal joint, allows greater range of motion
for the thumb. The actions of the thumb are described by their relation to
the hand itself. Figures 1–45, 1–46, and 1–47 illustrate the actions of the
thumb at the first carpometacarpal joint, which include:

- Flexion: moving the thumb toward the hand, and slightly
  forward.
- Extension: moving the thumb away from the hand and slightly
  backward.
- Abduction: moving the thumb toward the anterior of the wrist.
- Adduction: moving the thumb toward the posterior of the wrist.
- **Opposition**: diagonal movement of the thumb across the hand,
  making contact with the other digits.

> ### HERE'S A TIP
>
> The actions of the thumb can be difficult to understand. Don't give up! Practice
> the actions until they make sense to you, keeping these factors in mind:
>
> - From anatomical position, extension of the thumb must occur before
>   flexion.
> - From anatomical position, abduction must occur before adduction.
>
> Look at—and palpate—the actions of the thumb at the first carpometacarpal
> joint itself. Ignore what the tip of the thumb appears to be doing.

Joint actions rarely occur singularly. Movement is complex, with a
multitude of variations. You might flex your forearm and radially deviate your hand during medial rotation of the arm at the glenohumeral
joint, or plantarflex your foot at the talocrural joint while flexing your
leg at the tibiofemoral joint and extending your thigh at the acetabulofemoral joint. Complex movements are discussed and deconstructed in
Chapter 4, Deconstructing Complex Movements. Table 1–3 summarizes
the terms for joint actions.

MUSCLE STRUCTURE AND FUNCTION

Before you can effectively palpate and treat muscle, you must understand muscle structure, both gross (visible with the naked eye) and
microscopic (visible only when viewed under a microscope). When you
palpate or massage a muscle, you affect even its microscopic structures
(refer to Figures 1–61 and 1–62 on pages 52–53).

There are three types of muscle tissue, as shown in Figure 1–48.
Skeletal and cardiac muscle tissue is **striated** [STRY-ayt-ed]: when
viewed under a microscope, it has alternating light and dark bands.
Muscle-tissue control by the nervous system may be voluntary or

TABLE 1-3

TERMS FOR JOINT ACTIONS	
TERM FOR JOINT ACTION	**DESCRIPTION**
Flexion	A decrease in the angle between articulating bones in the sagittal plane.
Extension	An increase in the angle between articulating bones in the sagittal plane.
Lateral flexion	Bending of the head or the trunk to one side in the frontal plane.
Hyperextension	Extension of a body part beyond anatomical position.
Abduction	Movement of a limb away from the midline of the body, in the frontal plane.
Adduction	Movement of a limb toward the midline of the body, in the frontal plane.
Horizontal abduction	Movement of a flexed limb away from the midline of the body, in the horizontal or transverse plane.
Horizontal adduction	Movement of a flexed limb toward the midline of the body, in the horizontal or transverse plane.
Circumduction	Circular movement of the distal part of a limb while the proximal part of the limb remains stationary.
Rotation	Revolution of a bone around a single longitudinal axis.
Medial rotation	Rotation of the anterior surface of a long bone toward the midline of the body
Lateral rotation	Rotation of the anterior surface of a long bone away from the midline of the body.
Elevation	Movement of a body part upward, toward the head.
Depression	Movement of a body part downward, away from the head.
Protraction	Movement of the shoulder or the jaw forward, to the anterior.
Retraction	Movement of the shoulder or the jaw backward, to the posterior.
Inversion	Movement of the sole of the foot inward, toward the midline of the body.
Eversion	Movement of the sole of the foot outward, away from the midline of the body.
Dorsiflexion	Flexion of the dorsal aspect of the foot, pointing the toes toward the head.
Plantarflexion	Flexion of the plantar aspect of the foot, pointing the toes away from the head.
Pronation	Rotation of the forearm to turn the palm of the hand downward.
Supination	Rotation of the forearm to turn the palm of the hand upward.
Tilt	A slight movement of one aspect of a structure away from anatomical position.
Radial deviation	Abduction of the hand at the wrist, moving it away from the midline of the body.
Ulnar deviation	Adduction of the hand at the wrist, moving it toward the midline of the body.
Opposition	A diagonal movement of the thumb across the hand, making contact with the other digits.

© Milady, a part of Cengage Learning.

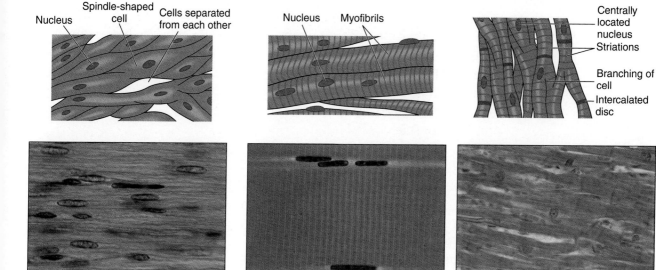

FIGURE 1-48 Skeletal, smooth, and cardiac muscle.

© Milady, a part of Cengage Learning.

involuntary. When muscle contraction is involuntary, it happens without your conscious participation. You do not have to remind your heart to beat or your blood vessels to dilate.

- **Smooth muscle** lines blood vessels and portions of the respiratory and digestive tracts. The contractions of smooth muscle tissue move substances through tracts. Smooth muscle is not striated and nervous system control of its contractions is not voluntary.
- **Cardiac muscle** is heart muscle. The contractions of cardiac muscle tissue pump blood through the chambers of the heart. Cardiac muscle is striated and its nervous system control is not voluntary.
- **Skeletal muscle** tissue is striated and for the most part, its nervous system control is voluntary.

DID YOU KNOW?

Although most skeletal muscles are consciously controlled by coordination with the nervous system, the actions of some skeletal muscles can be overridden by autonomic nervous system control. You don't have to remember to contract and relax your diaphragm in order to breathe, for example; normal respiration is under involuntary nervous system control. You can, however, override the involuntary control of the diaphragm and consciously control your breath to sigh, sneeze, cough, or to increase your intake of oxygen.

Muscle Anatomy

An examination of the anatomy of a skeletal muscle begins with the connective tissue wrappings that surround the multiple layers of gross and microscopic muscle components, shown in Figure 1–49.

Gross muscle anatomy

Superficial fascia lies deep to the dermis, the connective tissue layer of the skin, and is sometimes called the **hypodermis** [hy-poh-DUR-mis]. Superficial fascia separates muscles from the skin. Deep to superficial fascia is **deep fascia**, which lines the walls of the body and holds muscle groups together. Extensions of deep fascia, shown in Figure 1–49, form three layers of connective tissue that strengthen and protect a muscle:

- The outer **epimysium** [ep-i-MI-see-um] surrounds the entire muscle.
- The intermediate **perimysium** [payr-ih-MIS-ee-um] surrounds groups of muscle fibers called **fascicles** [FAS-ih-kuls].
- The inner **endomysium** [en-do-MY-see-um] extends into fascicles to surround and separate individual muscle fibers.

Microscopic muscle anatomy

A muscle fiber, called a **myofiber** [MY-oh-fy-bur], is a cell. It has the same components as most of the cells of the body: a cell membrane, cytoplasm, and nuclei and other organelles. As with all cells, proteins play

---

Superficial fascia

another term for the hypodermis.

Hypodermis

the layer of superficial fascia separating skin from muscles.

Deep fascia

dense connective tissue that lines the walls of the body and holds muscle groups together.

Epimysium

an extension of deep fascia that surrounds an entire skeletal muscle.

Perimysium

the intermediate layer of connective tissue within a skeletal muscle that surrounds groups of muscle fibers into fascicles.

Fascicle

a bundle of skeletal muscle fibers.

Endomysium

the inner layer of connective tissue that extends into the fascicles of a skeletal muscle to surround and separate individual muscle fibers.

Myofiber

a muscle cell.

FIGURE 1-49 Skeletal muscle-fiber structure.

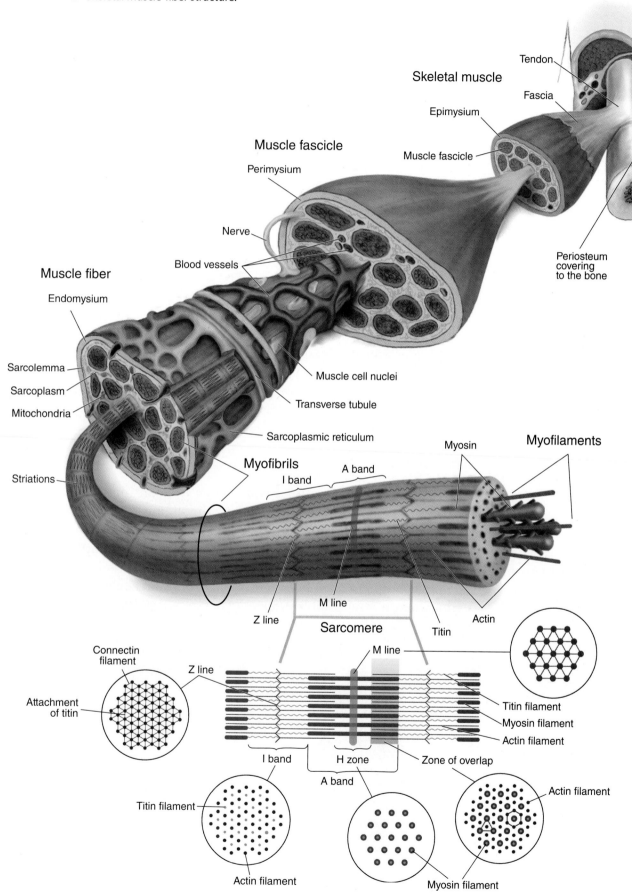

Myosin

a contractile protein within a myofiber that forms thick filaments.

Actin

a contractile protein within a myofiber that forms thin filaments.

Troponin

a regulatory protein within a myofiber whose action, governed by tropomyosin, allows or prohibits the slide of filaments to create skeletal muscle contraction.

Tropomyosin

a regulatory protein within a myofiber which governs the action of troponin.

DID YOU KNOW?

The function of the myofiber is contraction of the muscle.

Neurotransmitter

a chemical messenger from the nervous system that assists a nerve impulse across a gap, such as at the neuromuscular junction.

Neuromuscular junction

the functional junction between the nervous and muscular systems.

Neuron

a nerve cell.

vital roles in the myofiber's functioning. Components of the myofiber include:

- Proteins: **myosin** [MY-oh-sin] and **actin** [AK-tin], shown in Figure 1–49, are contractile proteins that compose the filaments within the myofiber that slide together during muscle contraction. **Troponin** [TROH-puh-nin] and **tropomyosin** [Troh-puh-MY-oh-sin], not shown in Figure 1–49, are regulatory proteins that regulate the slide of contractile proteins. The position of troponin and tropomyosin molecules allows or prevents the slide of actin filaments along filaments of myosin. It is the sliding of actin filaments that contracts the length of a skeletal muscle and moves the bones to which the muscle attaches closer together.

- Many nuclei: skeletal muscle contraction requires a ready supply of contractile and regulatory proteins. Because proteins play vital roles in muscle contraction and protein synthesis begins in the nucleus, a myofiber may contain as many as 100 nuclei, as shown in Figure 1–50. Also visible in Figure 1–49.

- Many mitochondria: sliding of filaments within the myofiber—and the resulting contraction of many myofibers—is powered by adenosine triphosphate (ATP), the body's energy currency. Mitochondria are the organelles that produce ATP. Where more ATP is required for general cellular work, greater numbers of mitochondria, shown in Figure 1–50, shown in Figure 1–49 are found nearby.

The Neuromuscular Junction

Skeletal muscle contraction results when the contractile protein filaments within a myofiber slide together. The sliding together of filaments is initiated by the action of **neurotransmitters**, chemical messengers from the nervous system. Neurotransmitters assist nerve impulses across gaps along the route they travel, such as at the **neuromuscular junction**, the functional junction between the nervous and skeletal muscle systems, where a single motor **neuron** (a nerve cell) stimulates many myofibers, as seen in Figure 1–50.

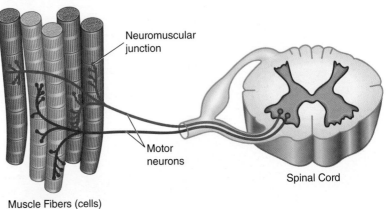

Neuromuscular junction

Motor neurons

Spinal Cord

Muscle Fibers (cells)

Motor Unit

FIGURE 1–50 A motor unit consists of a single motor neuron and the muscle fibers it stimulates at the neuromuscular junction.

Actions of neurotransmitters

Neurotransmitters at the neuromuscular junction initiate and control the slide of filaments in a myofiber:

- The neurotransmitter **acetylcholine (ACh)** [uh-SEET-ul-koh-leen] is released at the neuromuscular junction.
- The presence of ACh triggers mechanisms that result in a change in the electrical charge inside the myofiber.
- The change in the myofiber's electrical charge initiates a chemical change that triggers regulatory proteins to allow contractile protein filaments to slide together.
- An enzyme, **acetylcholinesterase (AChE)**, [uh-seet-ul-koh-luh-NESS-tur-ays] inactivates ACh, ensuring a single, complete filament slide before another can be triggered by the presence of ACh.

Motor units and recruitment

Each skeletal muscle has one neuromuscular junction, though that single motor neuron may stimulate many hundreds of myofibers. A **motor unit**, shown in Figure 1–50, is made up of a single motor neuron and all the myofibers it comes in contact with and can stimulate to contract. All the myofibers in a single motor unit contract simultaneously. The size and capacity of motor units, however, varies widely:

- A motor unit in a muscle controlling movement of the eye may contain fewer than 20 myofibers.
- A motor unit in a large, powerful muscle of the thigh may contain more than 1,000 myofibers.
- Muscles with many small motor units create precise, controlled contractions.
- Muscles with fewer, larger motor units create stronger, more powerful contractions.

DID YOU KNOW?

A single motor unit stimulates all its myofibers to contract completely. When greater force of contraction is needed, additional motor units must be called on to participate. Called **motor unit recruitment**, this process ensures safe, smooth muscle contraction and delays muscle fatigue: it allows some motor units to relieve strain on others by alternating contraction.

TYPES OF MUSCLE CONTRACTION

Skeletal muscle contraction creates action at a joint: the articulating bones may move closer together, farther apart, or around each other. A skeletal muscle attaches to the bones on either side of a joint via its tendons. The attachment of a skeletal muscle to the bone that is usually mobile during contraction is called its **insertion,** shown in Figure 1–51. The attachment to the bone that is fixed or not usually mobile during contraction is called its **origin.** There are various types of skeletal muscle contraction.

Acetylcholine or ACh

a neurotransmitter that triggers mechanisms at the neuromuscular junction that change the electrical charge inside the myofiber.

Acetylcholinesterase or AChE

an enzyme that inactivates acetylcholine (ACh), ensuring a single and complete filament slide before another can be triggered by the presence of ACh.

Motor unit

a motor neuron and all the myofibers it stimulates.

Motor unit recruitment

the process which allows some motor units to relieve strain on other motor units by alternating contraction or enlisting additional motor units when greater force of contraction is required.

Insertion

the skeletal muscle attachment on the bone that is usually mobile during contraction.

Origin

the skeletal muscle attachment on the bone that usually remains fixed during contraction.

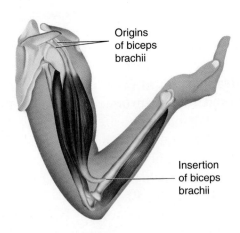

FIGURE 1–51 The origin usually attaches to the bone that is immobile during an action; the insertion of a muscle is usually on the bone that is mobile during an action.

Isotonic Contractions

During an **isotonic** [eye-soh-THAN-ik] **contraction**, the length of the muscle changes. The muscle may lengthen or it may shorten, but the result is movement of the bones to which the muscle attaches. Isotonic contractions result in skeletal movement and are categorized as follows.

Concentric contractions

During a **concentric** [kahn-SEN-trik] **contraction**, the muscle fibers shorten toward the center of the muscle: toward the belly of the muscle, *not* toward the origin. The result is shortening of the muscle. For example:

- You lift a book from a table: the fibers of Biceps brachii, a primary flexor of the forearm at the humeroulnar joint, contract toward the center on the anterior of the humeroulnar joint, shortening the distance between the anterior aspects of the humerus and the radius and ulna. In Figure 1–52, Biceps brachii is shown as it concentrically contracts during flexion of the forearm at the humeroulnar joint.

| **Isotonic**
a skeletal muscle contraction which changes the length of the muscle.

| **Concentric**
a skeletal muscle contraction that shortens the muscle.

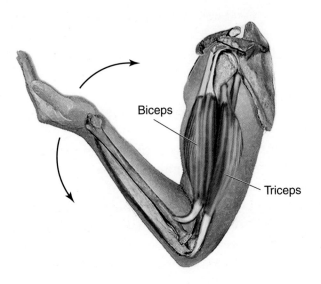

FIGURE 1–52 Contractions of Biceps brachii and Triceps brachii create flexion and extension of the forearm at the elbow.

Eccentric contractions

During an **eccentric** [ek-SEN-trik] **contraction**, the muscle fibers lengthen or slacken. The result is that the muscle length increases. For example:

- You lift a book from a table: the fibers of Triceps brachii, a primary extensor of the forearm at the humeroulnar joint, slacken to lengthen on the posterior of the humeroulnar joint, allowing the distance between the posterior aspects of the humerus the radius and ulna to lengthen. In Figure 1–52, Triceps brachii is shown as it eccentrically contracts during flexion of the forearm at the humeroulnar joint.

Eccentric contraction

a skeletal muscle contraction that slackens muscle fibers and lengthens the muscle.

DID YOU KNOW?

A muscle that eccentrically contracts in an action is said to oppose the muscle that concentrically contracts in the action. The interaction between concentric and eccentric contractions ensures smooth, safe, and effective muscle action. Muscle fibers in an eccentric contraction both allow concentric contraction and limit its range: the capacity of the muscle to completely slacken allows a complete concentric contraction in the opposing muscle, but its **resting length**, the normal length of the non-contracting muscle maintained by its tone, limits the concentric contraction to its natural range. Because of the dual actions of allowing and limiting by slackening and contracting a muscle in eccentric contraction can be more vulnerable to injury.

Resting length

the length of the non-contracting muscle, maintained by its tone.

Lab Activity 1–6 on page 50 is designed to help you learn how to demonstrate and identify concentric and eccentric muscle contractions.

Isometric Contractions

During an **isometric** [eye-soh-MET-rik] **contraction**, some fibers of a muscle contract, but the length of the muscle does not change and the distance between articulating bones is unaffected. Isometric contractions result in rapid muscle fatigue, because the contraction is sustained, demanding greater energy use.

For example:

You hold a book in one hand, your arm outstretched, immobile.

Isometric

a skeletal muscle contraction which does not change the length of the muscle.

Lab Activity 1–7 on page 51 is designed to help you learn how to demonstrate and identify isometric muscle contraction.

DID YOU KNOW?

Upright posture, created by the persistent state of contraction in postural muscles, is the result of isometric contraction, among other factors.

Reverse Actions

During a **reverse action**, the structure that is usually mobile in an action is fixed, while the structure that is usually fixed in an action is mobile. For example, extension of the leg at the tibiofemoral joint can be two very different actions:

- When rising from a chair to a standing position, as seen in Figure 1–53, you are extending your leg at the tibiofemoral joint. The femur is the mobile structure, while the tibia remains fixed: the weight of the entire skeleton is moved.

Reverse action

an action during which the structure that is usually mobile is fixed, while the structure that is usually fixed is mobile.

Lab Activity 1–8 on page 51 is designed to help you learn how to demonstrate and identify reverse muscle action.

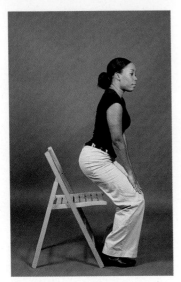

FIGURE 1–53 Rising from a seated position extends the leg at the knee while bearing the weight of the trunk; in a reverse action, this person might remain seated and swing her leg at the knee, also extending it, but with no weight-bearing component in the action.

Agonist

the prime skeletal mover in a muscle action.

Antagonist

a skeletal muscle that allows and limits the movement of an agonist in a muscle action.

Synergist

a skeletal muscle that assists an adjacent agonist or antagonist in an action.

Stabilizer

a skeletal muscle that fixes proximal joints in place during an action, so that distal limbs can bear weight more effectively.

■ When you remain seated, however, and swing your leg backward and forward, you are also extending your leg at the tibiofemoral joint: in this reverse action, the femur remains fixed while the tibia is mobile. The weight of the skeleton is not moved.

ROLES A MUSCLE CAN PLAY

The action of a muscle at a joint produces movement of the skeleton. Muscles play different roles in movement, depending on the action being performed, the type and shape of the muscle, and its fiber type.

Role by Muscle Action

Each skeletal muscle plays different roles, depending on the action required.

The agonist in an action

The **agonist** [AG-uh-nist] in an action is the prime mover, usually the muscle that is *concentrically contracting* or shortening the length of the muscle.
■ The agonist is usually the largest, most superficial muscle crossing the joint in motion.

The antagonist in an action

The **antagonist** [an-TAG-uh-nust] in an action is the muscle whose placement and fiber direction in relation to the agonist in the action requires it to *eccentrically contract*, or slacken to lengthen the muscle, in order for the action of the agonist at the joint to occur.
■ The antagonist is usually the largest, most superficial muscle that crosses the opposite aspect of the same joint as the agonist.
■ The agonist and antagonist are said to "oppose" each other in an action: concentric contraction of the agonist muscle is opposed by eccentric contraction of the antagonist muscle.

In flexion of the forearm at the humeroulnar joint, for example, shown in Figure 1–52, Biceps brachii is the agonist and Triceps brachii is the antagonist. In extension of the forearm at the humeroulnar joint, their roles are reversed: Triceps brachii is the agonist and Biceps brachii is the antagonist.

Synergists and stabilizers in actions

Movement of the skeleton is seldom the result of only agonist and antagonist muscle actions. A **synergist** [SIN-ur-jist] muscle is one that is adjacent to and assists the agonist or antagonist in an action, while other nearby muscles may act as **stabilizers**, fixing proximal joints or structures in place so that distal limbs can bear weight more effectively, unhindered by unnecessary movements. In flexion of the forearm at the humeroulnar joint, shown in Figure 1–52, adjacent muscles that may act as synergists and stabilizers include muscles in the forearm flexor and extensor groups, Anconeus, Brachialis, and Brachioradialis.

HERE'S A TIP

Note that the role assigned to one muscle participating in an action—agonist, antagonist, synergist, or stabilizer—refers to its *role in a given action*, not to the muscle itself. There is no list of muscles that are agonists or antagonists or synergists. While Biceps brachii may play the role of agonist in flexion of the forearm at the humeroulnar joint, for example, it switches roles to play the antagonist in extension of the forearm at the humeroulnar joint, and may be considered a synergist to supinator in supination of the forearm at the radioulnar joints.

As with many concepts in movement, there are varying opinions about which muscles play what roles in certain actions. Once again, in flexion of the forearm at the humeroulnar joint, Biceps brachii is the long, superficial muscle with vertical fibers that crosses the humeroulnar joint. Many sources consider Biceps brachii the agonist in flexion of the forearm at the humeroulnar joint. Other sources, however, name Brachialis as the agonist in flexion of the forearm at the humeroulnar joint because Brachialis, though it lies deep to Biceps brachii, has more fibers in its belly, has more vertical fibers crossing the same joint, and is a stronger flexor at that joint.

IN THE TREATMENT ROOM

Congenital skeletal and muscle formations, along with diseases or dysfunctions, also impact the roles muscles play in actions:

- A Rhomboid that is weak or injured may be assisted or even replaced in retraction of the scapula at the scapulocostal joints by the middle fibers of Trapezius, usually a weaker retractor.
- The action of a Deltoid that is poorly innervated by a congenitally malformed or injured motor nerve may have to be replaced by Infraspinatus and Teres minor in lateral rotation of the arm at the glenohumeral joint.
- Any adjacent muscle that crosses the same joint with some fibers in the same direction can serve as a synergist in an action. These factors make the strong case for utilizing skills in palpation and kinesiology for assessment of the client in your treatment room, not simply memorizing a list of agonists and antagonists in muscle actions.

Lab Activity 1–9 on page 51 is designed to help you learn how to demonstrate and identify the agonist and antagonist in an action.

Role by Muscle Function

Muscle roles can be created by their function: some types of muscles maintain the body's posture while others move the skeleton.

Phasic muscles

Phasic [FAY-zik] muscles are movers of the skeleton. They are used for quick, powerful movements. Phasic muscles usually respond to stress and dysfunction by becoming **hypotonic** [hy-poh-TAHN-ik]: weakening and losing tone. Table 1–4 lists the major phasic muscles and their main roles moving the skeleton.

Phasic

skeletal muscles that move the skeleton, used for quick, powerful movements.

TABLE 1-4

MAJOR PHASIC MUSCLES OF THE BODY AND THEIR ROLE IN MOVING THE SKELETON	
MAJOR PHASIC MUSCLES	**ROLE IN MOVING THE SKELETON**
The Scalene group	Flexes; laterally flexes and rotates the neck at the spinal joints.
Lower fibers of Pectoralis major	Adducts, horizontally adducts, flexes, and medially rotates the arm at the glenohumeral joint.
Trapezius (middle, lower fibers)	Retracts, depresses, and rotates the scapula at the scapulocostal joints.
Rhomboids	Retract the scapula at scapulocostal joints.
Serratus anterior	Stabilizes, protracts, and upwardly rotates the scapula at the scapulocostal joints.
Rectus abdominis	Flexes the trunk at the spinal joints.
Deltoid	Flexes and extends, medially and laterally rotates, and abducts the arm at the glenohumeral joint.
Forearm flexors and extensors	Flex or extend the forearm at the humeroulnar joint, or the hand at the radiocarpal joint.
The Gluteals: Gluteus maximus, medius, and minimus	Flexes or extends, medially or laterally rotates, and abducts or adducts the thigh at the acetabulofemoral joint.
Hamstrings	Extend the thigh at the acetabulofemoral joint and flex the leg at the tibiofemoral joint.
Vastus lateralis, medialis, and intermedius	Extend the leg at the tibiofemoral joint.
The Peroneal group: Peroneus longus, brevis, and tertius	All three peroneal muscles evert the foot at the intertarsal joints; Peroneus longus and brevis dorsiflex, but Peroneus tertius plantarflexes the foot at the talocrural joint.

Postural muscles

Postural

a skeletal muscle that stabilizes and supports the posture of the body.

Postural muscles stabilize and support the posture of the body. Postural muscles tend to respond to stress and dysfunction by becoming **hypertonic** [hy-pur-TAHN-ik], shortening and remaining in a partially contracted state. Table 1–5 lists the major postural muscles and their roles in maintaining posture.

TABLE 1-5

MAJOR POSTURAL MUSCLES OF THE BODY AND THEIR ROLES IN MAINTAINING POSTURE	
MAJOR POSTURAL MUSCLES	**ROLE IN MAINTAINING POSTURE**
Sternocleidomastoid (SCM)	Flexes the head at the spinal joints.
Trapezius (upper fibers)	Extends the neck at the spinal joints
Levator scapulae	Extends the neck at the spinal joints.
Upper Pectoralis major, Pectoralis minor	Adduct and horizontally adduct the arm at the glenohumeral joint.
Latissimus dorsi	Extends and adducts the arm at the glenohumeral joint.
Lumbar regions of the Erector spinae and Transversospinalis groups	Extend the trunk at the spinal joints.
Quadratus lumborum	Extends and laterally flexes the trunk at the spinal joints.
Psoas and Iliacus	Flex the trunk at the spinal joints.
Abdominal obliques	Flex the trunk at the spinal joints.
Piriformis	Laterally rotates the thigh at the acetabulofemoral joint.
Adductor longus and magnus	Adduct the thigh at the acetabulofemoral joint.
Tensor fasciae latae (TFL)	Medially rotates the thigh at the acetabulofemoral joint.
Medial hamstrings	Extend the thigh at the acetabulofemoral joint.
Gastrocnemius	Flexes the leg at the tibiofemoral joint.
Tibialis posterior	Plantarflexes and inverts the foot at the talocrural and intertarsal joints.

Postural muscles are found in the extremities as well as in the trunk. Their role in maintaining posture is often to extend and adduct muscles at a joint. Phasic muscles are also found throughout the body. Their role as movers of the skeleton requires a fuller range of actions at joints. Some muscles and muscle groups play roles in posture as well as movement of the skeleton: for example, while the upper fibers of Trapezius act as postural stabilizers by extending the head at spinal joints, its middle and lower fibers move the scapula to support the free movement of the arm at the glenohumeral joint. Figures 1–61 and 1–62 on pages 52–53 illustrate the major muscles of the body.

Lines of pull in muscles

A muscle's **line of pull** is an imaginary line drawn from its origin to its insertion that indicates the direction in which it will act on the joint it crosses, as shown in Figure 1–54. Each skeletal muscle crosses a joint and acts on that joint. If a muscle lies near to a joint, but does not actually cross it, it cannot act on that joint.

The direction of the muscle's fibers creates the action at the joint it crosses, its line of pull. In general terms:

- A muscle that crosses a joint with vertical fibers likely flexes and extends the bone at the joint.
- A muscle that crosses a joint with horizontal fibers likely abducts and adducts the bone at the joint.
- A muscle with fibers that wrap around a joint likely rotates the bone around the joint.

Muscle action at the joint is limited by several factors:

- The shape and orientation of the articulating bones: at the hinge humeroulnar joint, for example, the shape of the olecranon process of the ulna and the depth of the olecranon fossa of the humerus allow only flexion and extension.
- The condition of both the articulating bones and the muscle fibers: erosion or disease in the articulating bones and lack of tone or disease in the muscle limits action at the joint.

Of course, there are many variations and possibilities within these general rules. Some muscles cross more than one joint and can act on each. The fibers of other muscles are oriented in multiple directions, allowing them to create multiple actions.

Role by Muscle Shape

Although all skeletal muscles move the skeleton, a muscle's shape and the number and direction of its fibers—its grain—create its action at a joint. Understanding how the shape of a muscle creates its action furthers your understanding of its actions and potential injury patterns.

Some muscles are circular, such as the skeletal muscles that surround the eye and the mouth and the smooth muscles that form sphincters. Others are flat and attach to connective tissue structures, such as the attachment of the External obliques into the connective tissue of the abdomen.

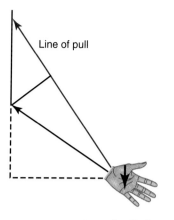
Line of pull

© Milady, a part of Cengage Learning.

FIGURE 1–54 Line of pull of a muscle indicates the direction in which it will act on the joint it crosses.

| **Line of pull**

an imaginary line drawn on a muscle from its origin to its insertion that indicates the direction in which it will act on the joint it crosses.

HERE'S A TIP

The actions of a muscle can be understood by knowing and palpating the joint it crosses and its line of pull. Understanding line of pull makes it unnecessary to memorize muscle actions!

Pennate muscles

A **pennate** [PEN-ayt] muscle has many fibers per motor unit. Pennate muscles are strong, but tire easily. The group is divided into:

- **Unipennate** [yoo-nih-PEN-ayt]: the fibers of these muscles are arranged to insert diagonally in a single direction into a strong tendon, which creates great strength. Extensor digitorum longus, shown in Figure 1–55, is an example of unipennate muscle.
- **Bipennate** [by-PEN-ayt]: these muscles have two rows of fibers that face in opposite diagonal directions, like the hairs of a feather. Bipennate muscles such as Rectus femoris, visible in Figure 1–56, create great power but have limited range of motion.
- **Multipennate** [mul-tih-PEN-ayt]: the fibers of multipennate muscles are arranged diagonally in multiple rows, with a central tendon that may itself branch into other tendons. Deltoid, Figure 1–57, is a multipennate muscle: it has anterior, middle, and posterior segments.

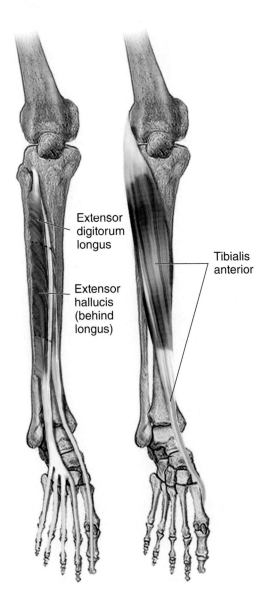

Extensor
digitorum
longus

Extensor
hallucis
(behind
longus)

Tibialis
anterior

FIGURE 1-55 Extensor digitorum longus is a unipennate muscle.

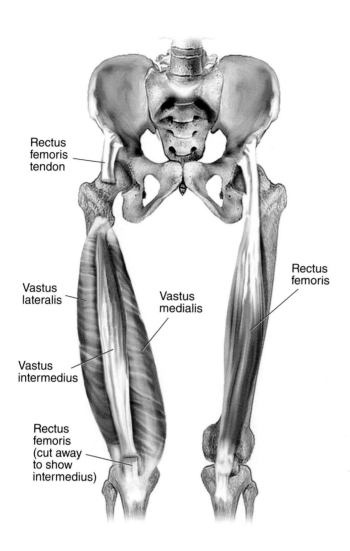

Rectus femoris tendon

Vastus lateralis

Vastus intermedius

Rectus femoris (cut away to show intermedius)

Vastus medialis

Rectus femoris

FIGURE 1-56 Rectus femoris is a bipennate muscle.

© Delmar, Cengage Learning.

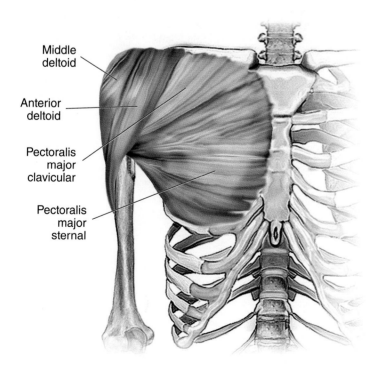

Middle deltoid

Anterior deltoid

Pectoralis major clavicular

Pectoralis major sternal

FIGURE 1-57 Deltoid is a multipennate muscle.

© Delmar, Cengage Learning.

Fusiform (fusiform= spindle-shaped)

A muscle shape; a spindle-shaped muscle which has a belly that is wider than either its origin or insertion.

Triangular

another name for convergent muscle shape.

Convergent

A muscle shape; the origin that is wider than the insertion. Also called triangular.

Fusiform muscles

Fusiform [FYOO-suh-form] muscles are spindle-shaped, with a belly that is wider than either the **origin** or the **insertion**. Fusiform muscles provide motion that is quicker rather than powerful, with a wide range. Biceps brachii, seen in Figure 1–58, is an example of a fusiform muscle.

Convergent muscles

Also known as **triangular** muscles, **convergent** [kun-VUR-jent] muscles have origins that are wider than their insertions, creating maximum force, such as in Pectoralis major, visible in Figure 1–57.

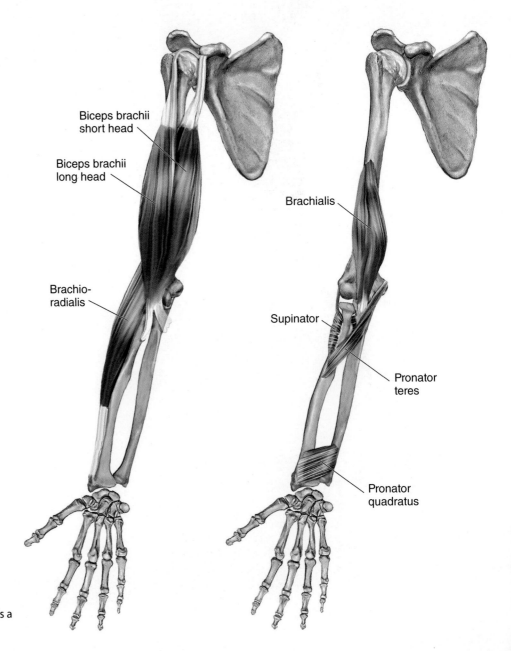

Biceps brachii short head

Biceps brachii long head

Brachialis

Brachio-radialis

Supinator

Pronator teres

Pronator quadratus

FIGURE 1–58 Biceps brachii is a fusiform muscle.

Parallel muscles

As the name suggests, the fibers of **parallel** muscles run parallel to each other. Also called **strap** muscles, these are usually long muscles that create large movements. They are not as strong as other muscles, but provide good endurance. An example of a parallel, or strap muscle is Sartorius, visible in Figure 1–59.

> **Parallel**
>
> a skeletal muscle shape with fibers that run parallel to each other; sometimes called a strap muscle.

> **Strap**
>
> another name for a parallel muscle.

> **DID YOU KNOW?**
>
> A subgroup is called "strap with tendinous intersections," exemplified by Rectus abdominis—the tendinous intersections create the "six-pack" look of highly developed abs.

Role by Fiber Type

Skeletal muscles are further characterized by their fiber type and the actions their fibers create: the fibers of some muscles create large

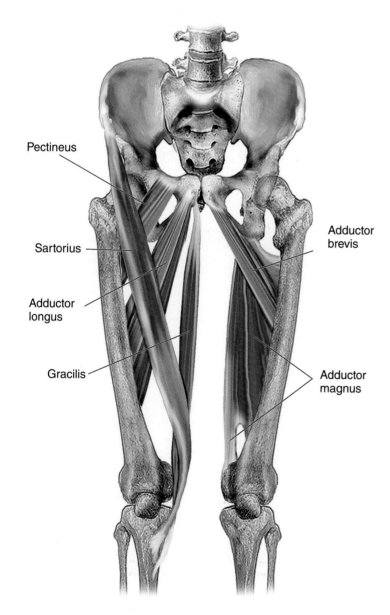

Pectineus

Sartorius

Adductor longus

Gracilis

Adductor brevis

Adductor magnus

FIGURE 1-59 Sartorius is a parallel, or strap, muscle.

DID YOU KNOW?

Postural muscles contain more Type I fibers, while phasic muscles contain a higher level of Type II fibers.

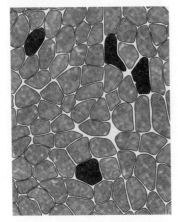

FIGURE 1–60 Type II fibers stain more darkly and are visible in this cross-section of a skeletal muscle. The lighter fibers are likely Type I fibers.

movements of the skeleton, while others support and maintain alignment of the skeleton. In many instances, these functions overlap. Muscle fibers vary by their size, the time it takes them to fatigue, their relative blood supply, and the velocity or speed of their contractions.

Type I muscle fibers

Type I muscle fibers, also called "slow twitch," are the smallest muscle fibers. They are slow to fatigue, have a rich blood supply, and the velocity of their contractions is slow. Type I muscle fibers are found in postural muscles, such as those in the neck, where they are used for maintaining posture and aerobic endurance activities.

Type IIA muscle fibers

Type IIA muscle fibers are larger than Type I. They are not as slow to fatigue, they also have a rich blood supply, and the velocity of their contractions is fast. Type IIA muscle fibers are found in leg muscles, where they are used for walking and sprinting.

Type IIB muscle fibers

Type IIB muscle fibers, also called "fast twitch," are the largest fibers. They are the quickest to fatigue; their blood supply is low and the velocity of their contractions is fast. Type IIB muscle fibers are found in arm muscles, where they are used for rapid, intense movements that are short in duration.

Most muscles contain both Type I and Type II fibers, as shown in Figure 1–60, and function as both movers and stabilizers. Table 1–6 summarizes muscle fiber characteristics and functions.

TABLE 1–6

MUSCLE FIBER CHARACTERISTICS				
MUSCLE FIBER TYPES	SIZE	FATIGUE TIME	BLOOD SUPPLY	CONTRACTION VELOCITY	LOCATIONS
Type I	Smallest	Slow	High	Slow	Postural muscles
Type IIA	Intermediate	Intermediate	High	Fast	Legs
Type IIB	Largest	Fast	Low	Fast	Arms

MUSCLE NAMES

The name of a muscle can reveal a great deal about its location and its action. Understanding the components of the name of a muscle can be a great help in predicting its location and action. For example, a muscle named "supinator" is probably located around the radioulnar joints, and its action is likely to be supination. The location and action of Flexor digitorum longus can be understood by examining each word in its name: "flexor" means this is a muscle that flexes, "digitorum" means that this is a muscle that acts on the digits of the hand or the foot, "longus" means that this is a long muscle, probably one with a shorter nearby counterpart.

Table 1–7 describes the components that make up the names of many muscles.

TABLE 1-7

MUSCLE NAME COMPONENTS	
MUSCLE NAME COMPONENT	**DEFINITION**
Flexor [FLEK-sur]	A muscle that flexes a joint.
Extensor [ik-STEN-sur]	A muscle that extends a joint.
Rotator [ROH-tayt-ur]	A muscle that moves a body part around a longitudinal axis.
Supinator [SOO-puh-nayt-ur]	A muscle that turns the hand upward.
Pronator [proh-NAY-tohr]	A muscle that turns the hand downward.
Abductor [ab-DUK-tur]	A muscle that moves a body part away from the midline of the body.
Adductor [ah-DUK-tur]	A muscle that moves a body part closer to the midline of the body.
Longus [LAWNG-us]	A muscle that is longer than another muscle in the same group; the name of a companion muscle may include the word "brevis."
Brevis [BREV-us]	A muscle that is shorter than another muscle in the same group; the name of a companion muscle may include the word "longus."
Magnus [MAG-nus]	A muscle that is the largest of muscles within a group; the name of the companion muscle in the same group may include the words "longus" and brevis."
Major	A muscle that is larger than another muscle in the same group; the name of a companion muscle may include the word "minor."
Minor	A muscle that is smaller than another muscle in the same group; the name of the companion muscle may include the word "major."
Profundus [proh-FUN-dus]	A muscle that is farther away from the surface of the body than another; the name of a companion muscle may include the word "superficialis."
Superficialis [soo-pur-fish-ee-AY-lis]	A muscle that is closer to the surface of the body than another; the name of the companion muscle may include the word "profundus."
Brachii; Brachialis [BRAY-kee-ee; bray-kih-AY-lis]	A muscle that attaches to the arm.
Radial; Radialis [RAY-dee-ul; RAY-dee-AY-lis]	A muscle that attaches to the thumb side of the forearm.
Ulnar; Ulnaris [UL-nur; ul-NAYR-us]	A muscle that attaches to the little-finger side of the forearm.
Carpal; Carpi [KAR-pul; KAR-pye]	A muscle that attaches to the wrist.
Digit; Digiti; Digitorum [DIJ-ut; DIJ-ih-ty; DIJ-ih-tore-um]	A muscle that attaches to the fingers or toes.
Pollix; Pollicis	A muscle that attaches to the thumb.
Femoral; Femoris [FEM-ur-ul; FEMU-ur-us]	A muscle that attaches to the femur or the thigh.
Tibialis [tib-ih-AL-is]	A muscle that attaches to the tibia.
Peroneal [payr-uh-NEE-ul]	A muscle that attaches to the fibula of the leg.
Fibularis; Fibulares [FIB-yuh-layr-is; FIB-yuh-layr-ees]	Another term for "peroneal."
Hallux; Hallucis [HAL-uks; HAL-yuh-sis]	A muscle that attaches to the big toe.
Scapulae [SKAP-yuh-lee]	A muscle that attaches to the scapula.
Levator [lih-VAYT-ur]	A muscle that lifts or elevates a body part or structure.
Spinae; Spinatus [SPY-nee; SPY-nuh-tus]	A muscle that attaches to a spiny process or to the spinal column.
Manus [MAN-us]	A muscle that attaches to the hand.
Pedis [PED-us]	A muscle that attaches to the foot.

Lab Activity 1–10 on page 51 is designed to help you learn how to demonstrate and identify muscle attachments and actions.

SUMMARY

This chapter introduced you to the concepts of client assessment—posture, gait assessment, and palpation—and to their roles in creating a client treatment plan. Client assessment is rooted in an understanding of how joints and muscles interact to create posture and gait. Effective palpation depends on knowledge of the actions of muscles during posture and gait. Chapter 2, Posture Assessment, introduces posture assessment techniques.

LAB ACTIVITIES

LAB ACTIVITY 1–1: PRELIMINARY POSTURE ASSESSMENT

1. Working in a triad, students take turns performing an initial visual assessment, answering the questions posed about the posture shown in Figure 1–2 on Page 4.
   - One partner acts as the client and is assessed.
   - A second partner performs the visual assessment.
   - The third partner quietly observes the assessment.
2. After each assessment, the assessing and observing partners compare their observations and discuss any discrepancies in their assessment of their partner's standing posture.
3. Switch partners and repeat until all partners have assessed and been assessed.

LAB ACTIVITY 1–2: PRELIMINARY GAIT ASSESSMENT

1. Working in a triad, one partner walks as far as she can in the space available as the assessing partner observes her usual gait, noting the following aspects of her gait, and the third partner observes the assessment:
   - Does she "lead" with her head or with her hips, with her arms or with her feet? Which part of her body enters the room first?
   - Is her spine straight as she walks, or is it "torqued" to one side?
   - Does she swing her arms equally or does one arm swing out wide?
   - Are her hips level or does one hip swing noticeably forward?
   - Do her feet point forward, inward or outward?
2. After each assessment, the assessing and observing partners compare their observations and discuss any discrepancies.
3. Switch partners and repeat until all partners have assessed and been assessed.

LAB ACTIVITY 1–3: DEMONSTRATING AND IDENTIFYING ANGULAR JOINT ACTIONS

1. Working with a partner, choose an activity of daily life that clearly demonstrates one of these joint actions:
    - Flexion of the head, the trunk, the arm, the elbow, the thigh, and the knee.
    - Extension of the arm and the thigh.
    - Lateral flexion of the head and the trunk.
    - Hyperextension of the head.
    - Abduction of the arm and the thigh.
    - Circumduction of the arm and the thigh. Keep in mind that circumduction can occur in more than one plane and may be a large or a small action.

2. Plan carefully how you can demonstrate your chosen action, but don't be afraid to use your imagination. Clearly demonstrate your chosen joint action, without superfluous movement.

3. Ask your partner to name the joint movement *at the large, proximal joint*, the body part being moved and the joint in motion, as in "_____ of the _____ at the _____."

4. Switch partners and repeat until all the joint movements have been demonstrated and correctly named.

LAB ACTIVITY 1–4: DEMONSTRATING AND IDENTIFYING ROTATIONAL JOINT ACTIONS

1. Working with a partner, choose an activity of daily life that clearly demonstrates one of these joint actions:
    - Rotation of the head and the trunk.
    - Medial rotation of the arm and the thigh.
    - Lateral rotation of the arm and the thigh.

2. Plan carefully how you can demonstrate your chosen action, but don't be afraid to use your imagination. Clearly demonstrate your chosen joint action, without superfluous movements.

3. Ask your partner to name the joint movement, the body part being moved and the joint in motion, as in "_____ of the _____ at the _____."

4. Switch partners and repeat until all the joint movements have been demonstrated and correctly named.

LAB ACTIVITY 1–5: DEMONSTRATING AND IDENTIFYING ADDITIONAL JOINT ACTIONS

1. Working with a partner, choose an activity of daily life that clearly demonstrates one of these joint actions:
   - Depression and elevation.
   - Protraction and retraction.
   - Inversion, eversion, dorsiflexion, and plantarflexion.
   - Pronation and supination of the forearm.
   - Anterior and posterior tilt of the pelvis.
   - Radial and ulnar deviation of the hand.
   - Opposition of the thumb.
2. Plan carefully how you can demonstrate your chosen action, but don't be afraid to use your imagination. Clearly demonstrate your chosen joint action, without superfluous movements.
3. Ask your partner to name the joint movement, the body part being moved and the joint in motion, as in "_____ of the _____ at the _____."
4. Switch partners and repeat until all the joint movements have been demonstrated and correctly named.

LAB ACTIVITY 1–6: DEMONSTRATING AND IDENTIFYING CONCENTRIC AND ECCENTRIC MUSCLE CONTRACTIONS

1. Working with a partner, demonstrate an action you perform every day in the classroom. Choose the large, proximal joint in this action. Decide with your partner:
   - Which bone is the structure that is mobile during the action and which bone is fixed or immobile during the action?
   - On which aspect of the joint was a skeletal muscle concentrically contracting?
   - On which aspect of the joint was a skeletal muscle eccentrically contracting?
2. Switch partners, choose and demonstrate another action, and repeat the action assessment.

LAB ACTIVITY 1–7: DEMONSTRATING AND IDENTIFYING ISOMETRIC MUSCLE CONTRACTION

1. Working with a partner, repeat the action you performed in the previous Lab Activity. Decide with your partner:
   - How would you change this action to create an isometric, rather than an isotonic, contraction?
   - Demonstrate the isometric contraction. Describe the difference in the sensation of the muscle during the isotonic and isometric contractions.
2. Switch partners, choose and demonstrate another action, and repeat the action assessment.

LAB ACTIVITY 1–8: DEMONSTRATING AND IDENTIFYING REVERSE MUSCLE ACTION

1. Working with a partner, demonstrate the reverse actions of extension of the leg at the knee.
2. Describe the difference in sensation in the muscles that are contracting during each action.
3. Discuss and demonstrate other reverse actions that you can think of.
4. Switch partners and repeat.

LAB ACTIVITY 1–9: DEMONSTRATING AND IDENTIFYING THE AGONIST AND ANTAGONIST IN AN ACTION

1. Working with a partner, flex and extend your leg at the knee as your partner places his hands around your thigh so that he is palpating both anterior and posterior thigh muscles.
2. In which action—flexion or extension—is muscle contraction palpable on the anterior aspect of your thigh? In which action is muscle contraction palpable on the posterior aspect?
3. Based on this palpation, name on which aspect of the thigh the agonist muscle lies, anterior or posterior, in flexion of the thigh and extension of the thigh at the acetabulofemoral joint.
4. Switch partners, choose a second action, and repeat.

LAB ACTIVITY 1–10: IDENTIFYING MUSCLE ATTACHMENTS AND ACTIONS

1. Using the information contained in Table 1-7, look at the muscles in Figures 1–61 and 1–62. What can you predict about the attachments and actions or the shape of each muscle, based on its name?
2. Refer to the attachments and actions of skeletal muscles listed in Chapters 8, 9, and 10 to see how you did!

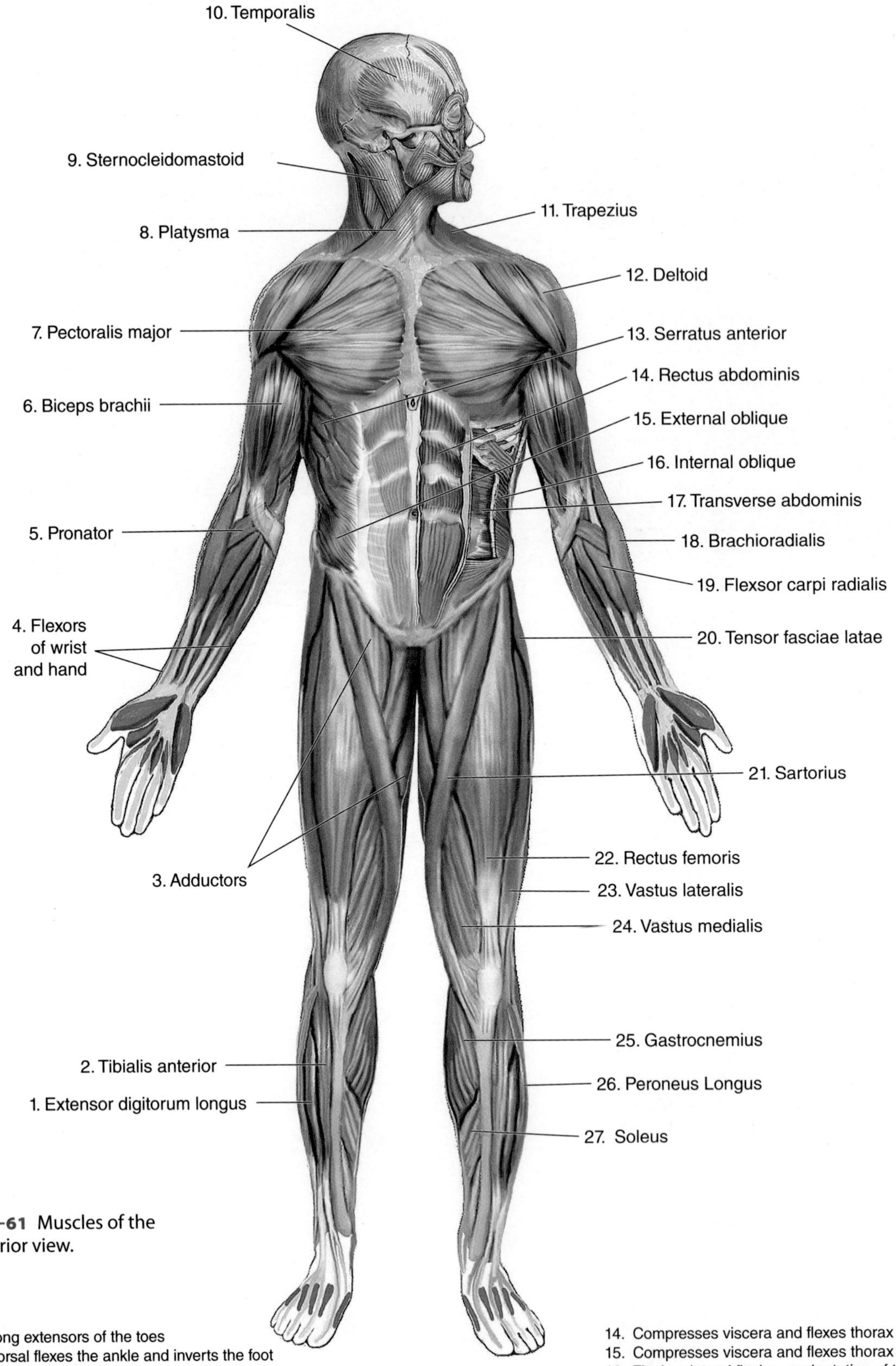

10. Temporalis
9. Sternocleidomastoid
8. Platysma
7. Pectoralis major
6. Biceps brachii
5. Pronator
4. Flexors of wrist and hand
3. Adductors
2. Tibialis anterior
1. Extensor digitorum longus

11. Trapezius
12. Deltoid
13. Serratus anterior
14. Rectus abdominis
15. External oblique
16. Internal oblique
17. Transverse abdominis
18. Brachioradialis
19. Flexsor carpi radialis
20. Tensor fasciae latae
21. Sartorius
22. Rectus femoris
23. Vastus lateralis
24. Vastus medialis
25. Gastrocnemius
26. Peroneus Longus
27. Soleus

FIGURE 1-61 Muscles of the body, anterior view.

1. Long extensors of the toes
2. Dorsal flexes the ankle and inverts the foot
3. Muscles that draw the leg toward the median line of the body
4. Muscles that flex the wrist and hand
5. Turns the hand from palm up to palm down
6. Flexes and supinates the forearm
7. Draws the arm forward and down
8. Subcutaneous muscle
9. Muscle that flexes and rotates the head
10. Closes and retracts the jaw
11. Assists in extension of the head and elevation and upward rotation of the scapula
12. Abducts and horizontally flexes the humerous
13. Elevates ribs in respiration and stabilizes the scapula

14. Compresses viscera and flexes thorax
15. Compresses viscera and flexes thorax
16. Flexion, lateral flexion, and rotation of trunk
17. Tenses abdominal wall
18. Flexes elbow
19. Wrist flexors
20. Assists in abduction, flexion, and rotation of femur
21. Flexes and laterally rotates the leg
22. Extends the knee
23. Extends the knee
24. Extends the knee. 22, 23, and 24 along with the Vastus Intermedius make up the Quadraceps Femoris
25. Plantar flexes the foot and assists in knee flexion
26. Everts the foot
27. Plantar flexes the foot

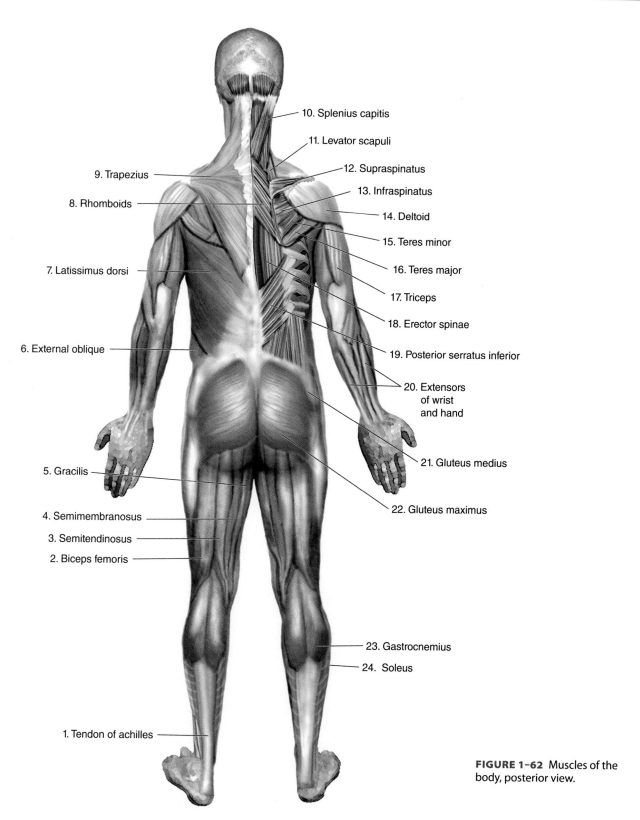

10. Splenius capitis
11. Levator scapuli
9. Trapezius
12. Supraspinatus
8. Rhomboids
13. Infraspinatus
14. Deltoid
15. Teres minor
7. Latissimus dorsi
16. Teres major
17. Triceps
18. Erector spinae
6. External oblique
19. Posterior serratus inferior
20. Extensors of wrist and hand
21. Gluteus medius
5. Gracilis
22. Gluteus maximus
4. Semimembranosus
3. Semitendinosus
2. Biceps femoris
23. Gastrocnemius
24. Soleus
1. Tendon of achilles

FIGURE 1-62 Muscles of the body, posterior view.

1. Attaches calf muscle to heel bone
2, 3, 4. Make up the hamstrings that flex the knee and assist in extension of the hip
5. Draws leg toward the mid-line
6. Supports abdominal viscera; flexes vertebral column
7. Draws arm backward and downward: rotates arm inward
8. Draws scapula toward the spine
9. Draws scapula toward the spine; rotates scapula either upward or downward; draws head backward
10. Draws head back or rotates the head
11. Elevation and/or downward rotation of scapula
12. Abducts the arm

13. Outward rotation and extension of arm
14. Abducts and rotates humerus
15. Lateral rotation of humerus
16. Inward rotation, abduction, and extension of humerus
17. Extends the forearm
18. Extension of the spine
19. Pulls ribs outward and down; opposes diaphragm
20. Extends the wrist and hand
21. Abducts and rotates the thigh
22. Extends, abducts, and rotates the thigh outward
23. Flexes the knee and plantar flexes the foot
24. Plantar flexes the foot

CASE PROFILES

Case Profile 1
Matt is a first-time client. When he made his appointment, he mentioned low-back pain after standing for more than 20 minutes or so. Will you assess Matt's standing or sitting posture, or both? What other assessments might you perform? What questions will you ask Matt?

Case Profile 2
Courtney, 21, is an avid skateboarder. She complains of pain in her right hip and knee. Will you assess Courtney's standing or seated posture, or both? Will you assess her gait? What other assessments might you perform? What questions will you ask Courtney?

Case Profile 3
Clem, 72, walks for 3 miles every morning. Recently, he has been suffering from a very sore right shoulder after his morning walk. Will you assess Clem's standing or sitting posture, or both? Will you assess his gait? What structures might you palpate? What questions will you ask Clem?

STUDY QUESTIONS

1. Which part of the skeleton, the axial or the appendicular, has more planar joints? How does the predominance of planar joints in this part of the skeleton affect its range of motion skeleton?
2. Which types of synovial joints allow circumduction? What other joints can allow movements that seem to duplicate circumduction?
3. At which joints does true rotation—rotation of a bone around a single axis—occur? What other joints allow movement that may be considered a type of rotation?
4. In which planes can abduction of the arm take place? Describe how the abduction of the arm differs in these planes.
5. List the factors that create joint fit.
6. Name the layers of connective tissue that wrap around the layers of a skeletal muscle, from superficial to deep.
7. How does the direction of fibers in a skeletal muscle create its line of pull?
8. Contrast isotonic and isometric muscle contractions. Which causes a muscle to fatigue more quickly?
9. Contrast the functions of phasic and postural muscles. Give an example of each type of muscle.
10. Contrast Type I and Type II muscle fibers. Which fiber type contracts faster? Which fatigues most quickly?

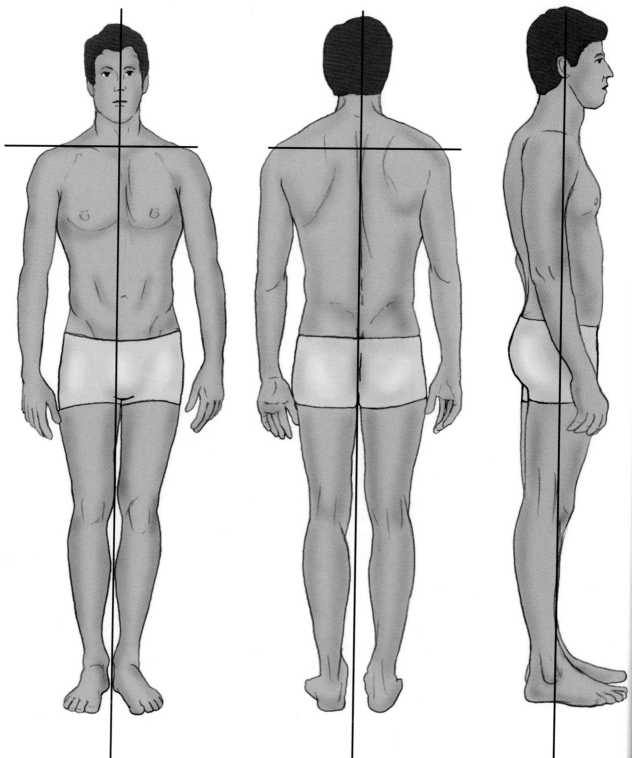

Posture Assessment

CHAPTER OUTLINE

- **SCOPE OF PRACTICE AND ASSESSMENT**
- **POSTURE ASSESSMENT GUIDELINES**
- **POSTURE ASSESSMENT**

LEARNING OBJECTIVES

- Identify normal standing, seated, and reclining postures.
- Understand common postural deviations and resulting compensation patterns in regions of the body.
- Compare pathologies that affect posture.
- Apply visual posture assessment techniques to locate common posture deviations and compensation patterns and to identify the structures involved.

INTRODUCTION

As massage therapists, we begin assessment of a client's condition by examining his posture, how he stands and sits, utilizing our understanding of joint and muscle actions. We assess posture before we palpate a client's structures because the results of posture assessment indicate the muscles and soft tissue structures that we will need to palpate. If assessment of your client's posture reveals a lateral curve in his thoracic region, for example, you will probably palpate the muscles that run along each side of his thoracic spine. Effective assessment of posture begins the treatment planning process.

SCOPE OF PRACTICE AND ASSESSMENT

When performing assessments, it is important that you stay within a defined scope of practice for massage therapy. This will ensure that your practice is ethical, credible, and professional, and that your clients are safe in your hands. Throughout your career, you will be presented with challenges to staying within this scope of practice. Complicating these challenges is the absence of a definition of scope of practice that is agreed upon throughout the profession. Some states and municipalities clearly define massage therapy within a statute governing its practitioners. Others do not specifically define the techniques or applications of massage therapy, even as they regulate its practitioners.

Margaret Avery-Moon, the founder and former owner of the Desert Institute of the Healing Arts in Tucson, Arizona (now Cortiva Institute-Tucson), and an active participant in national policy and curriculum formulation for nearly 30 years, offers this description of a massage therapy scope of practice.

"The scope of massage therapy includes the following:

- Visual and manual assessment of the balance in the musculoskeletal system and or energetic activities such as Meridians or Sens.

- Treatment and prevention of dysfunction in soft tissue, pain, joints, and energetic systems through the use of manual techniques such as compression, stretches, direct pressure, gliding and spreading of tissue, kneading, squeezing, percussive techniques, and hot and cold thermo-modalities.
- Massage therapists may use and are not limited to oils, liniments, essential oils, lotions, and the use of herbs for external purposes.
- Massage therapists may use tools to such as stones, Trigger Point tools, vibrators, moxibustion or other tools which do not puncture or breach the skin.
- Massage therapists are limited in scope through laws in their state or municipalities."

Challenges to scope of practice

In part because of the wide variety of venues where massage therapy is offered—chiropractic clinics, day spas, hair salons, health clubs, hospitals and rehabilitative facilities, and private offices such as that shown in Figure 2–1, which are all spaces sometimes shared with practitioners in allied health fields—clients may request or even expect services that are outside of either the statutory or informal scope of practice for massage therapy.

Because you care deeply about your clients' welfare and want to give them the best treatment possible, it may be tempting to step beyond the scope of practice

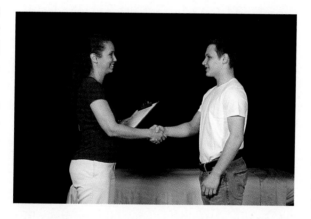

FIGURE 2–1 Therapeutic massage is offered in a wide variety of settings, including private clinics.

made possible by your training. Caring and self-confidence, however, do not expand the extent of your actual training and licensure. A physical therapist, for example, measures range of motion (ROM) at a joint to its exact degree, using a **goniometer** [go-ni-om-e-ter] shown in Figure 2–2, a device that precisely measures the range of a joint's motion. Although a massage therapist may also purchase a goniometer and may estimate the results of its use, he is not a physical therapist, whose training and licensure enables him to perform precise measurements of joint range of motion and to prescribe rehabilitative exercises.

Goniometer

a device for measuring range of joint movement.

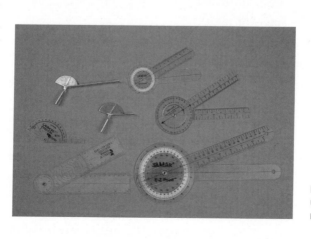

FIGURE 2–2 A physical therapist uses a goniometer to precisely measure joint range of motion.

There is wide agreement on these aspects of the scope of practice for massage therapy:

- A massage therapist provides services within the limits of his training, does not employ techniques for which he has not been adequately trained and represents his training and licensure truthfully and accurately.
- A massage therapist does not diagnose, prescribe, or perform any services or procedures that require a license under any other profession, such as osteopathy, physical therapy, chiropractic, podiatry, or others, unless he holds that specific license.

Scope of practice in posture assessment

The posture abnormalities described in this chapter for assessment are those that involve soft tissue weakness or hypotonicity, and for which massage therapy may be a valuable and effective treatment. If the soft tissue condition is secondary to another condition, such as a chronic neurological condition, or is an aftermath of a neurological event, such as cerebral hemorrhage caused by a stroke, massage therapy may be a valuable and effective adjunct to physical therapy and other care, under the supervision of a professional who holds the appropriate licensure.

Within the context of this chapter, the scope of practice for performing assessments includes

- Visual observation of the elements of posture, including the relative positions of joints and bony structures.
- Manual assessment of the movement of structures during range of joint motion.
- Recording of objective and subjective findings of assessments in written form, for the purposes of identifying treatment goals and procedures.

The results of our visual and manual assessments are tools for use in treatment planning. Discussions concerning scope of practice for massage therapy are ongoing and reflect the dynamic nature of the profession.

LEARNING ENHANCEMENT ACTIVITY

Use Margaret Avery-Moon's scope of practice definition as a starting point for group discussion, and consider drafting a scope of practice definition for your future practice.

POSTURE ASSESSMENT GUIDELINES

Throughout the assessment process, we focus our initial attention on the core of the client's body—his spine, head, and pelvis—for these reasons:

- The angle of the spinal vertebrae creates the position of the head and the pelvis.
- The limbs and associated muscles and soft tissue structures of the body must accommodate the position of the head and the pelvis, to keep us upright, balanced, and able to move about with ease.

- By examining the spine, the head and the pelvis—and how they behave in motion—we are able to predict patterns of strain in muscles and soft tissues that are targets for palpation and treatment.
- Therapeutic massage protocols typically begin by working on the trunk of the body first and then moving on to the extremities. This continuity of focused assessment from the core to the extremities is in line with that approach to treatment.

The Role of Posture

Posture is created and maintained by the interplay between the bones, joints, fascial structures, and muscles of the body and by the laws of gravity and other forces applied to the body as we stand, sit, bend, and move. The initial establishment of one's posture is influenced by several factors:

- Genetics: the size and shape of your skeleton is in large part determined by those of your parents.
- The health of growing body structures: nutritional deprivation can play a devastating role in altering growth and development of your skeleton and the soft tissues that create posture.
- The postures of those around you: children learn how to stand and walk by watching how others stand and walk. If either of your parents stands with one foot turned out or arms folded, chances are that you will stand that way, too. Genetics and structural health play a role here, too, of course: your parents stand the way they do because of their genetic make-up and the health of their structures (in addition to their having watched their own parents' postures).

The role of posture is to maintain the balance—the **equilibrium**—of the head. There are two types of equilibrium: **static equilibrium** is the maintenance of the position of your body in relation to your environment and reflects the force of gravity, while **dynamic equilibrium** maintains the position of your head in response to movement and keeps you balanced. Each type of equilibrium affects posture: moment to moment, we create the posture that allows us to maintain both static and dynamic equilibrium, as shown in Figure 2–3.

> **Equilibrium**
> the state of balance that maintains upright posture.

> **Static equilibrium**
> the maintenance of the position of the body in relation to the environment, or the force of gravity.

> **Dynamic equilibrium**
> the type of equilibrium that maintains the position of the head in response to movement in order to maintain balance.

Client Postures

Your client has more than one posture. He has a standing posture, during which the weight of his trunk is borne by the spine and the lower extremity; he has a seated posture, during which his head and the upper extremity must accommodate the tilt of the pelvis and flexion of the lower extremity in order to maintain equilibrium; and he has a reclining posture, during which his body's weight is borne by a horizontal surface and the musculature is in "neutral." Complete posture assessment includes viewing your client as he stands, sits, and reclines, and uses your skills in observation, touch, and comparison.

Balanced postures

We assess posture to discover postural **deviations or discrepancies**—variations from the standard or normal expectation for a particular

> **Deviation**
> a variation from the standard or normal expectation.

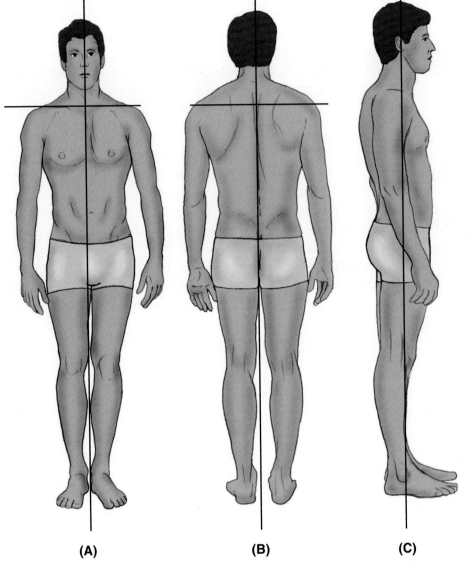

FIGURE 2-3 Anterior, posterior, and lateral views of posture in balance.

(A)   **(B)**   **(C)**

aspect of posture—that create patterns of muscle and soft tissue strain. Postural deviations are revealed by the degree of **asymmetry** [ay-SIM-uh-tree] or imbalance in body structure from one side to the other that they create in your client's posture.

Asymmetry

an imbalance in structure from one side of the body to the other.

- Ideal posture is symmetrical or and evenly balanced: the head, shoulders, and pelvis are level when seen from the front; the head and shoulders are in alignment; and the curves of the spine relate to a vertical line when seen from the side, as shown in Figure 2–3.

In order to define postural deviations, first we must define balanced postures. In the balanced standing posture, shown in Figures 2–3 and 2–4:

- The head is in a neutral position, directly atop the spine in all planes and not tilted or rotated to either side.
- The curves of the spine are to the anterior in the cervical and lumbar regions and to the posterior in the thoracic and sacral regions. The degree of each curve allows for equilibrium to be maintained without compensatory adjustments of other structures.

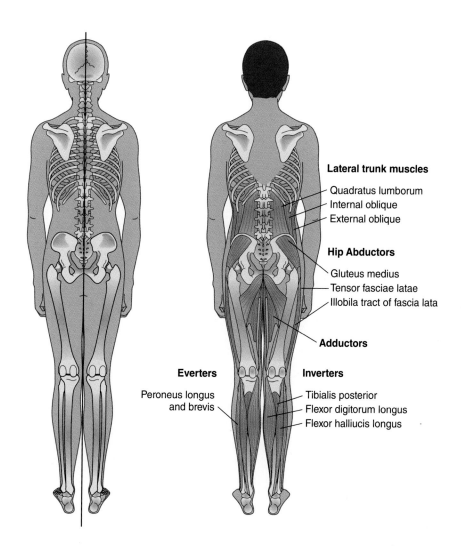

Lateral trunk muscles

- Quadratus lumborum
- Internal oblique
- External oblique

Hip Abductors

- Gluteus medius
- Tensor fasciae latae
- Illobila tract of fascia lata

Adductors

Everters

Peroneus longus and brevis

Inverters

- Tibialis posterior
- Flexor digitorum longus
- Flexor halliucis longus

FIGURE 2-4 Posterior view of ideal standing posture. Note that major postural muscles—in the lateral trunk, the Adductors and posterior leg muscles—are shaded for visibility.

© Delmar, Cengage Learning.

- The shoulders are level, with the head of each humerus aligned with the ear canal and the medial borders of the scapulae aligned with the spine and equal in distance from the surface of the posterior ribcage.
- The arms hang straight from the shoulder, with the forearms in alignment with the thighs and the dorsal surfaces of the hands facing laterally, not forward.
- The pelvis is in neutral, with both the anterior superior iliac spine (ASIS) and the posterior superior iliac spine (PSIS) equal in height.
- The hip and tibiofemoral joints are in neutral, with the kneecaps equal in height, pointing forward and at a distance that allows free movement between them.
- The ankles are in neutral, the feet point forward, and the arches of the feet are equal in degree, with no inversion or eversion.

In balanced seated posture:

- The head is in neutral.
- The shoulders are level and aligned with the ear canals.
- The back is straight, with the normal curves of the spine maintained.
- The lumbar region is in contact with the chair or another support.
- Weight is equally distributed on both hips.

© Delmar, Cengage Learning.

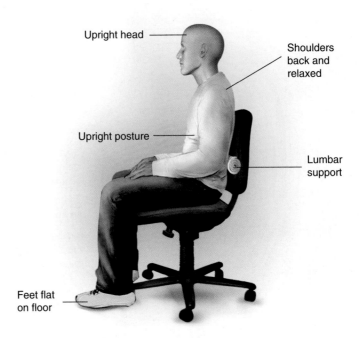

Upright head

Shoulders back and relaxed

Upright posture

Lumbar support

Feet flat on floor

FIGURE 2-5 In the ideal seated posture, joints are maintained and supported comfortably.

- The thighs are bent to 90° at the hips and the legs are bent to 90° at the knees so that both feet rest flat on the floor.

Figure 2–5 demonstrates many of the characteristics of the ideal seated posture.

In aligned supine, position, shown in Figure 2–6:
- The head is in neutral.
- The surface supports the normal curves of the spine so that they are maintained, by means of added support, if necessary.
- The arms are supported by the width of the surface.
- The surface prevents hyperflexion of the knees, by means of added support if necessary.

In aligned prone position, shown in Figure 2–7:
- The alignment of the head and the cervical region of the spine and easy, normal respiration are maintained.
- A properly placed bolster also supports the neutral alignment of the ankles.

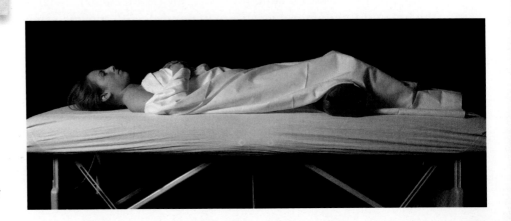

© Delmar, Cengage Learning

FIGURE 2-6 Elevating your client's knees in the supine position relieves strain on lower back muscles.

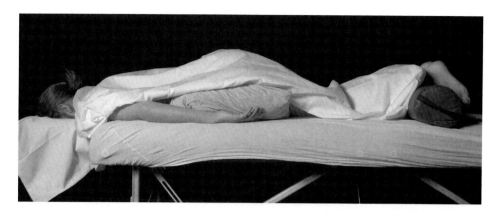

© Delmar, Cengage Learning

FIGURE 2–7 Placing a support beneath your client's abdomen in the prone position relieves strain on lower back structures.

Postural Deviations and Compensation Patterns

Postural deviations may be structural or functional, inborn or acquired:

- Structural deviations may be **congenital** [kahn-JEN-uh-tul], present at birth, or acquired, as the result of injury or illness. An example of a structural postural deviation is a leg that is anatomically shorter than its counterpart.
- Functional deviations may have many causes: poor posture habits, repetitive strain, injury, or illness. For example, a client's shoulders may functionally deviate upward and to the anterior as a result of habitually slumping forward while sitting at a computer.

Congenital

present at birth.

IN THE TREATMENT ROOM

Your client who works at a laptop or electronic notebook will experience a different pattern of strain from a client who uses a desktop PC (personal computer). On a PC, the monitor can be situated at eye level and the keyboard placed for ease while typing. On a laptop, the monitor and keyboard cannot be separated. If the keyboard is placed at a level to allow ease of typing, the user must lower his head to view the monitor. If the monitor is placed at eye level, the user must raise his hands unnaturally to type. Discuss the laptop setup your client normally uses and the duration of use, and then assess the resulting pattern of strain. You might suggest that your client invest in a separate monitor to attach to his laptop, so that he can achieve the same setup as a PC.

Posture compensations

The body does its best to maintain equilibrium by compensating for postural deviations. **Compensation** is the reactive accommodation by body structures to dysfunction that allows the body to maintain equilibrium. When an injury to your right foot prevents you from placing weight on it without pain, for example, your body compensates for the dysfunction by shifting your weight onto your left foot. This inequality of weight distribution then demands that other structures shift position or take on additional stress in order to maintain equilibrium. Postural compensations may be temporary, such as the one just described, or they may become chronic.

Compensation

the reactive accommodation by body structures to dysfunction in order to maintain equilibrium.

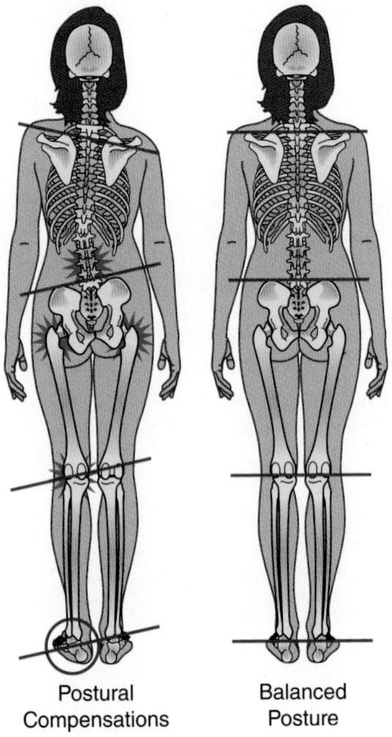

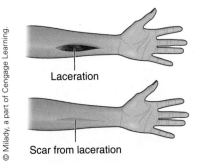

Postural   Balanced
Compensations   Posture

FIGURE 2–8 Postural compensations commonly cross the body, redistributing weight to maintain equilibrium, but occasionally they are found only on one side of the body.

© Milady, a part of Cengage Learning.

HERE'S A TIP

Structural postural deviations may cause muscle strain compensations, whereas functional postural deviations may be caused by muscle strain compensations. A twisting of your spine as it formed before you were born may elevate one hip in standing posture, causing chronic strain in the muscles supporting one side of the lumbar spine that compensate for the twisting. Your habit of sitting crookedly in a chair, however, may strain the muscles on one side of the lumbar spine, chronically shortening them and resulting in an elevation of that hip.

Compensations may occur in predictable patterns that cross over from one side of the body to the other, in order to maintain equilibrium. The left shoulder, for example, may elevate to compensate for an elevated right hip and the head may tilt toward the elevated shoulder in order to maintain its balance atop the spine, as shown in Figure 2–8. Compensation patterns are not always predictable, however: sometimes multiple compensations occur only on one side of the body. You must assess the body as it is, not as you assume it ought to be.

Pathologies affecting posture

Posture responds to changing conditions in the body, whether internal and external, temporary or ongoing, finite or progressive. Even our emotional state and common life events may be expressed in our posture. Such factors include:

- Surgery: a surgical incision disrupts the layers of connective tissue that line the body and body cavities and cover organs and structures. During healing, these layers of connective tissue may join in a dysfunctional pattern, forming scar tissue that disrupts normal posture and movement, such as that shown in Figure 2–9.
- Stress: stress is commonly expressed in posture. When under stress, we tend to hold our breath or take only quick, shallow breaths that tighten trunk and neck muscles and limit their ability to maintain ideal posture. Muscles that are deprived of adequate oxygen may be unable to contract or relax fully, limiting the ability of the circulatory system to rid muscles of the hormonal byproducts of chronic stress. Such tight muscles may restrict the free movement that maintains posture and equilibrium.
- Emotional distress: memories of painful or unresolved life events may be expressed in a variety of postures, for example, posture that hunches forward, as if to ward off life's blows or posture that is excessively rigid in order to maintain equilibrium in the face of adversity.

Various pathological conditions may alter posture. Treatment for some of these conditions is outside the scope of practice for massage therapists. We can, however, help these clients to:

Laceration

Scar from laceration

FIGURE 2–9 Surgical scarring may disrupt posture and movement.

© Milady, a part of Cengage Learning.

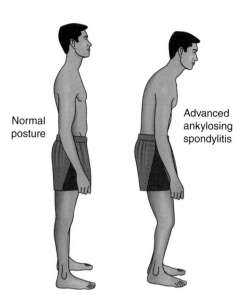

Normal posture

Advanced ankylosing spondylitis

FIGURE 2–10 Ankylosing spondylitis, shown here, is inflammatory and progressive.

© Milady, a part of Cengage Learning.

- Maintain their optimal level of function by temporarily alleviating muscle and other soft tissue contractures that may contribute to pain and dysfunction caused by postural deviations.
- Contribute to their overall functioning and sense of well-being by providing therapeutic touch.

Pathological conditions that may alter posture by affecting the musculoskeletal system include:

- **Ankylosing spondylitis** [ang-kih-LOH-sing spahn-dih-LYE-tis] is an inflammatory condition that is usually inherited and affects men far more often than women. Bony overgrowths on the anterior of vertebral bodies eventually join and fuse the vertebrae. The fusions usually begin in the lumbar region and proceed up the spine. The inflammation may spread to adjoining ligaments and other soft tissues. The posture of a client with ankylosing spondylitis will be stooped, with the trunk and head flexed, as shown in Figure 2–10.

- **Osteoporosis** [ahs-tee-oh-puh-ROH-sis] is a chronic, progressive condition that is the result of calcium being literally "pulled off" the bones. The bones of a client with osteoporosis, typically, a small-boned, Asian or Caucasian woman past menopause, are brittle and vulnerable to spontaneous fractures. They may break without any direct impact. Tiny fractures in the vertebrae may result in severe kyphosis, rounded shoulders, and a head forward posture, as shown in Figure 2–11. This client is at increased risk for fractures and falls, exacerbated by her stooped posture.

- **Parkinson's disease** is a neurological disorder in which dopamine-producing neurons in the brain are damaged or die. Dopamine is the neurotransmitter that is responsible for smooth muscle movement by balancing the contractions of agonists and antagonists. The muscle rigidity that results from neuronal damage or death produces a stiffly stooped posture and contractured extremities, as shown in Figure 2–12.

Ankylosing spondylitis (ankylosis=stiff joints; spondylitis=spinal inflammation)

an inflammatory condition, usually inherited, in which bony overgrowths on the anterior of vertebral bodies join and eventually fuses the vertebrae.

Osteoporosis (osteo= bone; -porosis=porous)

a chronic, progressive condition in which bones become increasingly brittle and vulnerable to spontaneous fracture; the result of calcium being literally "pulled off" the bones.

Parkinson's disease

a neurological disease in which neurons in the substantia nigra area of the brain that produces dopamine, the neurotransmitter which produces smooth muscle movement by balancing the contractions of agonists and antagonists, degenerate and eventually die.

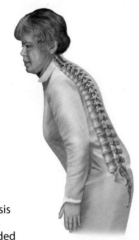

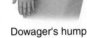

Dowager's hump

FIGURE 2-11 Osteoporosis fractures may result in the "dowager's hump"—rounded shoulders—seen here.

© Milady, a part of Cengage Learning.

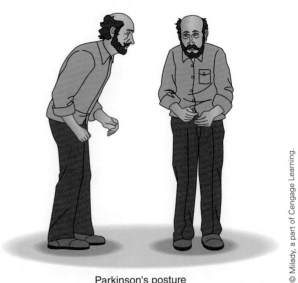

Parkinson's posture

FIGURE 2-12 The muscle rigidity caused by Parkinson's results in a frozen posture.

© Milady, a part of Cengage Learning.

Rheumatoid arthritis

a progressive, autoimmune disease in which the body's immune system attacks and destroys synovial membranes at multiple joints.

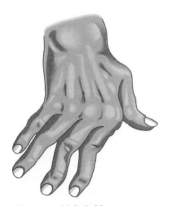

Rheumatoid Arthritis (late stage)

FIGURE 2-13 Disfigurement in the joints of the hands results from the progression of rheumatoid arthritis.

© Milady, a part of Cengage Learning.

Laminectomy

a surgical procedure in which the laminae of adjoining vertebrae may be trimmed or removed to relieve pressure on the spinal cord, or during which the vertebrae are fused together.

■ **Rheumatoid arthritis (RA)** is a progressive autoimmune disease in which the body's immune system attacks the synovial membranes of multiple joints. RA causes bilateral tenderness, inflammation, and contracture of multiple joints in the body. As the disease progresses, joints become disfigured, as shown in Figure 2–13. The posture of a client with RA may be altered by spinal deviations, disfigurement of weight-bearing joints, and by the strain it places on muscles and other soft tissues.

IN THE TREATMENT ROOM

Following back surgery, a client's posture may be significantly affected. In a **laminectomy** [lam-uh-NECK-tuh-mee], the laminae of adjoining vertebrae may be trimmed or removed to relieve pressure on the spinal cord by enlarging the spinal canal, as shown in Figure 2–14. The vertebrae may also be fused, rendering that segment of the spine immobile. Devices such as rods and screws may be inserted to provide stability in the lumbar spine, when the vertebrae are severely degenerated. Such procedures may therefore strictly limit the flexibility of the spine, resulting in a stiff, rigid posture; little movement at the articulation of the spine, the sacrum, and the pelvis; and the development of postural compensation and muscle-strain patterns. Be alert to these ramifications to the posture of a client after surgery on the spine.

POSTURE ASSESSMENT

Before assessing your client's posture, answer these questions:

■ What am I looking for? What information from my client's subjective reporting of symptoms has indicated posture assessment?

- What structures are the potential assessment targets? What specific deviations and compensation patterns are suggested by my client's subjective reporting of symptoms?

Use the answers to these questions as guidelines for posture assessment, but do not let them prejudice your assessment or lead you away from true discovery.

Posture Assessment Tools

Common recommendations for posture assessment include the use of a wall-mounted grid chart; a hanging plumb-bob, a lead weight suspended from a ceiling by a cord, which provides a true vertical line; and a camera and a client who is dressed in workout clothing in a brightly lit room, as shown in Figure 2–15.

This may be an ideal scenario for posture assessment, but it's one that is not present in most practice settings:

- Space set aside and the time required for this type of posture assessment are not always available.
- The client may not feel at ease—or stand in his usual posture—when lined up in front of a chart to be photographed from various angles.

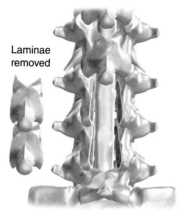

FIGURE 2–14 Laminae may be fused or even removed, as seen here, during a laminectomy.

© Milady, a part of Cengage Learning.

Postural Analysis Grid Chart

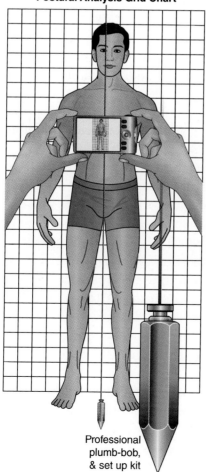

Professional plumb-bob, & set up kit

FIGURE 2–15 Standard postural assessment tools, such as the wall grid and plumb-bob are shown here. However, they are not available to massage therapists in all treatment settings.

© Milady, a part of Cengage Learning.

- Most clients come to their massage appointments dressed in work or street clothes, not workout clothing.

You can assess any client's posture in any setting, using the tools that are always available to you:

- Your interview and observation skills.
- Your hands, which can lightly trace the curves and angles of the body.
- Your practiced skill in comparing structures of the body.

You can also investigate the tools available in your setting that might help in posture assessment:

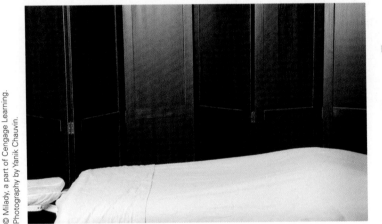

- A doorway, a corner of the room, a large painting, or a mirror can provide a vertical line for reference.
- The floor and ceiling, a desk or massage table, a large painting, or a mirror can provide a horizontal reference line.
- A light source that is behind your client may outline posture deviations better than overhead lighting.
- An uncrowded space for your client to stand and sit encourages his normal posture. Try to find a space large enough for your client to stand with both arms outstretched or sit with his arms and legs held naturally, as you move around him to observe his whole body. In Figure 2–16, the screens behind the massage table create both vertical and horizontal reference lines.

FIGURE 2–16 Vertical and horizontal reference lines to aid in posture assessment are found in most treatment settings.

Initial considerations in posture assessment

These additional steps assure an accurate posture assessment, demonstrated in Figure 2–17:

- Ask your client to remove her shoes before the assessment. The change in posture necessitated by even a slight shoe-heel height impacts the position of the spine and creates compensatory strain patterns. Assessing your client's posture in bare feet is more likely to reveal structural postural deviations.
- After the initial posture assessment, ask your client to put his shoes back on, and assess his standing posture a second time. Note the compensation patterns created by the height of his shoes. If appropriate, discuss the heel height of the shoes your client wears daily. This second postural assessment may reveal functional postural deviations caused by a change in heel height.
- Ask your client to remove layers of outer clothing, for example, a tight jacket or heavy coat that may alter his natural posture. Although the client in Figure 2–17 wears an outer vest, the contrast between her white vest and her black sleeve creates visual clarity for the massage therapist.

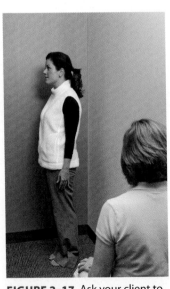

FIGURE 2–17 Ask your client to remove shoes or outer clothing that impede posture assessment, and make sure you can easily view both ears.

- Ask your client to tuck his hair behind his ears, so that you can view the external auditory meatus, the ear canal, to gauge the position of his head from the side.
- Ask your client if the room is warm enough. We tend to keep our shoulders raised and draw in our arms when we're chilly.

IN THE TREATMENT ROOM

Orthotics [or-THAWT-iks] are inserts that fit into one or both shoes, shown in Figure 2–18, and are designed to compensate for unequal leg length, dysfunctions in the arches, and other aspects of the foot. If your client wears orthotic inserts in his shoes, assess his standing posture with his orthotic inserts in place, then with his shoes and inserts removed, for comparison.

Advice about the effectiveness of orthotic inserts is not within the scope of practice of massage therapists. The choice to wear orthotic inserts is a personal one, made by the client with the advice or prescription of a foot specialist. Ideally, orthotic inserts are prescribed by a podiatrist, designed specifically for your client's feet, and evaluated regularly for effectiveness and for wear.

**Orthotics
(ortho=perpendicular)**

inserts that fit into one or both shoes, and are designed to compensate for unequal leg length, dysfunctions in the arches, and other dysfunctions of the foot that affect posture.

The order in which your client's postures are assessed is important:

- Assess your client's standing posture first. This assessment gives you information about the spine and the lower extremity as they bear the weight of the body and about the status of your client's posture generally.
- Assess your client's seated posture next. This assessment reveals strain patterns not present in standing posture. Assessing seated posture is indicated when assessing standing posture didn't reveal any strain patterns or postural deviations that could explain your client's reported symptoms.
- Assess your client's reclining postures last. Assessing the difference between your client's standing and reclining postures reveals the impact of weight-bearing on dysfunctions in his structure.

Your client's standing or seated posture at the beginning of your assessment is probably unnatural. Most of us try to stand or sit up "straight" when we know that we're being observed. Take your time performing a posture assessment, and engage your client in small talk as you perform your visual assessment. Allow your client time to relax into his normal posture.

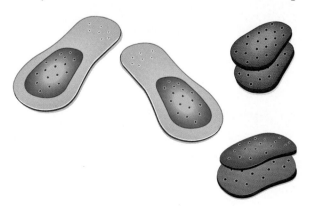

FIGURE 2–18 A client who wears an orthotic insert in one or both shoes should be assessed for deviations in the lumbar spine or the hip and for short leg syndrome, in addition to assessment of the arches of the feet.

© Milady, a part of Cengage Learning.

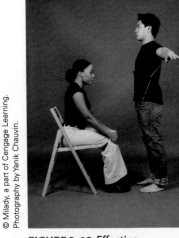

FIGURE 2–19 Effective assessment includes visual observation of structures at close eye level as well as from a distance.

Visual Assessment

Visual assessment serves as an initial posture assessment, alerting you to immediately visible postural deviations that you will explore during a more in-depth visual assessment of your client's posture, following these steps:

- Stand back: at first, stand far enough away from your client—at least five feet or so—that you can easily measure his standing posture against the room's reference points.
- Assess at eye level: next, step closer to your client and visually assess his postural landmarks at your eye level. Sit or kneel to assess his lumbar spine, pelvis, hips, and knees, as shown in Figure 2–19. Assessing posture at eye level allows you to gauge the true angle of structures.
- Assess from all aspects: viewing the 360° panorama of your client's posture gives you a complete assessment of the planes, curves, and angles of his standing posture.
- Highlight postural landmarks: postural landmarks are more evident if observed with the source of ambient light *behind* your client.

IN THE TREATMENT ROOM

Your visual assessment of your client's standing posture begins as you introduce yourself and shake his hand. The 60-second visual assessment described here is a quick, initial inventory that serves as a guide for further assessment. Sixty seconds may not seem enough time for any meaningful assessment, but with practice, you will find this an effective way to perform an initial visual assessment, such as on the client pictured in Figure 2–20:

- Observe your client's head position in relation to the spine: are the ears far in front of the shoulders? Is there a noticeable "hump" in her back, causing her shoulders to round?

  This step alerts you to potential deviations in the normal spinal curves and to the resulting strain on the muscles that flex and extend the neck.

- Observe the point of your client's chin in relation to the suprasternal notch, the notch where the manubrium of the sternum articulates with the sternal end of the clavicle: are these structures in alignment or is the chin pointing more toward one clavicle?

  This step alerts you to the possibility of dysfunction in the muscles that laterally flex the head on one side of the neck.

- Observe your client's hands as he faces you: are the thumbnails visible or do you see the back of one or both hands instead? Are the fingertips at an even level as her arms hang alongside her thighs?

  If you see the back of a hand, that arm may be pulled into medial rotation by tightness in one or more medial rotators or by "rounded shoulder." Asymmetry in the level of the fingertips may indicate an elevated shoulder.

- Observe your client's clothing: does the hem of a skirt or pants hang evenly or is it hitched up on one side? Does the neckline of her shirt drape more toward one shoulder or droop forward? Is a sleeve drooping over one wrist?

  These cues direct you toward compensation patterns that may have developed, in response to posture dysfunctions: for example, your client may lift one shoulder to compensate for an imbalance in the lumbar spine or hips.

- Observe your client's shoes: are the heels of one or both more noticeably worn on the medial or lateral sides?

  This step alerts you to possible inversion or eversion of your client's feet and guides you toward assessment of the arches of his foot and his leg muscles.

Lab Activity 2–1 on page 95 is designed to help you develop skills in visual posture assessment.

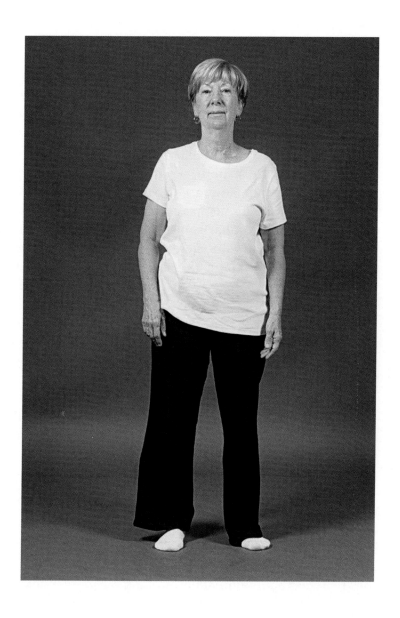

FIGURE 2-20 The drape of your client's clothing reveals obvious postural deviations and guides you toward closer assessment of certain structures.

© Milady, a part of Cengage Learning. Photography by Yanik Chauvin.

LEARNING ENHANCEMENT ACTIVITY

You develop proficiency in posture assessment by doing it over and over again. There is no substitute for repetition. Try performing a posture assessment on a classmate whenever you can: before a class, after a class, during break time. Assess the postures of your friends, your family, the people you work with. You learn something from each posture assessment you perform.

Find a comfortable seat in an open public space—a shopping mall or a school campus, for example—where you can easily observe a large number of people standing, sitting, and walking. Practice performing "stealth" visual assessments. Note head positions, hip positions, the placement of hands and feet. If you can make notes on your findings without offending those you observe or drawing the attention of security officers, so much the better.

Touch and comparison

Adding touch to visual assessment of posture—utilizing both visual and tactile input—engages different areas of your brain and deepens your critical thinking skills. As you see a deviation in normal posture, such as an exaggerated spinal curve, lightly run your hands along the area, getting a tactile sense of its range and degree. If the deviation you see has a contralateral counterpart, use light touch to compare both sides of your client's body. Touching postural landmarks can either reinforce or correct your visual observations.

Comparison is key in postural assessment. Is one shoulder elevated more than the other? Are both kneecaps level? Is one foot everted more than the other? Comparing structures with their counterparts and to your visual reference points facilitates postural assessment. Note any asymmetry as an indication for further assessment.

As you perform visual comparisons of the elements of your client's posture, consider comparing your client's range of motion (ROM) at the large proximal joints: at the spine, the shoulder and the hip, and then

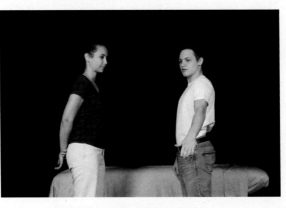

at the elbow and the knee. Limitations in joint range of motion can affect posture. Assessing ROM may include:

- **AROM:** active range of motion, during which your client demonstrates his range of motion at a joint, unassisted. To assess abduction of his arm at the shoulder, for example, your client raises his arm to the side, as shown in Figure 2–21, as you observe.
- **PROM:** passive range of motion, during which you move your client's joint through its range of motion, without his active participation. To assess abduction of his arm at the shoulder, for example,

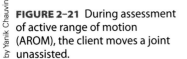

AROM

active range of motion; the client demonstrates the range of motion at a joint, unassisted.

FIGURE 2–21 During assessment of active range of motion (AROM), the client moves a joint unassisted.

© Miliady, a part of Cengage Learning. Photography by Yanik Chauvin.

PROM

passive range of motion: a therapist moves a client's joint through its range of motion without the client's participation.

you raise your client's arm to the side, as shown in Figure 2–22, taking care to support the joints.

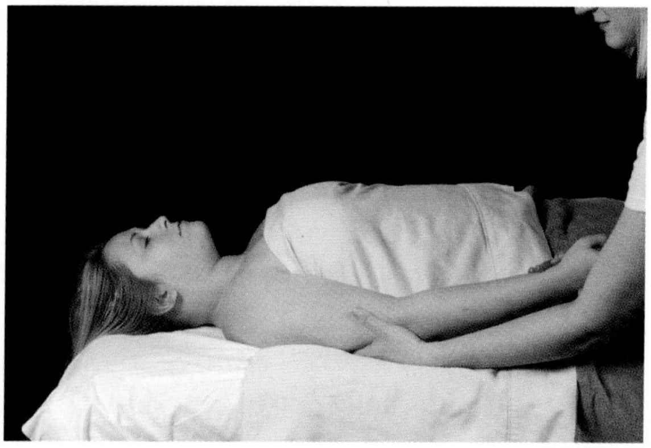

For massage therapy treatment planning, ROM at joints is assessed by comparing:

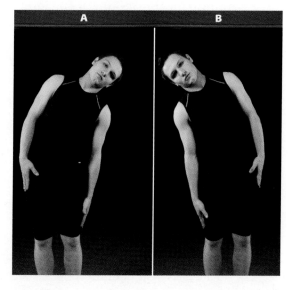

- ROM at a joint in comparison to its counterpart: does Jim's torso laterally flex as far to the right as it does to the left, as shown by the model in Figure 2–23? Can Sue flex her left thigh as high as she does her right?

- ROM at a joint in comparison to an expected functional range: is Sam able to flex either thigh enough to step onto a curb? Is Jill able to rotate her head enough, as shown in Figure 2–24, to see if someone is behind her?

- ROM that is without pain: perhaps Jeff can flex his left arm to its full range of 180°. He feels pain on the anterior of the arm, however, when he flexes it beyond 90° of flexion.

FIGURE 2-22 During assessment of passive range of motion (PROM), the massage therapist moves the joint through its range, without participation by the client.

© Milady, a part of Cengage Learning. Photography by Yanik Chauvin.

FIGURE 2-23A-B Assessment of range of motion is always performed bilaterally, to compare the range on each side of the body.

© Milady, a part of Cengage Learning. Photography by Yanik Chauvin.

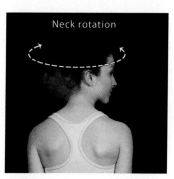

FIGURE 2-24 Assess whether the range of motion at a joint allows for movement within the functional expectation.

© Milady, a part of Cengage Learning. Photography by Yanik Chauvin.

HERE'S A TIP

Compare your client's range of motion at joints using the same vertical and horizontal reference lines you use to assess his posture. You may also use your own joint range of motion as a reference: ask your client, for example, to abduct each arm to your demonstrated 90° of abduction. You will find it useful to repeat range of motion comparisons as treatment progresses.

To assess ROM at a joint:

- Demonstrate for your client the joint action to be assessed.
- Supporting your client's joint, move it unassisted (PROM) through the range of motion that is possible for each action at this joint, as shown in Figure 2–25. Move the joint slowly, to assess the functional range of motion that is safe for this client's joint in each

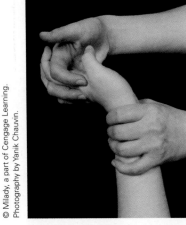

FIGURE 2–25 Gently assess the passive range of motion (PROM) at a joint that your client can perform, and then gently assess the passive range of motion (PROM) at the joint that is pain-free.

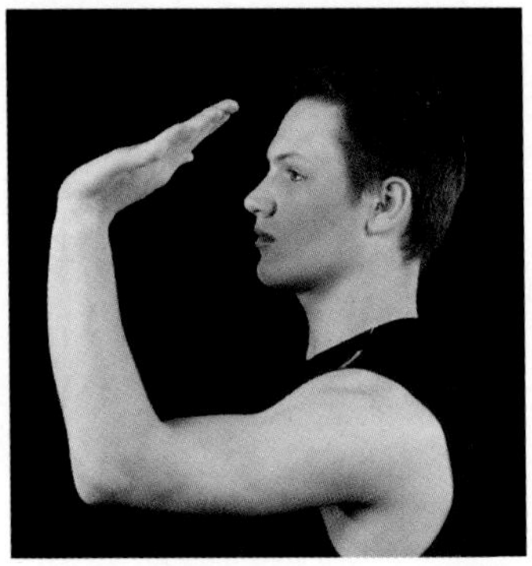

FIGURE 2–26 Ask your client to perform both the functional and pain-free active range of motion (AROM) at a joint.

End feel

the palpation feedback during passive range of joint motion which indicates the limitation of that joint's range of motion.

Lab Activity 2–2 on page 95 is designed to help you develop skills in range of motion assessment.

action. Ask your client to tell you the point in an action where pain is first felt, to assess the pain-free range of motion for this client's joint in the action.

■ Supporting your client's joint, move it unassisted by the client (PROM) through the range of pain-free motion for each action at this joint. Ask your client to tell you the point in the action where pain is first felt in any action, to assess the pain-free range of motion for this client's joint in each action.

■ Ask your client to move his joint unassisted by you (AROM) through the range of functional and pain-free motion for each action at this joint, as shown in Figure 2–26.

■ Duplicate the actions on the contralateral joint, using PROM and AROM; compare the range of functional and pain-free motion for each action at each joint.

■ Compare the assessed range of functional and pain-free range of motion for the actions at the joint. Create and maintain a written record of assessed ROM to gauge treatment progress.

DID YOU KNOW?

End feel is the palpation feedback detected by a massage therapist during PROM that indicates the limitation of a joint's ROM by one of these factors:

■ The structure of the articulating bones: the shape of the end of a bone limits ROM at a joint to prevent injury.

■ The strength and tension of the ligaments: taut, strong ligaments surrounding a joint help to maintain and limit ROM to prevent injury.

■ The tension of the muscles crossing the joint: hypertonic muscle fibers limit ROM at the joint where they cross.

■ Contact with soft body parts: excess adipose tissue or other factors, such as the size of a pregnant woman's abdomen, limit full ROM at joints.

■ Joint pathology or disuse: diseases such as osteoarthritis, decreased hormone and synovial fluid levels, and chronic immobility result in limited ROM at joints.

Variation in end feel at contralateral joints is one strong indicator of a need for further assessment and a compelling justification for contralateral ROM assessment.

The Spine, the Pelvis and the Head

Begin your postural assessment by examining the core of the body: the spine. Deviations in the curvatures of the spine are reflected in the positions of the pelvis and the head. In turn, the curves of the spine may compensate for structural deviations in the pelvis or the extremities. Assessing the spine points you toward additional deviations and compensations to investigate throughout the body.

The spine

Before an infant begins to stand—to bear the weight of the body along his spine—the spine is flat or slightly curved in a "C" shape toward the posterior. The curves of the spine develop over the first year of life to accommodate weight-bearing stress on the spine, absorb shock, and provide

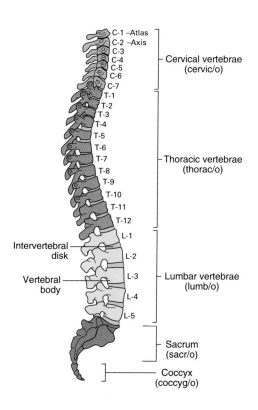

C-1 –Atlas
C-2 –Axis
C-3
C-4
C-5
C-6
C-7
Cervical vertebrae
(cervic/o)

T-1
T-2
T-3
T-4
T-5
T-6
T-7
T-8
T-9
T-10
T-11
T-12
Thoracic vertebrae
(thorac/o)

Intervertebral
disk

Vertebral
body

L-1
L-2
L-3
L-4
L-5
Lumbar vertebrae
(lumb/o)

Sacrum
(sacr/o)

Coccyx
(coccyg/o)

FIGURE 2-27 The normal curves of the spine.

© Delmar, Cengage Learning.

flexibility for maintaining equilibrium and for movement. The normal curves of the spine, shown in Figure 2–27, are:

- Toward the anterior in the cervical region.
- Toward the posterior in the thoracic region.
- Toward the anterior in the lumbar region.
- Toward the posterior in the sacral region.
- The vertebrae are stacked squarely over one another along the midline from C1 to L5, when viewed from the posterior.

The spine exemplifies the individuality of movement: the curves of the spine accommodate our individual manner of standing, walking, dancing, running, sitting, and reclining. This accommodation results in the individual curvatures of each client's spine.

IN THE TREATMENT ROOM

Maintaining comfort during assessment procedures for a client with a spinal deviation means supporting his posture *as it is*, not as you hope it may be at some time in the future:

- Your client with a significant spinal deviation may experience discomfort after standing for any duration. Perform your assessments with your client's tolerance level in mind.
- When your client is on the table, use pillows, bolsters, and wedges to fully support his head, neck, and trunk in the reclining posture that is natural and comfortable for him. When this client is supine, place a bolster beneath his knees and a support beneath his neck.
- A client with significant structural scoliosis or kyphosis, described later in this chapter, may have difficulty breathing when lying supine for any duration. Use pillows or a wedge to raise his torso to an angle that facilitates easy breathing.

The thoracic spine

Assessing the thoracic region of the spine first provides you with a baseline assessment of the core of the spine. The thoracic spine articulates with the ribs to form a closed cage around the thorax. Flexibility and movement, therefore, are somewhat limited in the thoracic region, making deviations in the thoracic region of the spine as likely to be structural as functional. Deviations in the cervical and lumbar regions of the spine often develop as compensations for deviations in the thoracic curve. Assess the thoracic region of the spine laterally and from the posterior.

Ask yourself the following:

- Are the shoulders level?
- Are the thoracic spinous processes oriented squarely over each other along the midline?
- Is the thoracic curve exaggerated or diminished?

Postural landmarks, shown in Figures 2–28 to 2–31:

- The acromion process of each scapula, visible in Figure 2–28.
- Thoracic spinous processes, shown in Figure 2–29.
- Midline orientation of the spinous processes during forward flexion of the trunk, as in Figure 2–31.
- Skin wrinkling on either side of the thoracic spine, visible in Figure 2–32.
- Placement of the inferior angles of the scapulae relative to the thoracic spine, shown in Figure 2–29.
- Anterior placement of the head of the humerus, visible in Figure 2–30.

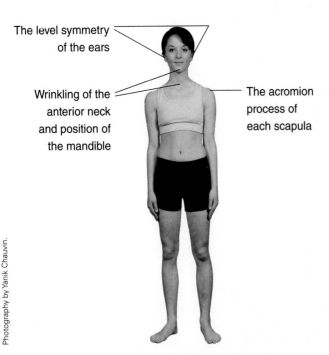

The level symmetry of the ears

Wrinkling of the anterior neck and position of the mandible

The acromion process of each scapula

FIGURE 2-28 Postural landmarks of the trunk, anterior view.

© Milady, a part of Cengage Learning. Photography by Yanik Chauvin.

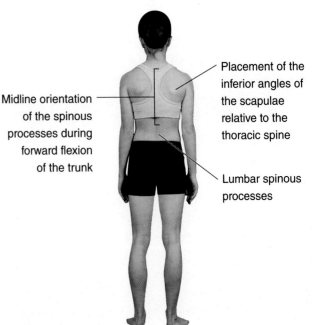

Midline orientation of the spinous processes during forward flexion of the trunk

Placement of the inferior angles of the scapulae relative to the thoracic spine

Lumbar spinous processes

FIGURE 2-29 Postural landmarks of the trunk, posterior view.

© Milady, a part of Cengage Learning. Photography by Yanik Chauvin.

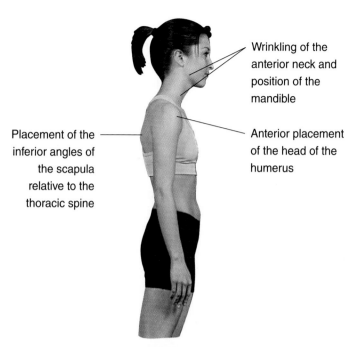

Wrinkling of the anterior neck and position of the mandible

Anterior placement of the head of the humerus

Placement of the inferior angles of the scapula relative to the thoracic spine

FIGURE 2-30 Postural landmarks of the trunk, lateral view.

© Milady, a part of Cengage Learning. Photography by Yanik Chauvin.

Common deviations in the thoracic spine

Scoliosis [skoh-lee-OH-sus] refers to a spinal curvature that is laterally S-shaped, as seen in Figure 2–32, or C-shaped, usually in the thoracic and lumbar regions. The vertebrae are not stacked squarely over one another at the midline. About half the U.S. population is affected to some degree by scoliosis. It can be so mild that it goes unnoticed or so severe that it becomes disabling. Scoliosis may be structural or functional:

- Structural scoliosis may be congenital or may develop later in childhood or adolescence and usually affects the thoracic or thoracolumbar regions of the spine. The vertebrae are not only curved laterally but are also rotated in a fixed position, elevating one side of the ribcage, as seen in Figure 2–32. Structural

> **Scoliosis**
> **(skolios=crooked)**
>
> a spinal curvature that is laterally S-shaped or C-shaped, usually in the thoracic and lumbar regions. The vertebrae are not stacked squarely over one another at the midline.

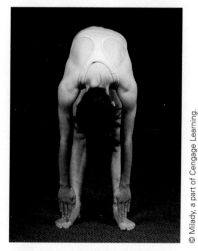

FIGURE 2-31 Assess the midline orientation of the spinous processes as your client flexes her spine.

© Milady, a part of Cengage Learning. Photography by Yanik Chauvin.

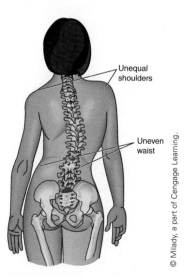

Unequal shoulders

Uneven waist

FIGURE 2-32 The scoliosis posture.

© Milady, a part of Cengage Learning.

scoliosis may resolve as the spine develops, but it may also progress. The adolescent form, which may be detected between the ages of 9 and 13, when growth in height intensifies, is the most common and affects girls far more than boys. Severe structural scoliosis may be disabling and can result in compression of organs in the thoracic and abdominopelvic cavities, requiring surgical intervention. Structural scoliosis is most visibly apparent during forward flexion of the trunk.

■ Functional or compensatory scoliosis is not congenital, is usually not progressive, and does not include fixed rotation of the vertebrae. Functional scoliosis can arise from, or can cause, the body's compensation for a dysfunction in posture or soft tissues, such as functional short leg syndrome, described later in this chapter. Because it does not arise from a structural malformation of the spine, functional scoliosis is not usually visibly apparent during forward flexion of the trunk.

IN THE TREATMENT ROOM

The lateral curves and rotated vertebrae of severe scoliosis result in convex regions on one side of the spine and concave regions on the other. The skin in the concave regions will be folded, as seen in Figure 2–32.

To assess for scoliosis:

■ Ask your client to slowly bend forward from his waist, as seen in Figure 2–31. He may be standing or seated.

■ As he bends forward, lightly trace the spinous processes with your fingertips and assess them along the midline: are the spinous processes aligned evenly over one another, or is there a palpable curve in the thoracic or lumbar region or in both regions? Does each spinous process point toward the posterior, or is there a rotational aspect in any region of the spine?

Kyphosis [ky-FOH-sus], sometimes called hyperkyphosis, is an exaggerated thoracic curve, as seen in Figure 2–33. Kyphosis, too, can be structural or functional:

■ In congenital kyphosis, the rate of development of the vertebral bodies results in wedge-shaped rather than rectangular vertebrae, which in turn results in the exaggerated curve.

■ Structural kyphosis may be caused by another condition, such as arthritis or osteoporosis. Kyphosis caused by osteoporosis is the result of progressive weakening and tiny fractures in thoracic vertebrae. The curve caused by structural kyphosis is angular and sharp.

■ Functional kyphosis can result from or can cause chronic hypotonicity and strain in the muscles that attach to the spine, the scapulae, and the ribcage, such as the Rhomboids, Pectoralis minor, Levator scapulae, and the thoracic Erector spinae and

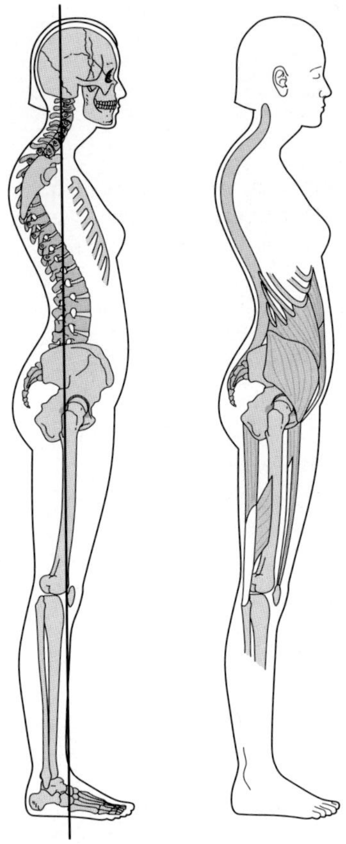

© Delmar, Cengage Learning.

FIGURE 2-33 The kyphosis-lordosis posture.

Kyphosis (kyphos=hunchbacked)

an exaggeration of the posterior thoracic curve of the spine.

Rounded shoulders

one result of a kyphotic thoracic curve. The scapulae are moved laterally, altering the position of the glenohumeral joint and bringing the head of the humerus down and toward the anterior.

Transversospinalis muscle groups. Habitual slumping of the trunk, common among clients who spend long hours at a poorly designed computer workstation, can also cause a kyphotic thoracic curve. The curve caused by functional kyphosis tends to be more rounded and less sharp.

HERE'S A TIP

A common compensation for kyphosis is an exaggeration of the lumbar curve called lordosis, described later in this chapter, which can be seen in Figure 2–33.

Rounded shoulders are one result of a kyphotic thoracic curve: the scapulae are moved laterally, affecting the position of the glenohumeral joint and bringing the head of the humerus down and toward the anterior.

A flat or upright thoracic curve may produce compensations that are opposite from those initiated by a kyphotic curve: the cervical curve may be flat or diminished, in order to maintain equilibrium of the head and the lumbar curve. The scapulae may be retracted closer to the spine, bringing the shoulders back toward the posterior, giving this posture its nickname, "military posture." A flat or diminished thoracic curve may also be structural and congenital. Shown in Figure 2–34, this straight posture is often mistaken for ideal posture.

The cervical spine and the head

The positions of the cervical spine and the head often accommodate deviations in the thoracic curve. Assess the cervical region of the spine laterally, from the anterior and from the posterior.

Ask yourself the following:

- Is the cervical curve exaggerated or diminished?
- Is the head held forward or tilted to one side?

Postural landmarks, including those shown in Figures 2–28, 2–29, and 2–30: and:

- The occiput and spinous process of C7.
- The level of the ears and their alignment on the trunk in lateral view.
- Wrinkling of the anterior neck .
- The angle of the mandible, relative to the suprasternal notch.

Common deviations in the cervical spine

As a result of a **head-forward posture**, shown in Figure 2–35, the lower cervical spine is maintained in a flexed position, while the upper cervical spine is extended, in order to maintain the equilibrium of the head. This posture forces the head forward and places stress on the posterior neck muscles.

A client who spends lots of time at a computer may develop a head-forward posture: as he focuses on the screen, his head moves forward and his posterior neck muscles must strain to accommodate the shifted weight of his head, which is now anterior to the spine instead of over it.

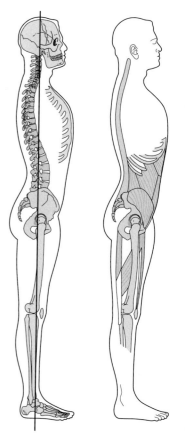

FIGURE 2–34 The "military" posture.

© Delmar, Cengage Learning.

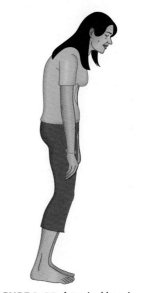

FIGURE 2–35 A typical head-forward posture.

© Milady, a part of Cengage Learning.

IN THE TREATMENT ROOM

A thoracic kyphotic curve may also result in compensatory hyperflexion of the lower cervical vertebrae and hyperextension of the upper cervical vertebrae, visible in Figure 2–34. When this happens, the skin of the posterior neck may have several deep, horizontal wrinkles.

A functionally exaggerated thoracic curve, rounded shoulders, head-forward posture, and a posteriorly tilted pelvis may result from accommodating the weight of a heavy backpack. Look for this group of compensations as the source of mid-back or neck pain in a client who is a student.

If a client has a **flat or diminished cervical curve**, his chin may appear to be retracted, the anterior neck is laterally wrinkled and his posture is military-like, as if standing at attention, rather than at ease, shown in Figure 2–34. A flat or diminished anterior curve makes the cervical spine appear rigidly straight, from the occiput to C7.

Head tilted or tilted and rotated posture: this posture may be caused by unilateral hypertonicity or hypotonicity in muscles that flex, laterally flex, and rotate the head at the neck, such as Sternocleidomastoid (SCM), Trapezius, and Splenius capitis and cervicis. **Torticollis**, [tort-uh-KAHL-us] also called "wry neck," Figure 2–36, is a condition in which the neck is kept in a twisted position. Torticollis may be congenital, but is more commonly caused by sleeping with the neck in an awkward position or by holding a telephone between the head and shoulder, chronically straining Trapezius, Levator scapulae, Sternocleidomastoid (SCM), the Scalenes, and Splenius capitis and cervicis.

The lumbar spine

The lumbar spine supports the weight of the head, the ribcage, the cervical and thoracic spines, and the upper extremity. Assess the lumbar curve as a window into the pelvis and the lower extremity, laterally and from the posterior.

Ask yourself the following:
- Are the lumbar spinous processes oriented along the midline?
- Is the lumbar curve exaggerated or diminished?

Postural landmarks, shown in Figure 2–31:
- Lumbar spinous processes.

Common deviations in the lumbar spine

Lordosis [lor-DOH-sis], also called hyperlordosis, is an exaggerated lumbar curve of the spine toward the anterior, shown as a compensation for kyphosis in Figure 2–33. Lordosis is not usually congenital or permanent. A compensating lumbar curve may result in tilting the pelvis to the anterior, creating strain patterns in Psoas and Iliacus, the lumbar Erector spinae and Transversospinalis muscle groups and the Hamstrings. Lordosis may be caused by many factors:
- The strain on the lumbar spine of obesity or pregnancy.
- Compensation in the thoracic spine for a significant kyphotic curve.

Torticollis

a condition in which the neck is kept in a laterally flexed or rotated position by hypertonic muscles and/or postural compensation patterns. Also called wry neck.

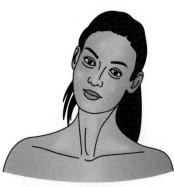

FIGURE 2–36 Torticollis, or wry neck, may afflict a client who spends his workday on the phone without using a headset.

Lordosis (lordos=bent backward)

an exaggeration of the anterior lumbar curve of the spine.

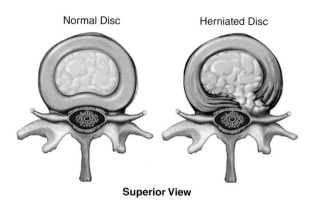

Normal Disc   Herniated Disc

Superior View

FIGURE 2–37 A herniated disc may cause pain, numbness, tingling, and postural dysfunction.

- Lordosis may be caused by arthritis, or by a **herniated disc**, which occurs when some of the disc material extrudes from between the bodies of adjacent vertebrae, as shown in Figure 2–37; or other disc problem.
- Lordosis may develop to maintain equilibrium while wearing high-heeled shoes.

Herniated disc

a condition in which disc material extrudes from between the bodies of adjacent vertebrae.

IN THE TREATMENT ROOM

If your client with a hyperlordotic curve wears high-heeled shoes, also assess the muscles that plantarflex the foot or extend the toes. These muscles may be strained by the effort to distribute weight equally onto the feet.

A **flat or decreased lumbar curve** may tilt the pelvis to the posterior, straining the lumbar Erector spinae and Transversospinalis muscle groups. A flat or diminished lumbar curve also limits the flexibility of the lumbar spine. The lack of an adequate anterior lumbar curve of the spine may be congenital or caused by habitual slumping while sitting. This posture is called "swayback," a term sometimes misapplied to lordosis, and is shown in Figure 2–38.

IN THE TREATMENT ROOM

These additional steps aid in assessing spinal curvatures and compensation patterns, as shown in Figures 2–39 and 2–40:

- With your client seated: standing beside your client, note any alterations in the curves of the spine from his standing to his seated posture. Slide your hand between your client's lumbar spine and the back of the chair. If your hand slides easily past the spine with room to spare, the lumbar curve may be exaggerated. If you are unable to slide your hand toward the spine to any degree, the lumbar spine may be flat or diminished from slumping in the chair.
- With your client supine: slide your hands laterally beneath both the cervical and lumbar regions of the spine. If you are unable to slide your hand beneath his neck to any degree, his cervical curve may be flat or diminished.
- With your client seated: slide your fist laterally between his lumbar spine and the chair. If your fist can pass easily and unimpeded between the chair and your client's spine, the lumbar curve may be exaggerated.

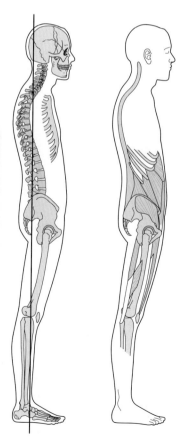

FIGURE 2–38 A swayback posture.

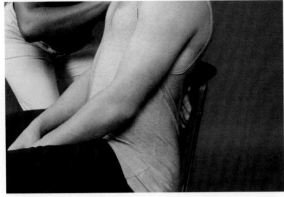

FIGURE 2–39 Slide your hand or your fist between your client's lumbar spine and the back of the chair to assess the degree of the lumbar curve.

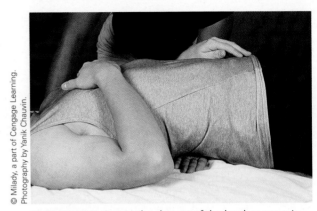

FIGURE 2–40 Assess the degree of the lumbar curve in supine as well as standing or seated position.

HERE'S A TIP

Ask your client to demonstrate his usual sitting positions, at his school or work desk, at home watching TV, or at his computer. Wait a few moments for him to become comfortable enough to assume his usual seated posture. Visually assess the positions of his head and shoulders and his spine: does he tuck one leg under the other, requiring compensations at the head, shoulders, and lumbar spine? Does he slump forward in his seat, rounding his shoulders and sending his head forward? Does he slump backward in his chair, rounding his lumbar curve, as shown in Figure 2–41? Compare the strains placed on his body by seated postures to those you observed in his standing posture.

Lab Activity 2–3 on page 96 is designed to help you develop skills in visually assessing the regions of the spine.

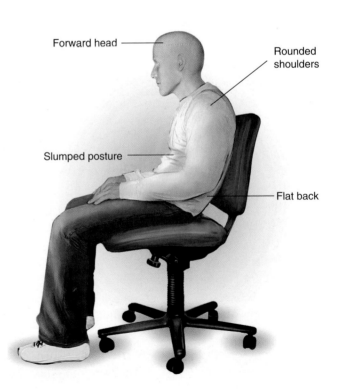

Forward head

Rounded shoulders

Slumped posture

Flat back

FIGURE 2–41 A slouching seated position, especially when sustained over hours at a computer, may result in functional postural deviations.

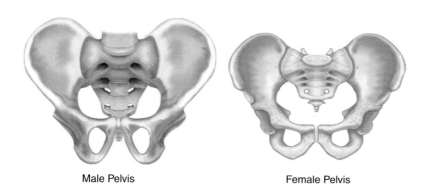

Male Pelvis   Female Pelvis

© Milady, a part of Cengage Learning.

FIGURE 2–42 The female pelvis is deeper and wider than the male pelvis, altering the position of assessment landmarks.

The pelvis

The female pelvis is wider and shallower than the male pelvis, as seen in Figure 2–42. Keep this difference in mind when locating the lateral iliac crest to assess the degree of level balance of the pelvis on your client.

Ask yourself the following:

- Is the iliac crest symmetrical when viewed from the anterior or posterior?
- Is the ASIS symmetrical or does either side seem to rotate to the anterior or posterior?

Postural landmarks, shown in Figures 2–43 and 2–44:

- The high point of the iliac crest.
- The anterior superior iliac spine (ASIS).
- Dimpling of the skin over the sacroiliac joints at the posterior superior iliac spine (PSIS), if visible.

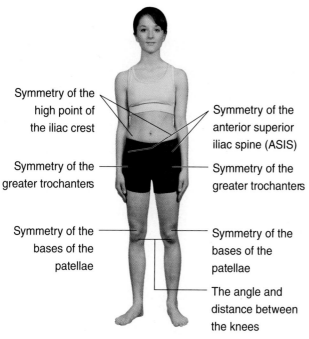

Symmetry of the high point of the iliac crest

Symmetry of the anterior superior iliac spine (ASIS)

Symmetry of the greater trochanters

Symmetry of the greater trochanters

Symmetry of the bases of the patellae

Symmetry of the bases of the patellae

The angle and distance between the knees

© Milady, a part of Cengage Learning. Photography by Yanik Chauvin.

FIGURE 2–43 Postural landmarks of the pelvis and the lower extremity, anterior view.

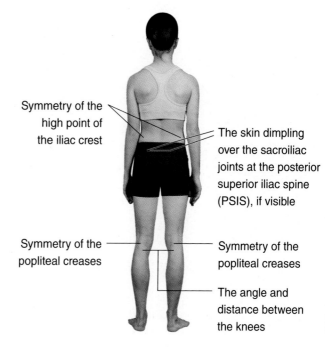

Symmetry of the high point of the iliac crest

The skin dimpling over the sacroiliac joints at the posterior superior iliac spine (PSIS), if visible

Symmetry of the popliteal creases

Symmetry of the popliteal creases

The angle and distance between the knees

© Milady, a part of Cengage Learning. Photography by Yanik Chauvin.

FIGURE 2–44 Postural landmarks of the pelvis and the lower extremity, posterior view.

Common deviations in the pelvis

Postural deviations at the pelvis may compensate for or be caused by deviations in the spine.

Unilateral elevation of the pelvis: unilateral elevation of the pelvis is one cause of functional **short leg syndrome**, the name given to a discrepancy in leg length. Structural short leg syndrome occurs when one leg is truly anatomically shorter than the other. Functional short leg syndrome may be a compensation for scoliosis: the lateral lumbar curve unilaterally elevates the pelvis, as seen in Figure 2–45, lengthening one leg and shortening the other leg.

Short leg syndrome

a discrepancy in leg length that may be structural, in which one leg is truly anatomically shorter than the other, or functional, perhaps a compensation for scoliosis.

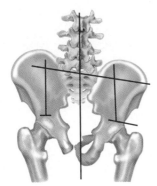

FIGURE 2–45 Short leg syndrome may be caused by structural or functional factors.

Lab Activity 2–4 on page 96 is designed to help you develop skills in visually assessing the pelvis.

> ### IN THE TREATMENT ROOM
>
> A client who habitually stands with one leg bent, shifting all his body weight onto the straight leg, may do so to unconsciously correct for the unilateral elevation of the hip on the bent-leg side of his body, possibly the result of short leg syndrome or as a compensation for scoliosis. Assess this client for both conditions.

Anterior tilt of the pelvis: the pelvis may be chronically tilted toward the anterior by a lordotic lumbar curve, as seen in Figure 2–33, or by chronic hypertonicity in the lumbar Erector spinae and Transversospinalis muscle groups and a corresponding hypotonicity in Rectus Abdominis.

Posterior tilt of the pelvis: an opposite scenario, one in which the lumbar curve is flat or diminished as in swayback posture, shown in Figure 2–38, the lumbar Erector spinae and Transversospinalis muscles are hypotonic, and Rectus abdominis is chronically hypertonic, may tilt the pelvis to the posterior.

> ### IN THE TREATMENT ROOM
>
> The pelvis may be unilaterally tilted toward the anterior or posterior, which may be revealed by kneeling in front of your client to compare the height of each ASIS, as in Figure 2–46, or by assessing the symmetry of the dimples found on the posterior pelvis, over the posterior superior iliac spine (PSIS).

The Lower Extremity

The lower extremity transfers the weight of the head, the trunk, and the upper extremity from the spine and the pelvis through the femur, onto the tibia and then onto the feet. Assess the lower extremity after assessing the pelvis.

The thigh and the leg

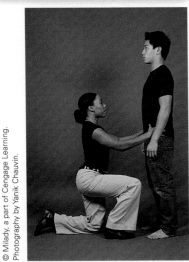

FIGURE 2–46 Assess the symmetry of the anterior superior iliac spines (ASIS) at eye level for greatest accuracy.

The gender difference in the width and depth of the pelvis creates a gender-related difference in the angle of the femur. The head of female femur articulates into a wider acetabulum, giving the greater trochanter greater visual and palpable prominence and increasing the medial angle of the femur toward the tibia. Assess the thigh and leg laterally and from the anterior and posterior.

© Milady, a part of Cengage Learning.

© Milady, a part of Cengage Learning. Photography by Yanik Chauvin.

Ask yourself the following:

- Are the greater trochanters level and pointing laterally?
- Are the angles of the femur equal?
- Are the kneecaps symmetrical and pointing forward?
- Is the distance between the knees sufficient to allow for free movement of the legs but close enough to provide upright support for the upper body?
- Are the knees hyperextended, or is either chronically flexed, throwing more of the body's weight onto the other leg?
- Kneeling behind your client to observe the popliteal creases, are they symmetrical?

Postural landmarks, visible in Figures 2–43 and 2–44:

- The greater trochanters
- The bases of the patellae
- The popliteal creases
- The angle and distance between the knees

Common deviations in the thigh and the leg

In knock-knees, **Genu valgum** [JEE-noo VAL-gum], seen in Figure 2–47, the shaft of the femur angles toward the midline, while the tibia and fibula angle away from the midline. Genu valgum is often a normal phase of development in young children, but occasionally persists into adulthood. The wider female pelvis means that females are more prone to the condition of knock-knees, which is usually self-correcting by adolescence.

In bow-legs, **Genu varum** [JEE-noo VAYR-um], also shown in Figure 2–47, the shaft of the femur angles away from the midline, while the tibia and fibula angle toward the midline. Genu varum may be developmental, or may be caused by an arthritic erosion of the cartilage at the inner knee, fracture of the proximal tibia, or unequal activity at the growth plate at the knee.

> **Genu valgum (genu= knee; valgum=turned or bent)**
>
> a condition in which the shaft of the femur angles toward the midline, while the tibia and fibula angle away from the midline.

> **Genu varum (genu=knee; varum=varied)**
>
> a condition in which the shaft of the femur angles away from the midline, while the tibia and fibula angle toward the midline.

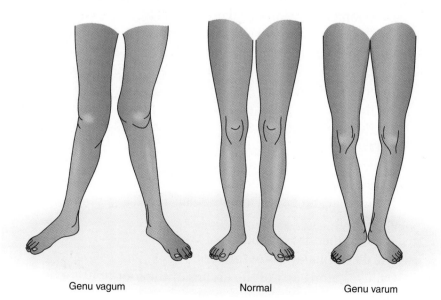

Genu vagum   Normal   Genu varum

FIGURE 2–47 Genu valgum or knock-knees, left, normal knee position, middle, and Genu varum or bow-legs, right.

Genu recurvatum (genu=knee; recurvatum= curved back):

a condition in which the shaft of the femur angles toward the posterior, while the tibia and fibula angle toward the anterior, hyperextending the leg at the knee.

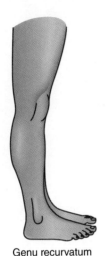

Genu recurvatum

FIGURE 2–48 Genu recurvatum (hyperextended knees).

Sometimes the knee is hyperextended: in **Genu recurvatum** [JEE-noo ree-kur-VAYT-um], the shaft of the femur angles toward the posterior, while the tibia and fibula angle toward the anterior, shown in Figure 2–48. Genu recurvatum is usually a congenital condition that results in a pattern of postural compensations, including anterior tilt of the pelvis and lordosis.

IN THE TREATMENT ROOM

A client with functional short leg syndrome may compensate for the difference in leg length by keeping the longer leg flexed in standing posture, to level the pelvis. This compensation shifts most of the weight of the body unequally onto the short leg. You can easily assess unequal weight bearing as follows.

Place two inexpensive digital scales side by side on the floor. For the most accurate finding, use a set of identical scales. Ask your client to stand with one foot on each scale, as shown in Figure 2–49:

- View the weight registered on each scale.
- If the result is more than a one or two pounds difference, ask your client if he can shift his weight to equalize it between the two scales. Note the postural changes he must make and the compensations each may create in adjusting his weight to achieve balance.
- A result of more than a few pounds may indicate an unequal distribution of weight to compensate for short leg syndrome.

The ankle and the foot

The orientation of your client's feet and the angle and degree of each arch reflects and is reflected in the position of the knees, the pelvis, the spine, and the head. Assess the legs and feet from the anterior and posterior. Assess the arches of each foot medially and from the anterior.

Ask yourself the following:

- Are the feet supinated (inverted) or pronated (everted)? Is any inversion or eversion equal on both feet?
- Are the toes facing forward or are they rotated toward the midline? Does any toe overlap another?
- Are the arches of the foot symmetrical? Is either arch higher or lower than the other?
- Are the toes relaxed or do they remain flexed in standing posture?
- Are there calluses that point toward an assessment of this client's gait?

Postural landmarks, shown in Figure 2–50:

- Medial and lateral malleoli, the "ankles."
- The medial and lateral longitudinal arches and the transverse arch of the foot.
- The first metatarsophalangeal joint.
- The distal phalanges of the toes.
- Calluses along any of the arches of the foot or at metatarsophalangeal or interphalangeal joints.

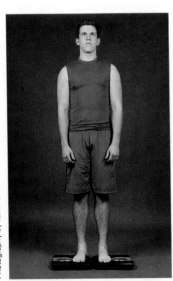

FIGURE 2–49 Assess unequal weight bearing by asking your client to stand with each foot on a separate scale.

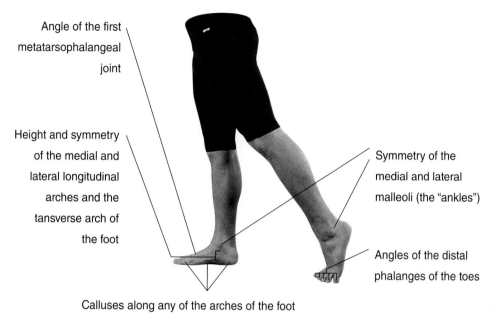

Angle of the first metatarsophalangeal joint

Height and symmetry of the medial and lateral longitudinal arches and the tansverse arch of the foot

Symmetry of the medial and lateral malleoli (the "ankles")

Angles of the distal phalanges of the toes

Calluses along any of the arches of the foot or at metatarsophalangeal or interphalangeal joints

© Milady, a part of Cengage Learning. Photography by Yanik Chauvin.

FIGURE 2–50 Postural landmarks on the ankle and foot, lateral views.

Gait

one's style or manner of walking.

Flat feet

the result of chronic eversion of the foot which transfers the weight of the body unequally onto the medial aspect of the plantar foot, flattening the medial longitudinal arch.

Bunion

another name for hallux valgus.

Hallux valgus (hallux=big toe; valgus=turned or bent)

a condition in which a bony prominence develops at the first metatarsophalangeal joint, pushing the big toe (the hallux) toward and sometimes over the second toe. Also called bunion.

Common deviations in the ankle and the foot

Chronic inversion: when the foot is **inverted**, as seen in Figure 1-37, it cannot adequately absorb shock during **gait,** one's style or manner of walking. Instability in the ankle may increase the risk of sprain. Inversion of the foot is sometimes congenital, the result of the baby's position in the womb. Weight distribution on an inverted foot is transferred unequally to the lateral longitudinal arch, which cannot provide an adequate level of shock absorption or postural support. The peroneal muscles of the lateral leg are strained, and the risk of an inversion sprain, the most common ankle sprain, is increased.

Chronic eversion, also called **flat feet:** when the foot is **everted,** also seen in Figure 1-37, stress transfers to the medial longitudinal arch of the foot and the deep muscles of the leg. Chronic, excessive eversion is a common condition, which can be caused by the stress of obesity, pregnancy, or injury to the foot or ankle. Chronic eversion may be related to short leg syndrome: to compensate for the leg-length discrepancy, the body drops the medial longitudinal arch on the foot of the longer leg, somewhat shortening it to equalize leg length.

Bunion or **hallux valgus** [BUN-yun, HAL-uks VAL-gus]: a bunion is a bony prominence that develops at the first metatarsophalangeal joint, pushing the big toe, the hallux, toward and sometimes over the second toe (Figure 2-51). When the big toe overlaps the second toe, stress is placed on the remaining toes and on the medial longitudinal and transverse arches. Often caused by wearing shoes that are too narrow or high heels that push the weight of the body forward on the foot, a bunion can be excruciatingly painful, disturbs normal gait, and may require surgical repair.

Partial, persistent toe flexion: when the weight of the body is transferred forward, by pregnancy, excess abdominal fat, or wearing high heels, the toes must remain flexed to try to maintain equilibrium.

Bunion —

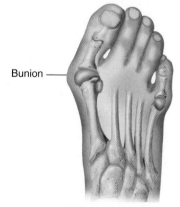

© Milady, a part of Cengage Learning.

FIGURE 2–51 A bunion may be painful, disturbing both posture and gait.

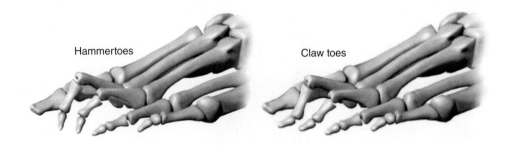

FIGURE 2–52 The unequal transfer of weight onto the toes may result in claw-toe or hammertoe, which affect both posture and gait.

Claw toe

contracture of extensor muscles in the leg that attach to toes which may buckle the toes upward, giving them a claw-like appearance.

Hammertoe

the result of chronic contraction the distal tendons of flexor muscles toes which buckles the toes upward proximally and downward distally, giving them a hammer-like appearance.

Claw toe and **hammertoe:** while many people suffer no consequences from chronic foot eversion other than excessive wear on their shoes, for others the arches can literally collapse, resulting in pain and altered gait. When the foot is chronically everted, as in flat feet, the weight of the body is transferred unequally to the medial aspect of the plantar foot, flattening the medial longitudinal arch. This flattening of the foot lengthens it slightly, persistently contracting the distal tendons of flexor and extensor muscles that attach to the distal phalanges of the toes. Depending on exactly which muscles are contracted first, the toes may buckle upward, called **claw toe**, or buckle upward proximally and then downward distally, called **hammertoe,** both shown in Figure 2–52.

DID YOU KNOW?

As shown in Figure 2–53, the foot has three arches, of which the medial longitudinal arch is the highest. The tarsal and metatarsal bones create the arches of the foot, and the intrinsic foot muscles and the distal tendons of Tibialis anterior and Peroneus longus help to maintain them. The arches of the foot absorb shock; provide flexibility, or the "spring" in your walk; and distribute weight across the foot.

Assessment of your client's arches is important: are they equal in height, length, and angle? Are there calluses at either end of one of the arches that might indicate a deviation in that arch?

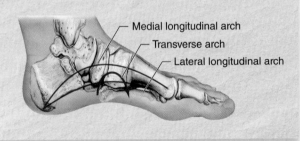

FIGURE 2–53 The arches of the foot.

The Upper Extremity

Because the glenohumeral joint has the combination of range of movement allowed at a ball-and-socket joint and a non-weight-bearing function, as compared to the weight-bearing ball-and-socket acetabulofemoral joint, it has a complex structure that depends heavily on the soft tissues—muscles, tendons and ligaments—for security during movement. Assess the non-weight-bearing upper extremities last.

Lab Activity 2–5 on page 97 is designed to help you develop skills in visually assessing the lower extremities.

The shoulder and the arm

The degree of the thoracic curve of the spine and the condition of the soft tissues that surround the glenohumeral joint create the placement and orientation of the head of the humerus as it articulates with the glenoid fossa at the glenohumeral joint. Assess the shoulder and arm laterally and from the anterior and posterior.

Ask yourself the following:

- Are either or both shoulders rounded downward and to the anterior?
- As standing posture is viewed from the side, do the hands hang along the length of the femur or anterior to it?
- Are the shoulders symmetrical? Is either shoulder elevated in relation to a horizontal reference line and to its counterpart?

Postural landmarks, visible in Figures 2–54 and 2–55:

- Position of the head of the humerus relative to the external ear canal.
- Position of one acromion relative to the other.
- Position of the hands relative to the femur.

Common deviations in the shoulder and the arm

Rounded shoulders: an exaggerated thoracic curve and head-forward position bring the shoulders forward and downward, as seen in Figures 2–34 and 2–36. The hands may hang far in front of the femur, rather than in alignment with it, when seen from the side.

- When both shoulders are rounded, the cause may be structural, perhaps caused by kyphosis, or functional, for example, from sitting at a computer in a slumped posture.

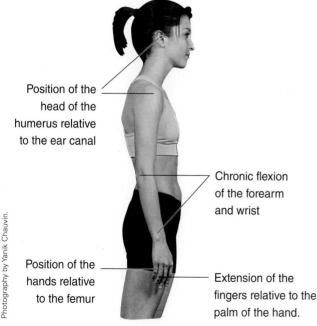

FIGURE 2–54 Postural landmarks of the arm, forearm, and hand, lateral view.

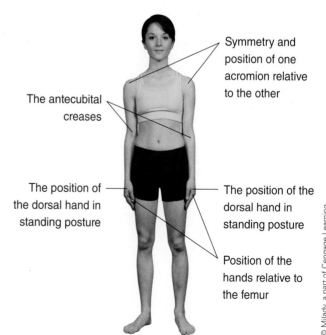

FIGURE 2–55 Postural landmarks of the arm, forearm, and hand, anterior view.

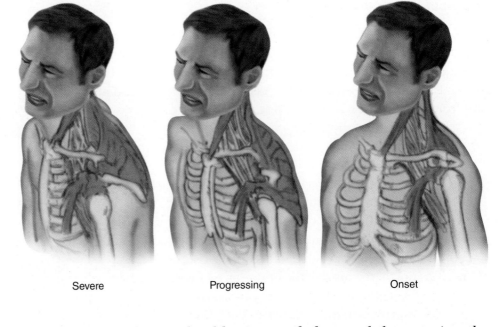

Severe   Progressing   Onset

FIGURE 2–56 Pectoralis Minor Syndrome is a type of Thoracic Outlet Syndrome that may become progressively more disabling, as shown here.

**| Pectoralis Minor
| Syndrome**

a type of thoracic outlet syndrome in which a chronically hypertonic pectoralis minor entraps nearby nerves, ligaments and blood vessels.

**| Thoracic Outlet
| Syndrome**

compression or entrapment of nerves and/or blood vessels by hypertonic muscles in the neck or chest.

- When only one shoulder is rounded toward the anterior, the cause is probably functional: a hypertonic Pectoralis minor pulls the scapula forward and downward, and a hypotonic Rhomboid is unable to counter its pull.

- A rounded shoulder that is accompanied by pain, numbness, or tingling that travels down into the arm may by symptomatic of **Pectoralis Minor Syndrome**, a type of **Thoracic Outlet Syndrome** in which a chronically hypertonic Pectoralis minor entraps nearby nerves, ligaments, and blood vessels, as in Figure 2–56. The hypertonic Pectoralis minor also pulls the coracoid process of the scapula down and toward the anterior, pushing the inferior angle of that scapula to the posterior, giving it a "winged" appearance in relation to its counterpart when seen from behind.

Rounded shoulders may also reflect chronic hypertonicity in the muscles that medially rotate the arm at the shoulder: Latissimus dorsi, Teres major, Subscapularis, and Pectoralis major.

Elevated shoulder: the acromion of one shoulder is visibly higher than the other. An elevated shoulder may be compensation for structural or functional scoliosis, as seen in Figure 2–33, or it may reflect chronic hypertonicity in a Rhomboid or Levator scapulae.

DID YOU KNOW?

An elevated shoulder may be the result of habitually carrying a heavy purse or backpack on that shoulder or wedging a telephone between that shoulder and the chin, or it may be caused by chronically poor seated posture, such as sitting with one leg tucked under the other, unilaterally elevating the pelvis. The opposite shoulder may have to be chronically elevated to maintain equilibrium of the head.

The forearm, wrist, and hand

Assess the forearm, wrist, and hand from all aspects: anterior and posterior and palmar and dorsal. Assess pronation and supination of the forearm with the forearm in flexion, to eliminate interference from movements of the shoulder.

Assess the following, referring to Figure 2–20 as a guide:

■ Are the antecubital creases symmetrical?
■ Are the elbows flexed when viewed in anatomical position?
■ When the client lies supine, do his forearms and wrists lie flat on the table surface?
■ When viewed from the anterior, are the dorsal surfaces of your standing client's hands visible, instead of his thumbs?
■ Do any of your client's fingers remain flexed when the hand is in a resting state?

Postural landmarks, visible in Figures 2–54 and 2–55:

■ Chronic flexion of the forearm and wrist, relative to anatomical position in standing posture and relative to the table surface in supine posture.
■ The position of the dorsal hand in standing posture.
■ Extension of the fingers relative to the palm of the hand.

Common deviations in the forearm, wrist and hand

Partial, chronic flexion of the forearm: this deviation may be most visible when your client is lying supine, as shown in Figure 2–57. His forearm and wrist do not lie on the table, but instead are raised at an angle off the table surface, forcing the fingers to curl to support the hand on a surface. In standing posture, the elbow remains partially flexed, not naturally extended. Chronic flexion of the forearm may be caused by chronic hypertonicity in the forearm flexor muscles or in Brachioradialis, Brachialis, and Biceps brachii.

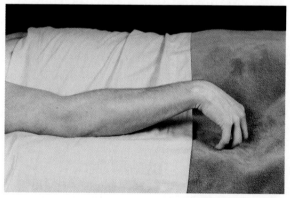

© Milady, a part of Cengage Learning. Photography by Yanik Chauvin.

FIGURE 2–57 Chronic forearm flexion is readily apparent in a supine client.

Partial, chronic pronation of the forearm: rounded shoulders may bring the dorsal surface of the hand to the anterior, or chronic hypertonicity in the muscles that pronate the forearm may keep the forearm persistently pronated.

Partial, chronic flexion of the fingers: one or more fingers may remain flexed at the metacarpophalangeal or interphalangeal joints, or may extend only with difficulty.

■ **Dupuytren's contracture** [doo-pwee-TRANS kun-TRAK-shur]: named by Dr. Dupuytren, this condition occurs when either the fascia of the palmar aponeurosis itself or one of the tendons that

Dupuytren's contracture

a condition in which either the palmar aponeurosis itself or one of the tendons deep to it, contracts, puckering the palm of the hand and maintaining one or more fingers in a flexed position.

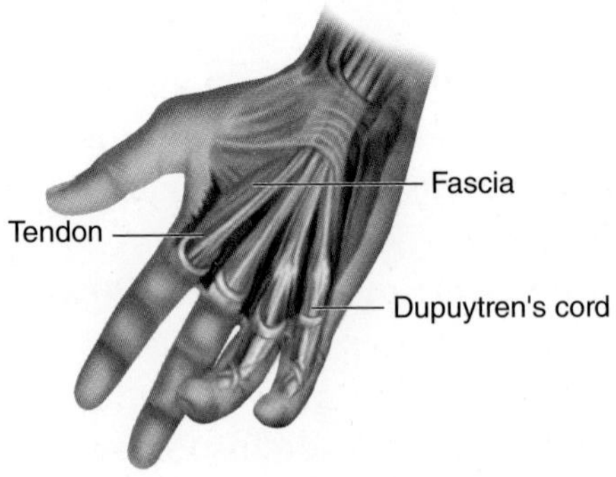

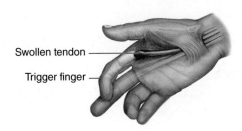

FIGURE 2–58 Dupuytren's contracture.

FIGURE 2–59 Stenosing Tenosynovitis, or "trigger finger."

Stenosing Tenosynovitis (stenosing=narrowing; teno-=tendon; synovitis=synovial inflammation)

when one or more fingers or the thumb is chronically flexed, or extends only with difficulty in a "snap," like pulling a trigger; caused by a narrowing of the tendon sheath surrounding either Flexor digitorum superficialis or Flexor digitorum profundus as it travels to the distal phalanx Also called "trigger finger."

Trigger finger

another name for Stenosing Tenosynovitis.

run deep to it contracts, puckering the palm of the hand and maintaining one or more fingers in a flexed position. Dupuytren's contracture, seen in Figure 2–58, may result from adhesions in the palm that form due to scarring, though there appears to be a genetic link in contractures that are not the result of injury. The contracture may be progressive, but may also respond to a variety of treatments, including massage.

- **Stenosing Tenosynovitis** [steh-NOH-sing ten-oh-sin-uh-VYTE], shown in Figure 2–59, is another term used when one or more fingers or the thumb is chronically flexed, or extends only with difficulty in a "snap," like pulling a trigger. Also known as **trigger finger**, this condition is caused by a narrowing of the sheath surrounding the tendon of either Flexor digitorum superficialis or Flexor digitorum profundus as it travels to the distal phalanx.

Table 2–1 briefly describes some common postural deviations and compensation patterns.

Utilizing Posture Assessment Findings

Record your posture assessment findings regularly and consistently:

- Develop a standardized list of terms to be used for posture assessments on all clients and a list of assessments to be performed in each individual client that reflects the both initial findings and the treatment goals.
- Create a visual representation of your client's initial posture assessment and of subsequent posture assessments, as a record of treatment progress.

The recorded results of posture assessment are a roadmap for the next steps—gait assessment and palpation—and for creating a treatment

TABLE 2-1

COMMON POSTURAL DEVIATIONS AND COMPENSATION PATTERNS		
POSTURAL DEVIATION	**DESCRIPTION**	**POSSIBLE COMPENSATIONS**
Scoliosis	A spinal curvature that is laterally S-shaped or C-shaped, usually in the thoracic and lumbar regions. The vertebrae are not stacked squarely over one another at the midline.	Unilateral elevation of the opposite side of the pelvis, unilateral elevation of the opposite or same-side shoulder, compensation for functional short leg syndrome. Psoas and Quadratus lumborum may be lengthened on one side of the spine and shortened on the other.
Kyphosis	An exaggerated posterior curve in the thoracic region of the spine.	Rounded shoulders, head-forward posture, an exaggerated anterior curve in the lumbar region of the spine. Rhomboids may be lengthened and Serratus anterior shortened. Flexors and extensors of the neck may be strained.
Lordosis	An exaggerated anterior curve in the lumbar region of the spine.	The anterior tilt of the pelvis in increased, straining the Hamstrings muscles and shortening the Erector spinae muscles.
Functional short leg syndrome	Unilateral elevation of one side of the pelvis, possibly as a result of scoliosis, lengthening the same-side leg and shortening the opposite leg.	Elevation of the same-side or opposite shoulder, lateral flexion of the head toward the elevated shoulder. The weight of the body is unequally borne by the short leg and the longer leg may remain flexed in standing posture.
Knock-knees	The shaft of the femur angles toward the midline, while the tibia and fibula angle away from the midline.	The medial longitudinal arch of the foot pronates as the weight of the body is unequally distributed onto the medial longitudinal arch. The medial leg and lateral thigh muscles may become hypertonic as they try to maintain equilibrium in the lower extremity.
Bow-legs	The shaft of the femur angles away from the midline, while the tibia and fibula angle toward the midline.	The foot supinates as the weight if the body is unequally distributed onto the lateral longitudinal arch; the lateral leg and medial thigh muscles may become hypertonic as they try to maintain equilibrium in the lower extremity.
Hyperextended knees	The shaft of the femur angles toward the posterior, while the tibia and fibula angle toward the anterior.	Exaggeration of the anterior curve of the lumbar region of the spine. Anterior tilt of the pelvis in increased, straining the Hamstrings muscles and shortening the Erector spinae muscles

© Milady, a part of Cengage Learning.

plan. As you review the recorded findings from a posture assessment, answer these questions:

■ Is a specific deviation or discrepancy from normal posture likely to be structural or functional? In other words, does the deviation arise from the skeleton or from the muscles or fascia overlaying the bones?

■ Is the specific deviation a compensation for another structural or functional deviation?

■ What other deviations may have been created to compensate for this one?

Whether the deviation from normal posture appears to be structural or functional:

■ Assess the effects on the other parts of the skeleton and on the muscles and fascial structures that attach to or may be overtaxed by compensating for the deviation.

■ Identify the postural and phasic muscles that act as agonists or antagonists at the deviating structures.

■ Define further assessments, such as gait assessment and palpation that will clarify patterns of compensation and strain.

Lab Activity 2–6 on page 98 is designed to help you develop skills in visually assessing the upper extremities.

■ For example, if the thoracic curve of your client's spine is exaggerated, additional posture assessments might include the position of his head, which may be pitched forward, and his shoulders, which may be rounded downward and toward the anterior. The results of these additional posture assessments may point you toward assessing the effects of these deviations on his gait and palpation of the muscles that extend the head and retract the scapulae.

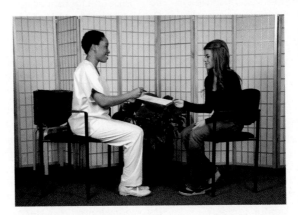

© Milady, a part of Cengage Learning. Photography by Yanik Chauvin.

FIGURE 2-60 Clients' involvement in treatment planning helps to ensure their participation and the eventual success of treatment.

Involve your client in creating and implementing the treatment plan, as shown in Figure 2–60. Client involvement in treatment planning contributes to the success of treatment!

IN THE TREATMENT ROOM

Creating a treatment plan for structural posture deviations may have to be more limited in scope than for postural deviations that are functional in origin. Congenital structural deviations and those caused by chronic bone disease cannot be reversed by massage, though massage may alleviate their effects on muscles, fascia, and other tissues:

■ Use the medical history information listed on your client's intake form for information about any chronic conditions that may contribute to the posture deviation.

■ Study your client's conditions to assess the appropriateness and effectiveness of massage and specific massage techniques for his condition.

■ Involve your client in creating a treatment plan that acknowledges the scope of practice of massage therapy and supports other forms of treatment your client receives.

The effects of functional postural deviations, because they often arise from muscle and fascial strain, and are not present at birth or pathological, may be more successfully treated by massage.

Lab Activity 2–7 on page 99 is designed to help you develop skills in utilizing visual assessment results in treatment planning.

SUMMARY

Understanding the development of postural deviations contributes to effective assessment of your client's structure. Visual assessment posture, coupled with an understanding of joint and muscle actions and your knowledge of the specific agonists and antagonists active in a specific action, sets the stage for analyzing your client's movements and their potential for dysfunction, described in Chapter 3, Gait Assessment.

LAB ACTIVITIES

LAB ACTIVITY 2–1: VISUAL POSTURE ASSESSMENT

1. Working in triads, one partner assesses and records his findings regarding the posture of another partner, while the third partner observes the assessment and records his findings regarding the posture being assessed and the assessment procedure.

2. Prepare for the visual observation:
   - Establish or create visible horizontal and vertical reference lines in the classroom.
   - Stand far enough from your partner to be able to observe posture in the context of the size of the classroom.
   - Ask your partner to remove shoes, tuck hair, etc. (you will ask for shoes to be put back on after your initial assessment).

3. Characterize your visual observations of these components of your partner's standing posture:
   - Observe your client's head position in relation to his spine.
   - Observe the point of your client's chin in relation to his suprasternal notch.
   - Observe your client's hands as he faces you.
   - Observe your client's clothing.
   - Observe your client's shoes.

4. Share and compare the findings recorded by the assessor and the observer; switch places and repeat until each partner has participated in all three roles.

LAB ACTIVITY 2–2: RANGE OF MOTION ASSESSMENT

1. Working in pairs, one partner assesses range of motion at large proximal joints as the other partner takes the role of the client.

2. Demonstrate each of the following joint actions for your partner and then ask him to perform AROM of each action at each joint. Finally, perform PROM of each action at each joint.
   - At each shoulder and hip joint: flexion and extension, abduction and adduction, medial and lateral rotation.
   - At each elbow and knee joint: flexion and extension.

3. Ask your partner to describe any differences in possible and pain free range of motion during AROM of each action.

4. Characterize the end feel you experienced during PROM of each action.

5. Share and compare the findings recorded by the assessor and the observer; switch places and repeat until each partner has performed all the tasks.

LAB ACTIVITY 2-3: VISUAL ASSESSMENT OF THE SPINE

Working in triads, one partner assesses and records his findings regarding the posture of another partner, while the third partner observes the assessment and records his findings regarding the posture being assessed and the assessment procedure.

1. Follow the steps outlined above for visual assessment of the regions of the spine, answering the following questions.

   In the thoracic region of the spine:
   - Are the shoulders level?
   - Are the thoracic spinous processes oriented squarely over each other along the midline?
   - Is the thoracic curve exaggerated or diminished?

   In the cervical region of the spine:
   - Is the cervical curve exaggerated or diminished?
   - Is the head held forward or tilted to one side?

   In the lumbar region of the spine:
   - Are the lumbar spinous processes oriented along the midline?
   - Is the lumbar curve exaggerated or diminished?

2. Characterize any visible deviations in the curves of the spine, using these terms:
   - Scoliosis
   - Kyphosis
   - Rounded shoulders
   - Flat or diminished lumbar curve
   - Head-forward posture
   - Flat or diminished cervical curve
   - Head tilted or tilted and rotated posture
   - Lordosis

3. Characterize any additional findings from this assessment of the spine.

4. Share and compare the findings recorded by the assessor and the observer; switch places and repeat until each partner has participated in all three roles.

LAB ACTIVITY 2-4: VISUAL ASSESSMENT OF THE PELVIS

1. Working in triads, one partner assesses and records her findings regarding the spinal curvatures and spinal alignment of another partner, while the third partner observes the assessment and records his findings regarding the posture being assessed and the assessment procedure. Looking at the regions of the spine from all angles at eye level, answer the following questions:
   - Is each iliac crest symmetrical when viewed from the anterior or posterior?

- Is each ASIS symmetrical or does one side seem to rotate to the anterior or posterior?

2. Characterize any visible deviations in the pelvis, using these terms:
   - Unilateral elevation of the pelvis
   - Short leg syndrome
   - Anterior tilt of the pelvis
   - Posterior tilt of the pelvis
3. Characterize any additional findings from this assessment of the pelvis.
4. Share and compare the findings recorded by the assessor and the observer. Switch places and repeat until each partner has participated in all three roles.

LAB ACTIVITY 2–5: VISUAL ASSESSMENT OF THE LOWER EXTREMITIES

1. Working in triads, one partner assesses and records his findings regarding the each lower extremity of another partner, while the third partner observes the assessment and records his findings regarding the posture being assessed and the assessment procedure. Looking at each lower extremity from all angles at eye level, answer the following questions:
   - Are the greater trochanters level and pointing laterally?
   - Are the angles of the femur equal?
   - Are the kneecaps level and pointing forward?
   - Is the distance between the knees sufficient to allow for free movement of the legs but close enough to provide upright support for the upper body?
   - Are the knees hyperextended or is either chronically flexed, throwing more of the body's weight onto the other leg?
   - If you can see the popliteal creases, are they symmetrical?
   - Are the feet supinated (inverted) or pronated (everted)? Is any inversion or eversion equal on both feet?
   - Are the toes facing forward or are the feet rotated toward the midline? Does any toe overlap another?
   - Are the arches of the foot symmetrical? Is either arch higher or lower than the other?
   - Are the toes relaxed or do they remain flexed in standing posture?
   - Are there calluses that point toward an assessment of this client's gait?
2. Characterize any visible deviations in the lower extremity, using these terms:
   - Knock-knees
   - Bow-legs
   - Knee hyperextension
   - Foot inversion
   - Foot eversion, or flat feet

- Bunion
- Partial, persistent toe flexion
- Claw toe and hammertoe

3. Characterize any additional findings from this assessment of the lower extremity.

4. Share and compare the findings recorded by the assessor and the observer. Switch places and repeat until each partner has participated in all three roles.

LAB ACTIVITY 2–6: VISUAL ASSESSMENT OF THE UPPER EXTREMITIES

1. Working in triads, one partner assesses and records his findings regarding the posture of another partner, while the third partner observes the assessment and records his findings regarding the posture being assessed and the assessment procedure. Follow the steps outlined above for visual assessment of each upper extremity, answering these questions:

   - Are either or both shoulders rounded downward and to the anterior?
   - In standing posture, do the hands hang along the length of the femur or anterior to it?
   - Are the shoulders level? Is either shoulder elevated in relation to a horizontal reference line and to its counterpart?
   - Are the antecubital creases symmetrical?
   - Are the hands in alignment with the elbows in anatomical position?
   - When the client lies supine, do his forearms and wrists lie flat on the table surface?
   - When viewed from the anterior, are the dorsal surfaces of your standing client's hands visible, instead of his thumbs?
   - Do any of your client's fingers remain flexed when the hand is in a resting state?

2. Characterize any visible deviations in the upper extremity, using these terms:

   - Rounded shoulders
   - Elevated shoulder
   - Partial, persistent flexion of the forearm
   - Partial, persistent eversion of the forearm
   - Partial, persistent flexion of the fingers
   - Dupuytren's contracture
   - Trigger finger

3. Characterize any additional findings from this assessment of the upper extremity.

4. Share and compare the findings recorded by the assessor and the observer. Switch places and repeat until each partner has participated in all three roles.

LAB ACTIVITY 2–7: UTILIZING VISUAL ASSESSMENT RESULTS IN TREATMENT PLANNING

1. Working with a partner whose posture you assessed during one of the previous labs in this chapter, use your recorded assessment results to create a visual representation of your postural assessment.

2. Using your recorded assessment results and the visual representation, answer these questions:

   - Is a specific deviation or discrepancy from normal posture likely to be structural or functional? In other words, does the deviation arise from the skeleton or from the muscles or fascia overlaying the bones?
   - Is the specific deviation a compensation for another structural or functional deviation?
   - What other deviations may have been created to compensate for this one?

3. Using your recorded assessment results, the visual representation and the answers to the questions posed in Question 2:

   - Assess the effects on the other parts of the skeleton and on the muscles and fascial structures that attach to or may be overtaxed by compensating for the deviation.
   - Identify the postural and phasic muscles that act as agonists or antagonists at the deviating structures.
   - Define further assessments, such as gait assessment and palpation that will clarify patterns of compensation and strain.

4. Switch partners and repeat the activity.

CASE PROFILES

Case Profile 1

Megan is a healthy, 36-year-old stay-at-home mother of young children who complains of constant soreness in her right lumbar area, especially after a long walk. Her left shoulder and neck are also often sore. Your initial visual assessment shows that the hem of Megan's T-shirt is hiked up on the right and that her head is slightly tilted toward her left shoulder. What postural assessments will you perform next? What do you suspect is the source of Megan's neck, shoulder, and low-back pain?

Case Profile 2

Sid, 27, is the editor of an online e-zine. He says his neck, shoulders, and upper back give him constant pain. In his downtime, Sid plays video poker while talking on his phone. What postural assessments will you perform on Sid? What do you immediately expect to find? What work habits may be contributing to Sid's back and neck problems?

Case Profile 3

Janice, 47, is otherwise in great shape but complains of an aching pain in her left thigh and hip after standing all day at her job in a rare-book store. In visually assessing Janice's posture, you notice that her right leg remains slightly bent as she stands. What postural assessments will you perform next? What do you suspect is the source of Janice's left thigh and hip pain?

STUDY QUESTIONS

1. Why do postural compensations develop?
2. Describe the postural landmarks you look for in an initial, 60-second visual assessment of your client's posture.
3. Describe two potential postural compensations that may result from scoliosis.
4. What is one potential lifestyle habit that may result in functional kyphosis?
5. Describe two pathological conditions that may impact posture.
6. Describe the three arches of the foot and the impact of flat feet.
7. How do you assess a client for swayback when he is seated or supine on your table?
8. Compare and contrast AROM and PROM.
9. Name two possible causes for an elevated shoulder.
10. Describe the appropriate scope of practice for a massage therapist in performing posture assessments.

Gait Assessment

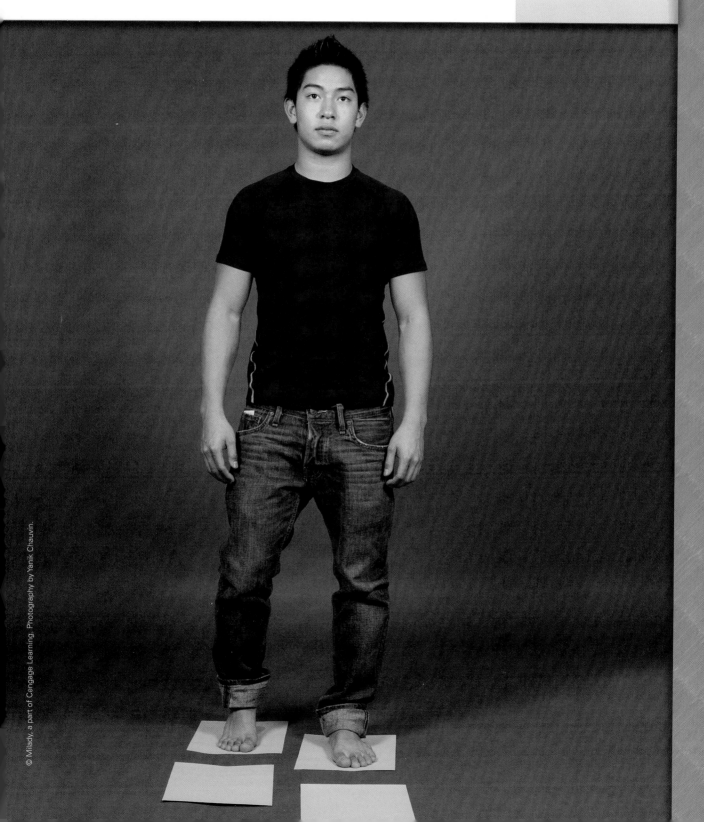

CHAPTER OUTLINE

- **GAIT ASSESSMENT GUIDELINES**
- **GAIT ASSESSMENT**

LEARNING OBJECTIVES

- **Define the phases and stages of normal gait.**
- **Describe the postural deviations, muscle dysfunctions, and pathologies that may alter gait.**
- **Apply visual assessment techniques to locate common altered gait patterns and to identify the structures involved.**

INTRODUCTION

Gait is as individual as posture and is intimately linked to it: postural deviations almost always affect gait. A head held forward, an elevated shoulder, an exaggerated lumbar curve, a shortened leg, a pronated or everted foot: each may alter a client's normal pattern of walking. Once you have assessed your client's posture—her body at rest—use the results of postural assessment to assess your client's gait—her body in motion.

GAIT ASSESSMENT GUIDELINES

Gait is a complex process, comprising multiple movements both in concert and in sequence, multiple structures from the head to the feet, and the external force of gravity and the internal force of equilibrium. Our goal in this chapter is to simplify gait by describing it and breaking it down into its broad components. Within this context, the scope of practice for performing gait assessments includes:

- Visual observation of the elements of gait, including the relative positions of joints and bony structures.
- Recording of objective and subjective findings of assessments in written form, for the purposes of identifying treatment goals and procedures.

The results of our visual gait assessments are tools for use in treatment planning. As noted in Chapter 2, Posture Assessment, discussions concerning scope of practice for massage therapy are ongoing and reflect the dynamic nature of the profession.

Components of Normal Gait

Stance phase

the period of time during gait when one or both limbs are in contact with the ground; the weight-bearing phase of the gait cycle.

Gait is divided into two distinct phases that are cyclic:

- The **stance phase**: the period of time during which one or both limbs are in contact with the ground. The stance phase constitutes about 60 percent of the gait cycle.

■ The **swing phase**: the period of time during which one limb is off the ground and swinging forward. The swing phase constitutes about 40 percent of the gait cycle.

The **gait cycle** is the stance and swing phases together. The gait cycle is equivalent to one **stride**, also known as **stride length**.

Swing phase

the period of time during gait when one limb is off the ground and swinging forward during the gait cycle.

Gait cycle

the stance and swing phases together equivalent to one stride.

Stride

the distance between one heel strike and the subsequent heel strike of the same foot. Also called stride length.

DID YOU KNOW?

Stride length is the distance between one heel strike and the subsequent heel strike of the same foot, as shown in Figure 3–1.

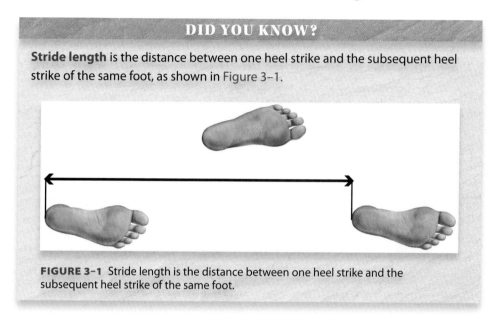

FIGURE 3-1 Stride length is the distance between one heel strike and the subsequent heel strike of the same foot.

Stance Phase

The stance phase refers to the weight-bearing phase of gait: it begins as one foot touches the ground and continues until that foot leaves the ground. The stance phase can be divided into five separate stages, which describe the actions of the foot as it is on the ground, as shown in Figure 3–2.

Heel strike

Heel strike: heel strike, also called **initial contact,** occurs as the heel of your front foot first makes contact with the ground, labeled "A" in

Heel strike

the beginning of the stance phase of gait occurs as the heel first makes contact with the ground. Also called initial contact.

Initial contact

another term for heel strike.

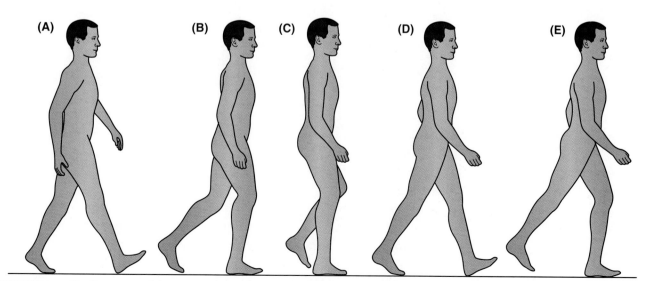

(A)   **(B)**   **(C)**   **(D)**   **(E)**

FIGURE 3-2 The five stages of the stance phase of gait: (a) Heel strike; (b) Foot flat; (c) Midstance; (d) Heel off; (e) Toe off.

© Delmar/Cengage Learning.

Figure 3–2. Heel strike is the beginning of the stance phase and involves actions throughout the body, starting at that foot:

- The foot and ankle are in neutral, slightly dorsiflexed.
- The leg is extended and the thigh is slightly flexed.
- The trunk is erect and contralaterally rotated.
- The pelvis on the opposite side is anteriorly tilted.
- The arm on the same side is hyperextended, while the opposite arm is flexed.
- The weight of the body shifts onto the other limb, which remains in contact with the ground, called **single support**.

Single support

the stage during the stance phase of gait when the entire weight of the body is on the limb that is in contact with the ground.

Step length

the distance between the heel strikes of the left and right feet.

LEARNING ENHANCEMENT ACTIVITY

Step length is the distance between the heel strikes of the left and right feet, different from stride length, which is the distance between heel strikes of the same foot. Step length is shown in Figure 3–3. Compare your step length on each foot:

- Take one normal step forward, keeping your rear foot on the floor. Place a mark on the floor to indicate the distance between the heel strike of the mobile foot and the position of the heel of the planted foot. This is your step length on this side of your body.
- Repeat the normal step, this time leading off with the opposite foot, keeping the foot that is now in the rear planted on the floor. Place a mark on the floor to indicate the distance between the heel strike of the mobile foot and the position of the heel of the planted foot. This is your step length on the other side of your body.
- Comparing step length on each side of the body may reveal dysfunction in the muscles that are active during heel strike (see Table 3–3).

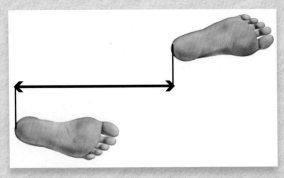

FIGURE 3–3 Step length is the distance between the heel strikes of the left and right feet.

Actions during the heel-strike stage of the stance phase involve multiple muscles:

- Dorsiflexors of the foot.
- Extensors of the leg.
- Flexors of the thigh.
- Extensors of the trunk.
- Contralateral rotators of the trunk: the Transversospinalis group, Psoas major, and the External abdominal obliques.
- Muscles that anteriorly tilt the pelvis.
- Flexors and extensors of the arm.

DID YOU KNOW?

Double support, the amount of time during gait when both limbs are touching the ground at the same time, occurs at the very beginning and the very end of each gait cycle. The amount of time spent in double support reflects the **cadence** [KAYD-ins], the speed of your gait: the faster you walk, the less time you spend in double support. **Single** support is the time during gait when only one foot is in contact with the ground. **Non-support** is the term for the time when both feet are off the ground, usually only during a running gait. Double and single support during gait is shown in Figure 3–4:

Double support

the time during gait when both limbs are touching the ground at the same time.

Cadence

the speed of one's gait.

Non-support

the period of time during gait when both feet are off the ground, usually only during a running gait.

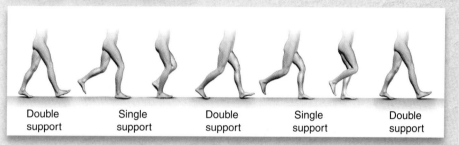

| Double support | Single support | Double support | Single support | Double support |

FIGURE 3–4 Double and single support during gait.

© Delmar/Cengage Learning.

DID YOU KNOW?

The synchronized pattern of **arm swing**, seen in Figure 3–5, contributes to an even gait: during the heel strike phase, the opposite arm is in flexion and the same side arm is extended or hyperextended, maintaining equilibrium and forward momentum. The usual range of arm swing matches step length, again contributing to equilibrium and forward momentum. Performing the following exercises will help you to understand the role of arm swing in gait:

Arm swing

the synchronized pattern arm movements that contributes to an even gait during the heel strike stage.

Exercise #1:

■ Walk across the room as you normally do, focusing on the natural arm swing that synchronizes with your step. Usually, the left arm swings as the right leg strides.

■ Next, walk across the room again—but this time, swing the arm that is on the same side as your mobile limb. Now, the left arm swings as the left leg strides.

■ Characterize the effect of the same side arm swing on your gait. Does changing the synchronicity of arm swing widen the distance between your feet in order to maintain equilibrium?

Exercise #2:

■ Walk across the room, focusing on the range of your arm swing, comparing it to the length of your step.

■ Now, walk across the room again—but this time, keep one arm held immobile by your side.

■ Walk across the room a third time, with both arms held immobile at your sides.

■ Characterize the effects of an unbalanced and absent arm swing on your gait. Does the restriction or removal of arm swing shorten your step length in order to maintain equilibrium?

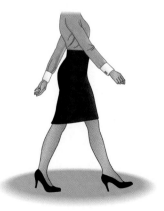

© Milady, a part of Cengage Learning.

FIGURE 3–5 Synchronized arm swing contributes to an even gait pattern and matches step length.

Foot flat

The **foot flat** or **loading response** stage of the stance phase, labeled "B" in Figure 3–2, follows the heel strike. The mobile front foot is now flat on the ground, accompanied by these actions:

- The foot slightly plantarflexes, although dorsiflexors maintain the position of the foot, so that it does not slap on the ground.
- The leg remains slightly extended as the thigh moves into extension.
- The trunk remains erect and the weight of the body continues to shift to the opposite, planted limb.

These actions involve muscles in addition to those active in heel strike:

- Plantarflexors of the foot.

DID YOU KNOW?

Step width, seen in Figure 3–6, is the distance between feet during stance phase of gait. Normal step width allows free movement of both feet without the medial malleoli or the calcaneus touching. Sometimes step width is unconsciously widened to increase balance and stability during gait, for example:

- An obese person may increase step width to maintain balance and distribute excess weight onto the lower extremity.
- A pregnant woman may increase step width due to softening of the pubic symphysis and weight gain, creating the "waddling" gait of late pregnancy.
- An elder may increase step width to compensate for deficits in balance, vision, and space perception.

Increased step width is sometimes accompanied by a decrease in cadence—the speed of the gait cycle—and by chronic strain in the adductor muscles.

Sometimes step width is narrowed, for example:

- When walking through a space that does not allow for normal step width, such as the aisle in an airplane or in a crowded supermarket.
- When walking on a treadmill. The strip of moveable tread where the walker must remain may inhibit normal step width, as does the intrusion of side support bars. Treadmill gait also inhibits normal step length because most people hold on to the support bars with both hands, eliminating natural arm swing from their gait. Normal cadence may also be disrupted by the automatic cadence of the treadmill.

Decreased step width increases the risk of falling and may result in chronic strain in the lateral thigh and leg—usually, the iliotibial band (ITB) and the Peroneal muscles.

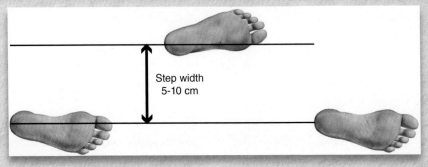

Step width
5-10 cm

FIGURE 3-6 Normal step width allows free movement of both feet.

Midstance

During the **midstance** stage of the stance phase, labeled "C" in Figure 3–2, the weight of the body has entirely shifted onto the limb that has been mobile and is now in stance. The body can now balance completely on that planted limb, the second occurrence of single support during the gait cycle, though the body remains in motion:

- Muscles that plantarflex the foot control the rate at which the leg travels over the ankle to begin to dorsiflex.
- The pelvis is now posteriorly tilted.
- The arms are now both extended.

This now also involves:

- Muscles that posteriorly tilt the pelvis.

Heel off

Stage four of the stance phase is called **heel off,** or **terminal stance,** labeled "D" in Figure 3–2. The weight of the body, which shifted entirely onto this planted limb during midstance, now begins to transfer again as the foot prepares to become mobile and leave the ground. Included in this stage is the preparatory **push off,** during which the body is propelled forward by the muscles that plantarflex the foot. Actions during heel off and push-off:

- The toes of the mobile foot are extended.
- The foot is quickly dorsiflexed, then plantarflexed.
- The leg is slightly flexed.
- The thigh is hyperextended, adducted, and medially rotated.
- The trunk begins to ipsilaterally rotate.
- The opposite arm begins to flex.

These muscles are now engaged:

- Extensors of the toes.
- Plantarflexors of the foot.
- Flexors of the leg.
- Ipsilateral rotators of the trunk.
- Flexors of the arm.

Toe off

The last stage of the stance phase, labeled "E" in Figure 3–2 and sometimes called **preswing**, represents the snippet of time before and during which the toes of the mobile foot leave the ground. This stage ends the stance phase and signals the beginning of the swing phase. During this stage:

- The foot plantarflexes.
- The leg and thigh flex.

These muscles remain active:

- Plantarflexors of the foot.
- Flexors of the leg.
- Flexors of the thigh.

Midstance

a stage of the stance phase during which the weight of the body has entirely shifted onto the limb that has been mobile and is now in stance.

Heel off

stage four of the stance phase. The weight of the body begins its transfer as the foot prepares to leave the ground. Also called terminal stance.

Terminal stance

another term for the heel off stage of the stance phase of gait.

Push off

a part of stage four of the stance phase during which the body is strongly propelled forward by the muscles that plantarflex the foot.

Toe off

Another term for preswing.

Preswing

the last stage of the stance phase, representing the snippet of time before and during which the toes leave the ground. Also called toe off.

TABLE 3–1

STANCE PHASE STRUCTURES AND THEIR ACTIONS					
STRUCTURE	DURING HEEL STRIKE	DURING FOOT FLAT	DURING MIDSTANCE	DURING HEEL OFF	DURING TOE OFF
Toes				Extended at the metatarsophalangeal joints.	
Foot	In neutral.	Slightly plantarflexes at the ankle. Dorsiflexors maintain the position of the foot at the ankle.	Plantarflexors control the rate at which the leg travels over the ankle to begin to dorsiflex the foot at the ankle.	Briefly dorsiflexes, then plantarflexes at the ankle.	Plantarflexes the foot at the ankle.
Leg	Slightly extended at the knee.	Slightly extended at the knee.		Slightly flexed at the knee.	Flexed at the knee.
Thigh	Slightly flexed at the hip.	Moves into extension at the hip.		Hyperextended, adducted, and medially rotated at the hip.	Flexed at the hip.
Pelvis	Anteriorly tilted or rotated on the opposite side at spinal joints.		Posteriorly tilted or rotated at spinal joints.		
Trunk	Erect but contralaterally rotated at spinal joints.	Remains erect.		Begins to ipsilaterally rotate at spinal joints.	
Arms	Hyperextended at the shoulder on the same side, flexed at the shoulder on the opposite side.	Both arms extended at the shoulder.		Opposite arm begins to flex at the shoulder.	

Table 3–1 summarizes the structures and their actions during the stance phase of gait.

Lab Activity 3–1 on page 125 is designed to help you assess the stance phase of gait.

LEARNING ENHANCEMENT ACTIVITY

The following exercise may help you to separate the stages of the stance phase:

- Walk across the room at your normal cadence, focusing on your heel strike and toe off, the first and final stages of stance.
- Now, walk across the room again, in slow motion. Focus your attention on what is happening between heel strike and toe off: the foot-flat stage, midstance, the shifting of body weight, and the rise of your heel off the ground as you prepare to push off your toes leave the ground.
- Walk across the room a third time at your normal cadence, bringing your focus to all five stages of the stance phase of gait. Repeat as often as it takes for you to easily identify the stages of stance.

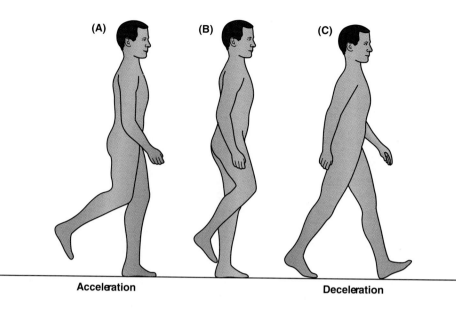

Acceleration   Deceleration

FIGURE 3-7 The swing phase of gait: (a) Acceleration; (b) Midswing; (c) Deceleration.

Swing Phase

The swing phase composes the non-weight-bearing phase of gait: the mobile foot is not in contact with the ground. The swing phase is divided into three stages: acceleration, midswing, and deceleration, seen in Figure 3–7.

Acceleration

In the acceleration stage of the swing phase:
- The foot dorsiflexes.
- Both the thigh and the leg rapidly flex.
- The pelvis is posteriorly tilted.

Muscles active during acceleration include
- Dorsiflexors of the foot.
- Flexors of the leg.
- Flexors of the thigh.
- Muscles that posteriorly tilt the pelvis.

During the acceleration stage, the rear limb catches up with the body.

Midswing

In midswing, the mobile limb moves close to the stance limb that is on the ground, as it swings through. The joint and muscle actions of acceleration continue, each to a lesser degree.

Deceleration

Deceleration prepares for heel strike, the first stage of the stance phase:
- The foot is held in neutral, slight dorsiflexion.
- The leg extends.
- The pelvis moves toward anterior tilt.

These muscles are active:
- Dorsiflexors of the foot.
- Extensors of the leg.
- Muscles that anteriorly tilt the pelvis.

Table 3–2 summarizes the structures and actions during the swing phase of gait.

TABLE 3–2

	SWING PHASE STRUCTURES AND THEIR ACTIONS		
STRUCTURE	DURING ACCELERATION	DURING MIDSWING	DURING DECELERATION
Foot	Dorsiflexes at the ankle.	Dorsiflexes at the ankle.	In neutral dorsiflexion at the ankle.
Leg	Rapidly flexes at the knee.	Flexes at the knee. The mobile leg moves closer to the stance leg.	Extends at the knee.
Thigh	Rapidly flexes at the hip.	Flexes at the hip.	
Pelvis	Posterior tilt at spinal joints.	Posterior tilt at spinal joints lessens.	Moves toward anterior tilt at spinal joints.

Table 3–3 summarizes the major muscles active during the normal gait cycle.

TABLE 3–3

MUSCLE ACTIONS DURING THE GAIT CYCLE	
GAIT ACTION	MUSCLES
Extension of the toes at the tarsometatarsal joints	Extensor hallucis longus and brevis and Extensor digitorum longus and brevis
Dorsiflexion of the foot at the ankle	Tibialis anterior, Extensor digitorum longus, Extensor hallucis longus, and Peroneus tertius
Plantarflexion of the foot at the ankle	Gastrocnemius and Soleus, Peroneus longus and brevis, Tibialis posterior, Flexor digitorum longus, Flexor hallucis longus, and Plantaris
Flexors of the leg at the knee	The Hamstrings group, Sartorius, Gracilis, Gastrocnemius, Plantaris, and Popliteus
Flexors of the thigh at the hip	Psoas and Iliacus, Sartorius, Tensor fasciae latae (TFL), Rectus femoris of the Quadriceps group, Pectineus, Adductor longus and brevis, and Gracilis and Gluteus medius and minimus
Extensors of the thigh at the hip	Gluteus maximus, posterior Gluteus medius and minimus, the Hamstrings, and Adductor magnus
Adductors of the thigh at the hip	Lower Gluteus maximus, the Adductor group, Biceps femoris and Quadratus femoris
Medial Rotators of the thigh at the hip	Anterior Gluteus medius and minimus, TFL, Semimembranosus and Semitendinosus, and Piriformis
Anterior tilt of the pelvis at spinal joints	The Erector spinae and Transversospinalis groups, Quadratus lumborum, Psoas and Iliacus, Latissimus dorsi, Rectus femoris of the Quadriceps group, Sartorius, TFL, Pectineus, Gracilis, and Adductor longus and brevis
Posterior tilt of the pelvis at spinal joints	Rectus abdominis, the External and Internal obliques, the Hamstrings group, the Gluteals, Adductor magnus, and Psoas
Ipsilateral rotators of the trunk at spinal joints	The Erector spinae muscle group and Internal abdominal oblique
Contralateral rotators of the trunk at spinal joints	The Transversospinalis group, Psoas, and the External abdominal obliques
Extensors of the trunk at spinal joints	The Erector spinae and Transversospinalis groups and Quadratus lumborum
Flexors of the arm at the shoulder	Anterior deltoid, Pectoralis major, Coracobrachialis, and Biceps brachii
Extensors of the arm at the shoulder	Posterior deltoid, Triceps brachii, Teres major and Latissimus dorsi

HERE'S A TIP

Keep in mind that those muscles listed above as active in the phases and stages of gait are agonists, and are concentrically contracting. Skeletal movement also requires the action of antagonists that eccentrically contract. Concentric contraction of muscles that dorsiflex the foot, for example, is allowed and also limited by the eccentric contraction of muscles that plantarflex the foot. When assessing gait, pay close attention to *all* the muscles and muscle groups involved in an action.

The entire body, not just the legs and feet, participates in gait:

- The pelvis and the shoulders may unilaterally elevate to a greater or lesser degree.
- The arms may abduct and adduct, in addition to flexing and extending, during arm swing.
- The head may tilt to adjust for changes in equilibrium, with each step.

Variations in Gait Patterns

The stance and swing phases of gait occur in every gait pattern, but they adjust to accommodate the pace and angle of gait when running or walking on an inclined surface.

Running gait

During running gait, shown in Figure 3–8, adjustments are made to accommodate the period of non-support, when both feet are off the ground, and the resulting impact on joints as one foot hits the ground and bears the full weight of the body:

- Postural muscles contract during non-support in order to maintain equilibrium, in the absence of ground support.
- Postural muscles also contract as one foot hits the ground, to accommodate the shifting of the full weight of the body onto that side.

Consider assessment of postural muscles as well as phasic muscles in clients who run regularly.

Lab Activity 3–2 on page 126 is designed to help you assess the swing phase of gait.

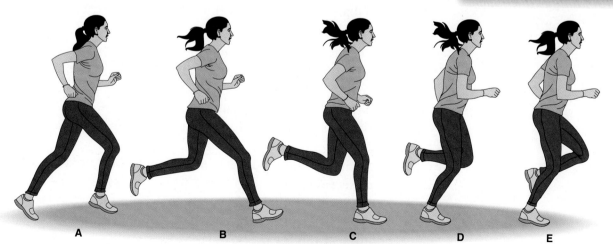

A   B   C   D   E

© Milady, a part of Cengage Learning.

FIGURE 3–8 Running gait contains periods of non-support, when neither foot is in contact with the ground, as seen in "B," and single support, when only one limb is in contact with the ground, as seen in the other images.

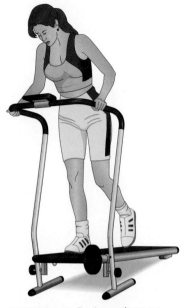

FIGURE 3-9 During gait on an uphill incline, the weight of the body shifts forward in order to maintain equilibrium.

© Milady, a part of Cengage Learning.

Inclined gait

When walking on an inclined surface rather than level ground, positional adjustments are made and the roles assumed by muscles active during gait change, to accommodate the shifting of body weight in order to maintain equilibrium:

- When walking on an uphill incline, shown in Figure 3–9, the weight of the body shifts forward. Posterior thigh and leg muscles may be strained during gait as they propel the body up the incline.
- When walking on a downhill incline, shown in Figure 3–10, the weight of the body shifts backward. Anterior thigh and leg muscles may be strained during gait as they keep the body from tumbling downhill.

Consider assessment of the appropriate postural muscles engaged in maintaining equilibrium on an incline in clients who hike or climb mountains—the abdominals, the lumbar erectors, the adductors, and the medial hamstrings.

Causes of Gait Dysfunctions

A gait dysfunction may be temporary, during recovery from toe surgery, for example, or permanent, such as following a stroke or other neurological event. Gait may be altered by an injury—a sprain, a break, an ingrown nail on the big toe, or by poorly fitting shoes—ones that are too short or too narrow, or with high heels that throw the weight of the body onto the toes during gait. Structural and functional postural deviations, muscle hypotonicity or hypertonicity, and some chronic health conditions can result in a range of gait dysfunctions.

Postural deviations

Assessment of your client's posture often yields clues that indicate assessment of specific components of her gait. Deviations in the curves of the spine, in the positions of the knees and ankles, and in the arches of the feet, will likely impact normal gait and create gait dysfunctions.

Scoliosis

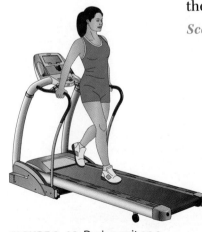

FIGURE 3-10 During gait on a downhill incline, the weight of the body shifts backward in order to maintain equilibrium.

© Milady, a part of Cengage Learning.

- The lateral and sometimes rotational curves in the thoracic and lumbar regions of the spine created by scoliosis, shown in Figure 2–34, often result in unilateral elevation of the pelvis and elevation of the opposite shoulder. These compensations may result in one functionally shorter leg and an unequal distribution of weight onto that leg.
- The gait of a client with scoliosis may or may not be affected to an observable degree, depending on the severity of the lateral and rotational curvatures and any accompanying conditions. The heel strike of a client with a functionally short leg, a common compensation for scoliosis, may be significantly harder on the long-leg side of her body, which may be reflected by the wear pattern on the shoe worn on that side.

Kyphosis

- The exaggerated thoracic curve of kyphosis, seen in Figure 2–36, may result in compensatory rounded shoulders, throwing the arms and hands toward the anterior and resulting in unequal distribution of the weight of the upper body toward the anterior. The posterior trunk muscles may be strained in the effort to counter this forward weight distribution. Because the arms are rounded to the anterior, arm swing during gait may intensify this strain.

- The gait of a client with kyphosis may or may not be visibly affected, depending on the severity of the kyphotic curve and any accompanying conditions.

Lordosis

- Lordosis may be a compensation for kyphosis, or it may be the result of poor posture habits or wearing shoes with high heels, as seen in Figure 3–5. The exaggerated lumbar curve of lordosis increases anterior tilt of the pelvis.

- The gait of a client with lordosis may be dysfunctional: the transition from heel strike (when the pelvis is tilted to the anterior) through foot flat to midstance (when the pelvis posteriorly tilts) may be stiff and incomplete.

IN THE TREATMENT ROOM

The force of heel strike varies. Some people contact the ground lightly, others strike with great force. The greater the force of the heel strike, the more its force is transmitted through the ankle and tibiofemoral joints to the acetabulofemoral joint and the pelvis.

- The shoes of people with an exceptionally hard heel strike wear out quickly and wear first at the heel, as shown in Figure 3–11. An uneven heel wear pattern on a client's shoes may indicate an unequal heel strike—possibly due to a leg-length discrepancy.

- To assess for uneven heel strike, check for pelvic symmetry or asymmetry, compensations for deviations in spinal curvatures, and hypertonicity in Quadratus Lumborum.

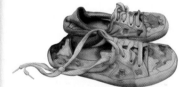

FIGURE 3–11 A forceful heel strike is revealed in the wear pattern of your client's shoes.

© Milady, a part of Cengage Learning.

Knock knees

- Because the knees may touch in a client with knock knees, shown in Figure 2–49, the ankles may also touch and the feet may be everted (pronated).

- The gait of a client with knock knees may be dysfunctional: she may swing her feet out during the swing phase of gait, to keep her ankles clear of each other, and may exaggerate her arm swing to maintain balance.

Bow legs

- The increased angle of the tibia in a client with bow legs, also seen in Figure 2–49, may invert (supinate) her feet, putting stress on the lateral longitudinal arches of her feet and distributing weight unequally onto the lateral foot.

- The gait of a client with bow legs may be dysfunctional: there may be a wider than normal distance between her feet in both stance and swing phases, resulting in a duck-like gait.

Hyperextended knees

- Hyperextension of the knees, seen in Figure 2–50, may result in a compensatory increase in anterior tilt of the pelvis.
- The gait of a client with hyperextended knees may be affected: the transition from heel strike, when the pelvis is tilted to the anterior, through foot flat to midstance, when the pelvis posteriorly tilts, may be stiff and incomplete, similar to the gait created by a lordotic spinal curve.

Deviations in the arches of the feet, shown in Figure 2–56:

- Excessive eversion of the arches of the feet, shown in Figure 2–53: during the push-off of the heel-off stage of stance, the weight of the body may be pushed onto the first and second toes, rather than across the foot. The gait of a client with excessive eversion may cause pain during push off. The unequal weight distribution may cause calluses and bunions to form.
- Excessive inversion of the arches of the feet, also shown in Figure 2–53: chronic inversion may place stress on the lateral longitudinal arches of the feet, distributing weight unequally onto the lateral foot. The gait of a client with excessive inversion may be dysfunctional: the inversion of the foot increases the risk for an inversion sprain of the ankle during normal gait on even a slightly inclined surface.

Bunion, claw toe, hammertoe

- A bunion, shown in Figure 2–54, alters the angle of the first toe, crowding the toe box of the shoe. A bunion may also become angled over or under the second toe, resulting in pain during gait that may alter weight distribution onto the unaffected foot.
- The toe extension required during the push-off of this stage of stance may be disrupted by a bunion, a claw toe, or a hammertoe, seen in Figure 2–55.

IN THE TREATMENT ROOM

The gait of a client who has had back surgery may be significantly affected. In a **laminectomy**, the laminae of adjoining vertebrae may be trimmed or removed, as seen in Figure 2–14, to relieve pressure on the spinal cord by enlarging the spinal canal. The vertebrae may also be surgically fused. Devices such as rods and screws may be inserted to provide stability in the lumbar spine when the vertebrae are severely degenerated. Such procedures may therefore strictly limit the flexibility of the spine, resulting in a stiff, rigid gait, little movement at the pelvis, postural compensation, and muscle strain patterns that affect gait, such as a flexed trunk, unequal weight distribution, and strain in the muscles that extend the trunk. Be alert to these ramifications to the gait of a client following surgery on the spine.

Muscle dysfunctions

Strained, hypertonic or weak, hypotonic muscles in either the trunk or the extremities may substantially affect gait.

Dysfunctions in muscles that act on the toes:

- Hypotonic or hypertonic Extensor digitorum longus, Extensor hallucis longus, or the intrinsic foot muscles may disrupt gait at push-off, during the heel-off stage of stance.

Dorsiflexor dysfunctions:

- Weak or hypotonic dorsiflexors: during heel strike, weak dorsiflexor muscles may fail to keep the foot from slapping the ground, a condition called **foot slap**. The body may compensate by flexing the thigh higher, so that instead of a heel strike, there is a toe strike. Weak dorsiflexors may also cause the toes to fail to clear the ground during the swing phase, called **foot drop**, as shown in Figure 3–12.
- Strained or hypertonic dorsiflexors: at the end of heel strike, strained or hypertonic dorsiflexors prevent a comfortable or efficient foot-flat stage, sending force toward the knee and restricting thigh extension.
- Unilateral dysfunction in the dorsiflexors results in an uneven gait.

Plantarflexion dysfunctions:

- Weak or hypotonic plantarflexors: when Gastrocnemius and Soleus are weak, the strong plantarflexion needed for push-off is weak, more noticeably when walking up an incline.
- Strained or hypertonic plantarflexors: when the plantarflexors are strained or hypertonic, heel strike is painful and weak. The inability to counter dorsiflexion may result in a toe strike or foot drop.
- Unilateral dysfunction in the plantarflexors results in an uneven gait.

Quadriceps dysfunctions:

- Weak or hypotonic Quadriceps (Quads): weak Quads can fail to extend the leg completely during the stance phase, requiring forward flexion of the trunk in compensation. This forward flexion, added to plantarflexion, can hyperextend the knee.

HERE'S A TIP

An elder client may be more prone to foot drop. Loss of muscle mass, balance problems, and the worsening of postural deviations over time all contribute to an increased risk of foot drop. Short leg syndrome, whether structural or functional, may also contribute to what may seem to be foot drop: the foot on the longer leg may simply encounter the floor too soon during gait, increasing the risk of tripping and falling.

Foot slap

occurs during the stance phase of gait, if weak dorsiflexor muscles fail to keep the foot from slapping the ground.

Foot drop

occurs during the swing phase of gait, if weak dorsiflexor muscles cause the toes to fail to clear the ground.

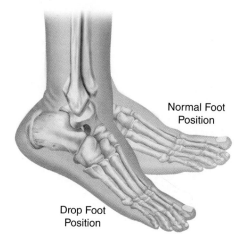

Normal Foot Position

Drop Foot Position

FIGURE 3–12 Weak, hypotonic dorsiflexors may allow the foot to drop during the swing phase of gait.

- Strained or hypertonic Quadriceps: tight Quads may restrict extension of the leg and the thigh, causing swing-phase disruptions.
- Unilateral dysfunction in the Quadriceps results in an uneven gait.

Hamstrings dysfunctions:

- Weak or hypotonic Hamstrings: weak Hamstrings can cause hyperextension of the knee during the stance phase and be unable to slow the forward extension of the leg during the swing phase.
- Strained or hypertonic Hamstrings: hypertonic Hamstrings resist full extension of the leg and the thigh, creating swing-phase disruptions.
- Unilateral dysfunction in the Hamstrings results in an uneven gait.

Dysfunctions in the Gluteals:

- Weak or hypotonic Gluteus maximus: a weak Gluteus maximus leaves the thigh in continuing extension during the stance phase. As the trunk shifts toward the posterior to compensate, gait takes on a forward to backward shifting that gives this gait its name: **rocking horse gait.**
- Strained or hypertonic Gluteus maximus: a hypertonic Gluteus maximus fails to allow complete extension of the thigh during the stance phase, shifting the trunk into flexion to compensate, and inhibits any lateral rotation of the thigh that may be needed to turn direction.
- Weak or hypotonic Gluteus medius: a weak Gluteus medius on one side of the hip causes the opposite hip to drop during the swing phase of gait, shifting the trunk toward the weakened Gluteus medius during the stance phase in compensation. This gait alteration is called **Trendelenbuerg** [TREN-duh-len-burg] **gait,** seen in Figure 3–13.

Rocking horse gait

a type of gait created when a weak Gluteus maximus keeps the thigh in persistent extension during the stance phase. As the trunk shifts toward the posterior to compensate, gait takes on a forward-to-backward shifting, like a rocking horse.

Trendelenberg gait

a type of gait created when a weak Gluteus medius on one hip causes the opposite hip to drop during the swing phase and shifts the trunk toward the weakened Gluteus medius during the stance phase.

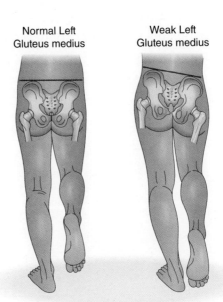

Normal Left
Gluteus medius

Weak Left
Gluteus medius

FIGURE 3-13 Trendelenburg gait, in which a weak Gluteus medius on one side of the hip causes the opposite hip to drop during the swing phase of gait.

- Strained or hypertonic Gluteus medius: a hypertonic Gluteus medius fails to allow complete extension of the thigh during the stance phase and inhibits any medial rotation of the thigh that may be needed to turn direction.
- Unilateral dysfunction in the Gluteals results in an uneven gait.

Dysfunctions in muscles that act on the pelvis:

- Hypotonicity or hypertonicity in muscles that tilt or elevate the pelvis a smooth transition between the heel-strike, foot-flat, and midstance stages of stance, creating a hobbled gait.

Dysfunctions in muscles that flex and extend the arm:

- Hypotonicity in arm flexors and extensors fails to produce the free and complete arm movements that maintain balance during the phases of gait.
- Hypertonicity in arm flexors and extensors does not allow adequate range of flexion or extension to maintain balance during the phases of gait.
- Unilateral dysfunction in arm flexors or extensors results in an uneven gait.

Pathologies affecting gait

Various pathological conditions may result in a dysfunctional gait, sometimes permanently. Treatment for some of these conditions is outside the scope of treatment for massage therapists. For these clients, we can help to:

- Maintain their optimal level of gait function by temporarily alleviating muscle and other soft tissue contractures that may contribute to the gait dysfunction.
- Contribute to their overall functioning and sense of well-being by providing therapeutic touch.

Pathological conditions that may result in dysfunctional gait because they affect the musculoskeletal system include:

- Fibromyalgia [fy-broh-my-ALG-a]: this syndrome is characterized by pain, fatigue, and stiffness in the connective tissue of the muscles, tendons, and ligaments. More common in women than men, it is associated with stress, poor sleep habits, and repetitive strain. People with fibromyalgia have tender points that occur in an identifiable pattern and may perceive pain or numbness that has no obvious cause and that does not respond within the usual expectations from touch. This client's tissues may be so painful and rigid that gait is slow and tortuous.
- **Myasthenia Gravis (MG)** [my-us-THEE-nee-uh GRAV-us]: MG is an autoimmune disease in which neurotransmitter receptor sites at the neuromuscular junction degenerate or are destroyed, interfering with muscle contraction and progressively weakening muscles. This client's gait may be significantly affected by the progressive muscle weakness.
- **Osteoarthritis (OA)** [ahs-tee-oh-arth-RY-tis]: this type of arthritis is characterized by degeneration of the articular cartilage

Myasthenia Gravis (my=muscle; asthenia=weakness)

an autoimmune disease in which neurotransmitter receptor sites at the neuromuscular junction degenerate or are destroyed, interfering with muscle contraction and progressively weakening muscles.

Osteoarthritis (osteo-bone; arthr-=joint; -itis=inflammation)

degeneration of the articular cartilage around synovial joints, due to age-related wear and tear on the joints.

around synovial joints, due to age-related wear and tear on the joints. The symptoms are usually unilateral and occur at the site of overuse. The gait of a client with osteoarthritis in her hips, knees, ankles, or feet may be stiff and painful. The muscles and other soft tissues may be strained by the degeneration of tissue at the joint. A client whose severe osteoarthritis has affected weight-bearing joints may have undergone joint replacement surgery, further impacting gait, at least during recovery and rehabilitation.

- **Osteoporosis**: the gait of a client with osteoporosis may be stiff and rigid. Tiny fractures in the vertebrae may result in severe kyphosis, altering gait. This client is at high risk for fractures. Her altered gait and vulnerability to falls may increase that risk.
- **Rheumatoid arthritis (RA)**: this type of arthritis is an autoimmune condition, characterized by the progressive destruction of synovial membranes. The symptoms are bilateral. The gait of a client with RA may be altered by disfigurement at weight-bearing joints and by the strain it places on muscles and other soft tissues.

Pathological conditions that may result in dysfunctional gait, such as those shown in Figure 3–14, because they affect nervous system function include:

- **Alzheimer's Disease** [AHLTS-hye-murs dih-ZEEZ]: Alzheimer's is one form of **dementia** [dih-MEN-chuh], a group of progressive, degenerative neurological disorders that affect memory and cognition, in which plaques—sticky deposits of a protein called beta amyloid—accumulate in the brain and result in the death of brain cells. Gait may be affected by the confusion and uncertainty that accompany Alzheimer's disease, along with the loss of balance

Alzheimer's disease (dementia=out of mind)

one form of dementia, a group of progressive, degenerative neurological disorders that affect memory and cognition, in which plaques, sticky deposits of a protein called beta amyloid, accumulate in the brain and result in the death of brain cells.

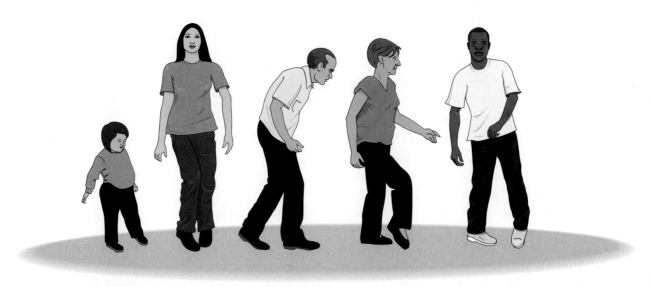

FIGURE 3–14 Altered gait patterns due to pathological conditions.

and muscle control that occur in its later stages. A client with Alzheimer's disease is also at greater risk of falling.

- **Amyotrophic Lateral Sclerosis (ALS)** [ay-mye-oh-TROH-fik LAT-ur-ul skluh-ROH-sus] is a neurological disease characterized by the degeneration of motor neurons and atrophy of voluntary muscles. The gait of a client with ALS may be slow and not well controlled and will progressively degenerate over time.

- **Dystonia** [dis-TOH-nee-uh] is a neurological disorder that seems to affect the ability of the brain to process certain neurotransmitters. The resulting bursts of stimulation to certain skeletal muscles cause involuntary movements, muscle strain, and contractures that disrupt gait.

- **Multiple Sclerosis (MS)** [MUL-tih-pul skluh-ROH-sus] is a neurological disease characterized by progressive destruction of the myelin sheaths that surround sensory and motor neurons in the central nervous system. Its symptoms include tremors, muscle spasticity, and loss of motor control. A client with MS is at risk for falls. As MS progresses, gait may become progressively weaker and balance more severely affected.

- **Parkinson's Disease:** the gait of a client with Parkinson's is usually shuffling, to a greater or lesser degree. Muscles are rigid and spastic. The stooped posture caused by Parkinson's disrupts balance, increasing the risk of falls.

- **Stroke** is also called a CVA, cerebrovascular accident. When a stroke occurs, an area of the brain is deprived of oxygen, either because a blood clot has blocked an artery—an ischemic stroke—or because there has been bleeding in the brain—a hemorrhagic stroke. Neurons die very quickly if deprived of oxygen. If the affected neurons are those that send motor impulses to skeletal muscles, movement and gait will be disrupted. The gait of a client who has had a stroke may be shuffling or stiff. Balance may be severely disrupted by unilateral loss of motor function, muscle atrophy or spasticity.

Amyotrophic Lateral Sclerosis (ALS) (myo=muscle; -trophy= atrophy or weakness; sclerosis=hardening)

a progressive neurological disease characterized by the degeneration of motor neurons and progressive atrophy of voluntary muscles. Also called Lou Gehrig's disease.

Dystonia (dys=loss of function; -tonia=tone)

a neurological disorder that affects the brain's ability to process certain neurotransmitters, initiating a series of events that disrupt gait.

Stroke

oxygen deprivation to an area of the brain caused by a blood clot blocking an artery, called an ischemic stroke, or by bleeding in an area of the brain, called a hemorrhagic stroke. Also called a CVA or cerebrovascular accident.

GAIT ASSESSMENT

The gait cycle described in the first part of this chapter presumes an unhurried cadence, on flat ground, with no dysfunctions that would alter normal gait. Not only is the use of the gate cycle concept essential to our understanding of normal gait, it is also a benchmark for deconstructing and understanding the causes of abnormal gait.

Gait Assessment Tools

As in posture assessment, the best tools for assessing gait are your interview and observation skills, your skilled touch, and your practice in comparing structures and movements of the body.

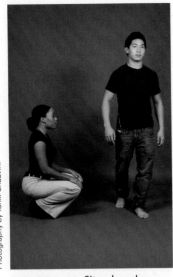

FIGURE 3–15 Sit or kneel so as to assess your client's gait at hip level.

Initial considerations in gait assessment

Take these steps to enhance assessment of your client's gait:

- Perform your assessments within the limits of your client's comfort. If walking is painful for her, interview your client to gain information about structures and movements involved in her dysfunction and perform non-demanding assessments, such as seated or reclining posture assessment and palpation.
- Assess your client's gait in the shoes she customarily wears and then without shoes, for comparison. If your client wears orthotic inserts in her shoes, assess her gait with her orthotic inserts in place and with her shoes and inserts removed, for comparison.
- Sit or kneel so that your eyes are at the level of your client's hips, as shown in Figure 3–15, to better gauge the angle and degree of movement in the core of the body during gait.
- Assess your client's gait from each side as she walks past you, and from in front of and behind, as she walks toward you and as she walks away from you, to see a complete picture of her gait.
- Perform each assessment more than once, to assure accuracy. So many variables may affect your client's gait. Only by assessing aspects of gait more than once can you be sure that the picture of her gait is an accurate one.

HERE'S A TIP

If your client is obese, heavily pregnant, or elderly, step width may be widened to accommodate the transfer of increased weight-bearing onto the lower extremities. Observing from infront of your client, assess the angle from the greater trochanter to the ankle on each leg: is the angle on each leg symmetrical? Does the angle allow maintenance of the torso in equilibrium during gait, or must the torso sway and shift body weight in order to maintain equilibrium? Does the distance between the feet during gait look natural to you, or is it affected by one of the conditions mentioned?

Use these tools, in addition to your observation skills:

- A tape measure, yard stick, or other means of measurement, such as marks placed in a wall every foot and yard.
- Vertical and horizontal reference lines in the room along the gait-assessment route.

In addition:

- Provide a space for gait assessment for your client that is sufficient in length for a minimum of six full strides and wide enough for an unhampered arm swing.
- Allow sufficient space for you to be able to measure your client's stride length and arm swing from each side.
- Observing gait with the main source of ambient lighting *behind* your visual field highlights the individual components of your assessment.

IN THE TREATMENT ROOM

Normal stride length, shown in Figure 3–1, is 2.2 feet (about 67 cm) for a woman and 2.5 feet (about 76 cm) for a man. To estimate normal stride length, multiply your female client's height in inches by .413 and divide the result by 12 to state the estimate in inches. For example, for a 5' 4" woman, multiply 64 by .413. Divide the result, 26.43, by 12 to get an estimated stride length of 2.2 feet. To estimate this same woman's stride length in metric measurement, multiply 162.5 cm by .413 to get an estimated stride length of 67 cm. To estimate the stride length of a male, as shown in Figure 3–16, use .415 as the multiplier.

In assessing stride length, it is the comparison of stride length for each leg that is significant. An unequal stride length is a signal that you should assess the muscles and other soft tissues on the short- stride side of the body.

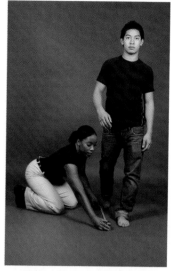

FIGURE 3-16 An unequal stride length signals assessment of the muscles and other soft tissues on the short stride side of the body.

© Milady, a part of Cengage Learning. Photography by Yanik Chauvin.

LEARNING ENHANCEMENT ACTIVITY

Use construction paper and talcum powder (talc), cornstarch, or massage oil to assess the degree of foot eversion or inversion during the foot-flat stage of the stance phase:

- Coat the plantar surfaces of your client's bare feet with talc, cornstarch, or massage oil.
- Place sheets of colored construction along a pathway for your client to walk on. Use dark paper if you are using talc or cornstarch and light-colored paper you if using oil, as shown in Figure 3–17.
- Making certain that the floor surface beneath the paper is not slippery, ask your client to stride naturally for a few steps onto the sheets of construction paper.
- Compare the footprint left on each sheet of paper: are the outlines of the soles of the feet equal? *Mark the papers "left" and "right" before picking them up.* Is the medial arch visible on either sheet of paper? The shape of the arch will help assess the degree of eversion or inversion and the comparison of the two feet can help you to notice any postural deviations.
- Be sure to remove any residue of powder or oil from your client's feet!

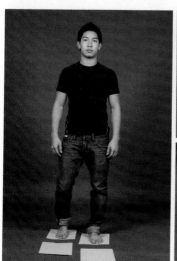
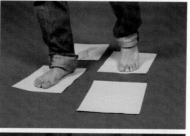
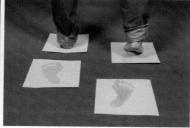

FIGURE 3-17 Assess the degree of foot eversion or inversion during the foot flat stage of the stance phase by visually recording your client's stride, using construction paper and talcum powder, cornstarch, or massage oil.

© Milady, a part of Cengage Learning. Photography by Yanik Chauvin.

Visual assessment

Sitting as far from your client as space allows, visually assess these aspects of her gait during the stance and swing phases as she walks toward you:

- Level of the head. Tilt of the head to one side during gait may indicate, among other things, compensation for a postural deviation in the spine.
- Level of the shoulders. An elevated shoulder affects both balance and arm swing during gait.
- The swing of each arm, relative to the other. Do both hands "clear" the body during arm swing? Chronic medial or lateral rotation of the shoulder turns the hand so that the thumb or little finger may brush against the body during arm swing.
- Level of the hips. Elevation of one hip affects both step width and stride length during gait.
- Distance between the knees. A wider distance may indicate Genu varum, a narrower distance may indicate Genu valgum.
- Distance between the ankles, step width. An exaggerated step width may indicate, among other things, compensation for a balance dysfunction.
- Eversion or inversion of the feet.

Sitting midway along the length of your client's assessment pathway, visually assess these aspects of her gait during the stance and swing phases as she passes in front of you from each side:

- The position of the head, relative to a vertical reference line.
- The position of the shoulders, relative to a vertical reference line.
- The swing of each arm, relative to the other. Does one arm swing farther to the anterior or posterior than the other? One cause of uneven arm swing may be excessive rotation of the spine during gait, in compensation for limited ROM of one thigh.
- The curvatures of the spine, relative to a vertical reference line.
- The tilt of the pelvis, relative to the position of the trunk. Pelvic tilt affects stride length during gait.
- The degree of thigh and knee flexion of each limb, relative to the other. Unequal thigh or leg flexion may indicate, among other causes, hypertonicity in thigh or leg extensors or hypotonicity in the thigh or leg flexors.
- The degree of dorsiflexion of each foot, relative to the floor, which may indicate weakness or hypotonicity in muscles that dorsiflex the leg.
- The degree of extension of the toes, relative to the floor. Chronic medial or lateral rotation of the thigh may alter the placement of the foot during the stance phase of gait, as observed in the direction in which the toes point.

Sitting as far from your client as space allows, visually assess these aspects of her gait during the stance and swing phases as she walks away from you, keeping in mind the potential causes of gait dysfunctions just described:

- Level of the head.
- Level of the shoulders.
- Level of the hips.
- Distance between the knees.
- Distance between the ankles.
- Eversion or inversion of the feet.

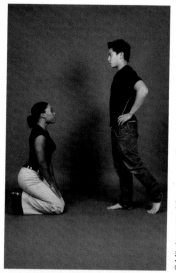

FIGURE 3–18 Walking with hands on hips reveals pelvic elevation and movement during gait.

© Milady a part of Cengage Learning. Photography by Yanik Chauvin.

IN THE TREATMENT ROOM

If your first visual assessment leads you to suspect unilateral elevation of your client's pelvis, ask him to walk toward you a second time, this time with his hands on his hips, which should better reveal unilateral elevation of the pelvis, as shown in Figure 3–18. Use a horizontal reference line to help you assess unilateral elevation of the pelvis.

HERE'S A TIP

You develop proficiency in gait assessment by doing it over and over again. There is no substitute for repetition. Try performing a gait assessment on a classmate whenever you can: before a class, after a class, during break-time. Assess the gait of your friends, your family, the people you work with. Repeat the mall-watching exercise recommended earlier in this chapter, this time focusing your attention on people's gait as they pass by. You learn something from each gait assessment you perform.

If your posture assessment revealed specific postural deviations, perform your gait assessment with your client's postural deviation in mind:

Scoliosis (Figure 2–35)

- Assess your client's gait by focusing on the elevation of the pelvis on the longer-leg side and unilateral elevation of the shoulder on either side.

Kyphosis (Figure 2–36)

- Assess your client's gait by focusing on the distribution of the weight of the upper body and the position of the trunk and the arms during gait.

Lordosis (Figure 2–36)

- Assess your client's gait by focusing on the ease of the transitions between the stages of the stance phase.

Knock knees and Bow legs (Figure 2–49)

- Assess your client's gait by focusing on the distance between her ankles during the swing phase of gait and the width of her arm-swing.

Hyperextended knees (Figure 2–50)

- Assess your client's gait by focusing on the ease of transition between the stages of the stance phase.

Deviations in the arches of the feet (Figure 2–56)

- Excessive eversion of the arches of the feet (flat feet): visually assess the degree of foot eversion, including examining shoes for wear patterns on the medial side, and look for the formation of calluses and bunions.
- Excessive inversion of the feet: visually assess the degree of foot inversion, examine her shoes for wear patterns on the lateral side, and compare the stability of her inverted ankles during the stance phase of gait.

Bunion, claw toe, and hammertoe (Figures 2–54 and 2–55)

- Examine your client's shoes for fit and for heel angle; ask her about the heel height of the shoes she wears daily, and if the heel height of her shoes is changed often (the persistent use of high heels causes significant functional postural deviations, described in the previous chapter, and resulting gait dysfunctions).
- Assess the level of circulation and sensation in your client's toes. Reduced sensation or circulation in the extremities may cause dysfunctions in movements of the toes.

Utilizing Gait-Assessment Findings

Record your gait-assessment findings regularly and consistently:

- Develop a standardized list of terms to be used for gait assessments on all clients and a list of assessments to be performed in each individual client that reflects both the initial findings and the treatment goals.
- Create a visual representation of your client's initial and subsequent gait assessments, as a record of treatment progress.
- Use the video function on your cell phone or computer to create a permanent record of your client's gait that reflects the progress of treatment of conditions that have affected gait. Create a series of videos, uploading or preserving each on your computer for storage and comparison, with your client's permission.

The recorded results of gait assessment are a roadmap for the next steps—palpation of your client's structures—and for creating a treatment plan. As you review the recorded findings from a gait assessment, answer these questions:

- What are the dysfunctions I noted in my client's gait?
- What is the role of postural deviations in any dysfunctions in my client's gait?
- Based on my assessment of my client's gait, what muscle, muscle groups, and other soft tissue structures are likely to be involved in any dysfunction that I found?

Lab Activity 3–3 on page 126 is designed to help you assess postural deviations that affect gait.

Lab Activity 3–4 on page 127 is designed to help you assess muscle dysfunctions that affect gait.

Whether or not the gait dysfunction appears to be related to a postural deviation, complete the following:

- Assess the effects on the other parts of the skeleton and on the muscles and fascial structures that attach to or may be overtaxed by compensating for the deviation.
- Identify the postural and phasic muscles that act on the deviating structures.
- Define further assessments, such as palpation, that will clarify patterns of compensation and strain and provide you with information to use in drafting a treatment plan.

Lab Activity 3–5 on page 127 is designed to help you utilize the results of gait assessment in treatment planning.

SUMMARY

Many clients seek therapeutic massage to treat the symptoms caused by dysfunctions or strains that occur during everyday movements, which may seem simple but which are, in fact, complex. Your understanding of the elements of posture and gait and how they both create and reflect dysfunction or strain is critical to the next assessment skill: taking apart complex movements to study the joint and muscle actions contained within them, described in Chapter 4, Deconstructing Complex Movements.

LAB ACTIVITIES

LAB ACTIVITY 3–1: ASSESSING THE STANCE PHASE OF GAIT

1. Working in a triad, one partner assesses and records her findings regarding the gait of another partner, while the third partner observes the assessment and records her findings regarding the gait being assessed and the assessment procedure. Follow the steps outlined above for visual assessment of the stance phase of gait, noting any asymmetry or discrepancies in these stages of the stance phase:
   - Heel strike
   - Foot flat
   - Midstance
   - Heel off
   - Toe off
2. Characterize any additional findings from this assessment of the stance phase.
3. Share and compare the findings recorded by the assessor and the observer. Switch places and repeat until each partner has participated in all three roles.

LAB ACTIVITY 3-2: ASSESSING THE SWING PHASE OF GAIT

1. Working in a triad, one partner assesses and records her findings regarding the gait of another partner, while the third partner observes the assessment and records her findings regarding the gait being assessed and the assessment procedure. Follow the steps outlined for visual assessment of the swing phase of gait, noting any asymmetry or discrepancies in these stages of the swing phase:
   - Acceleration
   - Midswing
   - Deceleration
2. Characterize any additional findings from this assessment of the swing phase.
3. Share and compare the findings recorded by the assessor and the observer. Switch places and repeat until each partner has participated in all three roles.

LAB ACTIVITY 3-3: ASSESSING POSTURAL DEVIATIONS THAT AFFECT GAIT

1. Working in a triad, one partner assesses and records her findings regarding the gait of another partner, while the third partner observes the assessment and records her findings regarding the gait being assessed and the assessment procedure. Follow the steps outlined above for visual assessment of the stance and swing phases of gait and the information presented about postural deviations, noting which, if any, of the following postural deviations may be involved in your partner's gait:
   - Scoliosis
   - Kyphosis
   - Lordosis
   - Knock knees
   - Bow legs
   - Hyperextended knees
   - Deviations in the arches of the feet
   - Bunion, claw toe, or hammertoe
2. Characterize any additional findings from this assessment of the causes of an altered gait.
3. Share and compare the findings recorded by the assessor and the observer. Switch places and repeat until each partner has participated in all three roles.

LAB ACTIVITY 3–4: ASSESSING MUSCLE DYSFUNCTIONS THAT AFFECT GAIT

1. Working in a triad, one partner assesses and records her findings regarding the gait of another partner, while the third partner observes the assessment and records her findings regarding the gait being assessed and the assessment procedure. Follow the steps outlined above for visual assessment of the stance and swing phases of gait and the information about muscle dysfunctions, noting which, if any, of the following muscle dysfunctions may be involved in your partner's gait:
   - Dysfunctions in muscles that act on the toes.
   - Dorsiflexor dysfunctions.
   - Plantarflexion dysfunctions.
   - Quadriceps dysfunctions.
   - Hamstrings dysfunctions.
   - Dysfunctions in the Gluteals.
   - Dysfunctions in muscles that act on the pelvis.
   - Dysfunctions in muscles that flex and extend the arm.
2. Characterize any additional findings from this assessment of the possible causes of an altered gait.
3. Share and compare the findings recorded by the assessor and the observer. Switch places and repeat until each partner has participated in all three roles.

LAB ACTIVITY 3–5: USING GAIT–ASSESSMENT RESULTS IN TREATMENT PLANNING

1. Working with a partner whose gait you assessed during one of the previous labs in this chapter, use your recorded assessment results to answer these questions:
   - What are the dysfunctions I noted in my partner's gait?
   - What is the role of postural deviations in any dysfunctions in my partner's gait?
   - Based on my assessment of my partner's gait, what muscle, muscle groups and other sift tissue structures are likely to be involved in any found dysfunction?
2. Using your recorded assessment results, your characterization of your partner's gait and the answers to the questions posed in #2:
   - Assess the effects on the other parts of the skeleton and on the muscles and fascial structures that attach to or may be overtaxed by compensating for the gait.
   - Identify the postural and phasic muscles act on the deviation in gait.
   - Define further assessments, such as palpation, that will clarify patterns of compensation and strain and provide you with information to use in drafting a treatment plan.
3. Switch partners and repeat the activity.

CASE PROFILES

Case Profile 1

Bethany, 31, is a flight attendant who works long shifts on intercontinental flights. She reports to you that she is experiencing pain and sometimes even numbness down the outside of both her thighs. What dysfunction of Bethany's gait may be resulting in this pain? What could be the cause of the dysfunction?

Case Profile 2

Joe, 38, just bought a new treadmill and has been walking five miles each day. Dissatisfied with the weight loss he's had in the past month, he has raised the angle of his treadmill to increase the difficulty of his workout. Now, Joe tells you he is having pain, stiffness, and some cramping in the muscles in the back of his legs and in his hips. What alteration of Joe's gait may be resulting in Joe's symptoms? What could be the cause of the alteration in gait?

Case Profile 3

Jeanette, 63, has osteoporosis. She tells you that sometimes her right foot catches on the ground while she's walking, and she's very afraid she might fall. What postural and/or gait assessments will you perform on Jeanette? What postural deviations and muscle dysfunctions may account for her walking problem?

STUDY QUESTIONS

1. How does arm swing or lack of arm swing impact gait?
2. During which stages of the stance phase of gait does the pelvis tilt (a) anteriorly and (b) posteriorly?
3. What muscle dysfunctions may disturb these actions of pelvic tilt?
4. Describe two pathological conditions that may impact gait.
5. Describe two postural deviations that may impact gait and what that gait might look like.
6. Describe the relationship between heel strike and short leg syndrome.
7. How might walking on a treadmill alter someone's gait?
8. Contrast the time spent in non-support during walking gait and running gait.
9. Describe the most effective way to assess unilateral hip elevation during gait.
10. Foot slap may be caused by weakness in what muscles?

Deconstructing Complex Movements

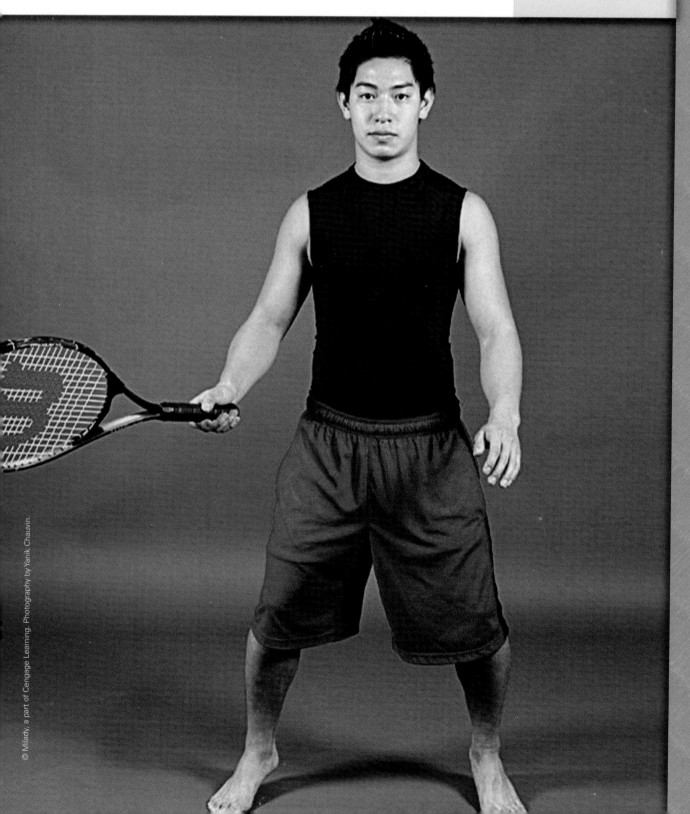

CHAPTER OUTLINE

- ■ MOVEMENT DECONSTRUCTION
- ■ DECONSTRUCTING A COMPLEX MOVEMENT
- ■ COMMON COMPLEX MOVEMENTS

LEARNING OBJECTIVES

- ■ Apply an understanding of joint and muscle actions, posture, and gait to the elements of complex movements.

- ■ Apply an understanding of joint and muscle actions, posture, and gait to the identification of dysfunctions that may cause or occur during complex movements.

- ■ Develop a systematic procedure for deconstructing complex movements.

INTRODUCTION

Complex movement is created by the interplay of posture and gait. Understanding complex movements is essential to identifying the causes of the strains and injuries that complex movements create in your clients. Deconstructing complex movements utilizes your understanding of joint and muscle actions, posture, and gait and applies it to the sequence of the individual actions that make up a complex movement. Once you grasp the elements of a complex action, you understand its potential for the dysfunction or strain that brought your client in for treatment. You are prepared to form an effective treatment plan that may include suggestions for altering complex movements intended to prevent reinjury and referring your client to an additional practitioner, such as a physical or occupational therapist.

Complex movement

movement that involves multiple joint and muscle actions in both the axial and appendicular skeleton.

MOVEMENT DECONSTRUCTION

Most movements of the body are complex in nature and in execution. For the purposes of this chapter, a **complex movement** is one that involves multiple joint and muscle actions in both the axial and appendicular skeleton.

Movement is highly individual and rarely symmetrical. No two people hit a golf ball or throw a football or climb a rock in exactly the same way. Factors that create the individuality of movement include strength and innate side dominance, deviations in posture, and dysfunctions in joints or muscles or in how they are used during gait. Even mood plays a role: whacking a tennis ball in anger doesn't much resemble a well-crafted, controlled slice of the ball. Each human body, however, is built of the same bones, joints, and muscles. At some point, everyone hitting a tennis ball abducts an arm, as shown in Figure 4–1.

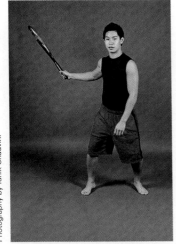

© Milady, a part of Cengage Learning.
Photography by Yanik Chauvin.

FIGURE 4–1 Opening the racket face to hit a forehand shot requires abduction of the arm at the shoulder, whatever the individual style.

Staging Complex Movements

Complex movements contain various actions by groups of muscles at multiple joints throughout the skeleton. It's easy to forget that rock climbing entails not only the joint and muscle actions on the thigh at the acetabulofemoral joint and the arm at the glenohumeral joint, but intricate movements of the fingers and toes, too. Assessing joint and muscle actions in any complex movement may be simplified by using a staging procedure. Most complex movements can be divided into three stages:

Initiation stage

The **initiation stage** begins when joints and muscles in the trunk and at the head and pelvis are being arranged to carry out the active stage of movement:

- Initiation includes the beginning posture from which action occurs.
- During this stage, postural muscles use both isotonic and isometric contractions to create and maintain the core posture from which an action will occur.
- The initiation stage, as shown in Figure 4–2, may last only a second or two. It may be intentional and smooth or it may be sudden, reactive, and jerky. Hypotonic or hypertonic postural muscles and preexisting postural deviations may result in strain or injury during initiation of movement.

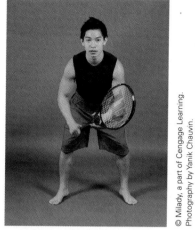

FIGURE 4–2 The initiation stage of a complex movement may be smooth or sudden.

Initiation stage

the first stage of a complex movement, when joints and muscles within the trunk and at the shoulder and hip are being arranged to carry out the active stages of movement. Initiation includes the beginning posture from which action occurs.

HERE'S A TIP

Extension is a typical joint action in the axial skeleton during the initiation stage of movement: the trunk is held erect by postural muscles at spinal joints to maintain equilibrium as action is initiated.

Action stage

the second stage of a complex movement, during which multiple joints and muscles in the axial and appendicular skeleton are engaged.

Action stage

During the **action stage**, multiple joints and muscles in the trunk and the extremities are engaged:

- The action stage includes the aspects of movement that occur immediately after initiation. The stage may be quick and intense, or it may be lengthy and sustained.
- The action stage may include a burst of power by phasic muscles that create the speed, strength, and endurance required for the movement.
- During the action stage, as shown in Figure 4–3, isotonic contractions create movements of the skeleton, while isometric contractions sustain weight bearing.
- Hypotonic or hypertonic phasic muscles may be unable to deliver the burst of activity or the sustained contraction required for the desired movement, resulting in strain or injury.

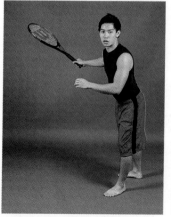

FIGURE 4–3 The action stage includes many joint and muscle actions throughout the body.

HERE'S A TIP

The full range of joint and muscle actions may occur during the action stage of movement.

Transition stage

the third stage of a complex movement, during which the movement is concluding or has ended.

HERE'S A TIP

Muscles may return the trunk to extension at the spinal joints during transition.

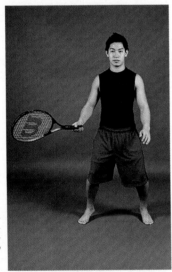

FIGURE 4-4 Following a burst of activity, moving into the transition stage may require phasic muscles to cease actions and postural muscles to maintain the return to static equilibrium.

Lab Activity 4-1 on page 154 is designed to help you identify the initiation, action, and transition stages of complex movement.

Transition stage

During the **transition stage**, the movement is concluding or has ended:

- In transition, the body may prepare to rest, to repeat the movement, or to create another movement.
- Phasic muscles enter a period of recovery, while postural muscles oversee the transition of posture from the active stage to either rest or the initiation stage of a repetition of movement, or to a subsequent movement, by adjusting the core of the body to reestablish equilibrium.
- Isometric contractions restore core posture.
- Hypotonic or hypertonic phasic muscles may spasm or cramp during the transition stage.
- The transition stage, as shown in Figure 4–4, may last only a second or two, depending on what posture or movement is to come next.

Not all complex movements are so simple that they can fit neatly into these stages—they're called complex for a reason! This staging system, however, can simplify complex movements by reducing them to identifiable elements.

DID YOU KNOW?

Complex movements may include a set sequence of actions or repetitions of actions. Washing a window includes spraying and wiping, again and again. When deconstructing a complex movement, make note of actions that are performed in a predictable sequence or that are repeated. The joint or muscle position from which an action is initiated may explain its injury, but sustained repetition of actions within a movement is in itself a cause of joint and muscle strain.

Describing Joint Actions

When describing assessments of posture and gait, and again for palpation of body structures, we began with the core of the body, not the extremities. For deconstructing complex movements, we also begin with the core by identifying the actions at spinal joints. Remember that when describing joint actions, we're referring to movement, not to posture. The following steps will help you to clarify the joint actions contained in a complex movement:

1. Designate a starting point for the movement. The starting point may be easy to select, such as the stance adopted before hitting a softball, or it may be arbitrary—for example, at what point does the ordinary cadence of walking become that of race walking? Designate the starting point that makes sense to you, then place the joint actions in the sequence in which they occur. Some actions, of course, are simultaneous—again, your decision may have to be arbitrary.

2. Describe the actions at the spinal joints first. Although they may not always be visible, most complex movements begin with actions in the trunk, however small. In Figure 4–5, for example, a tennis player rotates his spine slightly before moving to strike the ball.

3. Describe the actions at the head and the pelvis. What actions here are likely to maintain equilibrium?

4. Describe the actions at the proximal joints next: the joints of the pelvis, each hip and each shoulder, and each knee and each elbow.

5. Describe the actions at distal joints: each wrist and ankle, actions within each hand and its fingers, and each foot and its toes.

6. Describe the joint actions that are necessary to prepare to repeat the movement.

Table 4–1 reviews joint actions:

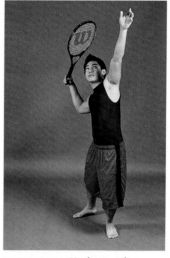

FIGURE 4–5 Understanding the actions at spinal joints is key to deconstructing a complex movement.

© Milady, a part of Cengage Learning. Photography by Yanik Chauvin.

TABLE 4–1

JOINT NAME	ACTIONS
Temporomandibular (TMJ): the jaw.	Depression and elevation, protraction and retraction, lateral deviation of the jaw
Atlanto-occipital: the joint between the occiput and C1.	Flexion and extension, slight lateral rotation
Atlanto-axial: the joint between C1 and C2.	Rotation
Intervertebral: the joints between vertebrae.	Flexion and extension, lateral flexion, rotation
Vertebrocostal: the joints between the vertebrae and the ribs.	Slight gliding
Sternoclavicular: the joint between the scapula and the medial clavicle.	Slight gliding
Acromioclavicular: the joint between the sternum and the lateral clavicle.	Slight gliding
Glenohumeral: the shoulder joint.	Flexion and extension, abduction and adduction, medial and lateral rotation, circumduction
Humeroulnar: the elbow joint.	Flexion and extension
Radioulnar: the joints between the radius and the ulna.	Rotation (pronation and supination)
Radiocarpal: the wrist joint.	Flexion and extension, abduction and adduction
Intercarpal: the joints between the carpal bones.	Gliding; flexion and abduction between the rows of carpals
Carpometacarpal: the joints between the wrist and the hand.	Gliding; flexion and extension, abduction and adduction, and circumduction at the thumb
Metacarpophalangeal (MCP): the joints between the hand and the fingers.	Flexion and extension, abduction and adduction, circumduction
Interphalangeal (IP): the joints of the fingers.	Flexion and extension
Sacroiliac: the joint between the sacrum and the pelvis.	Slight gliding
Pubic symphysis: the joint between the pubic bones.	Slight; more during pregnancy and childbirth
Acetabulofemoral: the hip joint.	Flexion and extension, abduction and adduction, medial and lateral rotation, circumduction
Tibiofemoral: the knee joint.	Flexion and extension
Talocrural: the joint between the tibia and the talus of the tarsals.	Dorsiflexion and plantarflexion
Intertarsal: the joints between the tarsal bones.	Inversion and eversion of the foot
Tarsometatarsal: the joints between the tarsal bones and the foot.	Slight gliding
Metatarsophalangeal (MTP): the joints between the foot and the toes.	Flexion and extension, abduction and adduction, circumduction
Interphalangeal: the joints of the toes.	Flexion and extension

© Milady, a part of Cengage Learning.

Lab Activity 4–2 on page 155 is designed to help you identify joint actions within complex movements.

Individual joint actions aren't always easy to discern during a complex movement. When lifting your arm to wave to a friend, for example, at what point does flexion of the arm at the shoulder become abduction? In deconstructing a movement, one way to answer this question is to palpate the large, superficial muscles acting at the joint during the actions. Palpation of the Deltoid will demonstrate that its anterior fibers flex the arm at the shoulder, while only the middle fibers abduct it.

Describing Muscle Actions

Once you have identified the joint actions contained in a complex movement, focus your attention on the types of muscles involved and the specific muscles and their roles as agonists or antagonists when acting on those joints to produce the movement. Let's review some terms describing muscle types, muscle roles, and muscle contractions:

- Phasic muscles are movers: they are used for quick, powerful movement of the skeleton. The tennis player in Figure 4–3 is moving quickly and generating power in phasic muscle to strike the ball.
- Postural muscles stabilize and support the posture of the body. The tennis player in Figure 4–2 uses postural muscles to maintain his stance while awaiting a serve from his partner.

Table 4–2 lists major phasic and postural muscles:

- The agonist in an action is the prime mover, or the muscle that is *concentrically contracting*, shortening the length of the muscle. The agonist is usually the largest, most superficial muscle crossing the joint in motion. The agonist in abduction of our tennis player's the arm, shown in Figure 4–1 is middle Deltoid.
- The antagonist in an action is the muscle whose placement and fiber direction in relation to the agonist in the action require it

TABLE 4–2

MAJOR POSTURAL MUSCLES	MAJOR PHASIC MUSCLES
Sternocleidomastoid (SCM)	The Scalene group
Trapezius (upper fibers)	Lower fibers of Pectoralis major
Levator scapulae	Trapezius (middle, lower fibers)
Upper pectoralis major, Pectoralis minor	Rhomboids
Latissimus dorsi	Serratus anterior
Lumbar erector spinae and Transversospinalis groups	Rectus abdominis
Quadratus lumborum	Deltoid
Psoas and Iliacus	Forearm flexors and extensors
Abdominal Obliques	The Gluteals: Gluteus maximus, medius, and minimus
Piriformis	Hamstrings
Adductor longus and magnus	Vastus lateralis, medialis, and intermedius
Tensor fasciae latae (TFL)	The Peroneal group: Peroneus longus, brevis, and tertius
Medial hamstrings	
Gastrocnemius and Soleus	
Tibialis posterior	

to *eccentrically contract*, lengthening the muscle, in order for the action to occur. As it lengthens, the antagonist muscle both allows and limits the action of the agonist muscle in a particular movement. The antagonist is usually the largest, most superficial muscle that crosses the opposite aspect of the same joint as the agonist. In the abduction of the arm at the shoulder shown in Figure 4–1, Latissimus dorsi is likely the antagonist.

- The agonist and antagonist are said to "oppose" each other in an action: concentric contraction of the agonist muscle is opposed by eccentric contraction of the antagonist muscle.

- A synergist muscle is one that is adjacent to and assists the agonist or antagonist in an action, while other nearby muscles may act as stabilizers, fixing proximal joints in place so that distal limbs can bear weight more effectively. A synergist muscle assisting in the tennis player's arm abduction shown in Figure 4–1 may be Supraspinatus, a smaller abductor of the arm, while the rotator cuff muscles stabilize the head of the humerus during abduction of the arm.

HERE'S A TIP

Review the information in Chapter 3, Gait Assessment, and apply it to deconstructing complex movements, many of which include a measure of gait. Pay attention to the transfer of weight from one limb to the other during complex movements, because this is a common point for dysfunction or injury to occur. The tennis player shown in Figure 4–2 keeps his body weight equally distributed and to the anterior on each foot as he awaits the ball, then quickly transfers his body weight onto his left limb to strike the ball, as in Figure 4–3.

Lab Activity 4–3 on page 156 is designed to help you identify the actions of agonist and antagonist muscles within complex movements.

Once you have identified the joints and their actions in the stages of a complex movement, use your knowledge of muscle actions to identify the agonists, antagonists, and possible synergists that are acting on the joints.

Identifying Dysfunctions

Structural or functional postural deviations may alter how a complex movement is performed and result in strain and dysfunction, while functional postural deviations, strain and dysfunction may also result from habitually poor postures when performing a complex movement.

Use the information in Chapter 2, Posture Assessment, and Chapter 3, Gait Assessment, to identify postural deviations or alterations in gait that may either cause or result from strain or dysfunction, when deconstructing a complex movement. Focus on deviations at the spine, at the head, at the pelvis, and at the shoulder and the hip. In Figure 4–6, for example, a tennis player with an elevated shoulder caused by scoliosis must create postural compensations in order to strike the ball and maintain equilibrium.

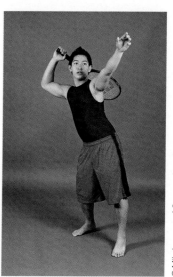

FIGURE 4–6 Postural deviations may significantly alter how a complex movement is performed.

Lab Activity 4–4 on page 157 is designed to help you identify potential posture and gait dysfunctions within complex movements.

Next, use the identified possible strains and dysfunctions to select target structures for assessment and palpation. Does your partner's movement, for example, suggest a functional short leg? What muscles may be involved in an apparent functional short leg syndrome or a compensatory elevated shoulder? How will you palpate these muscles?

DECONSTRUCTING A COMPLEX MOVEMENT

The best way to deconstruct a complex movement is to experience it yourself. To understand how your client uses his body to swing a golf club, swing one yourself or just imagine that you're swinging one. You may assume that you know how to throw a football because you've seen it done, but you cannot deconstruct throwing a football until your body has experienced it. Your body can most fully recreate and deconstruct what it has experienced. However, you may love golf or football but have zero desire to climb a rock, so even imagining rock climbing wouldn't work for you—and that's fine. Another effective approach is to research the elements of a complex movement that is new to you—for example, playing the piano, throwing a football, or practicing Tai-chi or Pilates. Use the Internet as a resource. Consult with an experienced massage therapist or other practitioner. Follow a football player, a pianist, or a Pilates instructor as he practices. Acquiring knowledge about the elements of movements that are unfamiliar to you enriches your assessment skills. You can also observe the actions of your rock-climbing client by asking him to recreate them for you as part of your assessment. Store this knowledge in your bank of understanding of complex movements. It's a less in-depth method for deconstructing a movement than doing it yourself, but perhaps a safer one for you!

HERE'S A TIP

Complex movements often include holding, lifting, throwing, or releasing an object, all of which have an impact on a joint at some point during the movement. Be aware that performing a given movement without the actual object fails to re-create the true experience. Mimicking throwing a football without the weight of the ball or the release of that weight or skateboarding without the impact of hitting the board after getting some airtime do not reflect the true effect on the joint of the full re-creation of the action.

Let's deconstruct a complex movement that you perform during just about every massage: effleurage. As you know, effleurage can be applied nearly anywhere on your client's body. Effleurage can be done with the forearms; with the full, flat hand or with a soft fist; or with the backs of the fingers, the thumbs, or the fingertips. Effleurage can be applied with deep pressure or it can be feather light. When effleurage is done well, it is a complex movement that uses all of your body and includes movement across a certain defined area.

Performing Effleurage

The effleurage deconstructed here is applied to a prone client's undraped lower extremity, using the moderate pressure of the therapist's full hands. This is a description of how the therapist shown in Figure 4–7 is performing effleurage. It is not the only way to perform effleurage, it is simply how she performs it.

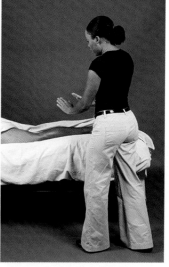

FIGURE 4-7 A massage therapist prepares to perform full hand effleurage on a prone client's lower extremity.

> ### DID YOU KNOW?
>
> Deconstructing a complex movement is not about correcting how a movement is done. It is about describing and understanding how it has been or can be performed.

Initiation stage

During the short initiation stage, the massage therapist is assuming the posture from which she will perform effleurage over her client's lower extremity. Figure 4–8 illustrates the initiation stage of the complex movement of effleurage.

We will begin by looking at the joint actions and major agonist and antagonists muscles, postural and phasic, acting during initiation.

At the trunk:

- **Joint actions at the spinal joints:** slight flexion of the lumbar spine.
- **Muscles acting on the trunk:** Rectus abdominis, the abdominal Obliques, and Psoas are agonists in flexion of the trunk at the spinal joints. The lumbar region of the Erector spinae muscle group and Quadratus lumborum are antagonists in flexion of the trunk at the spinal joints in the lumbar region.
- **Joint actions at cervical spinal joints:** extension or slight hyperextension of the head at the spinal joints.
- **Muscles acting on the head:** the upper fibers of Trapezius, Splenius capitis and cervicis, and the cervical region of the Erector spinae muscle group are agonists in extension of the head and neck at the spinal joints. SCM and the anterior and middle Scalenes are antagonists in extension of the head and neck at the spinal joints.
- **Joint actions at the lumbosacral joint:** slight anterior tilt of the pelvis.
- **Muscles acting on the pelvis:** the lumbar region of the Erector spinae muscle group, Quadratus lumborum, Latissimus dorsi, and Psoas are agonists in anterior tilt of the pelvis at the lumbosacral joint. Rectus abdominis, the Abdominal obliques, and the Hamstrings are antagonists in anterior tilt of the pelvis at the lumbosacral joint.

At the proximal joints:

- **Joint actions at each acetabulofemoral joint:** the left thigh is slightly flexed. The right thigh is extended.

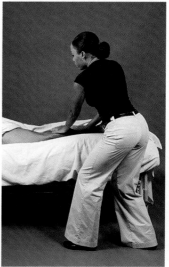

FIGURE 4-8 The initiation stage of effleurage. The massage therapist's spine is slightly flexed, while her head is slightly extended.

- **Muscles acting on each thigh:** Psoas, TFL, Rectus femoris, Gracilis, and Gluteus medius are agonists in flexion of the thigh at the acetabulofemoral joint. Gluteus maximus, the Hamstrings, and Adductor magnus, are antagonists in flexion of the thigh at the acetabulofemoral joint.
- **Joint actions at each glenohumeral joint:** the left arm is slightly flexed. The right arm is in neutral.
- **Muscles acting on each arm:** Anterior deltoid, Pectoralis major, Coracobrachialis, and Biceps brachii are agonists in flexion of the arm at the glenohumeral joint. Posterior deltoid, Latissimus dorsi, and Triceps brachii are antagonists in flexion of the arm at the glenohumeral joint.
- **Joint actions at each tibiofemoral joint:** the left leg is slightly flexed. The right leg is in neutral.
- **Muscles acting on each leg:** Gastrocnemius, the Hamstrings, and Sartorius are agonists in flexion of the leg at the tibiofemoral joint. The Quadriceps group is an antagonist in flexion of the leg at the tibiofemoral joint.
- **Joint actions at each humeroulnar joint:** both forearms are flexed.
- **Muscles acting on each forearm:** Brachialis, Biceps brachii, Brachioradialis, and the Forearm flexor group are agonists in flexion of the forearm at the humeroulnar joint. Triceps brachii, Anconeus, and the Forearm extensor group are antagonists in flexion of the forearm at the humeroulnar joint.

At the distal joints:

- **Joint actions at each talocrural joint:** The right foot is slightly dorsiflexed. The left foot is in neutral.
- **Muscles acting on each foot:** Tibialis anterior and Extensor digitorum longus are agonists in dorsiflexion of the foot at the talocrural joint. Gastrocnemius, Soleus, and Peroneus longus and brevis and antagonists in dorsiflexion of the foot at the talocrural joint.
- **Joint actions at each radiocarpal joint:** the left hand is slightly abducted, or in radial deviation. The right hand is slightly adducted, or in ulnar deviation.
- **Muscles acting on each hand:** Flexor carpi radialis and Extensor carpi radialis longus are agonists in abduction of the hand and antagonists in adduction of the hand at the radiocarpal joint. Flexor carpi ulnaris and Extensor carpi ulnaris are agonists in adduction and antagonists in abduction of the hand at the radiocarpal joint.
- **Joint actions within the hands and feet:** the toes are in neutral. The fingers are slightly flexed at the carpometacarpal (CMC) and interphalangeal (IP) joints.
- **Muscles acting on the hands and feet:** Flexor digitorum superficialis and profundus are agonists in flexion of the fingers at the CMC and IP joints. Extensor digitorum is an antagonist in flexion of the fingers at the CMC and IP joints.

Action stage

During the action stage of effleurage, the massage therapist performs long, fluid effleurage strokes with both hands over her client's entire lower extremity, working from foot up toward the hip and from the hip back down to the foot. Rather than a sudden burst of activity calling for speed or strength, the complex movement of effleurage requires controlled, sustained actions at multiple joints throughout the body. Figures 4–9 and 4–10 illustrate the action stage of the complex movement of effleurage.

Look at the joint actions and major agonist and antagonists muscles, postural and phasic, that are engaged during the action stage:

At the trunk:

- **Joint actions at the spinal joints:** flexion of the lumbar spine and extension of the neck increase as effleurage is applied toward the trunk, *followed by* extension of the lumbar spine and return to neutral of the neck as the hands move back down toward the feet.

- **Muscles acting on the trunk:** Rectus abdominis, the Abdominal obliques, and Psoas are agonists in flexion of the trunk and antagonists in extension of the trunk at spinal joints. The lumbar region of the Erector spinae muscle group and Quadratus lumborum are agonists in extension of the trunk and antagonists in flexion of the trunk in the lumbar region at spinal joints.

- **Joint actions at cervical spinal joints:** extension of the head at the spinal joints moves into flexion as the massage therapists looks down at her moving hands.

- **Muscles acting on the head:** the upper fibers of Trapezius, Splenius capitis and cervicis, and the cervical region of the Erector spinae muscle group are agonists in extension of the head and neck and antagonists in flexion of the head and neck at spinal joints. SCM and the anterior and middle scalenes are agonists in flexion of the head and neck and antagonists in extension of the head and neck at spinal joints.

- **Joint actions at the lumbosacral joint:** slight anterior tilt of the pelvis as effleurage is applied toward the trunk, *followed by* slight posterior tilt of the pelvis as the hands move back down toward the feet.

- **Muscles acting on the pelvis:** the lumbar region of the Erector spinae muscle group, Quadratus lumborum, Latissimus dorsi, and Psoas are agonists in anterior tilt of the pelvis and antagonists in posterior tilt at the lumbosacral joint. Rectus abdominis, the Abdominal obliques, and the Hamstrings are agonists in posterior tilt of the pelvis and antagonists in anterior tilt at the lumbosacral joint.

At the proximal joints:

- **Joint actions at each acetabulofemoral joint:** the left thigh increasingly flexes and the right thigh increasingly hyperextends as effleurage is applied from the foot toward the hip. Weight is transferred onto the left thigh, leg and foot, *followed*

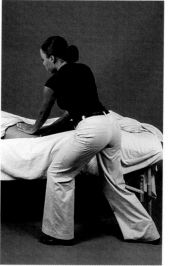

FIGURE 4–9 When performing effleurage toward the heart, the massage therapist's pressure is deeper and she supports less of her own weight.

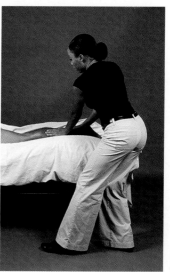

FIGURE 4–10 When stroking back down the leg toward the foot, the massage therapist's pressure is lighter and greater weight is borne by her body as the spine moves into extension.

by non-weight-bearing flexion of the left thigh and flexion of the right thigh. Weight is now transferred onto the right thigh, leg, and foot and the hands move back down toward the feet. As the stroke is completed, each thigh may flex, extend, and hyperextend more than once, as weight is transferred from limb to limb, walking along the side of the table to follow the stroke.

- **Muscles acting on each thigh:** Psoas, TFL, Rectus femoris, Gracilis, and Gluteus medius are agonists in flexion of the thigh and antagonists in extension of the thigh at the acetabulofemoral joint. Gluteus maximus, the Hamstrings, and Adductor magnus are agonists in extension of the thigh and antagonists in flexion of the thigh at the acetabulofemoral joint.

- **Joint actions at each glenohumeral joint:** each arm flexes as effleurage is applied from the foot toward the hip. The left arm laterally rotates and the right arm medially rotates as the hands round the hip. Each arm extends as the hands move back down toward the feet.

- **Muscles acting on each arm:** Anterior deltoid, Pectoralis major, Coracobrachialis, and Biceps brachii are agonists in flexion of the arm and antagonists in extension of the arm at the glenohumeral joint. Posterior deltoid, Latissimus dorsi, and Triceps brachii are agonists in extension of the arm and antagonists in flexion of the arm at the glenohumeral joint. Anterior deltoid, Latissimus dorsi, Teres major, and Subscapularis are agonists in medial rotation of the arm and antagonists in lateral rotation of the arm at the glenohumeral joint. Posterior deltoid, Infraspinatus, and Teres minor are agonists in lateral rotation of the arm and antagonists in medial rotation of the arm at the glenohumeral joint.

- **Joint actions at each tibiofemoral joint:** the left leg flexes and the right leg extends as effleurage is applied from the foot toward the hip. Each leg may flex and extend several times more as the stroke is completed.

- **Muscles acting on each leg:** Gastrocnemius, the Hamstrings, and Sartorius are agonists in flexion of the leg and antagonists in extension of the leg at the tibiofemoral joint. The Quadriceps group is an agonist in extension of the leg and antagonists in flexion of the leg at the tibiofemoral joint.

- **Joint actions at each humeroulnar joint:** both forearms extend as effleurage is applied from the foot toward the hip *followed by* flexion of both forearms as the hands move back down toward the foot. Each forearm may extend and flex several times more as the stroke is completed.

- **Muscles acting on each forearm:** Brachialis, Biceps brachii, Brachioradialis, and the Forearm flexor group are agonists in flexion of the forearm and antagonists in extension of the forearm at the humeroulnar joint. Triceps brachii, Anconeus, and the Forearm extensor group are agonists in extension of the forearm and antagonists in flexion of the forearm at the humeroulnar joint.

At the distal joints:

- **Joint actions at each talocrural joint:** the left foot dorsiflexes with weight-bearing as effleurage is applied from the foot toward the hip, then dorsiflexes without weight-bearing as weight is transferred onto the right limb during completion of the stroke back down toward the client's foot. The right foot plantarflexes with no weight-bearing as effleurage is applied from the client's foot toward the hip, then dorsiflexes with weight-bearing as weight is transferred onto the right limb during completion of the stroke back down toward the foot. Weight-bearing and non-weight-bearing dorsiflexion and non-weight-bearing plantarflexion may be repeated several times more as the stroke is completed.

- **Muscles acting on each foot:** Tibialis anterior and Extensor digitorum longus are agonists in dorsiflexion and antagonists in plantarflexion of the foot at the talocrural joint. Gastrocnemius, Soleus, and Peroneus longus and brevis are agonists in plantarflexion and antagonists in dorsiflexion of the foot at the talocrural joint.

- **Joint actions at each radiocarpal joint:** each hand flexes and extends, abducts, and adducts as effleurage is applied toward the hip from the foot, rounding the hip and stroking back down toward the hip.

- **Muscles acting on each hand:** the muscles of the Forearm flexor group are agonists in flexion and antagonists in extension of the hand at the radiocarpal joint. The muscles of the Forearm extensor group are agonists in extension and antagonists in flexion of the hand at the radiocarpal joint. Flexor carpi radialis and Extensor carpi radialis longus are agonists in abduction and antagonists in adduction of the hand at the radiocarpal joint. Flexor carpi ulnaris and Extensor carpi ulnaris are agonists in adduction and antagonists in abduction of the hand at the radiocarpal joint.

- **Joint actions within the hands and feet:** during full-hand effleurage with relaxed hands, there is slight flexion and extension of the fingers at the MCP and IP joints and abduction and adduction of the thumb at the CMC joint. During gait, there is slight flexion and extension of the toes at the MTP and IP joints.

- **Muscles acting on the hands and feet:** Flexor digitorum superficialis and profundus are agonists in flexion and antagonists in extension of the fingers at the MCP and IP joints. Extensor digitorum is an agonist in extension and an antagonist in flexion of the fingers at the MCP and IP joints. Abductor pollicis longus and brevis are agonists in abduction and antagonists in adduction of the thumb at the first CMC joint. Adductor pollicis is an agonist in adduction and an antagonist in abduction of the thumb at the first CMC joint. Flexor digitorum longus and brevis and Flexor hallucis longus are agonists in flexion and antagonists in extension of the toes at the MTP and IP joints. Extensor digitorum longus and brevis and Extensor hallucis longus are agonists in extension and antagonists in flexion of the toes at the MTP and IP joints.

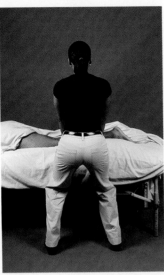

FIGURE 4-11 When the massage therapist turns to face the table, her weight is equally distributed and her head is extended.

Transition stage

During the transition stage of the complex movement of effleurage, our massage therapist has choices. She may continue performing effleurage on the lower extremity, using another hand position and perhaps deeper pressure, requiring postural adjustments by joints and muscles in the trunk. She may decide to turn her attention to her client's foot, working from the end of the table, standing or seated. Or, she may decide to perform petrissage on her client's lower extremity, requiring her to turn to face the table. Any of these subsequent complex movements require our therapist to transition away from the posture she used during the action phase of the complex movement of effleurage. In Figure 4–11, our therapist positions herself to perform petrissage by turning to face the table.

Look at the joint actions and major agonist and antagonists muscles, postural and phasic, acting during the transition stage.

At the trunk:

- **Joint actions at the spinal joints:** the spine moves into extension.
- **Muscles acting on the trunk:** the Erector spinae muscle group and Quadratus lumborum are agonists in extension of the trunk at the spinal joints. Rectus abdominis, the Abdominal obliques, and Psoas are antagonists in extension of the trunk at the spinal joints.
- **Joint actions at cervical spinal joints:** the head moves into extension.
- **Muscles acting on the head:** the upper fibers of Trapezius, Splenius capitis and cervicis, and the cervical region of the Erector spinae muscle group are agonists in extension of the head and neck at the spinal joints. SCM and the anterior and middle Scalenes are antagonists in extension of the head and neck at the spinal joints.
- **Joint actions at the lumbosacral joint:** the pelvis is in neutral.

At the proximal joints:

- **Joint actions at each acetabulofemoral joint:** the thighs move into extension.
- **Muscles acting on each thigh:** Gluteus maximus, the Hamstrings, and Adductor magnus are agonists in extension of the thigh at the acetabulofemoral joint. Psoas, TFL, Rectus femoris, Gracilis, and Gluteus medius are antagonists in extension of the thigh at the acetabulofemoral joint.
- **Joint actions at each glenohumeral joint:** the arms move into extension.
- **Muscles acting on each arm:** Posterior deltoid, Latissimus dorsi, and Triceps brachii are agonists in extension and antagonists in flexion of the arm at the glenohumeral joint. Anterior deltoid, Pectoralis major, Coracobrachialis, and Biceps brachii are agonists in flexion and antagonists in extension of the arm at the glenohumeral joint.
- **Joint actions at each tibiofemoral joint:** the legs move into extension.
- **Muscles acting on each leg:** the Quadriceps group is an agonist in extension of the leg at the tibiofemoral joint. Gastrocnemius,

the Hamstrings, and Sartorius are antagonists in extension of the leg at the tibiofemoral joint.

- **Joint actions at each humeroulnar joint:** the forearms move into extension.
- **Muscles acting on each forearm:** Triceps brachii, Anconeus, and the Forearm extensor group are agonists in extension of the forearm at the humeroulnar joint. Brachialis, Biceps brachii, Brachioradialis, and the Forearm flexor group are antagonists in extension of the forearm at the humeroulnar joint.

At the distal joints:

- **Joint actions at each talocrural joint:** the feet are in neutral.
- **Joint actions at each radiocarpal joint:** the hands move into extension.
- **Muscles acting on each hand:** the muscles of the Forearm extensor group are agonists in extension of the hand at the radiocarpal joint. The muscles of the Forearm flexor group are antagonists in extension of the hand at the radiocarpal joint.
- **Joint actions within the hands and feet:** the fingers and toes are in neutral.

Dysfunctions

- Structural or functional kyphosis and the resulting head-forward posture may cause strain in the muscles that extend the head and the spine at the spinal joints.
- Habitual slumping forward and dropping the head when performing effleurage may result in functional kyphosis and head-forward posture, straining those same muscles.
- Standing with the pelvis parallel to the table, rather than perpendicular to it, may result in twisting of the torso at the spinal joints while performing effleurage and subsequent strain in the muscles that rotate the trunk and act on the pelvis at the spinal joints.
- Recommended assessments include the curves of the spine, the position of the head and palpation of the muscles that extend the spine and head and those that rotate the trunk and act on the pelvis.

Deconstructing a complex movement may seem daunting at first. It becomes easier with each repetition. As you can see from the exercise of deconstructing effleurage:

- Knowledge of joint actions and the agonist and antagonist muscles that act at a specific joint is essential.
- Actions within a complex movement are often repeated and countered by an opposing action. Your same knowledge of the agonist and antagonist muscles in flexion of the arm at the shoulder is simply reapplied to the repetitions of an action or to its opposite action.

> **Lab Activity 4–5** on page 158 helps you to practice deconstructing a complex movement by applying the principles to a common massage technique you already know.

COMMON COMPLEX MOVEMENTS

The movements listed in this section are a small sample of the complex movements your clients will perform every day, any of which may result in strain or injury. Some of these movements are athletic, requiring skill and training, while others are routine, everyday movements that anyone can perform. To re-create most of these complex movements, the actual skill, setting, and equipment, although helpful, are unnecessary. The actions that make up the complex movement can still be performed in order to deconstruct it.

Choose one of the complex movements listed in this section to deconstruct. Include the following steps:

- Working with a partner, agree on how the movement will be portrayed. What elements will be included?
- Observe and assess your partner's complex movement, using the tools described in this chapter.
- Re-create the complex movement on your own, to experience the individual joint and muscle actions and to identify potential dysfunctions.
- Create a written record of your deconstruction of the complex movement to share with your classmates. Identify potential dysfunctions and outline postural and gait assessments and palpation target structures that you recommend.
- *This section contains one template for you to use in deconstructing the movement you select. Appendix D, Independent Study Activities, contains additional templates.*

Movement Deconstruction Template

Movement to be deconstructed: _____

Initiation stage

At the trunk:
- Joint actions at the spinal joints: _____
- Muscles acting on the trunk: _____
- Joint actions at cervical spinal joints: _____
- Muscles acting on the head: _____
- Joint actions at the lumbosacral joint: _____
- Muscles acting on the pelvis: _____

At the proximal joints:
- Joint actions at each acetabulofemoral joint: _____
- Muscles acting on each thigh: _____
- Joint actions at each glenohumeral joint: _____
- Muscles acting on each arm: _____
- Joint actions at each tibiofemoral joint: _____
- Muscles acting on each leg: _____
- Joint actions at each humeroulnar joint: _____
- Muscles acting on each forearm:_____

At the distal joints:
- Joint actions at each talocrural joint: _____
- Muscles acting on each foot: _____
- Joint actions at each radiocarpal joint: _____
- Muscles acting on each hand: _____

- Joint actions within the hands and feet: _____
- Muscles acting within the hands and feet: _____

Action stage

At the trunk:
- Joint actions at the spinal joints: _____
- Muscles acting on the trunk _____
- Joint actions at cervical spinal joints: _____
- Muscles acting on the head: _____
- Joint actions at the lumbosacral joint: _____
- Muscles acting on the pelvis: _____

At the proximal joints:
- Joint actions at each acetabulofemoral joint: _____
- Muscles acting on each thigh: _____
- Joint actions at each glenohumeral joint: _____
- Muscles acting on each arm: _____
- Joint actions at each tibiofemoral joint: _____
- Muscles acting on each leg: _____
- Joint actions at each humeroulnar joint: _____
- Muscles acting on each forearm: _____

At the distal joints:
- Joint actions at each talocrural joint: _____
- Muscles acting on each foot: _____
- Joint actions at each radiocarpal joint: _____
- Muscles acting on each hand: _____
- Joint actions within the hands and feet: _____
- Muscles acting within the hands and feet: _____

Transition stage

At the trunk:
- Joint actions at the spinal joints: _____
- Muscles acting on the trunk: _____
- Joint actions at cervical spinal joints: _____
- Muscles acting on the head: _____
- Joint actions at the lumbosacral joint: _____
- Muscles acting on the pelvis: _____

At the proximal joints:
- Joint actions at each acetabulofemoral joint: _____
- Muscles acting on each thigh: _____
- Joint actions at each glenohumeral joint: _____
- Muscles acting on each arm: _____
- Joint actions at each tibiofemoral joint: _____
- Muscles acting on each leg: _____
- Joint actions at each humeroulnar joint: _____
- Muscles acting on each forearm: _____

At the distal joints:
- Joint actions at each talocrural joint: _____
- Muscles acting on each foot: _____

- ■ Joint actions at each radiocarpal joint: _____
- ■ Muscles acting on each hand: _____
- ■ Joint actions within the hands and feet: _____
- ■ Muscles acting within the hands and feet: _____

What dysfunctions or patterns of strain were found? What additional assessments should be performed?

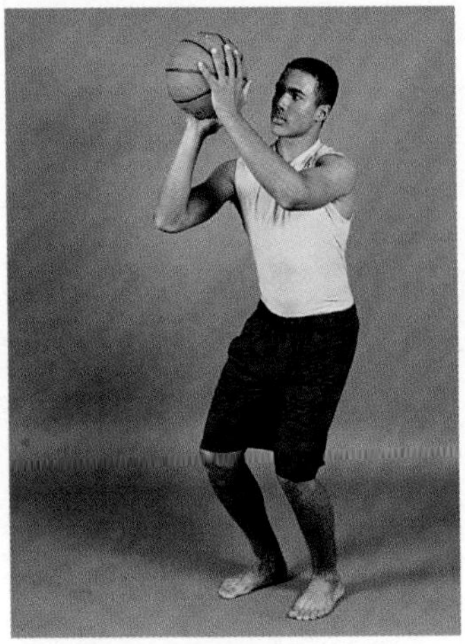

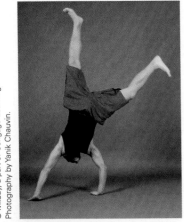

FIGURE 4–12 There is more than one way to hold the basketball for a free shot.

FIGURE 4–13 Keep the bowling ball's weight uppermost in your mind when deconstructing bowling.

FIGURE 4–14 Equilibrium takes a beating during a cartwheel!

Sample Movements for Deconstruction

Successfully deconstructing the variety of complex movements listed in this section will result in mastery of movement assessment and add significantly to your professional skills!

Basketball Free Shot

Decide how you'll hold the ball and whether or not you're taking a free shot before you begin the exercise of deconstruction. Figure 4–12, shows one way to perform a free shot.

Bowling

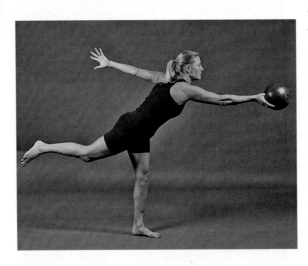

When deconstructing the complex movement of bowling, acknowledge that the weight of the bowling ball alters posture on the weight-bearing side of the body, while the release of the ball requires multiple adjustments in order to maintain equilibrium after the release. Figure 4–13 shows the action stage of the bowling movement.

HERE'S A TIP

If you're a novice bowler, be sure to get some guidance about the weight of the bowling ball that's right for you.

Cartwheel

The fully accomplished cartwheel demands a strong sense of equilibrium. Focus on the postural muscles that maintain equilibrium, even when the head is spinning. Figure 4–14 shows how a cartwheel is done.

HERE'S A TIP

Deconstructing a complex movement such as a cartwheel is easier if you can videotape someone doing a cartwheel and stop the action during replay, to focus on each element individually.

Cycling

To deconstruct the complex movement of cycling, you could include getting on or off a regular bicycle, riding a recumbent bicycle or a cycling machine in a health club, and trying out a tandem bicycle or even a unicycle. In Figure 4–15, our rider demonstrates riding a lightweight racing bike.

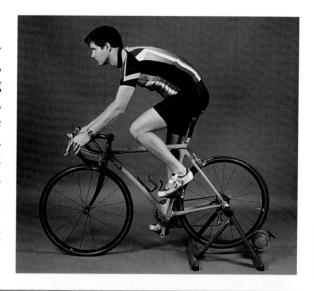

FIGURE 4–15 Riding a lightweight bicycle requires less thigh muscle strength than riding a heavier one.

HERE'S A TIP

Riding a bicycle that is the wrong size for your body causes strain and dysfunction. If you're borrowing a bike to deconstruct the complex movement of cycling, take its size into account.

Downhill Skiing

Skiing downhill can be done on a steep Alpine slope or on the bunny hill. No matter where you ski, turns are necessary for understanding the complex movement of skiing—include them in your deconstruction. In Figure 4–16, our skier models good downhill positioning: her body weight is forward, in front of her center of gravity.

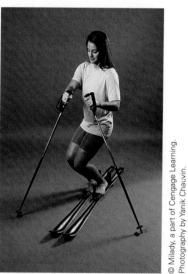

FIGURE 4–16 Advice from an avid skier: "Keep your arms and hands out in front at all times, to keep your weight forward. Don't ever get back on your heels!"

HERE'S A TIP

The actions incorporated in downhill skiing can be simulated on a downhill slope created on any surface—a treadmill or a steep driveway can stand in for a snow-covered slope in the mountains.

Getting On or Off a Massage Table

Climbing onto a massage table into the prone position is quite different from lying down on the table supine, as shown in Figure 4–17. Clients with restricted mobility may only be able to easily access the table from one

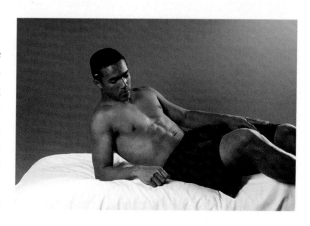

FIGURE 4–17 For some clients, getting onto the table into a supine rather than prone position is more difficult.

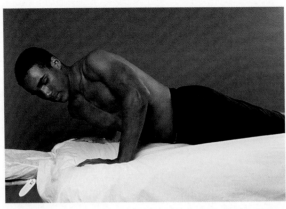

FIGURE 4-18 Deconstructing this complex movement demonstrates how getting off the table without instruction or aid may reinjure a client.

direction. Getting up from the massage table following an hour-long massage session, whether from a prone or supine position, as shown in Figure 4–18, can be a point of vulnerability and further injury for a client with postural or muscle strain dysfunctions. Deconstructing and understanding these particular complex movements adds to your ability to design a treatment session that addresses all the needs and vulnerabilities of your clients.

HERE'S A TIP

The height of the massage table can either ease or complicate the ease with which your client gets on and off it. Take the height of the particular massage table you are using into account in your deconstruction: you can choose to make the table too high, too low, or just right. You will learn something new from each configuration.

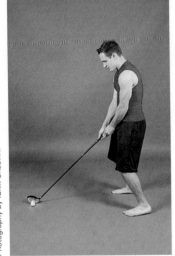

FIGURE 4-19 The initiation stage of a golf swing can create either a terrific or a horrible shot.

Golf Swing

The ability to competently deconstruct a golf swing may lead to a permanent position as a swing consultant to the PGA Tour! Even preparing for the golf swing, as shown in Figure 4–19, is a seemingly simple complex movement that requires multiple joint and muscle actions. Test your understanding of joint and muscle actions by deconstructing this "simply complex" movement. The complete golf swing is easy to divide into the stages of complex movement. Remember, however, that for a good swing, the follow-through is just as important as the stance.

HERE'S A TIP

Advice from an avid weekend golfer: "Keep your head down, your elbows in, and your knees loose. Or that's what I'm trying to do, anyway. . ."

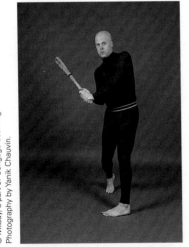

FIGURE 4-20 Trunk rotation is key in moving from the initiation stage to the action stage of batting.

Hitting a Softball

Do you hit from the left or from the right? Is the softball being thrown overhand or underhand? Are you trying to buy time for a runner or are you going for a home run? Deconstruct the at-bat of your dreams! In Figure 4–20, our model is considering his choices.

Making a Bed

This seemingly simple movement can be carried out any number of ways: the bed can be quite high, it can be a single mattress on the floor, or it can be a futon. It can have layers of heavy winter blankets or only a light summer sheet. The bed may have one light pillow or a virtual bevy of heavy ones. The person making the bed may be tall, short, strong, or frail. In Figure 4–21, our model makes a bed that sits low on the floor.

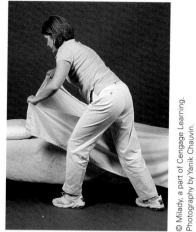

FIGURE 4–21 Making a bed that lies close to the floor may strain the muscles that extend the lumbar spine.

© Milady, a part of Cengage Learning. Photography by Yanik Chauvin.

> **HERE'S A TIP**
>
> Rather than just straightening the sheets and covers, you can opt to strip the bed and remake it from scratch—a complex series of complex movements!

Moving a Heavy Cabinet

A heavy cabinet may be pushed, pulled, or both. It may have doors or shelves that cannot be removed. It may have legs or sit flush with the floor, as shown in Figure 4–22. Decide beforehand what shape your cabinet is and what it will take to move it.

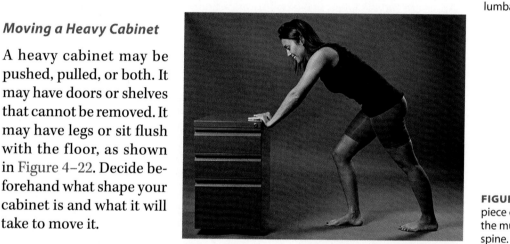

FIGURE 4–22 Pushing a heavy piece of furniture may also strain the muscles that extend the spine.

© Milady, a part of Cengage Learning. Photography by Yanik Chauvin.

> **HERE'S A TIP**
>
> Are you moving the cabinet on a wood floor, tile, or carpet? Are you moving it a few feet or into another room? These choices may considerably alter the complex movement and its potential for strain.

Painting a Wall

Painting an entire wall usually involves climbing a ladder, carrying a brush or roller, and reaching into high corners, as shown in Figure 4–23. Include all these actions when you deconstruct this complex movement.

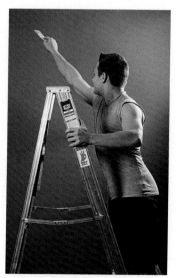

FIGURE 4–23 Painting a wall may require stooping, bending, and stretching of the lower body and repetitive reaching with the upper body.

© Milady, a part of Cengage Learning. Photography by Yanik Chauvin.

> **HERE'S A TIP**
>
> Repetitive actions, such as those demonstrated when painting a wall, carry a high risk for strain. While this movement may include fewer actions than some others, address the concept of repetitive strain in deconstructing it.

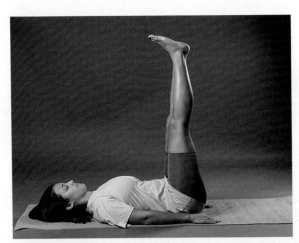

FIGURE 4–24 Pilates is designed to be beneficial for practitioners of all ages and mobility levels.

Performing Pilates

Pilates is a system of exercises to develop strength, flexibility, and balance by focusing on the core muscles of the back and the abdomen. Some Pilates exercises are done on a mat, as in Figure 4–24, or on the floor, while others involve the use of exercise equipment.

HERE'S A TIP

There are varying levels of Pilates for various populations, from elders with limited flexibility or range of motion to active, highly trained athletes. Deconstructing Pilates with a particular client in mind can help you to focus on the relevant movements.

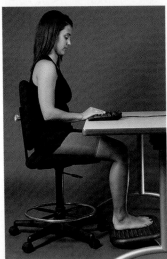
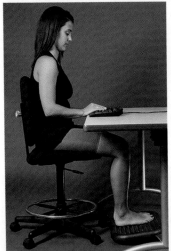

FIGURE 4–25 Sitting in an improper position or for long periods at a desktop computer or electronic music keyboard may create patterns of strain throughout the body.

Playing a Piano or Electronic Keyboard

The complex movement of playing a piano or electronic keyboard includes actions throughout the body, not just in the hands: some keyboards have pedals and other hand or foot controls. The model in Figure 4–25 is sitting in a chair, using a computer keyboard. If she were sitting on a backless piano bench, constant balancing of the trunk to maintain equilibrium would be required. Decide which scenario you will deconstruct.

Putting On a Jacket

There are so many ways to put on a jacket! A child, for example, may be taught to zip up his jacket, lay it front side down on the floor, and tunnel into it from a prone position. Some people slide into both sleeves at once, others one at a time. A person with limited arm strength may drape his jacket over the back of a straight chair, sit in the chair to slide his arms into its sleeves, then stand up again, bringing the jacket along. In Figure 4–26, the jacket wearer chooses her own style.

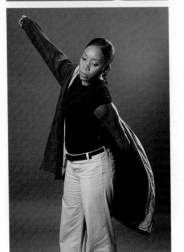

FIGURE 4–26 Most people slide their dominant-side arm in first when putting on a jacket.

Race Walking

Use the information in Chapter 2, Gait Assessment, to help you deconstruct race walking, which includes repetition of significant upper extremity as well as lower extremity actions, as shown in Figure 4–27.

Rock Climbing

Rock climbing has become an indoor activity, as shown in Figure 4–28, making it available to people who live far from mountain trails or cliffs. However, when done out in nature, rock climbers will probably be carrying backpacks and tools. Be sure to account for this factor in your deconstruction.

Rowing

To someone who has never rowed a boat or tried out a rowing machine, rowing may appear to be an upper-body activity. However, the complex movement of rowing involves the entire body—especially when rowing against a measure of resistance, which involves a great deal of action in the leg and core muscles. You may decide to deconstruct rowing of a small rowboat, the actions of a rower on a four-man scull, or those of a client at the rowing machine in her health club, as shown in Figure 4–29.

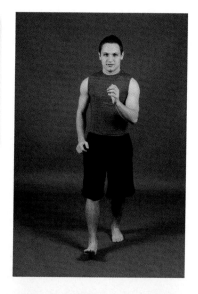

FIGURE 4–27 Remember: racewalking, like running, may include periods of non-support, when both feet are off the ground at the same time.

© Milady, a part of Cengage Learning. Photography by Yanik Chauvin.

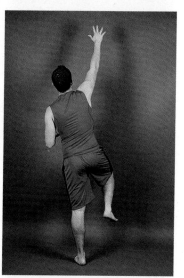

FIGURE 4–28 Rock climbing uses all your joints and muscles—and includes transferring all your weight from limb to limb.

© Milady, a part of Cengage Learning. Photography by Yanik Chauvin.

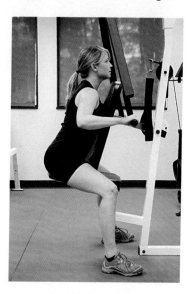

FIGURE 4–29 Rowing utilizes core muscles as well as those in the arms and forearms.

© Milady, a part of Cengage Learning. Photography by Yanik Chauvin.

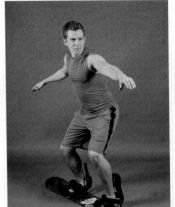

FIGURE 4–30 Snowboarders and skateboarders use their arms to create the lift they need to go airborne, and to maintain balance during direction changes.

Skateboarding or Snowboarding

Although the postures of skateboarders and snowboarders are similar, there is a big difference between being able to jump off the skateboard surface and being snapped onto a snowboard. Speed, agility, and balance, however, are required to stay upright on either board, as shown in Figure 4–30.

Swimming a Forward Crawl

If you try to recreate this complex movement anywhere but in a body of water, you will lack the factor of the resistance of water against your moving body. You can do a fair approximation, however, by "swimming" on a narrow bench or massage table (just remember to breathe . . .), as shown in Figure 4–31.

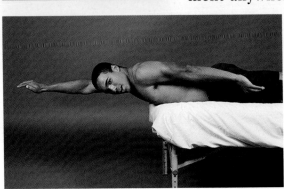

FIGURE 4–31 If you are simulating a forward crawl in the classroom, don't forget to turn your head to breathe.

Tai-chi

The slow, gentle movements of Tai-chi are superb for enhancing a massage therapist's tableside posture and body mechanics, as shown in Figure 4–32.

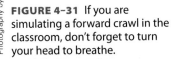
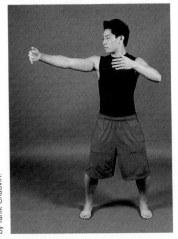

FIGURE 4–32 The slowness of Tai-chi movements contributes to building strength in core muscles and to maintaining balance.

HERE'S A TIP

Observing a Tai-chi class or renting a Tai-chi DVD from the library will help you to choose one movement to deconstruct from the series of complex movements contained within a Tai-chi session.

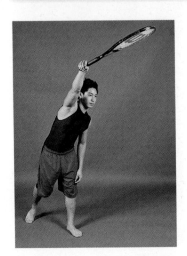

FIGURE 4–33 Advice from an avid tennis player: "Toss the ball to the left, rather than straight up: by the time you turn your body to hit it, the ball will be directly in front of you."

Tennis Serve

A tennis ball can be served overhead (as shown in Figure 4–33) or side-arm, or it can even be served by bouncing it off the ground before striking it. The overhead serve is an elegant complex movement, involving a multitude of individual actions. Most people hold the racket and hit the ball with their dominant hand, but some others choose toss the ball with their dominant hand, then switch their racket hand after the serve.

Throwing a Football

A football can be thrown forward or toward a corner of the field. It may be headed toward a receiver who is close by or far down the field. A football may be thrown when the thrower is planted securely in place, as shown in Figure 4–34, or on the run. Each throw has to be delivered at just the right angle and with just the right amount of speed and spin to find its target.

Tossing a Frisbee

As with the pass of a football, the Frisbee toss can be done from a still position or on the run, as shown in Figure 4–35. The receiver may be a six-foot tall friend or a six pound terrier who refuses to jump for it. Decide how and to whom your Frisbee is flying.

Unloading the Trunk of a Car

When deconstructing this complex movement, you can decide to unload 16 bags of groceries in plastic bags and carry them into the house, or you can unload one giant plasma TV box and set it on the ground. Either complex movement involves bending, lifting, turning, and transferring weight, as shown in Figure 4–36.

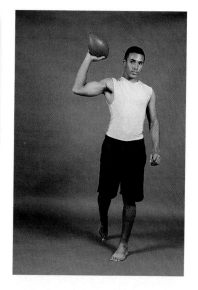

FIGURE 4–34 Postural muscles are especially important in "setting" the thrower's stance during the initiation stage.

© Milady, a part of Cengage Learning. Photography by Yanik Chauvin.

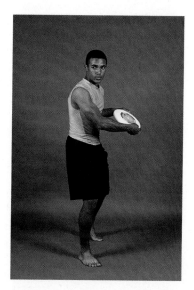

FIGURE 4–35 Tossing a Frisbee is a great example of abduction in the horizontal plane.

© Milady, a part of Cengage Learning. Photography by Yanik Chauvin.

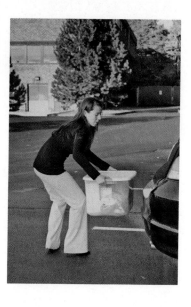

FIGURE 4–36 The height of car trunks varies, depending on the age of the vehicle: older models have lower, deeper trunks while newer cars are more likely to have hatchbacks with higher, shallower rear cargo areas.

© Milady, a part of Cengage Learning. Photography by Yanik Chauvin.

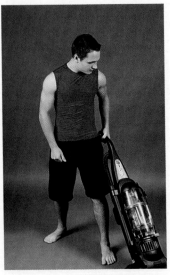

FIGURE 4–37 The muscles that extend the lumbar spine are vulnerable to strain when pulling a heavy vacuum cleaner back toward your body.

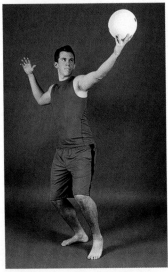

FIGURE 4–38 The transition phase of a volleyball serve may need to ready the body for a subsequent burst of speed.

Vacuuming

Many surfaces require cleaning with a vacuum cleaner: bare floors, carpets, stairs, window blinds, and your car's interior. Some vacuum cleaners have canisters and flexible hoses. Others are upright with shorter hoses, as shown in Figure 4–37. Pick your tool and your dirty surface to deconstruct vacuuming.

Volleyball Serve

Volleyball may be played on a sandy beach or in a wood-floored school gym. As with other complex movements that entail throwing a ball, the target recipient's location is variable, as is the desired speed and velocity of the serve. Preparation to serve is shown in Figure 4-38.

HERE'S A TIP

Keep in mind that the volleyball server in her school gym will no doubt be wearing athletic shoes, while the server on the beach may be barefoot on sand, potentially altering her movement.

SUMMARY

An understanding of the elements of posture and gait and knowledge of fundamental joint and muscle anatomy and physiology can be brought together to deconstruct complex movements. Deconstructing a complex movement into its specific actions, as done in this chapter, is valuable experience that prepares you to target and assess potential dysfunctions and guides you toward palpation of the structures involved, described next in Chapter 5, The Science of Palpation and in Chapter 6, The Art of Palpation.

LAB ACTIVITIES

LAB ACTIVITY 4–1: IDENTIFYING STAGES OF COMPLEX MOVEMENTS

1. Working with a partner, ask him to rise from his seated position in a chair. After reading the descriptions outlined above, identify the initiation, action, and transition stages of his movement:

    ■ Initiation: the initiation stage of rising from a chair may involve leaning the trunk forward, placing both hands on the seat of the chair, spreading the feet, and other actions that prepare the sitter to rise.

    ■ Action: the action stage includes the actions of all the joints and muscles that result in your partner moving his body from a sitting to a standing posture.

■ Transition: the transition stage includes what your partner does once he has fully risen from his chair. He may move his trunk, head and feet to create and maintain equilibrium while standing. He may decide to sit down again, and will perform actions that prepare his body for another initiation stage of movement. He may decide to walk away, requiring another type of initiation stage.

2. Ask your partner to repeat the movement as many times as are necessary for you to focus on identifying the initiation, action, and transition stages.

3. Switch partners and repeat. Compare your results with each other and with the class.

LAB ACTIVITY 4–2: IDENTIFYING JOINT ACTIONS WITHIN COMPLEX MOVEMENTS

1. Working with a partner, ask him to rise from his seated position in a chair. Following the staging procedure outlined above, describe the actions at each of the joints listed below. Ask your partner to repeat his action as many times as are necessary for you to focus on the actions at each joint individually:

Initiation: joint actions during the initiation stage may be minimal, but are significant to movement.

Joint actions in the trunk
■ Actions at the spinal joints: _____
■ Actions at the head _____
■ Actions at the pelvis _____

Joint actions at the proximal joints:
■ Actions at each acetabulofemoral joint _____
■ Actions at each glenohumeral joint _____
■ Actions at each knee _____
■ Actions at each elbow _____

Joint actions at the distal joints:
■ Actions at each ankle _____
■ Actions at each wrist _____
■ Actions within the hands and the feet _____

Action stage: joint actions during the action stage may be multiple in numbers, large in range of motion, and simultaneous.

Joint actions on the trunk:
■ Actions at the spinal joints _____
■ Actions at the head _____
■ Actions at the pelvis _____

Joint actions at the proximal joints:
■ Actions at each acetabulofemoral joint _____
■ Actions at each glenohumeral joint _____
■ Actions at each knee _____
■ Actions at each elbow _____

Joint actions at the distal joints:

- Actions at each ankle _____
- Actions at each wrist _____
- Actions within the hands and the feet _____

Transition stage: joint actions during the transition stage may be minimal once more, and are created to ready the body for the posture or movement that is to come.

Joint actions on the trunk:

- Actions at the spinal joints _____
- Actions at the head _____
- Actions at the pelvis _____

Joint actions at the proximal joints:

- Actions at each acetabulofemoral joint _____
- Actions at each glenohumeral joint _____
- Actions at each knee _____
- Actions at each elbow _____   _____

Joint actions at the distal joints:

- Actions at each ankle _____
- Actions at each wrist _____
- Actions within the hands and the feet _____

2. Switch partners and repeat. Compare your results with each other and with the class.

LAB ACTIVITY 4–3: IDENTIFYING MUSCLE ACTIONS WITHIN COMPLEX MOVEMENTS

1. Working with a partner, ask him to rise from his seated position in a chair. Following the staging procedure outlined above, describe the agonist and antagonist muscles in the action at each of the joints listed below. Ask your partner to repeat his action as many times as are necessary for you to focus on the muscle actions individually:

Initiation stage

Muscles acting on the trunk:

- Muscles acting on the spinal joints _____
- Muscles acting on the head _____
- Muscles acting on the pelvis _____

Muscles acting on proximal joints:

- Muscles acting on each acetabulofemoral joint _____
- Muscles acting on each glenohumeral joint _____
- Muscles acting on each knee _____
- Muscles acting on each elbow _____

Muscles acting on distal joints:

- Muscles acting on each ankle _____
- Muscles acting on each wrist _____
- Muscles acting on the hands and feet _____

Action stage

Muscles acting on the trunk:

- Muscles acting on the spinal joints _____
- Muscles acting on the head _____
- Muscles acting on the pelvis _____

Muscles acting on proximal joints:

- Muscles acting on each acetabulofemoral joint _____
- Muscles acting on each glenohumeral joint _____
- Muscles acting on each knee _____
- Muscles acting on each elbow _____

Muscles acting on distal joints:

- Muscles acting on each ankle _____
- Muscles acting on each wrist _____
- Muscles acting on the hands and feet _____

Transition stage

Muscles acting on the trunk:

- Muscles acting on the spinal joints _____
- Muscles acting on the head _____
- Muscles acting on the pelvis _____

Muscles acting on proximal joints:

- Muscles acting on each acetabulofemoral joint _____
- Muscles acting on each glenohumeral joint _____
- Muscles acting on each knee _____
- Muscles acting on each elbow _____

Muscles acting on distal joints:

- Muscles acting on each ankle _____
- Muscles acting on each wrist _____
- Muscles acting on the hands and feet _____

2. Identify muscles that may act as synergists in actions at the large, proximal joints.
3. Switch partners and repeat. Compare your results with each other and with the class.

LAB ACTIVITY 4–4: IDENTIFYING POSTURE AND GAIT DYSFUNCTIONS WITHIN COMPLEX MOVEMENTS

1. Working with a partner, ask him to rise from his seated position in a chair. Following the staging procedure outlined above and your understanding of posture deviations and gait from the information presented in Chapter 2, identify potential strains and dysfunctions that may either cause or result from the manner in which your partner rises from his chair. Ask your partner to repeat his action as many times as are necessary for you to focus on potential dysfunctions individually.

2. Switch partners and repeat. Compare your results with each other and with the class.

LAB ACTIVITY 4–5: DECONSTRUCTING A MASSAGE TECHNIQUE

1. Working with a partner, deconstruct the complex movement of petrissage or another massage technique, using the following template.

Initiation stage

At the trunk:

- ■ Joint actions at the spinal joints: _____
- ■ Muscles acting on the trunk: _____
- ■ Joint actions at cervical spinal joints: _____
- ■ Muscles acting on the head: _____
- ■ Joint actions at the lumbosacral joint: _____
- ■ Muscles acting on the pelvis: _____

At the proximal joints:

- ■ Joint actions at each acetabulofemoral joint: _____
- ■ Muscles acting on each thigh: _____
- ■ Joint actions at each glenohumeral joint: _____
- ■ Muscles acting on each arm: _____
- ■ Joint actions at each tibiofemoral joint: _____
- ■ Muscles acting on each leg: _____
- ■ Joint actions at each humeroulnar joint: _____
- ■ Muscles acting on each forearm: _____

At the distal joints:

- ■ Joint actions at each talocrural joint: _____
- ■ Muscles acting on each foot: _____
- ■ Joint actions at each radiocarpal joint: _____
- ■ Muscles acting on each hand: _____
- ■ Joint actions within the hands and feet: _____
- ■ Muscles acting within the hands and feet: _____

Action stage:

At the trunk:

- ■ Joint actions at the spinal joints: _____
- ■ Muscles acting on the trunk _____
- ■ Joint actions at cervical spinal joints: _____
- ■ Muscles acting on the head: _____
- ■ Joint actions at the lumbosacral joint: _____
- ■ Muscles acting on the pelvis: _____

At the proximal joints:

- ■ Joint actions at each acetabulofemoral joint: _____
- ■ Muscles acting on each thigh: _____
- ■ Joint actions at each glenohumeral joint: _____
- ■ Muscles acting on each arm: _____
- ■ Joint actions at each tibiofemoral joint: _____
- ■ Muscles acting on each leg: _____
- ■ Joint actions at each humeroulnar joint: _____
- ■ Muscles acting on each forearm: _____

At the distal joints:

- Joint actions at each talocrural joint: _____
- Muscles acting on each foot: _____
- Joint actions at each radiocarpal joint: _____
- Muscles acting on each hand: _____
- Joint actions within the hands and feet: _____
- Muscles acting within the hands and feet: _____

Transition stage:

At the trunk:

- Joint actions at the spinal joints: _____
- Muscles acting on the trunk _____
- Joint actions at cervical spinal joints: _____
- Muscles acting on the head: _____
- Joint actions at the lumbosacral joint: _____
- Muscles acting on the pelvis: _____

At the proximal joints:

- Joint actions at each acetabulofemoral joint: _____
- Muscles acting on each thigh: _____
- Joint actions at each glenohumeral joint: _____
- Muscles acting on each arm: _____
- Joint actions at each tibiofemoral joint: _____
- Muscles acting on each leg: _____
- Joint actions at each humeroulnar joint: _____
- Muscles acting on each forearm: _____

At the distal joints:

- Joint actions at each talocrural joint: _____
- Muscles acting on each foot: _____
- Joint actions at each radiocarpal joint: _____
- Muscles acting on each hand: _____
- Joint actions within the hands and feet: _____
- Muscles acting within the hands and feet: _____

What dysfunctions or patterns of strain were found? What additional assessments should be performed?

2. Switch partners and repeat. Compare your deconstructions and discuss any differences you find: are the differences in the deconstructions due to the individuality of movement or to the interpretations of the movement?

CASE PROFILES

Case Profile 1

CJ, 24, reports that he's had pain in his left lower back ever since he had to stow his heavy backpack in the overhead compartment of the plane on his trip home last week. During which stage of this complex movement might CJ have strained his left lower back? During which joint actions? Which agonist and antagonist muscles may have been involved? Could any postural deviations have contributed to his injury? What assessments and palpations do you plan to perform?

Case Profile 2

Sara, a 36-year old waitress, had to miss her last massage appointment to work an extra shift. She is tired and tense today. Sara takes most of the session to relax, but toward the end seems to deeply relax and may even be asleep when you leave the room. When Sara comes out of your treatment room, she's limping and rubbing her right hip and tells you she hurt herself getting up from the table. During which stage of this complex movement might Sara have strained her right hip? During which joint actions? Which agonist and antagonist muscles may have been involved? Could any postural deviations or gait patterns have contributed to her injury? What assessments and palpations do you plan to perform?

Case Profile 3

Jennifer, 39, is a busy single mom and massage therapist who has recently started working out at a health club. Jen has pain in her mid-back and posterior cervical muscles. How do you assess the potential causes of Jen's pain? What complex movements might you ask her to perform? What posture deviations or gait dysfunctions might you look for, and how will you assess them?

STUDY QUESTIONS

1. Contrast complex movement and simple movement: what makes a movement complex? Give an example of a simple movement and a complex movement.
2. Describe why turning the pages of this textbook may be considered a complex movement.
3. Describe how the initiation and transition stages of a complex movement may resemble one another.
4. How do you differentiate one joint action from another on a structure during a complex movement?
5. Why is it important to identify antagonist muscles in complex movements?
6. Describe the role of postural deviations in deconstructing complex movements: do they cause or do they result from performing complex movements?
7. Describe the role of gait in deconstructing complex movements: do alterations or disruptions in gait cause or result from performing complex movements?
8. How does re-creating a complex movement contribute to deconstructing it?
9. How does deconstructing a complex movement contribute to selecting target structures for palpation?
10. How does deconstructing a complex movement contribute to planning subsequent assessments and creating a treatment plan?

The Science of Palpation

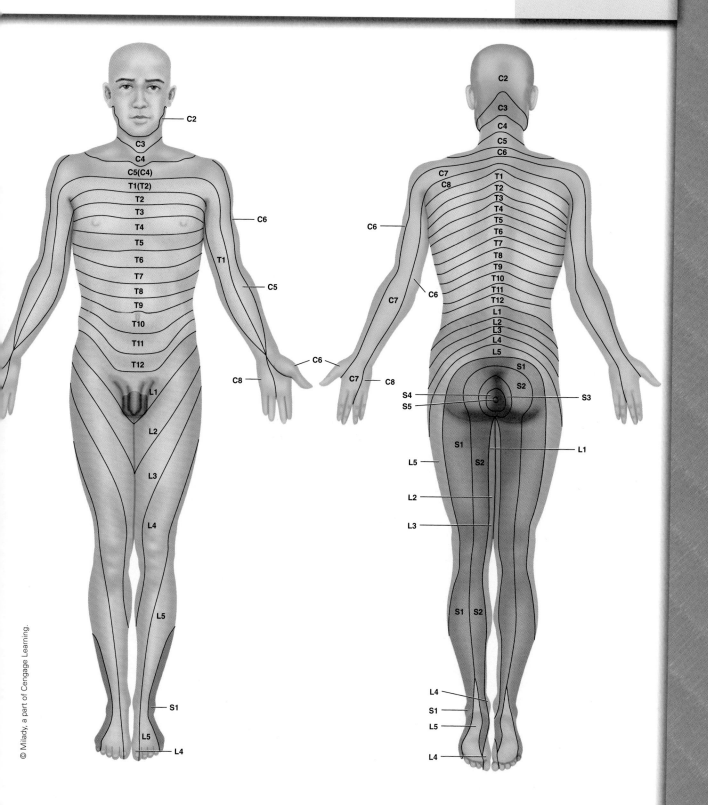

CHAPTER OUTLINE

- SENSATION
- PERCEPTION OF SENSATION
- ADAPTATION TO SENSATION
- DOMINANCE AND SENSATION
- APPLYING THE SCIENCE OF PALPATION

LEARNING OBJECTIVES

- Understand and apply the concepts of sensation, perception, dominance, and adaptation to palpation of the body's structures.
- Describe and identify endangerment sites on the body and cautions and contraindications to palpation.
- Apply the principles of cautions and contraindications to palpation of special client populations.

INTRODUCTION

Your relationship with your client embodies communication through touch. Meaningful touch—touch that is purposeful and skilled, that arises from knowledge of the body's structures and function, and that is applied with therapeutic intent—is both given and received during massage. Palpation provides objective feedback about tissue quality, mobility, temperature, and texture and subjective feedback about pressure and pain. A thorough understanding of the anatomy and physiology of touch—the science of palpation—is essential for effective therapeutic massage. In this chapter, the components and the mechanics of touch are described as they relate to the experience of the massage therapist and the client and as applied to endangerment sites of the body, cautions and contraindications to palpation, and palpation of special client populations.

SENSATION

Sensation

the awareness of change in a condition.

In order for touch to be perceived, sensation must occur. **Sensation** is the awareness of change in a condition. Sensation may be conscious or unconscious. The condition may be a change in the internal environment (you're suddenly hungry for pizza) or the external environment (raindrops are falling on your head).

How Sensation Occurs

Sensation occurs as the result of four conditions:

Stimulus

a change in the environment that invokes a nervous system response.

- Stimulation: a **stimulus**, a change in the environment, occurs that is strong enough to activate sensory neurons.

- Reception: a **sensory receptor**, a specialized neuron in the peripheral nervous system, converts the stimulus into an electrical signal strong enough to produce nerve impulses.
- Conduction: the nerve impulses are conducted from the sensory receptor to the brain, along nerve pathways.
- Integration: an area of the brain receives the nerve impulses and integrates them to produce sensation.

Sensory Receptors

Sensory receptors may be classified according to the type of stimulus they detect:

- **Mechanoreceptors** detect mechanical pressure and sense touch; pressure; vibration; **proprioception**, your perception of the position of your body parts without your looking at them; hearing; and equilibrium.
- **Thermoreceptors** detect changes in temperature.
- **Nociceptors** detect physical or chemical damage to tissues, which is what we call pain.

Somatic sensory receptors detect stimuli that arise from body structures rather than from internal organs. They are found in both the epidermis and the dermis and in the subcutaneous layer of tissue deep to the skin, as shown in Figure 5–1. **Tactile receptors** are the somatic sensory receptors for touch and pressure. Although the greatest concentration of touch receptors is found in the fingertips, the lips, and the eyes, tactile receptors are distributed throughout skin and the tissue deep to skin.

Sensory receptor

a specialized neuron in the peripheral nervous system that converts a stimulus into an electrical signal strong enough to produce nerve impulses.

Mechanoreceptor

a sensory receptor that detects mechanical pressure and senses touch, pressure, vibration, and proprioception and is involved in hearing and equilibrium.

Proprioception

the perception of the position of your body parts without your looking at them.

Thermoreceptors

sensory receptors that detect change in temperature.

Nociceptors

sensory receptors that detect physical or chemical damage to tissues (pain).

Somatic sensory receptors

sensory receptors that detect stimuli arising from body structures.

Tactile receptors

sensory receptors that detect touch and pressure.

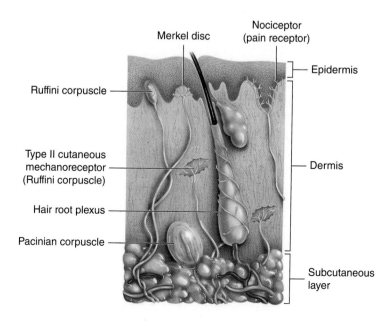

Merkel disc
Nociceptor (pain receptor)
Epidermis
Ruffini corpuscle
Type II cutaneous mechanoreceptor (Ruffini corpuscle)
Dermis
Hair root plexus
Pacinian corpuscle
Subcutaneous layer

FIGURE 5–1 Tactile receptors are found throughout the epidermis and the dermis.

TABLE 5-1

SOMATIC SENSORY RECEPTORS		
SOMATIC SENSORY RECEPTOR	SENSATIONS DETECTED	LOCATION
Tactile Receptors		
Free nerve endings	Touch, pressure	Throughout the epidermis
Meissner corpuscles	Fine touch, pressure, slow vibrations	Eyelids, lips, fingertips
Ruffini corpuscles	Skin stretching, pressure	Throughout the dermis
Pacinian corpuscles	Pressure, fast vibration, tickle	Throughout the skin, fingers, joint capsules
Merkel discs	Touch, pressure	Deep epidermis
Hair root plexuses	Touch (movement of hairs on skin)	Throughout the epidermis
Itch and tickle receptors	Itching, tickling	Throughout the epidermis
Thermoreceptors		
Cold and warm receptors	Cold or warmth	Skin layers
Pain receptors		
Nociceptors	Pain	Throughout all tissue except the brain

Table 5–1 summarizes the types of somatic sensory receptors, the sensations they detect, and where they are found.

Types of Sensations

Sensations may be visceral, arising from the body's organs, or somatic, arising from the body's structures. In this text, we focus on somatic sensations:

- **Tactile sensations** include touch, pressure, vibration, itch, and tickle.
- **Thermal sensations** include coldness and warmth.
- Pain can be both a somatic and a visceral sensation.

Tactile sensations

Touch sensations result from stimulation of the tactile sensory receptors found in the skin or in the subcutaneous layer of tissue:

- **Crude touch** senses that something has touched the skin. It does not perceive the exact location of the touch, nor the exact size, shape or texture of the stimulus, as may be the sensation felt by the client shown in Figure 5–2, as the massage therapist's fingertips make initial contact with her skin.
- **Fine touch** provides the detailed information lacking in crude touch: the exact location, the size, shape, and texture of the stimulating source, as shown in Figure 5–3, and may follow the sensation of crude touch.
- **Pressure** is both more sustained and applied over a larger area than crude or fine touch; tissue is displaced, as shown in Figure 5–4.

Tactile sensations

sensations that result from touch, including fine and crude touch, pressure, vibration, itching, and tickling.

Thermal sensations

sensations that result from warmth or coolness.

Crude touch

the type of touch that senses something has touched the skin, but which does not perceive the exact location of the touch, nor the exact size, shape, or texture of the stimulus.

Fine touch

touch that provides the detailed information lacking in crude touch, such as the exact location, size, shape, and texture of the stimulating source.

Pressure

touch that displaces tissue.

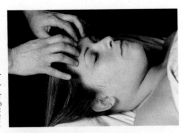

FIGURE 5-2 During crude touch, the client senses little about the details of your touch.

- **Vibration** sensations result from tactile receptor signals that are both rapid and repetitive.
- The sensation of **itching**, a local or generalized response in the skin that can arise from a variety of stimuli, including chemical irritants, and substances that elicit an allergic response by the immune system.
- **Tickling** is usually stimulated only by the touch of another person or an object, such as a feather—it is very difficult, it seems, to tickle yourself!

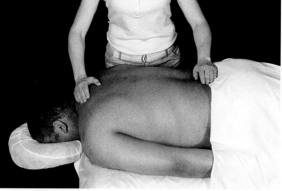

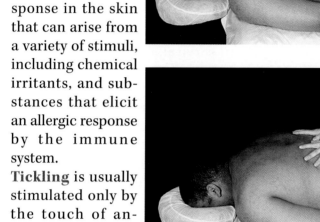

Vibration

sensations that result from tactile receptor signals that are both rapid and repetitive.

FIGURE 5-3 The sensation of fine touch provides more information about the nature and quality of touch.

FIGURE 5-4 Pressure is touch that displaces tissue.

IN THE TREATMENT ROOM

Try to minimize your client's ticklish response:

- Broaden and deepen your touch: light, fingertip touch is more likely to elicit a ticklish response.
- Place your other hand nearby, as shown in Figure 5-5: a secondary source of touch may diminish the ticklish response.
- Ask your client to place her hand over your hand: her own touch may discourage the ticklish response.

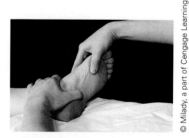

FIGURE 5-5 Placing both hands on your client may provide a distraction to the sensation of tickling.

Thermal sensations

Coolness and warmth are each detected by different thermoreceptors, which operate within a relatively narrow range of temperature: temperatures below 50 °F (10°C) and above 118 °F (47.8°C) stimulate receptors for pain, not for temperature. Thermoreceptors for coolness and for warmth are also found in different regions of the skin, as shown in Figure 5–1:

- Cold receptors are found in the stratum basale, the deepest layer of the epidermis. They are stimulated by temperatures between 50 °F (10°C) and 105 °F (40.5°C).
- Heat receptors are found in the dermis, and are stimulated by temperatures between 90 °F (32.2°C) and 118 °F (47.8°C).

Itching

a local or generalized response in the skin that can arise from a variety of stimuli, including chemical irritants, and substances that elicit an allergic response by the immune system

Tickling sensation

a sensory receptor response usually stimulated by the touch of another person or by an object, such as a feather.

Thermoregulation

the adjusting of body temperature to within the range of homeostasis.

Paradoxical cold

a "tactile illusion" which occurs when a usually warm stimulus is perceived as cold, or vice versa.

Visceral pain

pain that arises from a body organ.

Somatic pain

pain that arises from a body structure.

Acute pain

pain of less than six months' duration

Fast pain

pain that occurs in response to the stimulus in about 1/10th of a second

Slow pain

pain that develops about a second or so after the stimulating event and gradually increases in intensity.

DID YOU KNOW?

Thermoregulation, the adjusting of body temperature to normal range, is also a function of skin. The body is cooled by the evaporation of perspiration from the epidermis and warmed by an increase of blood flow in the dermis. In an example of "tactile illusion," some people experience a stimulus which is usually warm as cold, or vice versa. This is called **paradoxical cold** and explains why some clients may sense a heat-producing topical analgesic as chilling.

Pain sensations

The sensation of pain is vital for survival. Pain protects your body from further damage to tissues by alerting you, first rapidly and then continuously, to the source of the damage. Pain may be **visceral**, arising from a body organ, such as the stomach or **somatic**, arising from a body structure, such as the foot. Conditions that induce somatic pain include:

■ Overstretching of a structure
■ Sustained muscle contraction or spasm
■ Prolonged ischemia, interrupted blood flow

Nociceptors, visible in Figure 5–1, are found in all body tissue except the brain. Messages of the various types of pain are carried to the brain by different nerve fibers, resulting in a range of pain sensations. Table 5–2 describes types of pain sensations.

Pain may be short lived or long lasting, and may continue to occur after the initiating source of the pain has been eliminated or resolved.

■ **Acute pain** is pain of less than six months' duration. Stimulated by tissue damage, acute pain activates the sympathetic response

DID YOU KNOW?

Fast pain followed by slow pain is a pattern that often occurs following injury to a somatic structure. An ankle sprain is sharply painful for the first few seconds or minutes, then begins to ache deeply. Both sensations of pain are intense, but the sensations are reaching the brain via different nerve fibers and serve different functions.

TABLE 5–2

PAIN SENSATIONS	
PAIN SENSATION	**DESCRIPTION**
Fast pain	Occurs in response to the stimulus in about 1/10th of a second. Fast pain is felt in superficial, not deeper, tissues and serves to demand immediate attention to address the source of the damage. *A slap to the face results in fast pain.*
Slow pain	Develops about a second or so after the stimulating event and gradually increases in intensity. Slow pain may be as intense as fast pain, but is sensed in both superficial and deep tissue and in organs. Slow pain serves as a reminder that either the immediate attention called for by fast pain has not resolved the damage or that subsequent intervention is required. *A toothache or a knot in a muscle can be sensed as slow pain.*
Somatic pain	Sensed by receptors in muscles, joints, tendons, and fascia. *A sore shoulder is one example of somatic pain.*
Cutaneous pain	Sensed by nociceptors in the epidermis. *A paper cut results in cutaneous pain.*
Visceral pain	Sensed by nociceptors in the body's internal organs. *A stomach ache is visceral pain.*
Nociceptive pain	Results from damage to tissues. *A cat scratch that draws blood will cause nociceptive pain.*
Neuropathic pain	Results from damage to nervous system structures. *Pain resulting from impingement of the sciatic nerve by the Piriformis muscle is neuropathic pain.*

of the autonomic nervous system, which creates anxiety, rapid heart rate, and so on, and compels one toward relieving the source of the pain. This response makes acute pain highly functional.

- **Chronic pain**, on the other hand, may have begun as acute pain but has persisted for more than six months. Chronic pain is not well understood. It often appears to serve no purpose and may persist without any apparent or discoverable underlying cause. Chronic pain responds less well to treatment and may be the primary presenting condition for clients seeking bodywork treatment.

- **Breakthrough pain** occurs when chronic pain no longer is controlled by medication. Breakthrough pain may result in treatment by ever-stronger pain medications and is a risk for prescription drug or self-medication abuse.

Chronic pain

pain of more than six months duration.

Breakthrough pain

pain that occurs when chronic pain no longer is controlled by medication.

IN THE TREATMENT ROOM

The words your client uses to describe her pain are important:

- Acute pain is often described as breathtaking, sharp, intense, or prickling.
- Chronic pain is often described as deep, aching, throbbing, or burning pain.

- **Referred pain** is pain that is felt on or just deep to the skin, but which does not arise from the site where the pain sensation is perceived.

- Referred pain that is somatic in origin may indicate a myofascial trigger point that is "referring," or sending pain to the area where it is perceived. A myofascial trigger point in the Rhomboid, for example, may refer pain into the axilla.

- Referred pain that is visceral in origin may be perceived at predictable sites found over the organ affected, or in another superficial location served by the same segment of the spinal cord. Figure 5–6 illustrates this pattern of referred visceral pain.

Referred pain

pain that is felt on or just deep to the skin, but which does not arise from the site where the pain sensation is perceived.

IN THE TREATMENT ROOM

If your client reports superficial pain that does not seem to indicate a myofascial trigger point or that fails to respond as expected to therapeutic treatment, the pain may be referred visceral pain, a symptom that should be evaluated by your client's primary health care provider.

IN THE TREATMENT ROOM

Somatic pain may arise in response to temporary toxicity in tissues. A client who spends every Friday night overindulging in fatty and sweet food accompanied by alcohol, after sitting at a desk all week without exercising, may come for her Saturday morning massage appointment with tissues that are swollen, stressed, and painful to the touch from leftover toxins, especially around the iliotibial band (ITB), in the soles of the feet, around the abdomen, and the backs of her arms. Depth of touch may need to be altered for this client.

Nociceptive pain

pain that results from damage to tissues.

Neuropathic pain

pain that results from damage to nervous system structures.

Cutaneous pain

pain that is sensed by nociceptors in the epidermis.

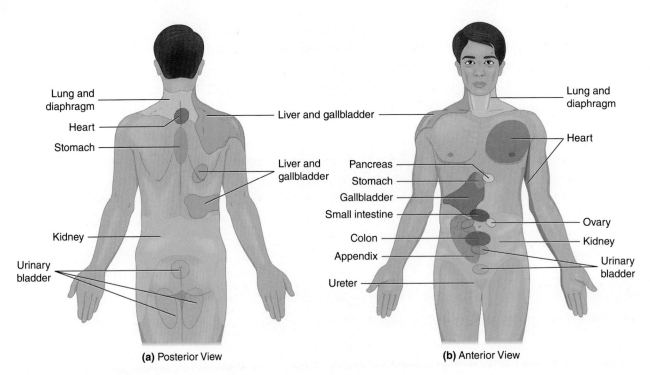

Lung and diaphragm
Heart
Stomach
Liver and gallbladder
Liver and gallbladder
Kidney
Urinary bladder

Lung and diaphragm
Heart
Pancreas
Stomach
Gallbladder
Small intestine
Colon
Appendix
Ureter
Ovary
Kidney
Urinary bladder

(a) Posterior View   **(b)** Anterior View

© Milady, a part of Cengage Learning.

FIGURE 5–6 Referred visceral pain may be sensed in a predictable area away from the point of origin (such as stomach pain that may be referred to the thoracic region of the spine).

| Perception
the conscious awareness and interpretation of sensations.

PERCEPTION OF SENSATION

Perception is the conscious awareness and interpretation of sensations. Perception can be as individual as each client's personality and is influenced by genetic and even cultural forces. Perception of sensation presents challenges for the massage therapist: touch that is perceived as too deep by one client may be perceived as annoyingly light by another. The temperature in your treatment room may be too warm for one client and too cool for the next. Pain that is excruciating to one client may be only moderately perceived by another.

IN THE TREATMENT ROOM

While the mechanics of sensation are universal, the experience of it is individual: the sensations of touch, pressure, temperature, and sometimes pain are experienced by the client as you first place your hand on her. With practice, you will learn to gauge the quality and texture of skin and its underlying structures, and the meaning of the temperature of the tissue you are palpating.

You will also develop your own palpation vocabulary:

- Is the tissue soft or hard, wooden or rigid, congested, or firm?
- Is it fragile, adhered, resistant, or unstable?
- Is the skin cool to the touch, warm, hot, or frigid?

Factors Altering Perception

Perception of sensation may be altered by many factors. Terms used to describe these dysfunctions are described in Table 5–3.

TABLE 5–3

TERMS FOR FACTORS ALTERING PERCEPTION	
TERMS	**FACTORS ALTERING PERCEPTION**
Neuropathy or peripheral neuropathy	Pain, numbness, or tingling caused by damage to peripheral nerves. The symptoms of neuropathy are exhibited along **dermatomes,** shown in Figure 5–7, areas on the skin that provide sensory input to the central nervous system via specific spinal nerves and correspond to the sensory nerve pathway.
Anesthesia	Suppression of perception of pain sensations, usually induced by prescribed medications called anesthetics, such as those administered be an anesthesiologist during surgery.
Paresthesia	Tingling, pricking, or burning (usually not painful) in one area. Similar to neuropathy, paresthesia does not usually involve symptoms along dermatomes.
Hyperesthesia	Increased sensitivity to touch, often involving dysfunction of touch or pain receptors in the skin.
Allodynia	Pain in response to a usually non-painful stimulus. Tactile allodynia is induced by very light touch. It may result from damage to the nervous system or as a side effect of some treatments for cancer.
Phantom pain	Pain that persists in a body limb that has been amputated. It is thought that the area of the brain that interpreted sensations from that limb remains responsive to stimuli proximal to the missing limb, or that the brain itself retains nerve cells that are responsive to that limb, even in the absence of actual sensory input. Although phantom limb pain usually disappears after six months or so, it can persist and remain chronic and resistant to drug treatment.

Neuropathy

pain, numbness, or tingling caused by damage to peripheral nerves, those that are outside the central nervous system.

Dermatomes

areas on the skin that provide sensory input to the central nervous system via specific spinal nerves and which correspond to the sensory nerve pathway.

Anesthesia

Suppression of perception of pain sensations, usually induced by prescribed medications called anesthetics, such as those administered be an anesthesiologist during surgery.

Paresthesia

tingling, pricking, or burning, usually not painful, in one area.

Hyperesthesia

increased sensitivity to touch, often involving dysfunction of touch or pain receptors in the skin.

Allodynia

pain in response to a usually non-painful stimulus.

Phantom pain

pain that persists in a body limb that has been amputated.

IN THE TREATMENT ROOM

Certain medications, especially those for pain or for treatment of mood disorders such as depression, may alter sensation and perception of sensation. A client who is taking prescribed medication for pain may be unable to accurately perceive—and provide feedback about—depth of touch or pressure. Other medications, such as muscle relaxants, antidepressants, and tranquilizers, for example, may also interfere with perception of touch, pressure, or pain sensations.

The list of such medications is both long and ever-changing. It is essential that you obtain a complete list of the names of all medications that your client is taking, that you research the possible sensation-inhibiting side effects of these medications, and that you obtain information about medication compliance and doses taken on the days of treatment. Good resources for this research include:

- A pharmacist with whom you forge an ongoing relationship and whom you can turn to with medication questions.
- Online sites listing information about medications and their side effects, such as www.webmd.com, www.drugs.com, or www.rxlist.com.

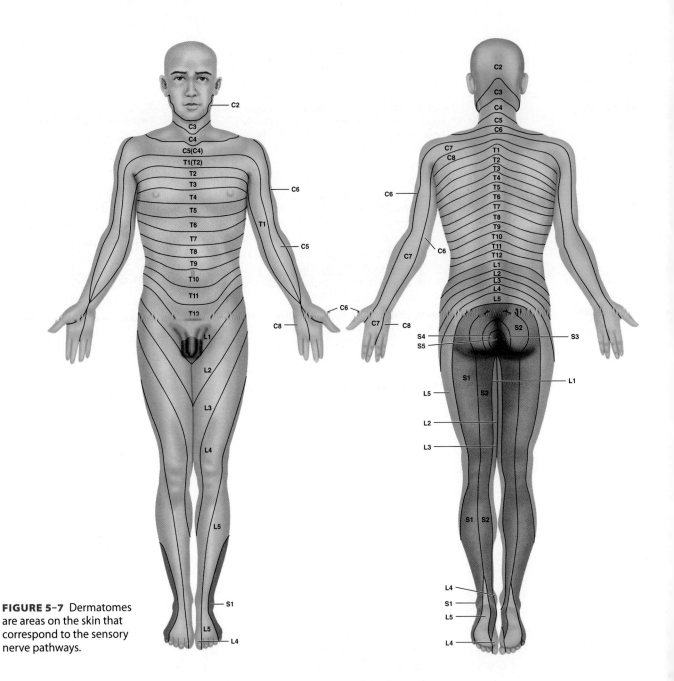

FIGURE 5-7 Dermatomes are areas on the skin that correspond to the sensory nerve pathways.

Conditions altering perception of touch

Conditions that may alter perception of touch, pressure, or pain sensations include damage to nervous system structures or the effects of chronic diseases on the nervous and circulatory systems. It is important to obtain complete and accurate information regarding your client's health history and current health status. Research client conditions to understand your client's potential disruption of sensation perception. Effective palpation technique requires focused attention to the health of your client's tissues and underlying structures and the expected level of sensation.

Great care should be taken when palpating clients with the conditions described in Table 5–4. Reports of sensations from these clients may be unreliable and at odds with your objective findings, due to the disruption of their sensory perception.

TABLE 5-4

CONDITIONS ALTERING PERCEPTION OF TOUCH	
CONDITION	**EFFECT ON SENSATION**
Cancer	Cancer itself does not usually disrupt sensation, but the treatments for cancer surely can. Long-term chemotherapy or radiation may damage the nervous system and cause local or systemic tactile allodynia, pain from a stimulus that is not ordinarily painful. A client with tactile allodynia may not be able to tolerate hands-on palpation and may require modalities that do not include direct touch, such as Reiki or healing touch.
Carpal tunnel syndrome (CTS)	CTS is caused by compression or entrapment of the median nerve as it travels beneath the transverse carpal ligament, the flexor retinaculum, of the wrist. Symptoms are often felt on the anterior aspect of the hand or wrist and include pain, numbness or tingling, and weakness in the affected hand.
Chronic pain syndrome	People with chronic pain syndrome experience a level of pain that is not supported by medical tests or examinations—in other words, their pain is out of proportion to their apparent condition. The perception of touch and pressure for someone with chronic pain syndrome may be contrary to palpatory expectation or experience. This client perceives pain or numbness that appears to be without any objective cause.
Circulatory disorders	People with heart disease or atherosclerosis, or clogged arteries, also known as "hardening of the arteries," have poor systemic circulation of blood and oxygen, placing their tissues under stress. As a result, they may experience varying degrees of numbness or pain in the affected areas.
Diabetic neuropathy	Many people with diabetes eventually experience the effects of long-term high levels of blood glucose: pain, numbness, or tingling, especially in the extremities.
Fibromyalgia	This syndrome is characterized by pain, fatigue, and stiffness in the connective tissue of the muscles, tendons, and ligaments. More common in women, it is thought to be associated with stress, poor sleep habits, and repetitive strain. People with fibromyalgia have tender points that occur in an identifiable pattern, and may perceive pain or numbness that appears to be without any objective cause and that does not respond within the usual expectations from touch.
Multiple sclerosis (MS)	MS involves the progressive destruction of myelin, the protective covering around sensory and motor neurons in the central nervous system. Symptoms include the progressive loss of motor control and sensation perceptions, including touch, pressure, and pain.
Nerve entrapment	Nerve function is disrupted wherever a nerve is compressed by nearby tissues, whether in the wrist, as in carpal tunnel syndrome, in the low back or hip, as in sciatica or Piriformis syndrome, described in Chapter 10, Palpating Deeper Muscles and Muscle Groups, or elsewhere. This disruption results in pain, tingling, numbness, weakness, and possible loss of function in the area served by that nerve.
Spinal cord injury	A complete severance of the spinal cord, called a transection, results in an absolute loss of motor and sensory nerve function to the organs and structures of the body, inferior to the level of the severance. There is no sensation in the affected region of the body.
Stroke	A stroke may cause temporary or permanent damage to sensory or motor nerves, resulting in loss of function and sensation to the affected areas.

Carpal tunnel syndrome

pain, tingling, or numbness caused by compression or entrapment of the median nerve as it travels beneath the transverse carpal ligament, the flexor retinaculum, of the wrist.

Fibromyalgia

a syndrome characterized by pain, fatigue, and stiffness in the connective tissue of the muscles, tendons and ligaments.

Multiple sclerosis

an autoimmune disease which causes the progressive destruction of myelin, the protective covering around sensory and motor neurons in the central nervous system. Symptoms include the progressive loss of motor control and perception of sensations, including touch, pressure, and pain.

Nerve entrapment

pain, tingling, numbness, weakness, and possible loss of sensory and motor function caused by compression of a nerve by nearby tissue.

IN THE TREATMENT ROOM

A client's perception of sensation—and her accurate description of sensation—may also be disrupted by past or continuing physical or emotional trauma. A client who has experienced trauma may disconnect from the sensations in her body, which may be reminders of the trauma and may bring up painful memories. This client may or may not disclose the past trauma to you. In some cases, the trauma has been deeply buried and the client's own awareness of it is limited or even nonexistent. Because she may be unable to accurately perceive or report sensations, it is critical that you stay focused during palpation and alert to any disparity in the level of pressure being applied and her response, or lack of response, to it. Be aware of the following possibilities in clients who have experienced trauma:

- A client who is completely out of touch with her body may be endangered by allowing a type of touch or depth of touch that is inappropriate or ill-advised. This client, for example, may request deeper palpation pressure than is beneficial for her at that time.
- A client who has experienced emotional or physical trauma may be unable to speak up for herself to stop touch that is painful. She may allow or encourage range of motion at a joint, for example, even though you observe signs of pain, such as clenching, breath holding, or stiffness.

It can be a challenge to provide caring, professional touch that is also appropriate for such a client. You can help this client by using nonjudgmental statements and by staying within your scope of practice. Some suggestions for communicating with her:

- Avoid statements that may be perceived as judgmental—"Wow, your leg is stiff!" or "Is that as far as you can move that thigh?" Be aware that statements that may seem positive to you, such as "Gee, you're lucky to be so thin," are in fact expressing a judgment and may be perceived as invasive and hurtful.
- Use active-listening skills and objective observations that reflect the client's words or actions—"So you're saying that your leg feels stiff today," or "Moving your thigh seems to be a little more difficult today. Is that right?"
- Avoid trying to "fix" this client or offering advice—statements such as "Well, did you tell him how you feel?" or "You'll get over it in time" are not helpful or within your scope of practice.
- Allow this client the space to experience or vent her emotions. The emotional release may be expressed in her body, making your work more effective. Offer paper tissues if needed, or offer to step outside the room, if that seems called for. You can honor your client's process best by not interfering with it or judging it.
- Stay mindful of your scope of practice. Occasionally, a client may turn to her massage therapist for therapy for emotional issues that are beyond our scope of practice. Be kind but firm in stating the boundaries of massage therapy.
- While being mindful of client confidentiality, talk with mentors and peers about boundaries and scope of practice issues, for support and guidance.

ADAPTATION TO SENSATION

Sensory receptors may also be classified by their rate of **adaptation**: the decrease, over time, in the perception of a sensation, even though the stimulus remains. Receptors are classified as either rapidly adapting or slowly adapting:

- **Rapidly adapting receptors** signal a *change* in a stimulus and include tactile receptors for touch and pressure. Rapid adaptation occurs in about 1/10th of a second.
- **Slowly adapting receptors** continue to trigger nerve impulses for as long as the stimulus persists and are associated with sensations of pain. Adaptation that takes one second or longer is considered slow adaptation—in other words, 10 times longer than a rapidly adapting receptor.

Adaptation Rates of Sensory Receptors

Receptors for different sensations have different adaptation rates:

- Sensory receptors for touch and pressure tend to be rapidly adapting. It is important for you to know whether what is touching you is a gentle breeze or the tail of a scorpion. Rapid adaptation allows a fast response keeps you safe, or in biological homeostasis. In the same way, you must be able to accurately gauge the pressure of touch, to prevent damage to tissues.
- Thermoreceptors tend to adapt rapidly at first and then slowly. Again, the rate of adaptation contributes to maintaining homeostasis by allowing you to decide if action is needed to warm or cool your body.
- Nociceptors, sensory receptors for pain, tend to adapt slowly. In addition, the chemicals released in response to pain may linger in tissues, contributing to the continuing sensation of pain. This slow adaptation rate, too, is functional: if you adapted rapidly to pain, taking steps to remedy the source of the pain would be less compelling and greater tissue damage or even death might occur. Table 5–5 list the adaptation rate of different types of sensory receptors.

Adaptation

the decrease, over time, in the perception of a sensation, even though the stimulus remains.

Rapidly adapting receptors

sensory receptors that signal a change in a stimulus and adapt to it in about 1/10th of a second.

Slowly adapting receptors

sensory receptors that continue to trigger nerve impulses for as long as a stimulus persists and are associated with sensations of pain. Adaptation that takes one second or longer is considered slow adaptation.

TABLE 5–5

ADAPTATION RATE OF SENSORY RECEPTORS	
RECEPTOR TYPE	ADAPTATION RATE
Tactile Receptors	
Free nerve endings	Rapid
Meissner corpuscles	Rapid
Ruffini corpuscles	Slow
Pacinian corpuscles	Rapid
Merkel discs	Slow
Hair-root plexuses	Rapid
Itch and tickle receptors	Rapid, then slow
Thermoreceptors	
Cold and warm receptors	Rapid, then slow
Pain receptors	
Nociceptors	Slow

IN THE TREATMENT ROOM

Adaptation and Palpation

Because rates of adaptation of receptors for touch and pressure tend to be rapid, the following occurs during massage:

- Your palpating fingertips adapt rapidly to sensations of touch and pressure, possibly resulting in less than accurate palpatory input if you leave your palpating fingertips in one specific location for a period of time.
- Your client's superficial sensory receptors in her skin adapt rapidly to the your touch and pressure, possibly resulting in unreliable feedback, especially in the presence of other factors—for example, chronic conditions and medications.

The rapid-then-slow adaptation rate of the thermoreceptors is important in gauging initial touch:

- Any great temperature variance between the client's skin and your skin will be quite evident at first touch, and then will seem to subside. Be aware that this subsiding may indicate adaptation to the sensation, not an actual change in temperature.

The slow adaptation rate of the nociceptors means that you must be cautious in your approach to palpation of structures that may become painful after initial touch:

- It is essential to monitor your client's level of pain sensation as you continue to palpate tissues: is it decreasing, increasing, or remaining constant in response to palpation?
- Pay close attention to your client's pain medication dosages. A recent or increased dose of pain medication may make it impossible to accurately assess the pressure of palpatory touch.

Lab Activity 5–1 on page 183 is designed to help you experience your rate of adaptation to a new stimulus.

DOMINANCE AND SENSATION

Dominance

the preference for using one hand over the other for reaching, grasping, holding, and manipulating objects.

An additional factor in perceiving and adapting to sensation is dominance. In this context, **dominance** refers to the preference for using one hand over the other as the tool of choice for reaching, grasping, holding, and manipulating objects. Sometimes called hand dominance, this phenomenon expresses itself early in life in the choosing of one hand over the other for most uses. In about 80 percent of the world's population, the choice is the right hand, and it does not usually change over a person's lifetime.

DID YOU KNOW?

Dominance extends to the feet and the eyes: most people who are right-handed are also right-foot dominant, in that they step out with their right foot first and use their right eye to "see with"—their right eye moves first and more rapidly than the left. Some people's dominance is so strong that they chew their food only on the dominant side of their jaw! However, a few people are cross-dominant: they reach first with their right hand, but step forward first with their left foot.

Dominance is an expression of **lateralization** in the brain: the left side of the brain sends messages to and is controlled by the right side of the brain, and vice versa. Dominance is not entirely static. Some people are relatively dexterous or adept with either hand. Those with equal facility are called **ambidextrous**. Others find having to use only their non-dominant hand overwhelming.

Most people are able to make the switch to the non-dominant member fairly quickly, if the dominant hand or foot can't be used for a period of time.

People who permanently lose the use of a dominant hand or foot eventually learn to use the remaining member. Left-handed people are daily faced with having to alter their preferred handedness in a right-handed world.

Dominance and Palpation

Understanding the role of dominance helps you anticipate patterns of use and strain in your client and can be a guide for selecting which tissues to palpate. Dominance has significance in palpation for both the client and the massage therapist:

- Somatic structures on the dominant side of your client's body may be slightly larger and more developed than on the non-dominant side.
- Perception of sensation may be more acute on the dominant side of the body, while the underused and slightly weaker structures on the non-dominant side may be more injury-prone. For these reasons, it is always wise to palpate structures on both sides of your client's body.
- Many massage therapy students must work hard to develop equal dexterity on both sides of their body, and especially to develop equal palpation sensitivity in both hands. Ambidextrous massage therapists are well-blessed!

APPLYING THE SCIENCE OF PALPATION

As with other therapeutic techniques, your skill and knowledge of sensation and perception, along with input from your client, ensures that palpation is safely and appropriate.

Endangerment Sites

Endangerment sites are specific sites on the body that are vulnerable to injury from direct or significant pressure. Your understanding of endangerment sites guides you in deciding where, when, and how palpation is safely and appropriately applied.

- Visually locate endangerment sites before beginning to palpate.
- Acknowledge the individuality of each client's anatomy when locating specific endangerment sites.
- Keep touch feather-light over endangerment sites.

Endangerment sites and the structures that may be affected by touch are outlined in Table 5-6.

Lateralization

a phenomenon of the brain in which the left side of the brain sends messages to and is controlled by the right side of the brain, and vice versa.

Ambidextrous

having equal facility with either hand.

Lab Activity 5–2 on page 183 is designed to help you experience the challenge of performing tasks with your non-dominant hand.

Endangerment site

a specific site on the body that is vulnerable to injury from direct or significant pressure.

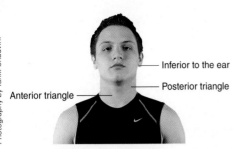

Anterior triangle — — Inferior to the ear
— Posterior triangle

FIGURE 5–8 Anterior view of endangerment sites on the head and neck.

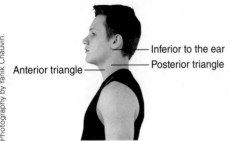

Anterior triangle — — Inferior to the ear
— Posterior triangle

FIGURE 5–9 Lateral view of endangerment sites on the head and neck.

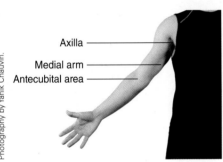

Axilla —
Medial arm —
Antecubital area —

FIGURE 5–10 Endangerment sites on the arm and forearm.

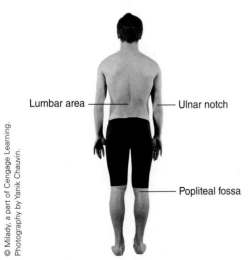

Lumbar area — — Ulnar notch

— Popliteal fossa

FIGURE 5–11 Posterior view of endangerment sites on the trunk and lower extremity.

TABLE 5–6

ENDANGERMENT SITE LOCATIONS AND STRUCTURES OF CONCERN		
ENDANGERMENT SITE	**LOCATION**	**STRUCTURES OF CONCERN**
Inferior to the ear (Figures 5–8 and 5–9)	The notch posterior to the angle of the mandible.	Facial nerve, external carotid artery, styloid process of the temporal bone.
Anterior triangle of the neck (Figures 5–8 and 5–9)	The area bordered by the angle of the mandible, both sides of the sternocleidomastoid (SCM) muscle and the trachea, which creates an inverted triangle.	Carotid artery, internal jugular vein, vagus nerve, lymph nodes.
Posterior triangle of the neck (Figure 5–9)	The area bordered by the posterior margin of the SCM, the anterior margin of the upper trapezius muscle, and the clavicle.	Brachial plexus, subclavian artery, brachiocephalic and external jugular veins, lymph nodes.
Axilla (Figure 5–10)	The armpit.	Axillary, median, musculocutaneous, and ulnar nerves, brachial artery, lymph nodes.
Medial Arm (Figure 5–10)	Upper, inner arm between the Biceps brachii and Triceps brachii muscle bellies.	Ulnar, musculocutaneous and median nerves, brachial artery, basilic vein, lymph nodes.
Antecubital area of the elbow (Figure 5–10)	Anterior bend of the elbow.	Median nerve, radial and ulnar arteries, median cubital vein.
Ulnar notch of the elbow (Figure 5–11)	The "funny bone" on the posterior of the elbow.	Ulnar nerve.
Femoral triangle (Figure 5–12)	Area bordered by the Sartorius and Adductor longus muscles and the inguinal ligament.	Femoral nerve, femoral artery, femoral and great saphenous vein, lymph nodes.
Popliteal fossa (Figure 5–11)	Posterior aspect of the knee; the area bordered by Gastrocnemius and the Hamstrings muscles.	Tibial and common peroneal nerves, popliteal artery, popliteal vein.
Abdomen (Figure 5–12)	Upper area of the abdomen, just deep to the ribs.	On the right: liver, gallbladder; on the left: spleen; deep center: abdominal aorta.
Upper lumbar area (Figure 5–11)	Area just inferior to the ribs, superior to the iliac crest, and lateral to the spine.	Kidneys.

TABLE 5-7

CONDITIONS THAT CONTRAINDICATE SYSTEMIC MASSAGE	
CONDITION	**CONTRAINDICATION**
Fever	Fever is a systemic contraindication: palpation is contraindicated for a client who has a fever: generally, a body temperature above 99.4°F (37.4°C).
Acute infectious disease	Active infection is a systemic contraindication: palpation is contraindicated for a client who has an active infection, for the safety of the client and of the therapist and her other clients.
Inflammation	Local inflammation is a local contraindication: palpation over an area of inflammation is contraindicated. Pressure over the area may intensify inflammation. If the client also shows signs of fever or active infection, inflammation is a systemic contraindication.
Edema (swelling)	Swelling is a local contraindication for palpation: do not apply direct pressure over an area of edema.

© Milady, a part of Cengage Learning.

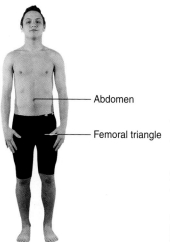

Abdomen

Femoral triangle

FIGURE 5-12 Anterior view of endangerment sites on the trunk and lower extremity

© Milady, a part of Cengage Learning. Photography by Yanik Chauvin.

Contraindications to Palpation

Contraindications to palpation are conditions that render massage treatment, including palpation, inadvisable. Contraindications may be local, confined to the area affected, or systemic, bodywide. General contraindications are summarized in Table 5–7.

Only intact skin should be touched. Contagious and some noncontagious skin conditions can be contraindications to touch. Table 5–8 describes skin conditions that indicate a local or systemic contraindication.

Cautions to palpation

Cautions to palpation don't necessarily mean that you can't palpate your client. **Cautions** to palpation mean that a client's local or systemic conditions indicate extra care before proceeding:

- Visually assess the tissue to be palpated. Verify that the skin is intact and that there are no varicosities, bruises, cuts, or scrapes that might be impacted by touch.
- Avoid palpating over or near any rash. Touch may intensify itching or spread the rash, either on the client or to the therapist.
- Whenever possible, perform a thorough intake interview before palpation. Is this client's tissue healthy enough for palpation? Are her joints stable enough for palpation and assisted or active movement? Does this client have a chronic condition that may be negatively impacted by palpation?

Lab Activity 5–3 on page 183 is designed to help you identify endangerment sites on the body.

Contraindication

a condition that renders massage treatment, including palpation, inadvisable, because it may cause injury to the client. Contraindications may be local, confined to the area affected, or systemic, meaning bodywide.

Caution

a client's local or systemic conditions that indicate extra care should be taken before proceeding with palpation or massage treatment.

IN THE TREATMENT ROOM

Use palpation over a client's clothing sparingly, because you have not visually assessed the underlying tissue.

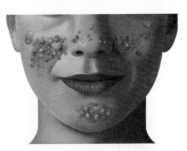

FIGURE 5–13 Adult acne can occur on the face or the trunk of the body.

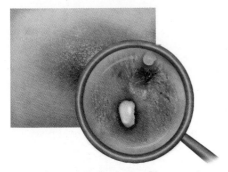

FIGURE 5–14 Boils on the skin may be one sign of poor immune system functioning.

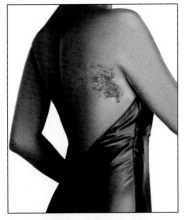

FIGURE 5–15 Herpes zoster is caused by the same virus that causes chicken pox; it remains dormant in the body and may recur as shingles later in life.

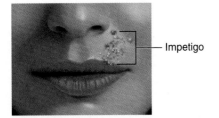
Impetigo

FIGURE 5–16 Impetigo is highly contagious.

TABLE 5–8

SKIN CONDITIONS THAT CONTRAINDICATE LOCAL OR SYSTEMIC MASSAGE	
SKIN CONDITION	**CONTRAINDICATION**
Acne (Figure 5–13)	Local
Boils (Figure 5–14)	Local; systemic, if the boils are widespread (a group of boils is called a carbuncle).
Broken blood vessels	Local
Bruises	Local
Burns and blisters	Local; systemic, if widespread.
Fungal infections (on skin, under nails)	Local; systemic if widespread.
Herpes simplex (cold sore)	Local
Herpes zoster (shingles; Figure 5–15)	Local; systemic if widespread or accompanied by fever.
Hypersensitive skin	Local; the cause of the hypersensitivity should be medically investigated.
Impetigo (Figure 5–16)	Systemic; this is a highly contagious condition.
Lacerations	Local, until completely healed.
Lumps	Local; the source of the lump should be medically investigated.
Rashes (eczema, psoriasis, etc.)	Systemic; local, if the rash has been diagnosed as non-contagious.
Scaly spots	Systemic; local if the condition has been diagnosed as non-contagious.
Scratches	Local, until completely healed.
Skin cancer (Figures 5–17 and 5–18)	For basal cell carcinoma: local. For squamous cell carcinoma or melanoma: systemic.
Skin tags	Local
Stings and bites	Local; systemic, if the client's reaction to the sting or bite is bodywide.
Tumors	Systemic, unless medical clearance for circulatory massage is given.
Varicose veins (Figure 5–19)	Local
Warts	Local; systemic, if widespread.
Wounds	Local, until completely healed; systemic, if the effects are widespread.

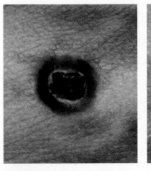
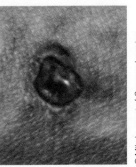

FIGURE 5–17 Left: Squamous cell carcinoma; right: Basal cell carcinoma

Palpating Special Client Populations

In addition to the contraindications and cautions described above, adjustments to palpation technique may be indicated with certain client populations.

 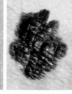

Asymmetry   Border Irregularity   Color   Diameter: ¼ inch or 6 mm

FIGURE 5–18 Remember the characteristics of melanoma as: ABCD, for Asymmetry, Border, Color and Diameter.

Palpating a client who is injured

Before palpating a client with an injury, obtain complete intake information and perform a thorough interview, to assess the appropriateness of palpation. Review palpation decisions at each subsequent appointment, until the injury has resolved, following these guidelines:

- How recent is the injury? If the injury is less than 48 hours old, you will need to proceed gently and with great caution.
- Has the injury been examined and/or treated by any health care provider? What was the diagnosis and treatment? Has that examiner given directions for follow-up care that would preclude palpation or bodywork? Avoid working near an injury that has not been medically evaluated, or reschedule treatment until after a medical evaluation.
- Is the skin surrounding the injury intact? Avoid any areas where skin is not intact.
- Are there any signs of inflammation? Signs of inflammation include local pain, heat, redness, and swelling. Avoid palpating areas that may be inflamed.
- Is your client taking pain medication? If so, she may not be able to give accurate feedback regarding pain and pressure. Proceed with extreme caution, keeping your pressure superficial.

Asymmetry

marked differences in the size or shape of contralateral structures.

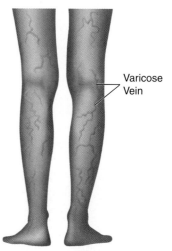

Varicose Vein

FIGURE 5–19 Varicose veins are a local contraindication to direct touch.

IN THE TREATMENT ROOM

If your client's answers to interview questions suggest that palpation over or near the site of an injury may be contraindicated, you can still palpate structures that may be developing compensation patterns in order to accommodate the effects of the injury, until palpation over the injury site is indicated by the progression of healing.

Palpating a client who is chronically ill

Assessment for the appropriateness of palpation may be a continuing process with a client who has a chronic illness, such as cancer, HIV/AIDS, or an autoimmune disorder. People with chronic illnesses experience varying levels of vitality and may fatigue easily. Palpation techniques that require active client participation may fatigue your client more than they provide input to guide your treatment plan.

- Regularly update medication information for your client: what medications is she taking, how much, and how often? Keep complete SOAP notes, described in Chapter 6, The Art of Palpation, regarding changes you observe in tissue health or level of sensation that may be related to changes in medications and dosages.
- Research the medications your client is taking, so that you have additional information to combine with your own observations in deciding the appropriateness of palpation for your client.
- Research to understand your client's chronic illness. If it is progressive, you must continue to make adjustments in your palpation techniques to accommodate your client's evolving condition.

IN THE TREATMENT ROOM

Obtain complete information about the medications your client takes, and research their potential side effects. A client with a chronic illness may be taking multiple medications, which may require frequent dosage changes and result in intensification of side effects. Some medication side effects may preclude certain massage or palpation techniques.

Palpating an elder client

We begin to lose muscle mass at about age 30. During each subsequent decade, 7–8 percent of muscle mass is lost, and its space is filled with adipose and fibrous connective tissue. Over the same decades, bone mass is also lost and tendons and ligaments become brittle. As a result, joints become increasingly unstable. Elder skin loses its firmness and elasticity, becomes dry and fragile, and bruises or tears easily.

IN THE TREATMENT ROOM

Small-boned, Caucasian, or Asian women are at risk in later years to osteoporosis, which is characterized by progressively brittle, fragile bones. The bones of a client with osteoporosis are vulnerable to spontaneous fracture. Osteoporosis is a progressive condition. Over time, the bones of a client with osteoporosis become more vulnerable to fracture. As time goes on, adjust your technique to accommodate the increased fragility of your client's bones.

Changes in somatic structures in elder clients may also be accompanied by additional chronic or debilitating conditions that potentially complicate palpation, including medications that may alter perceptions of sensation.

Palpating an elder client may require using the adjustments listed for clients with chronic illnesses, plus additional adjustments:

- Palpation pressure should be minimal, especially around joints and over areas of fragile skin. Figure 5–20 shows common sites of fragility on elder bodies. Use plenty of lubricant when palpating areas of fragile skin.

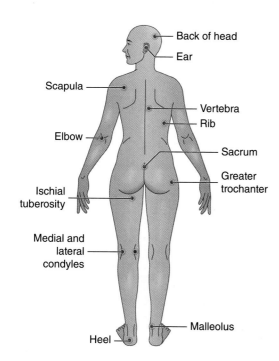

FIGURE 5-20 Use more lubricant around these fragile areas on your elder client.

- Flaccid muscle tissue fibers are easily damaged, and brittle tendons and ligaments are easily torn. Avoid exerting pressure across muscle fibers or against the line of pull of tendons and ligaments.
- Stabilize joints with a supporting hand during any palpation that requires joint movement.
- Avoid downward pressure over bones, especially near the hip joints and the spine. Use light pressure only, toward or away from the midline and at an oblique angle.

Palpating a client who is obese

Palpating a client who is significantly overweight—50 pounds or more—presents a challenge. How do you palpate through a dense layer of subcutaneous adipose tissue to reach fascia or muscle tissue? In many cases, it can't be done with great effectiveness. You must rely on other assessment skills, for example, visual assessment, information gathering, and performing range-of-motion tests, for treatment planning information.

> ### DID YOU KNOW?
>
> The distribution of subcutaneous adipose tissue varies with gender. Women tend to carry more in their breasts, hips, and thighs. Men tend to accumulate fat tissue in the abdomen. Tissue also changes with age throughout the body. Tissue spaces once filled by skeletal muscle are now filled with adipose and fibrous connective tissue. There are also, of course, individual differences in adipose distribution, and genetics plays a role.

Obesity has significant repercussions for somatic tissues:
- Tissue in the dermis and the subcutaneous layer is stretched and strained. This stressed tissue can be quite tender. Palpation pressure may need to be adjusted.

- The weight-bearing joints—hips, knees, ankles, and joints of the feet—are also under stress. Joint capsule components tend to spread laterally in response, especially in the ankles and feet.
- Excess interstitial fluid tends to gather in somatic tissues, which the lymphatic system may not be able to drain sufficiently.

These repercussions of obesity require adjustments in the approach to palpation:

- Avoid the urge to use deeper palpation pressure. Trying harder won't make palpation through dense tissue any more effective and may cause pain in your client's stressed tissues.
- Support joints that may be under strain and work within you client's comfortable range of motion.

IN THE TREATMENT ROOM

Make adjustments in table height, draping, propping, and positioning that will ensure safety and comfort for your client and for you. Placing your obese client in a side-lying position to allow adipose tissue to fall toward the table surface, for example, may allow you to palpate some structures more effectively, but may also require an adjustment in table height.

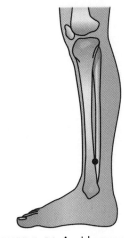

© Milady, a part of Cengage Learning.

FIGURE 5–21 Avoid pressure on the medial leg of a pregnant client.

Palpating a client who is pregnant

Relaxin is a hormone that progressively relaxes soft tissue during pregnancy, allowing the passage of the infant's head out of the birth canal during delivery. Because the effects of Relaxin are bodywide, exercise extra caution during palpation:

- Joints are less stable, and the ligaments around them are easily stretched. Carefully support your client's joints during palpation and avoid overtaxing ligaments.
- Muscle tissue is softer, or "mushier," during pregnancy. This is a natural phenomenon. No amount of exercise or deep bodywork can alter it. Because of this, the usual knots and trigger points in muscles and tendons often subside during pregnancy. Adjust your expectations of what this client's muscles "ought" to feel like.
- Edema in your client's extremities may be a pregnancy-related condition. Avoid palpating directly over any area of edema and refer this client to her obstetrician for evaluation of the cause of the edema.

IN THE TREATMENT ROOM

Avoid palpating the medial leg or the reproductive points, shown in Figure 5–21, around the ankle of a pregnant client.

Lab Activity 5–4 on page 185 is designed to help you accommodate the needs of special client populations during the assessment process.

SUMMARY

The art of palpation utilizes your understanding of sensation and perception, your skill in locating endangerment sites, your knowledge of the cautions and contraindications to palpation, and your comfort with the adjustments necessary for palpating clients in special populations. In Chapter 6, The Art of Palpation, you will learn to master effective palpation and the Four-Step Protocol, a systematic approach to palpating any structure of the body.

LAB ACTIVITIES

LAB ACTIVITY 5–1: RATE OF ADAPTATION

1. Working with a partner, note the rate of adaptation to touch for each of you by timing how long it takes to stop noticing that you are wearing a ring or a bracelet on a different hand or finger, or have removed a ring or bracelet you always wear, or have put on a ring or bracelet, if you usually don't wear one.
2. Next, note your rate of adaptation to temperature by timing how long it takes for each of you to adapt to the heat of water that is 110 °F (about 43°C) or warmer, that is, the time when you no longer perceive the water as warmer than your skin.
3. Compare the results of each exercise: what was the difference in adaptation time for each partner? Was the difference apparent in both exercises? Was the difference noticeable or negligible?

LAB ACTIVITY 5–2: HAND DOMINANCE

1. Working with a partner, time how much longer each task below takes when performed with your non-dominant hand:
   - Write your name on an index card.
   - Button or zip an item of clothing.
   - Find page 212 in this textbook.
   - Enter a phone number on a keypad.
2. Switch partners and repeat. Compare and share your experiences.

LAB ACTIVITY 5–3: LOCATING ENDANGERMENT SITES

1. Working with a partner, follow the directions below to locate, not palpate, these endangerment sites:
Position:
   - Supine partner. Undrape your partner's neck.
   - Stand or sit at the head of the table.
Endangerment sites on the neck:
   - Inferior to the ear: locate the angle of the mandible. *Gently* place your fingertips posterior to it, just below your partner's earlobe. Inch your fingertips progressively lower in this area until you feel the carotid pulse.
   - Anterior and posterior triangles of the neck: locate the angle of the mandible again. *Gently* place your fingertips anterior to it,

in between the vertical fibers of the Sternocleidomastoid (SCM) muscles, locating the anterior triangle of the neck, as shown in Figures 5–8 and 5–9. To locate the posterior triangle, move your fingertips laterally along the clavicle to the mass of muscle fibers at the attachment of Trapezius on the clavicle. The posterior triangle, also visible in Figures 5–8 and 5–9, lies superior to the clavicle and intermediate between SCM and Trapezius.

2. Locate endangerment sites on the arm:

Position:

- Supine partner. Undrape your partner's arm.
- Stand at the side of the table.

Endangerment sites on the arm:

- The axilla: abduct your partner's arm and support her elbow. *Gently* locate the twin masses of muscle and adipose tissue that create the anterior and posterior axillary folds. The axilla lies between these folds, as shown in Figure 5–10.
- The medial arm: *gently* move your fingertips medially and distally on your partner's arm, locating the depression between the bellies of Biceps brachii on the anterior and Triceps brachii on the posterior, shown in Figure 5–10.
- The antecubital area of the elbow: place your partner's arm along the table, with the forearm slightly flexed. *Gently* move your fingertips distally on the anterior arm to locate the anterior bend of the elbow, shown in Figure 5–10.
- The ulnar notch of the elbow: flex your partner's arm and forearm. Just proximal to the elbow joint, *gently* locate the depression on the distal posterior arm, shown in Figure 5–11.

3. Locate the endangerment site on the anterior trunk:

Position:

- Supine partner. Undrape your partner's abdomen and drape the breast area.
- Stand at the side of the table.

Endangerment site on the anterior trunk:

- The abdomen: *gently* place your hands on your partner's upper abdomen. Trace the angle of the anterior ribcage laterally to locate the sites of the underlying organs, shown in Figure 5–12.

4. Locate the endangerment sites on the anterior thigh:

Position:

- Supine partner. Undrape your partner's thigh and ask her to hold the drape securely so that privacy is assured during the work.
- Stand at the side of the table.

Endangerment site on the anterior thigh:

- The femoral triangle, indicated in Figure 5–12: place your partner's thigh in a "Figure 4" position, with the thigh flexed and abducted at the hip. *G*ently locate the depression in the proximal medial thigh between Sartorius on the anterior and the Adductors in the medial thigh with your fingertips.

5. Reposition your partner to locate the endangerment sites on the posterior leg:

Position:

■ Prone partner. Undrape your partner's thigh and leg.

■ Stand at the side of the table.

Endangerment site on the posterior leg:

■ The popliteal fossa: flex your partner's leg and support her ankle. With your fingertips, *gently* locate the depression that lies between the prominent tendons of the hamstring muscles and proximal to the prominent Gastrocnemius muscle in the leg, shown in Figure 5–11.

6. Locate the endangerment site on the posterior trunk:

Position:

■ Prone partner. Undrape your partner's back.

■ Stand at the side of the table.

Endangerment site on the posterior trunk:

■ Upper lumbar area, shown in Figure 5–11: locate the posterior iliac crest and the inferior posterior ribcage. With your fingertips, *gently* locate the area in between these structures, lateral to the spine.

7. Switch partners and repeat. Discuss your experiences and compare notes.

LAB ACTIVITY 5–4: ASSESSING SPECIAL CLIENT POPULATIONS

1. Working in a group, allow half the group members to choose one of the following roles to act out, demonstrating the salient characteristics of the client they are portraying:

■ A client with a recent injury.

■ A client with a chronic illness.

■ An elder client.

■ An obese client.

■ A client who is pregnant.

2. Remaining group members will work with these clients, performing the following tasks:

■ Discussing potential cautions and contraindications with the client.

■ Positioning and draping the client appropriately.

■ Noting to the client one step that will be taken or will be avoided to address her individual condition.

3. Switch partners and repeat until all the group members have played client roles and acted as massage therapists.

4. Exchange feedback on the experience and share the results of feedback with the group and the class.

CASE PROFILES

Case Profile 1

Juan, 45, is a new client who has never had a massage before. For months, he has had pain that travels from his right hip into his lateral leg. He says the pain is deep and aching. Sometimes taking an over the counter pain pill helps, but the pain now tends to return quickly, even after taking his usual dosage. Looking at Table 5–2, how would you characterize Juan's pain? In listening to the words Juan uses to describe his pain, is it likely to be acute, chronic, breakthrough pain, or a combination?

Case Profile 2

Emily, 27, is a nursing assistant in an assisted living facility where she cares for elder patients, sometimes helping them into and out of their wheelchairs. She tells you she has pain, tingling, and numbness in her right hip and sometimes in her right low back. Referring to Table 5–4, what condition could be causing Emily's symptoms? How may this condition impact Emily's perception of touch during palpation?

Case Profile 3

Suzanne, 57, has a chronic autoimmune disease—lupus. She takes multiple medications for her condition, including steroids and prescribed narcotics for pain. What steps will you take to ensure that your palpation of Suzanne's tissues is appropriate and takes into account the possible side effects of her medications that may interfere with her perception of touch?

STUDY QUESTIONS

1. How does the rate of perception of sensation affect palpation, from the standpoint of both the client and the therapist?
2. How does adaptation to sensation affect palpation, from the standpoint of both the client and the therapist?
3. How does dominance in your body affect your palpation findings?
4. What are three conditions that may alter perception of sensation? How might each condition impact the experience of palpation from the standpoint of both the client and the therapist?
5. Describe the location of endangerment sites on the head and neck.
6. Name three sites on the body that are potential areas of injury due to fragile skin, on an elder client.
7. What are two recommendations for safe palpation on a client who is obese?
8. What do you need to know about the medications and dosages taken by a client with a chronic illness?
9. Name two skin conditions that may be systemic contraindications to palpation or massage.
10. Contrast acute and chronic pain; describe words a client may use to describe each type of pain.

The Art of Palpation

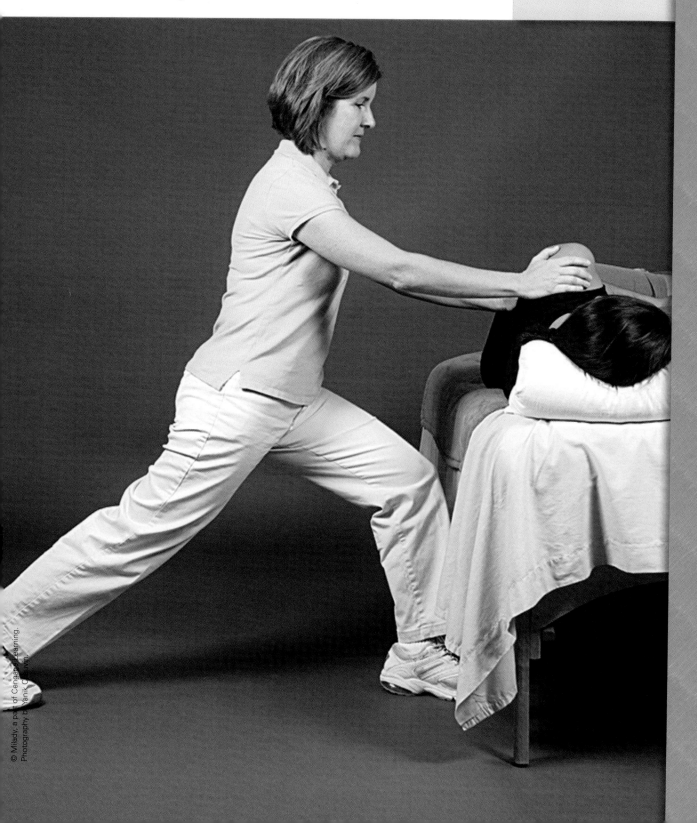

CHAPTER OUTLINE

- **ELEMENTS OF PALPATORY TOUCH**
- **INTEGRATING PALPATION INTO TREATMENT**
- **LAYERS OF PALPATION**
- **THE FOUR-STEP PALPATION PROTOCOL**

LEARNING OBJECTIVES

- Understand and apply exercises to enhance touch sensitivity.
- Apply and gauge the effectiveness of appropriate palpatory pressure on bony landmarks, soft tissue structures, and muscles.
- Describe and apply appropriate, safe, and comfortable palpation pressure.
- Apply appropriate client and self-positioning techniques to palpation.
- Apply techniques for locating target palpation tissues.
- Incorporate safe and effective client actions during muscle palpations.
- Understand and apply safe and effective resistance against client muscle movements.
- Compare and evaluate findings of palpations of bony landmarks, soft tissue structures, and muscles.

INTRODUCTION

Palpation brings together elements of science and art to create a thorough assessment that is also a complete therapeutic experience for the client. In this chapter, you will examine and develop the elements of effective palpation: touch sensitivity and pressure. You will also learn how to apply the Four-Step Palpation Protocol, a systematic approach to palpation of any body structure, which includes positioning yourself and the client, locating **target structures**, adding action and resistance to action, and, finally, evaluating palpation results for treatment planning.

Target structure

the bony landmark, soft tissue structure, or muscle that is selected as the primary palpation site.

ELEMENTS OF PALPATORY TOUCH

Elements that create meaningful palpation are highly developed touch sensitivity and comfortable, effective palpatory pressure.

Touch Sensitivity

Touch sensitivity is your ability to place your hand on your client's body and accurately perceive and characterize the temperature, tone, texture, health, and energy of the tissue layers.

Sensitivity to touch is more effective for palpation than deeper pressure: enhanced touch sensitivity lessens the need for deep palpation pressure.

Touch sensitivity

the ability to place the hand on a client's body and accurately perceive and characterize the temperature, tone, texture, health, and energy of the tissue layers.

Guidelines for enhancing touch sensitivity

Some people seem to be born with greater touch sensitivity than others, and most people have greater sensitivity in their dominant hand. Everyone, however, can work to enhance and equalize their sensitivity to touch by practicing activities such as those described below, and most massage therapists find that their touch sensitivity tends to increase as they gain experience in providing touch.

Guidelines for developing touch sensitivity:

- Use your whole hand for palpation. While the fingertips hold more sense receptors than the rest of the hand, the entire hand is sense-receptor–rich when compared to other areas of the body. Clients are accustomed to the touch of their therapist's whole hand. The touch of a relaxed hand, such as that shown in Figure 6–1, is comforting to the client. Palpating with only the fingertips can feel "pokey" to the client and fails to utilize the sensory input that is available from the whole hand.

- Explore the grain of each muscle, or the condition of bundles of muscle fibers called fascicles. Palpate the fibers in one direction, with the grain, and then at an angle, against the grain, as if strumming slowly across the strings of a guitar.

- Gauge the difference in sensitivity between your dominant and non-dominant hand, with each exercise below. Over time, these exercises will equalize dexterity and touch sensitivity in your non-dominant hand. Perform each exercise with both hands.

- Unless there are safety concerns, work blindfolded or with your eyes closed during these exercises, to eliminate visual distractions. Palpation is about *touch*. Most of the time, it doesn't matter what you're looking at!

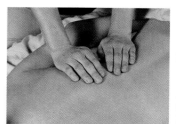

FIGURE 6–1 The still touch of your relaxed hand can be reassuring to your client.

© Milady, a part of Cengage Learning. Photography by Yanik Chauvin.

> **HERE'S A TIP**
>
> With experience, you will develop a sense for the feel of healthy muscle fibers.

> **Lab Activity 6–1** on page 222 is designed to help you develop your touch sensitivity.

IN THE TREATMENT ROOM

Should you use lubricant when palpating? Some therapists feel that lubricant interferes with touch sensitivity, while others are not bothered by palpating over a lubricant. Most therapists agree that applying a lubricant prior to palpation alters the temperature of any structure: water-based lotions tend to cool the skin, while oils tend to be warming. If you feel that lubricant interferes with your palpation, remove it from the area with witch hazel mixed with an equal amount of water on a soft cloth, or complete your palpations before applying lubricant.

Palpation Pressure

Applying appropriate palpation pressure seems to be one of the biggest challenges for the novice massage therapist: how much pressure is enough? How much is too much? There is no simple answer. The most effective level of palpation pressure and individual tolerance for palpation pressure varies from client to client, and from session to session. To develop skills in applying palpation pressure, consider these three factors.

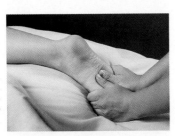

FIGURE 6–2 Palpating deeper bony landmarks, such as on the plantar surface of the foot, may require more palpatory pressure.

HERE'S A TIP

"Muscling" the palpation of a structure—using intense pressure—is almost never the best way to assess it.

Consider the target tissue

Palpating most bony landmarks requires less pressure than is needed to palpate muscle tissue. Often, there is little tissue between a bony landmark and the client's skin. The acromion of the scapula is superficial and easily palpable, but the plantar aspect of the metatarsals lie deep to multiple layers thick muscle fibers, as seen in Figure 6–2. Deeper muscles, such as the lateral rotators of the thigh are located beneath multiple layers of superficial tissue and other muscles.

Is deeper pressure the answer to locating these muscles? Should you push through these superficial muscles in order to palpate a deeper one?

Skilled palpation utilizes less pressure than unskilled palpation. Keep the condition of the target palpation structure in mind when applying pressure: pressure can be deepened, if necessary, but once palpation pressure has been too deep, tissue resistance to touch increases.

Palpation Pressure Guidelines:

- Deep palpation pressure used to locate a bony landmark may bruise the superficial soft tissue. Touch sensitivity, not deeper palpation pressure, results in more effective palpation of deeper bony landmarks and muscle tissue. While deeper pressure may be indicated over some areas of dense muscle tissue and may be tolerated by the client, protect superficial tissues while palpating deep muscles. Highly developed touch sensitivity takes the place of the urge to palpate more deeply than is comfortable or otherwise indicated for the client.

IN THE TREATMENT ROOM

Use gentle palpation pressure over bony landmarks that are just deep to the skin. The focus is on *locating* the landmark. Using deeper palpation pressure does not help you locate a bony landmark.

Mother hand

the non-palpating hand, which is used to stabilize the client's body, to provide secure touch, and to balance the therapist's body position.

- Pay attention to the pressure being applied by the **mother hand**. The mother hand is the non-palpating hand, which in Figure 6–3 is the therapist's left hand, resting on her client's low back. The mother hand may be used to stabilize the client's body, to provide secure touch, and to balance the therapist's body position. The mother hand may be the dominant or non-dominant hand. Which palpating hand is "mothering" may change, depending on what structure you are palpating and where you stand in relation to your client. Endeavor to rest your mother hand on the client's body at all times, even when moving your position.

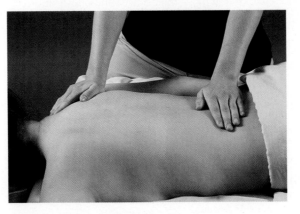

FIGURE 6–3 Your client's sense of security is increased by the touch of your mother hand. Use your whole hand, not just your fingertips, for client comfort and increased palpation feedback.

Effective palpation pressure results in useful palpation feedback. **Palpation feedback** includes the characteristics of the palpated tissue experienced, measured, and described for evaluation purposes, for example:

Palpation feedback

the characteristics of the palpated tissue experienced by the palpating massage therapist.

- Temperature: differences in temperature of tissue from one area or structure to another may indicate inflammation or congestion if the palpated tissue is warmer than surrounding tissue, or stagnation or impaired circulation if the palpated tissue is cooler than nearby tissue.

- Tone is the small amount of tension that remains in skeletal muscles in between contractions. In postural muscles, tone helps us maintain posture. Among the many possible causes, hypertonic muscles may indicate trigger points and fascial restrictions. A hypotonic muscle may be weakened by nerve impingement or because it opposes a hypertonic muscle.
- **Texture** refers to the "grain" of a muscle that reflects the condition of bundles of muscle fibers called fascicles, and may indicate the presence of trigger points and restrictions in the layers of deep fascia that surround muscle fibers and fascicles.

Texture

the palpatory feel of the "grain" of muscle fibers.

- Asymmetry: marked differences in the size or shape contralateral structures, known as asymmetry [ay-SIM-ut-ree], may be the result of repetitive stresses, congenital malformations, pathology, or unknown causes. Any notable asymmetry discovered during palpation indicates postural and gait assessment, as well as discussion with the client about possible repetitive strain due to their occupational and recreational activities.

Palpation feedback is an important assessment tool, one that develops with the application of focused attention. Your awareness of palpation feedback grows with each palpation you perform.

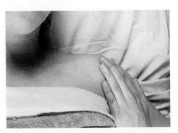

FIGURE 6–4 Effective palpation pressure does not inhibit tissue movement or engage tissue resistance.

IN THE TREATMENT ROOM

When palpating muscles or fascial tissue, use pressure that displaces the first layer of hands-on touch—the skin—and then "sinks" or "melts" gently through the subsequent layers of tissue, as shown in Figure 6–4. Effective palpation pressure *does not inhibit tissue movement or tissue nutrition (blood flow).*

Consider the client

Palpation of a 20-year-old marathon runner differs from palpation of a 60-year-old client with osteoarthritis. The condition of the skin, connective tissue, muscles, joints, and bones of these two very different clients requires adjustments in palpation pressure to guarantee their safety and comfort—the paramount factor in applying palpatory pressure. Younger, healthier tissue is not necessarily more effectively palpated by deeper pressure, however: even a healthy, active muscle will cringe from painfully deep pressure.

IN THE TREATMENT ROOM

Palpation pressure that is too deep may interfere with a muscle action you ask your client to perform, especially if her tactile perception is compromised for any reason.

Palpation Pressure Guidelines:
- Clients with special needs, such as the elderly, the chronically ill, and pregnant women require specific adjustments to palpation pressure. Consider the client's overall condition, including age and vitality level, the condition of target tissues, and both these factors as they appear on the day of treatment, when planning palpation pressure.

Consider soft tissue barriers

Tissue barrier

a pre-existing limitation on the manipulation of a tissue.

A **tissue barrier** is a preexisting limitation on the manipulation of a tissue. Each type of barrier represents a challenge to effective palpation:
- Anatomical barriers are the size and shape of a structure. A client's distribution of adipose tissue in the trunk, for example, may present a barrier to palpation of the abdominal muscles.
- Physiological barriers include the condition of a structure or tissue pathology. A client with severe osteoporosis, for example, may not be able to tolerate even moderate palpation pressure. A client with an inflamed shoulder joint may not be able to perform even a moderate range of motion at that joint.

■ Emotional barriers are those resulting from a client's past or present psychological experiences. They may be expressed by resistance to touch: a client may "guard" the site of past injury or a physical or emotional trauma, making the optimal degree of palpation pressure either inappropriate or ineffective. Another client may have had a negative experience with therapeutic touch and is reluctant to revisit the experience.

HERE'S A TIP

Deeper palpation pressure does not remove barriers to touch or resistance to touch and may, in fact, intensify them.

Palpation Pressure Guidelines:

■ Focus on slowly sinking or melting into tissue, as shown in Figure 6–5. Work with the tissue rather than forcing through it. Work within the client's current range of motion. Don't force more movement than is comfortable. Palpation is not arm wrestling!

IN THE TREATMENT ROOM

Avoid telling your client to relax. If it were that simple, he would have done it himself!

■ Work with your client's breath: suggest a deep breath, breathe along with him, and perform movement and palpation on your client's deep exhalation.

■ Gentle rocking, shown in Figure 6–6, and stabilized shaking may encourage less resistance.

■ If you sense resistance in the target muscle, palpate the contralateral muscle first. You may find less resistance on that side of the body.

■ Encourage receptivity to touch by your relaxed hands and open posture.

■ Use the value of stillness. Your reassuring, quiet touch, just by itself, may go far in helping to dissolve your client's resistance to touch.

■ Ask for feedback from your client about your palpation pressure, and look for signs from your client that your pressure may be too deep: clenching of muscles, breath holding, or increased resistance to movement.

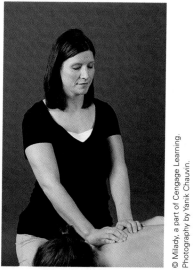

FIGURE 6–5 Deepen your palpation focus by working with your eyes closed.

© Milady, a part of Cengage Learning. Photography by Yanik Chauvin.

Lab Activity 6–2 on page 223 helps you to develop appropriate palpation pressure.

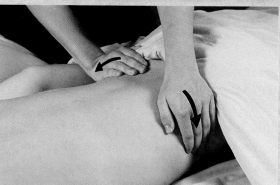

FIGURE 6–6 Work with your client's breath and stabilize his position as you work through tissue barriers or resistance to touch.

© Milady, a part of Cengage Learning. Photography by Yanik Chauvin.

INTEGRATING PALPATION INTO TREATMENT

Integrating palpation techniques into the therapeutic massage session often brings up questions in a new therapist: Do I palpate my client before treatment? Do I try to palpate during a massage, even though it might break the flow? Do I need to palpate again after the massage? Do I palpate a client seated or standing, or only when she's on the table? The answer to each of these questions is, Yes! Absolutely!

Palpating Before Treatment

Various assessments, including palpation, follow the intake interview during an initial appointment and then are repeated, usually after the first treatment and again just before the next treatment. Explain the purpose of palpation and describe the structures you plan to palpate, to include your client in the decision-making process.

Palpation prior to treatment may be done either while your client is clothed, seated, or standing, or once he is lying on the treatment table, disrobed, and fully draped.

- *Be aware that palpating over clothing deprives you of the opportunity to visually inspect your client's skin before palpating.*

Palpating your client's muscles prior to treatment provides:

- A baseline assessment of the condition of your client's muscle and soft tissue texture and tone before they are affected by treatment and as an aid in treatment planning.
- A point of comparison for assessing the effect of treatment by palpation both during and following the massage.
- Reassurance to a client who is new to your practice or new to massage.

Palpating During Treatment

Therapists sometimes worry that palpating individual muscles or soft tissue structures during a massage will interrupt the flow of the work, that palpation will feel "pokey" to the client, compared to soothing massage strokes, or that it might disrupt the session by requiring participation from a client who is deeply relaxed.

Most experienced massage therapists agree that palpation during a massage session can be easily and smoothly incorporated. Even directing muscle actions to your client for palpation during the massage can be done in a nonintrusive manner. With practice, palpation becomes a natural and fluid component of the therapeutic massage experience for both you and your client.

Palpating your client's muscles during treatment allows you to:

- Follow up on findings that were noted during the initial, superficial palpation that was done before treatment.
- Assess a discovery made during the massage that was not reported before the treatment began. Soreness, swelling, pain, or

> ### DID YOU KNOW?
>
> Palpatory touch communicates non-verbally to a new client: "you are safe in my hands."

restrictions in movement may have gone unnoticed by your client until they are revealed by your touch.

- Integrate palpation into your chosen treatment modality.

Palpating Following Treatment

Once the massage has been completed and your client is dressed, a final palpation of the target areas of treatment provides you with:

- An assessment of the effects of treatment.
- Information with which to plan for subsequent treatment.
- A tool for engaging your client in his own care: discussing the results of palpation and treatment leads naturally to educating your client about self-care steps he can take between appointments—stretches and changes in work habits, for example, that will support treatment.

LAYERS OF PALPATION

Once the appropriateness of palpation for your client is assessed and any special needs have been addressed, the next step is selecting the tissues to palpate—the palpation targets. In this section, our focus is on the palpable layers of the body that will yield the most valuable information for treatment planning.

Palpating the Energy Field

The first layer of touch communication with your client is found by resting your hand just above the body surface. You may sense the subtle presence of your client's energy field as slight pressure against the palpating hand, as a vibration, or as a density in the air. Temperature radiating from the surface of your client's body may also be felt at this level.

> **DID YOU KNOW?**
>
> Excessive warmth sensed just above the surface of the body may indicate inflammation in that area, while an area of distinct coolness may indicate poor blood circulation.

Palpating the Skin

The next level of palpation is the skin. Once your client's skin has been visually assessed to assure that it is intact and free of rashes, bruises, or varicosities, you are ready to perform a direct palpation that can reveal a great deal about your client's overall health and the health of his underlying tissues. This is the first level of direct palpatory touch.

- Palpation of the skin results in more accurate assessment of temperature than a visual examination. Potential signs of inflammation, such as heat, pain, and swelling, are more apparent from

> **HERE'S A TIP**
>
> Your initial palpatory touch should be firm, focused, and purposeful.

direct touch. Your client may become aware of sensation only when his skin itself is palpated. At this point, you can gauge his level of sensation: is it as expected, increased, decreased, or lacking? You can also gauge the condition of your client's skin: is it moist or dry, tensile or fragile?

Palpating Fascia

Palpation of the subcutaneous layer of tissue—superficial fascia—is the next layer of assessment. Superficial fascia separates and connects the skin and underlying muscles, and allows free movement between the layers of tissue. Light palpation pressure should allow you to feel fascia as a "springy" cushion.

- Palpation of superficial fascia reveals important assessment information: is movement between the skin and fascial tissue restricted or free? Does your client's skin have a "dimpled" appearance that may indicate structural adhesions between the skin and superficial fascia? Is there an even glide between the layers from one location to another, or is one area "stuck"? Palpation of fascia is described in detail in Chapter 7, Palpating Bony Landmarks and Fascial Structures.

> ### DID YOU KNOW?
>
> Deep fascia supports and surrounds muscle fibers, muscles and muscle groups, and organ compartments. Extensions of deep fascia form tendons, ligaments, and aponeuroses, flat sheets of fascia that connect structures where there is no bony attachment.

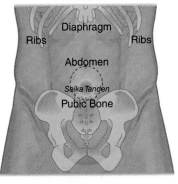

FIGURE 6–7 You may feel pulsing in the area of the *hara* as you palpate the abdomen.

Craniosacral system

the meninges and cerebrospinal fluid that surround and protect the brain and spinal cord, and the related bones of the skull, the spine, and the sacrum.

© Milady, a part of Cengage Learning.

IN THE TREATMENT ROOM

You may sense a pulsing in your client's body as you palpate at deeper levels, below the surface of the skin. Pulsing may indicate one of the following:

- Pulsing in the hara: in Traditional Chinese Medicine, the *hara* [HAR-uh] has great significance—it is considered the "center of being." Pulsing in the *hara* that relates to one of the body's meridians may appear during palpatory touch, intensify—sometimes strongly—and then subside. Anatomically, the *hara* is located where the abdominal aorta splits to become the femoral arteries. For palpation purposes, it encompasses the area of the abdomen bordered by the ribcage, the anterior superior iliac spine (ASIS), and the pubis, shown in Figure 6–7. *Pulsing in the hara that does not subside or is accompanied by pain may indicate an underlying pathology in your client's cardiovascular system that must be evaluated by his primary health care adviser.* The *hara* pulse is separate from and distinguishable from the cardiac pulse.

- Craniosacral pulsing: the **craniosacral system** [kray-nee-oh-SAY-krul SIS-tum] comprises the meninges and cerebrospinal fluid that surround and protect the brain and spinal cord and the related bones of the skull, the spine, and the sacrum. It has a rhythmic pulse, sometimes described as a "shimmering," that reflects the subtle and slightly rotational action of the body, from the midline out, in response to movements in the craniosacral system. The pulsing created by the movement within the semi-closed, craniosacral system is only evident during extremely light touch, approximately the weight of a nickel, and can be felt almost anywhere in the body. It is inhibited by deeper touch, The craniosacral pulse is separate from and distinguishable from the cardiac pulse.

- Cardiac pulse: the cardiac pulse reflects the alternating dilation and constriction of arterial walls that follows each contraction and relaxation of the left ventricle of the heart. The cardiac pulse is most evident in the large arteries near the heart and dissipates toward the periphery, disappearing completely in the capillaries. The pulse is most palpable where arteries are most superficial, such as the radial artery at the wrist or the carotid artery lateral to the larynx. Cardiac pulsing that is evident elsewhere, either visibly or during palpation, especially if accompanied by pain at the site, or which is irregular or unequal bilaterally, may indicate an underlying pathology in your client's cardiovascular system that must be evaluated by his primary health care adviser. *Always delay palpation or treatment of a client who may be put at risk by it until medical clearance has been given to proceed.*

- Pulsing from an unknown cause: we don't understand everything that transpires within the human body. Most bodyworkers have felt pulsing, movements, abrupt changes in temperature, and other phenomena during touch for which there is no adequate explanation. Such occurrences may not be understood, but they can be noted, appreciated, and stored as part of your catalog of palpatory experience.

Palpating Bony Landmarks

- Although bones lie deeper to the body surface than muscles, palpating bony landmarks can be considered the next layer of palpation. By locating bony landmarks, the origins and insertions of individual muscles are accurately defined for palpation. Palpating bony landmarks also reveals postural deviations or imbalances that point you toward palpation of related muscles and muscle groups. Palpation of bony landmarks is described in detail in Chapter 7, Palpating Bony Landmarks and Connective Tissue Structures.

Palpating Muscles

- Direct palpation of the muscle layer of tissue includes palpating the tendinous muscle attachments, the grain of the bundles of fibers of the muscle, and the muscle belly itself. Muscle palpation reveals the tone, texture, and quality of muscle tissue, revealing if the muscle is knotted, fibrotic, flaccid, or firm.

Effective muscle palpation involves locating the target muscle, positioning the client comfortably and applying appropriate pressure, and evaluating the results of effective muscle palpation to guide you in your choice of treatment modality. Palpation of superficial muscles is described in detail in Chapter 8, Palpating Superficial Muscles of the Axial Skeleton and in Chapter 9, Palpating Superficial Muscles of the Extremities. Palpation of deeper muscles is described in detail in Chapter 10, Palpating Deeper Muscles and Muscle Groups.

Trigger point

an extremely irritable nodule in muscle tissue—usually near a tendinous attachment—that elicits acute pain at the site or refers pain elsewhere when palpated directly.

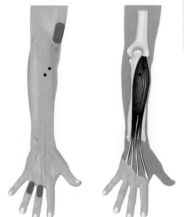

FIGURE 6-8 Trigger points tend to refer symptoms in a predictable pattern.

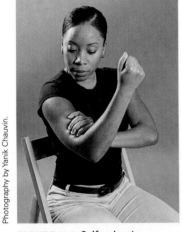

FIGURE 6-9 Self-palpation can be an important first step in learning to palpate layers of tissue.

Lab Activities 6–3 on page 224 and **6–4** on page 224 help you learn how to apply appropriate pressure for different layers of palpation target structures and for clients with barriers to touch.

IN THE TREATMENT ROOM

Your client may not be aware of pain or restrictions in movement until they arise during touch. Sometimes, your client's report of pain in one site is caused by a **trigger point**, an extremely irritable nodule in muscle tissue that causes acute pain at the site or refers pain elsewhere when palpated directly, as shown in Figure 6–8, or causes some restriction at an adjacent or even distant site. Pain, numbness, or tingling caused by the impingement of a nerve by a trigger point or fascial restriction, for example, is often sensed in an area distal to the site of the impingement.

Self-Palpation

Palpating your own structures may help you to accurately locate bony landmarks, connective tissue structures, and muscle bellies, as shown in Figure 6–9, Self-palpation can also be an important, comfortable first step in comparing tissue tone, temperature, and texture, and for learning how to apply palpation pressure:

- Designate your body structures realistically: is your tissue 23 or 65 years old? Are you obese, chronically ill, or pregnant? Self-palpation is most useful as a tool for comparison of tissues if you are comparing apples to apples, not apples to oranges.
- Use self-palpation to assess the comfortable level of pressure for locating bony landmarks; to experience the texture and mobility of ligaments, tendons, and aponeuroses; and to experience the orientation and depth of muscle fibers.
- Follow self-palpation with immediate palpation of another person's structures, whenever possible, to reap the benefits of tissue comparison.

DID YOU KNOW?

When you practice palpation techniques on your own body structures, sensory receptors in two locations, in your palpating hand and in the structure you are palpating, are stimulated to conduct impulses to two different areas of the brain, requiring two different types of integration: "Hey, my leg is being touched! What should I do?" and, "Hey, I'm touching my leg. What does that mean?" Perception of two simultaneous events occurs.

THE FOUR–STEP PALPATION PROTOCOL

The Four–Step Palpation Protocol is a systematic approach to palpation that creates dependable palpation results for treatment planning.

- First, you select and create the optimal positions for the client and for yourself for palpation of the palpation target structures.
- Second, you locate each palpation target, transferring your knowledge of anatomy into your hands to locate specific bony attachments, muscle attachments, and muscle fibers.

TABLE 6-1

THE FOUR-STEP PALPATION PROTOCOL
STEP #1
Position: you position your client for optimal comfort and access for palpation of target structures, and position yourself for comfort and effectiveness of technique.
STEP #2
Location: you use your knowledge of human anatomy to correctly and comfortably place your hands on the palpation target structure.
STEP #3
Action and resistance: you direct your client to perform an action of the muscle you are palpating. You may apply resistance in the form of gentle pressure on a body structure to prevent further muscle movement during palpation.
STEP #4
Evaluation: you characterize the results of your palpation and note the results for use in treatment planning.

- Third, if the palpation target is a muscle, you direct the client to perform that muscle's actions during palpation, transferring your knowledge of muscle actions into your hands to evaluate the movement of muscle fibers during the contraction–relaxation cycle. You may apply resistance to the action of the palpation target muscle, introducing an additional, controlled level of stress on the muscle that makes its action more apparent.
- Fourth, you evaluate the results of your palpations—name and quantify them—to create a specific and effective treatment plan for your client.

Table 6–1 summarizes the Four-Step Palpation Protocol.

IN THE TREATMENT ROOM

Ask yourself these questions before you palpate your client:

- What structures am I palpating? The choice of which bony landmarks, soft tissue structures and muscles to palpate is made with information from two sources: what your client tells you and what your eyes and hands tell you. Subjective reporting includes your client's description of his pain and his experience of what makes the pain worse and what makes it better. Objective findings are what your assessments of your client's posture and gait reveal and what your hands discover during the massage.
- What am I looking for? Your knowledge of the body and your experience as a practitioner provides you with an accumulation of information for decision-making, such as common locations for trigger points and predictable pain-referral patterns.

Palpation may show you something quite different from what you went looking for. This process of discovery is one of the great learning experiences for every massage therapist!

Step One: Positioning for Palpation

Positioning for palpation includes not only the position of the client's body relative to your stance but also the position of your hands.

Client positioning and draping

There is seldom only one "correct" draping procedure or client position for palpation of any structure. There are simply too many variables found in the real life treatment room to limit you to one choice of palpation position or drape. The client position and draping suggested in the subsequent chapters are those that experience has proven to be the safest, most comfortable and most effective. Alternate positions and draping are presented, and creativity within the bound of safety, comfort, and effectiveness is encouraged.

The choice of client position depends on the target structure to be palpated and whether the palpation is part of the initial assessment that occurs before the client is on the table or is performed during treatment, when the client is undressed and draped on the table. Take these factors into account when choosing a safe, comfortable, and effective position for palpation:

- The location of the target structure to be palpated, your client's size relative to yours, and the degree of your client's mobility.
- Ease of the position for your client: the palpation position should never cause pain or discomfort or place stress on your client's tissues or joints—even for a moment.
- Effectiveness of the position for your purpose: proper body mechanics don't place stress on your joints or muscles, either, or require you to assume a position that might result in strain or injury.

IN THE TREATMENT ROOM

Take the time to keep your client comfortable:

- Place or remove bolsters to facilitate properly aligned client positioning before palpating, as shown in Figure 6–10.
- Reposition your client for effective palpation without strain, if the target structure cannot be effectively palpated in his current position.
- Adjust positioning and draping to the needs of the client, not the needs of your technique.

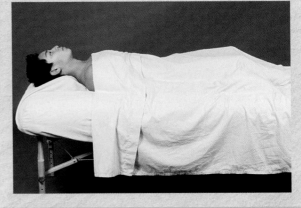

FIGURE 6–10 Take the time to place or remove bolsters to facilitate proper alignment for your client's body.

Draping maintains client security while allowing access to the target structure for palpation. Take these factors into account when draping for palpation:

- If you plan to palpate a target structure on both sides of the body, undrape and tuck the drape on both sides of the body before beginning the palpations.

- Tuck the drape securely, so that it remains in place during movement of your client's extremities, as shown in Figure 6–11.

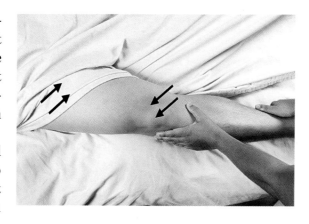

FIGURE 6–11 Secure draping allows your client to relax as you focus on performing effective palpations.

- Keep a full-sized sheet on hand to use as a top sheet during palpation of a client in side-lying position to avoid potential exposure of intimate body parts, and use a large towel or pillowcase to cover the breast area during supine palpations on your female client's torso.

- For palpation of some structures, such as the pectorals or the adductors, it is advisable to ask your client to grasp the drape and hold it securely, as shown in Figure 6–12.

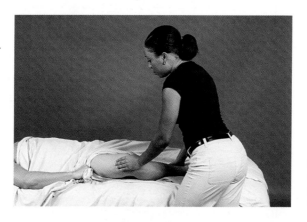

FIGURE 6–12 Palpating your client while standing allows for assessment of structures during weight-bearing.

- Palpate through the drape, if necessary to maintain client comfort. As your touch sensitivity develops, draping through the sheet or through clothing becomes more effective.

HERE'S A TIP

Throughout the text, draping recommendations are described with each individual palpation instruction.

Palpation may be done with the client standing or seated while clothed, or with the client supine, prone, or in side-lying position on the treatment table, under a drape.

Palpation with your client standing:

- As shown in Figure 6–13, this is a valuable tool for assessing skeletal structures while your client is weight-bearing and gives you simultaneous access to structures on both the anterior and posterior of the trunk.

- You can easily give verbal instructions for palpation actions to the client while he is in a standing position.

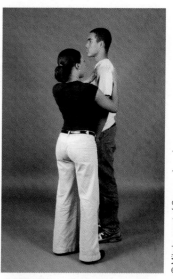

FIGURE 6–13 Palpating your client while standing allows for assessment of structures during weight-bearing.

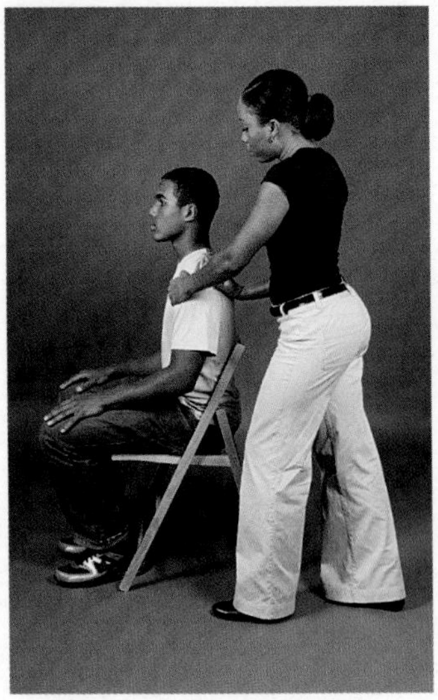

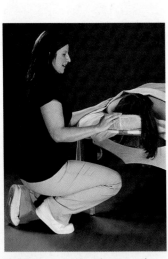

FIGURE 6-14 Palpating your client in a seated position that allows easy access to target structures while working comfortably.

© Milady, a part of Cengage Learning. Photography by Yanik Chauvin.

FIGURE 6-15 You can easily give verbal instructions for palpation actions to the client while she is in a supine position.

© Milady, a part of Cengage Learning. Photography by Yanik Chauvin.

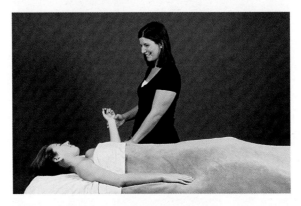

FIGURE 6-16 Kneel or crouch beside your prone client to facilitate verbal communication.

© Milady, a part of Cengage Learning. Photography by Yanik Chauvin.

IN THE TREATMENT ROOM

If your client is significantly taller or shorter than you, palpation of structures on his head, neck, or trunk may be more comfortably accomplished with one of you seated. Support his posture by placing your mother hand so that it counters palpation pressure and your client is not pushed off-balance. Ask your standing client to remove his shoes. Heel height and angle will impact your assessment of his skeletal structures. Even 1" to 2" (2.5–5 cm) heels can exaggerate a lordotic spinal curvature.

Palpation with your client seated:

■ As shown in Figure 6–14, this gives you simultaneous access to structures on both the anterior and posterior of your client's trunk, without the client bearing his weight. You can easily palpate opposing muscles that act on the trunk, the neck, and the arm, and gauge the full range of motion of the shoulder joint.

■ Seat your client at a level that allows easy access to target structures while working comfortably—without raising your shoulders or hunching over your client.

■ Support the client's posture by placing your mother hand so that it counters palpation pressure and your client is not pushed off-balance.

■ You can easily give verbal instructions for palpation actions to the client while he is in a seated position.

Palpation with your client lying supine on the treatment table:

■ As shown in Figure 6–15, this client position gives you access to all of your client's anterior structures, without the encumbrance of clothing. Since your client is not weight-bearing, it also allows palpation of thigh, leg, and foot structures in passive extension.

■ You can easily give verbal instructions for palpation actions to the client while she is in a supine position.

Palpating with your client lying prone on the treatment table:

■ As shown in Figure 6–16, palpating your prone client gives you access to all your client's posterior structures, without the encumbrance of clothing. Since the client is not weight-bearing, it also allows palpation of hip, thigh, leg, and foot structures in passive extension.

■ Verbal communication may be more difficult with your client lying prone. He may wish to turn his head to ease communication. If this is uncomfortable, you can squat or kneel to speak directly into his ear to give verbal instructions before you palpate.

Palpating with the client in side-lying position on the treatment table:

■ Palpating a side-lying client, as in Figure 6–17, allows you easy access to structures on the lateral aspect, such as Serratus anterior,

Tensor fasciae latae, the iliotibial band, and the peroneal muscles. The side-lying position facilitates palpation of some otherwise hard-to-access muscles, such as Subscapularis and allows easy, full range-of-motion assessment of the ball-and-socket joint at the shoulder.

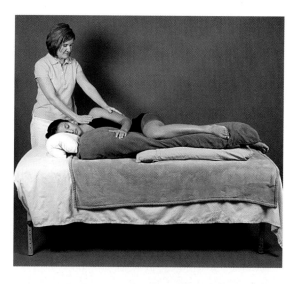

FIGURE 6–17 Placing your client in side-lying position opens up the lateral aspect of the body for palpation and treatment.

© Milady, a part of Cengage Learning. Photography by Yanik Chauvin.

IN THE TREATMENT ROOM

You can easily give verbal instructions for palpation actions to the client while he is in a side-lying position.

HERE'S A TIP

Take the time to create a comfortable, stable side-lying position for your client:

Setting up:

- Note that your client's shoulders and hips will be raised higher off the table in side-lying position. Lower the height of your table.
- Use a full-sized sheet as a top cover to provide complete draping security for a larger client.
- Place pillows, bolsters, or a full-body supporting system, pictured in Figure 6–17, to eliminate pressure or stress on joints and to support all the body's structures.

Positioning:

- Beginning with your client prone or supine, ask him to turn *toward you* to lie on his side to prevent him from rolling off the table. As an added cue, place your hand on the shoulder that you want to be turned toward you as you give the instruction.
- Once your client is lying on his side, place pillows under his head so that his spine is in alignment from the occiput to the sacrum, and pressure on his shoulder joint is eliminated.
- Suggest to your client that he place his upper arm, the arm not lying on the table, outside the sheet. This keeps the drape secure and allows access to the arm and shoulder. Ask him to bend both arms 90° at the elbow, for comfort. Offer your client a pillow to grasp in front of him, for added upper-body stability.

Aligning:

- Standing or kneeling beside the table, align your arm alongside your client's spine at his back, as in Figure 6–18. Ask him to adjust the position of

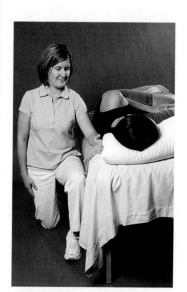

FIGURE 6–18 Align the position of your client's head to assure a straight line from the occiput to the sacrum.

© Milady, a part of Cengage Learning. Photography by Yanik Chauvin.

his head, usually backward, so that both the sacrum and the base of the skull lie against your arm and hand. Your client's spine should be aligned along the straight line of your arm, from his occiput to his sacrum.

■ Resting on your elbow, raise your forearm vertically from the table surface, to gauge the angle of your client's shoulders: they should be level at a 90° angle from the table, as in Figure 6–19. Suggest to your client the adjustment that will level his shoulders to that angle, or you can gently grasp the head of the humerus on his bottom shoulder to adjust his shoulder alignment yourself.

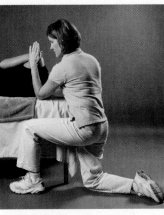

© Milady, a part of Cengage Learning. Photography by Yanik Chauvin.

FIGURE 6–19 Create a 90° angle at the shoulders to keep your client from slumping forward.

■ Ask your client to straighten his bottom leg, the leg that lies on the table, and flex his top leg to a 90° angle at both the hip and the knee. Place a large bolster or more pillows beneath that leg at the knee and ankle joints, so that the hip, knee, and ankle are level and equidistant above the table, as in Figure 6–20. Straighten the lower leg on the bolster from the knee to the ankle to the foot, and make sure the foot is supported on the bolster.

■ Verify that your client feels secure and comfortable in his position before you begin palpating.

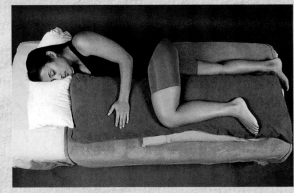

FIGURE 6–20 Keep the hip, knee and ankle level and equidistant above the table.

Additional tips for using the side-lying position:

■ Avoid bending your trunk laterally while working with your client in side-lying position. Bend your knees to work from your center of gravity.

■ Note that with your client in side-lying position, your pressure will be outward, as shown in Figure 6–21, not downward. Use your mother hand to counter palpation pressure, to keep your client's torso in alignment and to apply resistance to muscle actions.

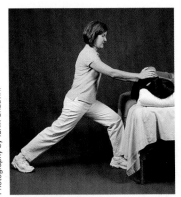

© Milady, a part of Cengage Learning. Photography by Yanik Chauvin.

FIGURE 6–21 Palpation pressure on a side-lying client is outward, not downward. Adjust your table height accordingly.

■ Consider lowering your table one or two notches to accommodate proper body mechanics when working with your client in side-lying position.

■ Recheck your client's alignment in side-lying position after each palpation, to ensure that his torso is not slumping forward or backward.

■ Remove all pillows and bolsters before repositioning your client into a supine or prone position or into the side-lying position on his opposite side.

Lab Activity 6–5 on page 225 helps you learn how to effectively position your client for palpation.

LEARNING ENHANCEMENT ACTIVITY

Commit to placing a "client" (practice with a friend) in the side-lying position on a massage table at least 10 times in the next 30 days. Practice moving your client from both supine and prone positions into side-lying. Practice moving the client from the side-lying position into a supine or prone position. Practice turning the client from lying on his left side to lying on his right side.

Massage Therapist Positioning

You will almost certainly move and reposition both yourself and your client frequently during palpation. You may even need to change positions during the palpation of a single structure, perhaps to palpate the grain of muscle tissue from more than one direction. Avoid staying planted in one position or working with a lowered head and hunched shoulders, as shown in Figure 6–22. Move whenever necessary to maintain body alignment, and make sure that changes in position accommodate proper body mechanics.

Maintaining good body mechanics during palpation calls for creativity and flexibility. Take the time to protect your best tool—your body. Good body mechanics, pictured in Figure 6–23, includes these posture adjustments:

- Keep your back straight, knees bent, the shoulders level, and the head up: no hunching or bending.
- Face the direction of your stroke or palpation: no contorting.
- Point your feet in the direction of force or movement: no twisting.
- Stand over your center of gravity: a low center of gravity ensures stability and less back strain.

Table 6–2 summarizes good palpation body mechanics.

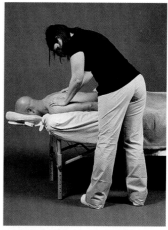

FIGURE 6–22 Poor body mechanics result in discomfort for you and poor quality of touch for your client.

IN THE TREATMENT ROOM

Palpation is highly focused work. It's easy to forget the basics of smart work habits:

- Keep breathing. Holding your breath while palpating tightens your muscles, interfering with effective palpation. Holding your breath relays a message of distress to your client, while deep, relaxed breathing loosens tight shoulders, arms, and hands and transmits a message of relaxation.
- Occasionally close your eyes. When you close your eyes, you raise your head and straighten your shoulders to stabilize your balance, contributing to good body mechanics.
- Value stillness. Although movement is important to maintain good body mechanics, stillness is invaluable for palpation. Use stillness to create space for your client to breathe and to experience his response to palpation. Use stillness as a tool for deepening your touch sensitivity and for listening to what your client's body has to say.

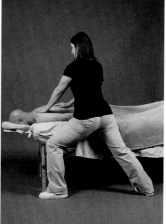

FIGURE 6–23 Good body mechanics are as important during palpation as they are during any other phase of your work.

TABLE 6–2

POOR AND PREFERRED PALPATION BODY MECHANICS	
POOR PALPATION BODY MECHANICS	PREFERRED PALPATION BODY MECHANICS
Head is down, looking closely at the palpation target structure.	Head is up, with eyes closed to help direct focus and maintain good posture.
One shoulder is lifted to accommodate the palpating hand position.	Shoulders are level, arms and hands are relaxed and in contact with the client.
Back is twisted to reach the target structure.	Back is straight, not twisted.
Hips face the table, no matter where the palpation pressure will be applied.	Hips face the direction of palpation pressure.
Weight is shifted to one side of the body.	Weight is evenly distributed on both feet.
Feet face the table, no matter where the palpation pressure will be applied.	Feet face the direction of palpation pressure.
Feet remain planted in one spot, regardless of the position of the palpating hands.	Feet are repositioned whenever necessary, to accommodate changes in the direction of the palpating hand.

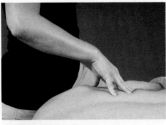

© Milady, a part of Cengage Learning. Photography by Yanik Chauvin.

FIGURE 6–24 Poor hand positions are uncomfortable for you and for your client.

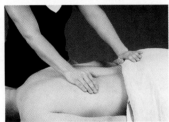

© Milady, a part of Cengage Learning. Photography by Yanik Chauvin.

FIGURE 6–25 Using your whole, relaxed hands with your wrists in "neutral" is smart for you and comfortable for your client.

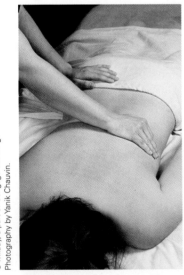

© Milady, a part of Cengage Learning. Photography by Yanik Chauvin.

FIGURE 6–26 As you work from medial to lateral on your client's trunk, alter the position of your palpating hand to accommodate the curves of the body

Lines of cleavage

the linear clefts in the skin that indicate the direction of its fibers.

TABLE 6–3

POOR AND PREFERRED PALPATING HAND POSITIONS	
POOR PALPATING HAND POSITIONS	**PREFERRED PALPATING HAND POSITIONS**
Palpating only with the fingertips.	Palpating with the whole hand.
Raising most of the hand off the client's body.	Resting the palpating hand on the client's body.
Hyperextending the wrist.	Keeping the wrist in "neutral".
Hyperextending the fingers.	Keeping the fingers only slightly flexed.
Positioning the palpating hand counter to the curve of a structure.	Positioning the palpating hand along the curve of a structure.
Tightening the hand to maintain fingertips-only touch.	Relaxing the hand to increase sensory input and reassure the client.
Maintaining touch with only one hand, not using the mother hand.	Maintaining touch with both hands, using the mother hand.

© Milady, a part of Cengage Learning.

Positioning for palpation includes attention to the positions of both the palpating hand and the mother hand. Working with relaxed hands and working with the whole hand is as important to palpation as it is to effleurage. The client should never feel that he is being poked or prodded.

The position of your palpating hand must be both comfortable for you and effective for palpation, while your mother hand rests on your client's body nearby or functions during palpation.

Table 6–3 compares poor palpating hand positions, shown in Figure 6–24, to preferred positions, shown in Figure 6–25.

Step Two: Locating Target Structures

Palpating a structure depends on accurately locating it. Each body is unique. Although almost everyone's spine has 24 vertebrae, if all our vertebrae were exactly the same size we'd all be exactly the same height! Your palpation skills deepen as you experience the variety of individual structures within the shared human anatomical framework.

Guidelines for locating target structures

With time and experience, you will develop the location methods that work best for you. Here are some useful guidelines.

Locating target structures on the trunk:

- Palpate from the medial aspect to the lateral aspect, as shown in Figure 6–26. Working from the midline out, following the rounded shape of the trunk, is more comfortable for the client.
- The flow of arterial systemic circulation and the direction of the fibers of most superficial trunk muscles.
- The pathway of dermatomes and the **lines of cleavage**, the linear clefts in the skin that indicate the direction of its fibers, illustrated in Figure 6–27.
- The direction of many Swedish massage strokes of the trunk.

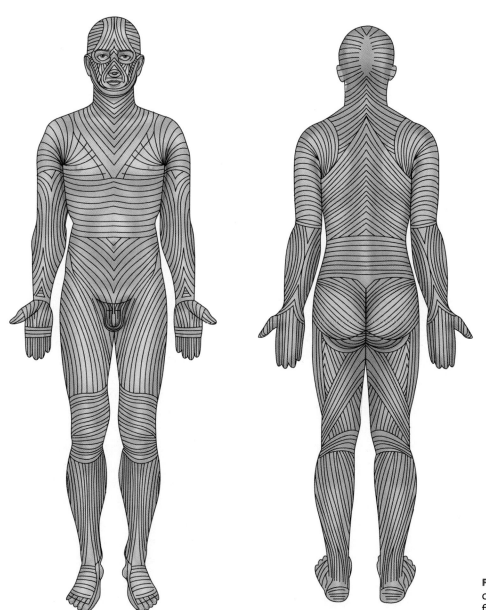

FIGURE 6–27 The lines of cleavage indicate the direction of fibers in the skin.

IN THE TREATMENT ROOM

You may find it easier to palpate some structures on the trunk from the opposite side of the table. This stance allows you to follow the roundedness of the trunk with ease, without hyperextending your wrist, and allows you to use your whole palpating hand. You may decide to use your mother hand to stabilize the trunk while palpating across the body. Using the range of positions—supine, prone, and side-lying—may be necessary to completely palpate all the structures on your client's trunk while he is on the table.

HERE'S A TIP

Working against the direction of the lines of cleavage may place stress on delicate skin.

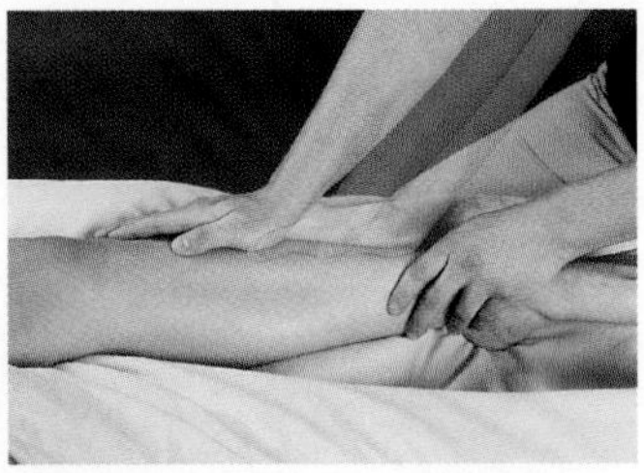

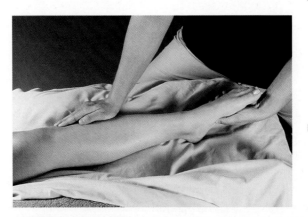

FIGURE 6–28 Palpating from distal to proximal on the limbs facilitates the location of bony landmarks.

Locating target structures on the extremities:

- Palpate from the distal aspect to the proximal aspect, as shown in Figure 6–28. Working in a proximal direction on the arms and the legs facilitates location of bony landmarks as your hands glide up the shaft of the long bones. This directional approach respects:
  1. The flow of arterial systemic circulation and the direction of the fibers of most superficial trunk muscles.
  2. The pathway of dermatomes and the lines of cleavage.
  3. The direction of many Swedish massage strokes of the extremities.

IN THE TREATMENT ROOM

You can easily locate most of the structures on the extremities with your client supine or prone. The structures on the lateral thigh and leg, such as the greater trochanter of the femur, the iliotibial band, tensor fasciae latae, and the peroneal muscles, are easier to locate with your client in side-lying position.

Procedures for locating target structures

The recommended order for locating structures for muscle palpation is:

- First: bony landmarks and sites of the origins and insertions of the target muscle.
- Next: fascial structures such as tendons, ligaments, and other connective tissue structures, for muscle palpation.
- Finally: the muscle itself—the belly and all the muscle's fibers.

Using Tibialis anterior as an example, with your partner supine on the massage table:

- Work with your eyes closed and your hands relaxed. Focus on your position and body mechanics and your palpation pressure and touch sensitivity. Remind yourself that palpation is meaningful touch.
- Position and drape your client appropriately.

FIGURE 6–29 Locating bone landmarks orients you to the attachment sites of Tibialis anterior, the target muscle in this palpation.

- Locate the bony landmarks: the insertion is the base of the first metatarsal and the origin is the lateral condyle and proximal surface of the tibia.
- Gently palpate each of the attachment sites by placing one hand at each location, as shown in Figure 6–29.

IN THE TREATMENT ROOM

The base of the first metatarsal is often quite tender. Palpate gently.

- Locate the muscle tendon: the lengthy and visible tendinous portion of Tibialis anterior extends from the muscle belly to its insertion. Follow the path of the tendon, shown in Figure 6–30, as it crosses from its insertion on the medial foot toward the muscle belly on the lateral aspect of the tibia.
- Locate the muscle belly and fibers: palpate proximally from the tendinous portion of Tibialis anterior, as shown in Figure 6–31, taking time to explore the grain of the muscle fibers and to note any fascial restrictions or trigger points in the muscle fibers.
- Seek feedback from your client: is the palpation pressure comfortable? Are there any areas of tenderness or pain in the palpated structure?

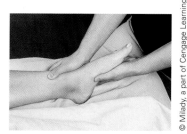

FIGURE 6–30 The distal tendon of Tibialis anterior crosses from the lateral tibia toward its insertion on the medial foot.

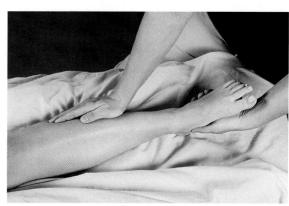

Palpate slowly and thoroughly, with these questions in mind:

- Temperature of the muscle tissue: is it warmer or cooler to the touch than surrounding tissue?
- Tone of the tissue: is it **hypertonic**, increased in muscle tone? Is it **hypotonic**, lacking in muscle tone?
- Texture of the tissue: is it flaccid? Rigid?

Having located the structural components of the target Tibialis anterior, complete the same procedure on the contralateral Tibialis anterior. Compare temperature, tone, and texture, while being alert to asymmetry in the muscles.

FIGURE 6–31 Explore the grain of the muscle belly of Tibialis anterior from all directions.

Hypertonic

an excess of tone in a skeletal muscle.

Hypotonic

a lack of functional tone in a skeletal muscle.

Lab Activity 6–6 on page 226 helps you learn how to locate palpation target structures.

Step Three: Directing Muscle Actions

Once you locate the palpation target components—the bony landmarks, tendons, and the tissue of the muscle—you can proceed with active palpation, palpating muscle fibers during contraction, by directing the client to perform a muscle action during the palpation.

Terminology for directing muscle actions

Massage therapists are trained to use correct terminology for anatomical structures and joint movements. It is the language of health care professions. In speaking with clients, however, everyday language is often more accessible. Develop a set of layperson's terms to use with clients: asked to "radially deviate" his right hand, your client is probably lost, and most people outside the health professions describe any muscle contraction as "flexing." It's up to you to adjust your language in order to communicate clearly:

- Be mindful of the client's ability to receive direction: most people depend on visual cues for complete communication. A client who is lying prone or supine in a darkened room, is deeply relaxed, or who is without his customary vision or hearing devices, may need additional prompting in order to follow directions.

■ Avoid giving more than one direction at once. Keep communication simple and straightforward. Check to make sure the client understands the direction.

■ Direct the action with the client's position in mind. "Lift" or "to the side" may mean something completely different to the client who is lying prone than it does to you, who is standing.

■ Consider the structure being moved. To direct actions of the arm at the shoulder, for example, the layperson's terms might include "lift" for flexion, "reach back" for extension, "raise to the side" for abduction, and "bring back to your side" for adduction. When directing rotational actions, using "turn your (or head, arm, or leg) toward . . ." is the clearest alternative.

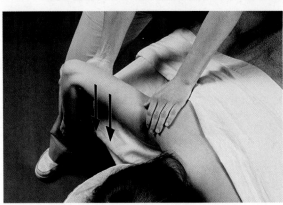

FIGURE 6-32 To clarify your desired action, first lead your client through passive movement before asking your client to perform the action.

■ Reinforce the direction, especially if you suspect that using a lay term may not be adequate. If the client is supine, demonstrate the desired action for him. If your client is prone, touch the structure to be moved and lead her through the action passively, as shown in Figure 6–32, before asking her to perform the action unassisted.

■ If the steps outlined above fail to communicate the requested action to your client, place your hands gently on the structure you want moved and gently press it *in the direction of the movement you want.* Say to your client, "Please move (or turn) away from my hand."

A list of terms for muscle actions that you develop yourself may more useful than memorizing a list of terms someone else has made up. Your clients know how you use words—they'll respond to language that is familiar to them. To begin with, however, try using the directions for movement listed in Table 6–4. Remember that these are suggestions for terms to use with your clients, and should be accompanied by gestures that clarify your intention.

LEARNING ENHANCEMENT ACTIVITY

Create a list of alternative terms for muscle actions that you feel will be easily understood by clients. Use as many terms from your list as you can with your classmates and practice clients when performing each of your next ten massages. Keep notes on your results, revise your list, and adopt the terms that work best for your clients.

TABLE 6-4

SUGGESTED LAY MOVEMENT TERMINOLOGY	
MOVEMENT	SUGGESTED DIRECTION
Flexion of the head at spinal joints	"Bring your chin down toward your chest."
Extension of the head at spinal joints	"Bring your head back up" or "Look up at the ceiling."
Lateral flexion of the head at spinal joints	"Bring your ear down toward your shoulder."
Rotation of the head at spinal joints	"Turn your head to look behind you."
Depression of the jaw at the temporomandibular joint	"Drop your jaw."
Elevation of the jaw at the temporomandibular joint	"Close your mouth."
Protraction of the jaw at the temporomandibular joint	"Stick your jaw out."
Retraction of the jaw at the temporomandibular joint	"Bring your jaw backward."
Lateral deviation of the jaw at the temporomandibular joint	"Move your jaw from side to side."
Flexion of the trunk at spinal joints	"Bend forward from your waist."
Extension of the trunk at spinal joints	"Stand back up straight" or "Bend backward at your waist."
Lateral flexion of the trunk at spinal joints	"Bend sideways from your waist."
Rotation of the trunk at spinal joints	"Turn from your shoulders to look behind you."
Elevation of the shoulder at scapulocostal joints	"Shrug your shoulders."
Depression of the shoulder at scapulocostal joints	"Bring your shoulders back down" or "Drop your shoulders down."
Protraction of the shoulder at scapulocostal joints	"Reach forward with your arm."
Retraction of the shoulder at scapulocostal joints	"Bring your shoulder back again" or "Move your shoulder backward."
Flexion of the arm at the glenohumeral joint	"Raise your arm to the front."
Extension of the arm at the glenohumeral joint	"Bring your arm back down" or "Reach straight back with your arm."
Abduction of the arm at the glenohumeral joint	"Raise your arm out to the side."
Adduction of the arm at the glenohumeral joint	"Bring your arm back down to your side" or "Reach across your chest."
Medial rotation of the arm at the glenohumeral joint	"Turn your arm in so you can see your elbow."
Lateral rotation of the arm at the glenohumeral joint	"Turn your arm out so you can reach behind."
Circumduction of the arm at the glenohumeral joint	"Make a circle with your arm."
Flexion of the forearm at the humeroulnar joint	"Bend your arm at the elbow."
Extension of the forearm at the humeroulnar joint	"Straighten your arm at the elbow."
Pronation of the forearm at the radioulnar joints	"Turn your hand down toward the floor."
Supination of the forearm at the radioulnar joints	"Turn your hand up toward the ceiling."
Flexion of the wrist at the radiocarpal joint	"Bend your wrist toward your elbow."
Extension of the wrist	"Straighten your wrist."
Radial deviation (abduction) of the wrist at the radiocarpal joint	"Move your hand toward your thumb."

(continued)

TABLE 6-4   *continued*

MOVEMENT	SUGGESTED DIRECTION
Ulnar deviation (adduction) of the wrist at the radiocarpal joint	"Move your hand away from your thumb."
Flexion of the fingers at the MCP and IP joints	"Bend your fingers."
Extension of the fingers at the MCP and IP joints	"Straighten your fingers."
Anterior tilt of the pelvis at the lumbosacral joint	"Stick your buttocks out."
Posterior tilt of the pelvis at the lumbosacral joint	"Pull your buttocks in."
Elevation of the pelvis at the lumbosacral joint	"Raise this hip."
Depression of the pelvis at the lumbosacral joint	"Push this hip down."
Flexion of the thigh at the acetabulofemoral joint	"Raise your leg to the front."
Extension of the thigh at the acetabulofemoral joint	"Bring your leg back down" or "Push your leg backward."
Medial rotation of the thigh at the acetabulofemoral joint	"Turn your knee inward."
Lateral rotation of the thigh at the acetabulofemoral joint	"Turn your knee out to the side."
Abduction of the thigh at the acetabulofemoral joint	"Lift your leg out to the side."
Adduction of the thigh at the acetabulofemoral joint	"Bring your leg back down" or "Bring your leg across your body."
Circumduction of the thigh at the acetabulofemoral joint	"Make a circle with your leg."
Flexion of the leg at the tibiofemoral joint	"Bend your leg at the knee."
Extension of the leg at the tibiofemoral joint	"Straighten your leg at the knee."
Dorsiflexion of the foot at the talocrural joint	"Point your foot toward your head."
Plantarflexion of the foot at the talocrural joint	"Point your foot away from your head."
Inversion of the foot at the intertarsal joints	"Turn your ankle in."
Eversion of the foot at the intertarsal joints	"Turn your ankle out."
Flexion of the toes at the MTP and IP joints	"Curl your toes under."
Extension of the toes at the MTP and IP joints	"Straighten your toes."

Guidelines for directing muscle actions

Complete muscle palpation includes:

- Palpating the fibers of both the target and contralateral muscles in their resting state.
- Palpating muscle fibers during contraction.
- Palpating the agonist, antagonist, and one or more synergists in a particular action.

Before directing a muscle action, perform these initial palpations:

- Palpate the resting target muscle first: assessing the temperature, tone, and texture of the muscle fibers in their resting state gives you a baseline of tactile input on the target muscle.
- Palpate the resting conralateral muscle next, to assess it in its resting state.
- When possible, palpate the resting target and contralateral muscles at the same time, as in Figure 6–33, to gain simultaneous input about any asymmetry in these muscles.

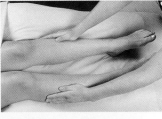

FIGURE 6-33 Palpate target muscles bilaterally to compare tone, temperature, and texture.

Follow these initial palpations by palpating the target muscle during different types of movement. Complete palpation includes assessment of all three types of movement:

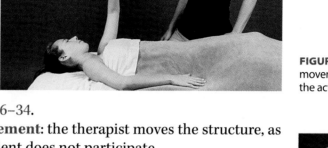

Milady, a part of Cengage Learning. Photography by Yanik Chauvin.

FIGURE 6–34 In active movement, your client performs the action unassisted.

- During **active movement**: the client makes the muscle action unassisted, as in Figure 6–34.
- During **passive movement**: the therapist moves the structure, as in Figure 6–35, the client does not participate.
- During **resisted movement**: the client makes the muscle action while the therapist provides resistance against the movement, as in Figure 6–36. Adding resistance to movement during palpation is described later in this chapter.

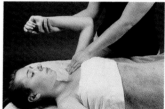

Milady, a part of Cengage Learning. Photography by Yanik Chauvin.

FIGURE 6–35 In passive movement, you manipulate your client's structure without his participation.

HERE'S A TIP

While almost all skeletal muscles are capable of multiple actions, there is nearly always one primary action in which the target muscle is the primary mover when its action is strongest. Although gluteus maximus extends, laterally rotates, abducts, and adducts the thigh, it is also the strongest extensor of the thigh. Extension of the thigh is the first action you would direct your client to do while you are palpating gluteus maximus.

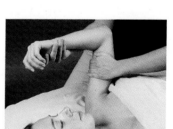

Milady, a part of Cengage Learning. Photography by Yanik Chauvin.

FIGURE 6–36 You may provide gentle resistance to an increase of active movement.

- Direct your client to perform the primary action of the target muscle first: ask him to perform the action *once* and then return to his neutral position. It's the *action* of the muscle, not its position, that is being assessed. Palpate during the action, not after it! Only by palpating the action of fibers *during the contraction* is the therapist able to gauge what is occurring in the muscle.

IN THE TREATMENT ROOM

Because they want to be helpful, clients sometimes repeat your directed muscle action again and again in rapid succession. This quickly fatigues the target muscle and yields inaccurate palpation results, not to mention causing unnecessary discomfort for your client! Ask your client to perform an action once, palpate during the action, and then move on to palpation of the action of the contralateral muscle. Return to the target muscle for subsequent palpations during a different directed action, if necessary, to assure a complete assessment.

Direct the client to perform other actions of the target muscle:
- If palpation during the primary action of the target muscle did not yield any useful information, ask the client to perform other

Active movement

the client makes a muscle action unassisted by the therapist.

Passive movement

the therapist moves the client's structure during an action; the client does not participate.

Resisted movement

the client makes the muscle action while the therapist provides resistance against the movement.

actions, including the opposing actions of the antagonist, to widen the pool of available palpation input.

IN THE TREATMENT ROOM

Work with your client's breath. Palpate on his exhalation. Make sure your client continues to breathe throughout the palpation, so that nearby muscles and structures don't tighten.

Allow your client to control the timing of the muscle action such as, "Sam, when you're ready, bend your head toward your right shoulder, and then bring it back to the center again." Thank your client for his help.

Direct the client to perform the same actions with the contralateral muscle:

- An essential component of palpation is comparison of tissues and structures on a particular client's body. Don't neglect this valuable source of information.

Direct the client to perform the desired actions of the target muscle and its contralateral partner simultaneously:

- Ask the client to do this only if he can do it easily and comfortably.

DID YOU KNOW?

Bilateral muscle actions allow simultaneous palpation of contralateral muscles. You can palpate both sides of Sternocleidomastoid (SCM), for example, during flexion of the head at the spinal joints. Unilateral actions, such as lateral flexion and rotation, of course, disallow simultaneous palpation. SCM laterally flexes and rotates the neck at spinal joints, but only one side is active during each unilateral action.

Obviously, simultaneous palpation of contralateral structures does not work with your client in side-lying position. And while some muscles that act on the extremities can be palpated in action simultaneously, your client may feel as if he's readying for take-off from the table. Use your understanding of muscle actions to decide when it's safe—or possible—to direct simultaneous actions for contralateral palpation.

Procedures for directing muscle actions

Again using Tibialis anterior as an example, perform the palpation as described, adding the direction of a muscle action:

- Recall that Tibialis anterior has two primary actions, and that these actions occur at two separate joints: dorsiflexion of the foot occurs at the talocrural joint, and inversion of the foot occurs at the intertarsal joints.
- Decide what terms you will use instead of "dorsiflexion" and "inversion" to direct these muscle actions to your client. Consider "point your foot toward your head" for dorsiflexion and "turn your foot in toward your body" for inversion. Using hand gestures to demonstrate the directed action, as shown in Figure 6–37, is helpful.

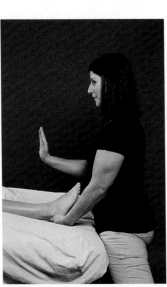

FIGURE 6-37 Demonstrate the action you wish your client to perform as you offer verbal instructions.

- Direct the client to perform each muscle action separately and with both the target and contralateral Tibialis anterior together. Palpate during each muscle action, allowing recovery time between each muscle action.
- Repeat the palpation during passive movement.
- Seek feedback from your client: for example, ask if there is pain or tenderness during any muscle action.
- Note during each action the position and prominence of the distal tendon and the muscle belly.
- Having palpated the structural components of the target Tibialis anterior, complete the same procedure on the contralateral Tibialis anterior, comparing temperature, tone, and texture, while being alert to asymmetry in structure and the quality of contraction during active and passive movement.
- Now, repeat the palpation of Tibialis anterior, adding the direction of muscle action.

Adding Resistance to Muscle Actions

Palpating a muscle during unresisted action does not always allow you to thoroughly assess the tone and texture of the muscle. Adding gentle resistance requires the muscle to strengthen the force of contraction, easing palpation of the muscle fibers during muscle action.

Resistance in the context of palpation is the application of gentle pressure on a structure during muscle action that elicits a stronger contraction in the muscle in order to perform the action. The resistance to increased movement places an additional, controlled, stress on the muscle, and the stronger contraction in response to that stress makes the muscle fibers more apparent for palpation.

Resistance to movement
the application of gentle pressure on a body structure to elicit stronger muscle contraction during palpation.

Comfortable, safe resistance does not prevent further movement. It simply requires greater effort from the muscle, making it more prominent for palpation. Keep these cautions in mind when applying resistance:

- Applying resistance should never cause discomfort. Very little resistance is usually needed in order to strengthen the contraction. Once again, palpation is not a wrestling match!
- Do not apply resistance to a muscle that is already strained. If adding resistance causes discomfort in the target muscle *or anywhere else*, stop immediately.

Guidelines for adding resistance to muscle actions

- Introduce resistance when palpation during unresisted action has not yielded a complete assessment of the target muscle during action. Use your mother hand to inhibit movement of the structure. Place your mother hand distal to the joint being acted upon, not on the target muscle itself. Note that the mother hand, which served as a guide while directing a muscle action, now stays in place to provide resistance to and counter the direction of additional movement during the action.

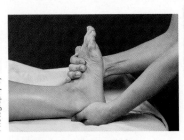

FIGURE 6–38 Your resisting mother hand inhibits further movement, without force.

HERE'S A TIP

Position your mother hand to resist the angle of movement to be directed, if the movement is rotational.

- Avoid squeezing or grasping with your mother hand. *Place* your mother hand—don't push with it—so as to require stronger muscle contraction without overtaxing the muscle. Your mother hand doesn't exert pressure. It simply acts as a barrier.
- Allow the client to control the action and the amount of resistance. Once your resisting mother hand is in place, direct the action and palpate during the resisted action, as in Figure 6–38.

Procedures for adding resistance to muscle actions

Still using Tibialis anterior as an example, perform the palpation described on page 208, adding resistance to the muscle action you directed:

- Place your mother hand on the foot, distal to the joint Tibialis anterior crosses, moving the position of your hand to directly resist each directed action, such as dorsiflexion at the talocrural joint or inversion at the intertarsal joints.

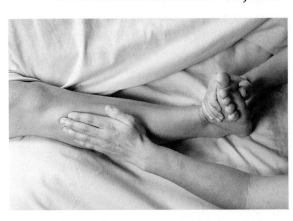

- Direct the client to perform each directed action against resistance. Palpate during the resisted action, as shown in Figure 6–39.
- Note the relative strength of the contraction during both the unresisted and resisted, active and passive actions, and the results of resistance on the success of the palpation.

FIGURE 6–39 Place your mother hand at an angle that resists, but does not prevent, movement.

LEARNING ENHANCEMENT ACTIVITY

Commit to integrating these palpation techniques into at least 10 massages over the next 30 days, to become at ease with the process of locating bony landmarks, tendons, and muscles and directing a muscle action without disrupting the flow of the session. Only by practicing this integration of palpation techniques into your work will you become comfortable with it. There is no substitute for the value of repetition in building hands-on skills. At some point, you must put this book down and turn to the table!

Lab Activity 6–7 on page 226 helps you learn how to direct an action and add resistance to movement during palpation.

Step Four: Evaluating Palpation Findings

Each palpation of bones, soft tissues, and muscles provides you with information that will guide you in the creation of a treatment plan. Evaluating palpation results is essential for client assessment, and works best when approached in a systematic manner. Weigh all factors when evaluating palpation results for treatment planning. Before evaluating palpation results, it's helpful to answer these questions:

- How did I choose which target muscles to palpate?
- What was I looking for?
- What did I find?

Evaluating palpation results is largely about making comparisons. After each palpation you perform, you may make several comparisons, each for its own reason. Many factors—gender, age, lifestyle, and overall conditioning—come into play when comparing individual tissues. As you gain experience, you will learn which comparisons are most valid for treatment planning purposes:

- Comparing Sophie's right Rhomboid to her left Rhomboid: comparing the temperature, tone, and texture of one muscle to the contralateral muscle yields good information for evaluation. Asymmetry in any of these factors is noted for treatment planning.
- Comparing Sophie's Rhomboids to Sam's Rhomboids: gender differences in most tissues are often readily apparent, so comparing Sophie's tissues to Sam's may not be the best indicator for treatment planning. If Sophie and Sam have worked in the same coal mine for the past 20 years and are the same size and age, however, comparing their rhomboids may be valid.
- Comparing Sophie's Rhomboids to Joan's Rhomboids: while Sophie was toiling in the coal mine, Joan was dictating sales figures to her secretary. Comparing Sophie's Rhomboids to Joan's may not yield great information for treatment planning, unless they share other traits, such as gender (they do) or age (they may).
- Comparing Sophie's Rhomboids to all the Rhomboids in the universe: well, maybe not the entire universe, maybe just all the Rhomboids you have ever palpated. Each palpation adds to your bank of palpatory knowledge and skill. Each subsequent palpation is more knowledgeable and more skilled, with the result that comparing Sophie's Rhomboids to those of all the others eventually makes sense for treatment planning.

Terminology for evaluation

Using standard terminology for palpation findings is helpful for several reasons: not only is consistency from client file to client file valuable for the therapist, but the use of terms that are recognized across allied health professions facilitates communication among practitioners and acceptance of massage therapist records by other practitioners. Table 6–5 summarizes terms commonly used to describe palpation findings.

TABLE 6–5

TERMS FOR PALPATION FINDINGS	
TERM FOR PALPATION FINDINGS	**DEFINITION**
Congestion	Excess fluid in the muscle. For the therapist, palpation feedback is a feeling of fullness or sponginess in the muscle. The client may complain of a feeling of tightness in the muscle.
Contracture	The permanent shortening of a muscle due to the replacement of destroyed muscle fibers by fibrous connective tissue. For the therapist, palpation feedback is a feeling of rigidity and hardness in the tissue. The client may lack sensation in the muscle.
Cramp	A painful, spasmodic contraction of a muscle. For the therapist, palpation feedback is a feeling of extreme tightness and immobility of the muscle. The client will report acute pain and a lack of voluntary control of the cramping muscle.
Flaccid	A muscle that is lacking in tone. For the therapist, palpation feedback is a feeling of flabby, soft tissue. The client may experience pain from light-to-moderate palpation pressure.
Hypertonic	Increased muscle tone, which may be rigid; the muscle itself is stiff, or spastic; muscle stiffness because of tendon nerve reflexes. For the therapist, palpation feedback is a feeling of stiffness and lack of mobility. The client may report acute or chronic pain and fatigue in the muscle.
Hypotonic	Decreased or lost muscle tone, perhaps from extended immobility or damage to motor neurons. For the therapist, palpation feedback is a feeling of softness and lack of responsiveness to palpatory touch.
Spasm	A sudden, involuntary contraction of a single muscle within a large group of muscles. For the therapist, palpation feedback is a feeling of extreme hardness and perhaps even tremor in the belly of the muscle. The client may report acute pain and lack of voluntary control over the muscle in spasm.
Tone	The small amount of tension remaining in a relaxed muscle. This minimal level of contraction in certain skeletal muscles helps us maintain posture.
Trigger point	An extremely irritable nodule in muscle tissue—usually near a tendinous attachment—that elicits acute pain at the site or refers pain elsewhere when palpated directly. For the therapist, palpation feedback is a hard nodule. The client may report acute pain at the site of the trigger point or at the referral site.

HERE'S A TIP

In addition to the terms defined in Table 6–5, some massage therapists choose self-defined terms to describe muscle tone and texture, such as:

- Brittle, elastic, or fibrotic.
- Flexible, hard, hot, or knotted.
- Rigid, stiff, thickened, tight.

Use self-defined terms consistently from client file to client file. It may be wise to create a chart of terms you use regularly, defining them in writing.

IN THE TREATMENT ROOM

You may choose to quantify your palpation results, in a manner that is meaningful to you. Although range of motion is measured in the degrees of a circle, palpation results may not be so objectively measurable. Here are some hints:

- Create a number system for evaluating palpation results. The system may relate to the level of pressure you are using, for example, "1" may mean minimal pressure and "4" may indicate firm, sustained pressure, or to the tone or texture of the muscle tissue being palpated, for example "1" may be hypotonic, "5" may be hypertonic, and "3" may indicate normal, healthy muscle tissue.
- Once you have developed your quantifying system, use it consistently.

Palpation findings from each treatment session are recorded in the SOAP notes, described in Table 6–6, for each session in the client's file. SOAP notes are a valuable tool for client recordkeeping and are widely used in massage therapy settings. Detailed SOAP charting is described in *Hands Heal: Documentation For Massage Therapy* by Diane L. Thompson, Lippincott, Williams and Wilkins.

Using palpation results in treatment planning

Once palpation has been completed, the basic questions posed above have been answered, and the palpation results have been characterized, you and your client will draft a treatment plan together. Client participation is integral to the planning process and critical to the success of any treatment plan. Educating your client and seeking his input in treatment decisions is part of treatment.

Set treatment goals:

- Include your client in planning by describing your objective findings, based on your assessments of his posture and gait, the palpations you performed, and his subjective reporting of symptoms such as pain.
- Once you both agree on the nature and extent of the objective and subjective findings, discuss treatment options. Describe treatment modalities and suggest the frequency of sessions and the duration of treatment that you recommend. Define and agree on your client's participation in his care, and agree on how progress will be measured and evaluated.

TABLE 6-6

THE SOAP CHART	
S: **Subjective**	What you heard—the client's report of symptoms: frequency, intensity, duration, and onset. Also, the client's report of relevant medical history.
O: **Objective**	What you found—the therapist's observations and findings from palpation and the results of other assessment tests.
A: **Application**	What you did—the treatment provided and the measurable and reported results of the treatment.
P: **Planning**	What comes next—the treatment plan for the next session and the long-term treatment goals, including homework for the client.

Subjective

the "S" in SOAP notes, describing the client's report of symptoms: frequency, intensity, duration, and onset, and the client's report of relevant medical history.

Objective

the "O" in SOAP notes, describing the therapist's observations and findings from palpation and the results of other assessment tests.

Application

the "A" in SOAP notes, describing the treatment provided and the measurable, reported results of the treatment

Planning

the "P" in SOAP notes, describing the treatment plan for the next session and the long-term treatment goals, including homework for the client.

Select treatment modalities:

- The tools you have in your tool bag of treatment modalities can either limit or expand the treatment options available for your clients. No single modality is appropriate for every client. The successful massage therapist continues to acquire additional competencies and certifications throughout his career.

- Practice describing treatment modality options in terms your client can understand. Using unfamiliar terms can create a barrier to communication. Few clients are looking for an anatomy lecture from you. Most clients just want to feel better and to trust that you know how to help them.

- Describe a modality in terms of how the client will experience it and what the anticipated benefit is, for example: "If we decide to use reflexology, you'll be reclining in this chair, you'll only need to remove your shoes and socks, and you should feel very relaxed and balanced by the end of the session." Or, "If we decide to use myofascial technique, I won't be using any lubricant, and you may feel a stretching or even a burning sensation as I focus on deeper tissues. You may feel sore for a few hours or a day after this treatment, but I'll give you some tips to alleviate the soreness."

- Present your client with treatment options that are appropriate for his age, overall health condition, and for the treatment goal. If you know your client has delicate, papery skin, for example, myofascial therapy is not the modality to recommend.

Negotiate treatment frequency and duration:

- In a perfect world, your client would always schedule his appointments per your recommendation, could afford to come as often as you deem necessary, and life would never intrude on your treatment plan.

- In the real world, describe for your client the ideal schedule of treatment frequency and duration, acknowledge that this is an ideal, and confirm that coming somewhere in the neighborhood of that would be optimal.

- Discuss with your client how the regularity of treatment relates to the consistency of progress.

Define client participation:

- In the days and hours in between care, your client can contribute to his treatment progress: with your guidance, he can alter work and play habits that contributed to his need for treatment. He can perform stretches and relaxation techniques to augment your therapy, and he can follow other suggestions you make to jump-start his recovery.

- Discuss and define the mutual expectations for client participation. Your client's participation may be limited to showing up for appointments twice a month, or it may involves extensive homework of stretches and changes in work habits. The important point is that the level of participation is achievable and agreed upon.

- After each treatment session, discuss the level of participation your client can realistically commit to.
- Accept that your client's intentions for following your suggestions may outstrip the actual attention he can devote to them.

Measure and evaluate treatment progress:

- Engaging your client in evaluating treatment results is essential for further planning.
- After each treatment session, discuss the progress you have observed in concrete terms, for example: "You were able to raise your arm above your shoulder this week" or "The knots in your mid-back seemed to be less tender this week." Check in with your client to make sure you are both seeing the same level of progress.
- Discuss any changes in the treatment plan that are the result of evaluating treatment progress, for example: "Since we're seeing great progress, I think we can scale back to one appointment a week," or "Since the progress isn't what we were hoping for, I'd like to suggest some additional stretches for you to do at home each day."

> **Lab Activity 6–8** on page 227 helps you learn how to utilize palpation findings in treatment planning.

IN THE TREATMENT ROOM

It's common to assume that your treatment goals and your client's treatment goals are the same: to alleviate pain and discomfort and to encourage the full range of motion and function. It may not always be so simple, however. Your client with chronic pain and dysfunction may be experiencing what is called **secondary gain** from his condition, wherein there is something to be gained from maintaining the status quo of his pain and dysfunction. Perhaps he is the receiving a great deal of positive, caring attention because of his condition. He may be relieved of the daily responsibilities of work, school, or family that he would face as a fully functioning person. Accepting treatment may endanger these secondary gains.

The body itself can be complicit, by creating compensation patterns to accommodate dysfunction. The changes that your treatment make in these physical patterns can be very uncomfortable at certain points during treatment, even though the end result will be enhanced functioning. Your client may decide to stop treatment or to reject a certain modality because of the physical and emotional challenges of letting go of his dysfunction. Family members may also have a stake in maintaining the dynamic created by your client's chronic dysfunction.

Working with a client who has a chronic condition and experiences secondary gains as a result of his condition is challenging. It is helpful to clarify your scope of practice and to engage allied health professionals—physicians or psychotherapists for example—in your client's recovery process. After obtaining your client's written permission to discuss her condition and your treatment, contact these professionals in writing, enclose a copy of your client's permission form and offer to share updates on your work with this client.

> **Secondary gain**
>
> the experience of reaping benefit from a usually negative experience, such as when a client gains physical or emotional benefit from maintaining the status quo of an injury or chronic condition.

SUMMARY

The Four-Step Palpation Protocol is a systematic approach to palpation that creates dependable palpation results for treatment planning. Steps include locating target structures, directing muscle actions, adding resistance to muscle actions, and evaluating palpation findings. In the next chapter, you will learn how to locate, palpate, and evaluate bony landmarks and fascial structures.

LAB ACTIVITIES

LAB ACTIVITY 6-1: TOUCH SENSITIVITY

The following Lab Activity is designed to enhance various components of touch sensitivity, such as sensitivity to temperature and texture, and to enhance your focus for palpation and equal handedness for palpation dexterity.

Practice these touch sensitivity enhancement activities often, to maintain your palpation skill level. Keep notes on your activity results, to help gauge your touch sensitivity as it progresses. *Appendix D, Independent Study Activities, contains additional exercises to enhance your touch sensitivity.*

Strategy

Strategy: squares of fabric of palpably different textures are placed in the hands of a blindfolded participant, who must correctly identify the fabric he is palpating by its texture, using both his dominant and non-dominant hand. Next, squares of fabric of distinctly variant colors and therefore, temperatures, are placed in his hands. He must correctly identify the color of the fabric he is palpating by its temperature, using both his dominant and non-dominant hand.

Exercise:

1. Working blindfolded and with a partner: your partner will place a square of fabric in your dominant hand. Palpate the cloth thoroughly, as shown in Figure 6–40, until you are certain which fabric you hold in your hand by your assessment of its texture. Tell your partner what your conclusion is.

2. Now, your partner will place a second fabric square in your non-dominant hand. It may or may not be the same fabric. Only your partner knows, at this point. Palpate the cloth thoroughly, until you are certain which fabric it is, by your assessment of its texture. Tell your partner what your conclusion is.

3. Next, your partner will place a square of fabric in your dominant hand. Palpate the cloth thoroughly. Store in your mind the sense you have of its temperature, in relation to your hand.

4. Now, your partner will place a second fabric square in your non-dominant hand. It may or may not be the same fabric. Only your partner knows, at this point. Palpate the cloth thoroughly, until you are certain whether or

not it is the same fabric as the first square, by assessing any difference in temperature. Is it warmer, cooler, or the same temperature as the first square? Tell your partner what your conclusion is.

5. Remove your blindfold and assess your results. Repeat this exercise with as many fabric squares as you can, always assessing your results in terms of which textures and temperatures you were most accurate about and how your dominant and non-dominant hand compare in sensitivity to texture.

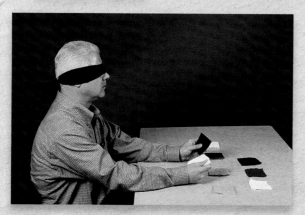

FIGURE 6–40
Palpating fabrics of varying textures and colors enhances touch sensitivity in both your dominant and non-dominant hand.

© Milady, a part of Cengage Learning.
Photography by Yanik Chauvin.

Repeat this exercise with as many fabric squares as you can, always assessing your results in terms of which temperatures you were most accurate about and how your dominant and non-dominant hand compare in sensitivity to temperature.

HERE'S A TIP

White fabric will feel the coolest, red will be much warmer than white, while black fabric will feel warmer than either white or red. Keep the factor of adaptation in mind: the longer you palpate the fabric square, the greater role adaptation, and the actual warming of the cloth by your body temperature, will play in your assessment!

LAB ACTIVITY 6–2: PALPATION PRESSURE

1. Working with a partner, palpate a superficial bony landmark, such as the olecranon of the ulna—the elbow, or the patella—the kneecap. Note the degree of pressure that was needed to effectively assess this landmark.

2. Next, palpate a bony landmark that is deeper from the surface of the body, such as the metatarsals of the foot from the plantar aspect, shown in Figure 6–2. How much more palpation pressure was needed to effectively assess the deeper structure?

3. Now, select a target muscle for the group to palpate on each other; choose a superficial muscle, such as Trapezius or the Quadriceps group. Take some time for each palpation; spend a minute or two between each palpation characterizing the previous one: what were

the qualities of the skin and the underlying layer of tissue? Was the target tissue firm or flaccid, tight, or knotted?

4. Compare the results of your palpations. What were the differences in the pressure you used and the results you experienced?

5. Switch partners and repeat steps 1–4.

LAB ACTIVITY 6-3: BARRIERS TO PALPATION

1. Working with a partner, choose an existing physiological or anatomical tissue barrier in each partner. It may be at the site of an old injury or it may be a sore shoulder from this morning's workout. It is highly unlikely that neither of you has some sort of tissue barrier. This is the target structure: the bony landmark, soft tissue structure, or muscle that is selected as the primary palpation site for palpation in this Lab Activity.

2. Working with your eyes closed and focusing on the target structure, slowly palpate through the superficial layers and be alert to the first sign of a tissue barrier. At this point, don't worry too much about the finer points of palpation technique—this is practice. How do you first sense the barrier? Name the change you feel. Would you characterize it as physiological, anatomical, or as a combination of barriers?

3. As you continue to gently palpate, how does the tissue barrier change? Does it dissipate? Does it become more resistant to your touch? If you palpated more deeply, what do you think would happen?

4. If you and your partner feel safe in the process and are communicating well, try increasing the palpation pressure in tiny increments. What changes, if any, occur as a result of the alteration of pressure?

5. Switch partners and repeat.

LAB ACTIVITY 6-4: LAYERS OF PALPATION

1. Working with a partner lying supine, place your hands about 2–3" (5–7.5 cm) above the surface of her abdomen. Close your eyes and be still for a few minutes, noting the input you receive from this level of contact with your partner's energy field.

2. Lower your hands to about 1 inch above your partner's abdomen. Open yourself to your partner's energy field and temperature as your hands receive the input from this distance above the abdomen. Repeat this procedure one more time, lowering your hands to just barely above actual contact. Close your eyes and be still for a few minutes, noting the input you receive from this level of contact with your partner's energy field.

3. Choose words that describe what the sensations at each level of the energy field felt like to you. Discuss with your partner what his awareness of your presence was during palpation of his energy field.

4. Undrape an area of the body. In this area, palpate your partner's skin. Note the following characteristics of your partner's skin:

    ■ Temperature: is the temperature of your partner's skin warmer or cooler than your hands? Is the temperature within the range of normal expectation, or is it noticeably warmer or cooler than normal expectation?

    ■ Condition: is the skin moist or dry? Is it brittle or flexible? Does the skin spring back following touch, or does your touch leave a depression in the tissue? Characterize its palpation feedback.

5. Turn your attention to the superficial fascia beneath your partner's skin:

    ■ How can you distinguish the superficial fascia from the skin?

    ■ Is the underlying layer of fascia mobile or does it feel "stuck"?

    ■ Is there dimpling in the skin that may indicate a restriction in the superficial fascia? Describe its palpation feedback.

6. Palpate a bony landmark in the same area:

    ■ How can you distinguish the bony landmark from the surrounding tissue?

    ■ Is its size and shape within normal expectation? Palpate its contralateral counterpart for comparison.

    ■ Is the landmark tender? Characterize its palpation feedback.

7. Briefly palpate a muscle that attaches to this landmark:

    ■ How can you distinguish the muscle tissue from the skin, fascia, bone, and other tissues, such as ligaments or tendons, in the area?

    ■ Is the muscle tight or relaxed, supple or perhaps grainy? Characterize its palpation feedback.

8. Switch partners and repeat the exercises. Discuss and share your experiences.

LAB ACTIVITY 6–5: POSITIONING FOR PALPATION

1. Working with a partner who is fully clothed and standing, choose three structures to palpate. Choose one each from the bony landmarks, soft tissue structures, and the muscles and palpate one on of each on his trunk, one on his upper extremity and one on his lower extremity.

2. Next, palpate the structures from different positions:

    ■ Standing, facing your partner from the front.

    ■ Standing behind him.

    ■ Kneeling to palpate the lower extremity at eye level, shown in Figure 6–41.

    ■ Facing your partner from the side.

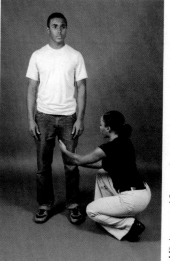

FIGURE 6–41 Changing your position to palpate structures at eye level maintains proper body mechanics.

3. Repeat the palpations with your partner fully clothed and seated, lying supine and draped on a massage table, and lying prone and draped on a massage table.
4. Discuss the advantages and disadvantages of each position, his as well as yours, with your partner. Which structures are best palpated with the client standing, seated, supine, or prone? Which are more difficult in the different positions?

LAB ACTIVITY 6–6: LOCATING PALPATION TARGETS

1. Working with a partner who is lying supine on the massage table, undrape one leg.
2. Palpate the bony landmarks, tendons, and muscle fibers of Tibialis anterior on each leg, following the procedures outlines above. Experiment with placement of your mother hand in each palpation. At this point, don't worry too much about the finer points of palpation technique—this is practice.
3. Discuss the results with your partner: how could the location procedures been improved? Was the process easier or more difficult on either leg? Was the palpation pressure at the insertion comfortable?
4. Switch partners and repeat.

LAB ACTIVITY 6–7: DIRECTING ACTIONS DURING PALPATION

1. Working with a partner who is lying supine on the massage table, undrape one leg.
2. Palpate the bony landmarks, tendons, and muscle fibers of Tibialis anterior on both of your partner's legs. Experiment with placement of your mother hand in each palpation.
3. Direct your partner in performing the primary actions of Tibialis anterior, following the procedure outlined above. Palpate the target Tibialis anterior during each muscle action.
4. Add resistance to each action of the target Tibialis anterior. Experiment with using your dominant and non-dominant hand as the resisting mother hand.
5. Discuss the results with your partner: was the application of resistance comfortable for your partner? Which was easier, using your dominant or non-dominant hand as the resisting mother hand? What were the differences in using resistance and in the results obtained in each of the actions of Tibialis anterior?
6. Switch partners and repeat.

LAB ACTIVITY 6–8: UTILIZING PALPATION RESULTS IN TREATMENT PLANNING

1. Working in a group, take turns role playing the following situations while the rest of the group observes and takes feedback notes to share:

   - Your client works at a computer all day, every day. Your palpation has revealed trigger points and adhesions in his Rhomboids. What are your treatment goals? What are the modalities that you will suggest to your client? What is the frequency and duration of treatment? How will the client participate in treatment? How will you measure and evaluate progress?

   - Another client has had a change in his work schedule and can't keep up with his weekly appointments. He says he can probably come in once a month. What changes in treatment goals, modalities, and client participation might you suggest to this client?

   - Your palpation and treatment evaluation shows some progress in your client's low-back problem, but he wants to see faster recovery. What changes in treatment goals, modalities, and client participation might you suggest to this client?

2. Continue until everyone in the group has participated. Share your notes and thoughts, and discuss the decisions and recommendations that were made.

CASE PROFILES

Case Profile #1

Phil is a 38-year-old mechanic who complains of pain and stiffness in his right shoulder that sometimes radiates all the way down his arm, into his hand. What target structures would you palpate on this client? What positions would you place this client in for palpation? Describe the structures you would locate and the procedure for locating them.

Case Profile #2

Amy is a 45-year-old dancer who has pain and stiffness in her right hip and the lateral side of her right thigh when she walks or climbs stairs. What target structures would you palpate on this client? What positions would you place this client in for palpation? Describe the structures you would locate, the muscle actions you would direct and your process for adding resistance to movement.

Case Profile #3

Carl is a 56-year-old writer who is quite sedentary and is overweight. He has come to a massage therapist because of persistent pain across his upper back. What target structures would you palpate on this client? What positions would you place this client in for palpation? Describe the structures you would locate, the muscle actions you would direct, and your process for adding resistance to movement. What palpation skills will help you meet the challenge of this client's body structure?

STUDY QUESTIONS

1. Why might you use less pressure when palpating a bony landmark than when palpating a muscle?
2. Name two strategies for working through tissue barriers.
3. Why is touch sensitivity important to effective palpation? Name three strategies for enhancing touch sensitivity.
4. Describe the role of the mother hand during palpation. How does using the mother hand contribute to good body mechanics?
5. Contrast poor and preferred hand positions. What are the benefits of maintaining good hand positions during palpation?
6. Name three structures that are more easily palpated with the client in side-lying position and describe two challenges for the massage therapist when working with a side-lying client.
7. Why is using lay terminology for directing client muscle actions important? Name four lay terms you have developed to replace anatomically correct terms for muscle actions.
8. What are two cautions to remember when applying resistance to movement during palpation?
9. When is adding resistance to movement beneficial during palpation? Where is the mother hand placed when adding resistance?
10. Contrast hypotonic and hypertonic muscle tone. List and describe three self-defined terms you plan to use in evaluating palpation results for treatment planning.

Palpating Bony Landmarks and Fascial Structures

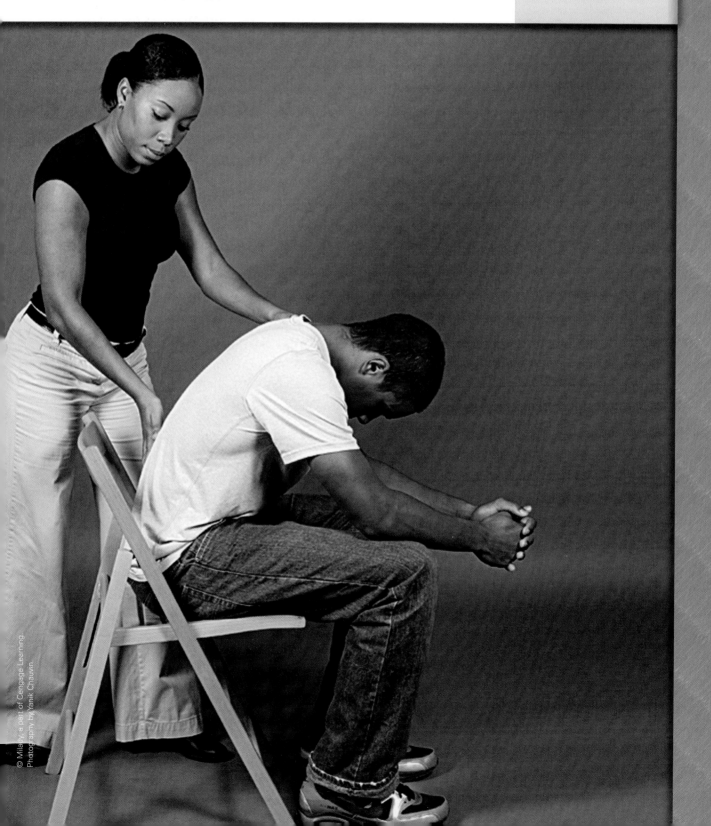

CHAPTER OUTLINE

- BONY LANDMARKS
- FASCIAL STRUCTURES
- PALPATION OF BONY LANDMARKS AND FASCIAL STRUCTURES
- PALPATING BONY LANDMARKS AND FASCIAL STRUCTURES ON THE AXIAL SKELETON
- PALPATING BONY LANDMARKS AND FASCIAL STRUCTURES ON THE UPPER EXTREMITY
- PALPATING BONY LANDMARKS AND FASCIAL STRUCTURES ON THE LOWER EXTREMITY

LEARNING OBJECTIVES

- Identify the types and functions of landmarks on bones and the types and functions of palpable fascial structures.
- Describe the properties of connective tissue and fascia.
- Locate and apply effective, comfortable palpation to bony landmarks and associated fascial structures on the axial and appendicular skeleton.

INTRODUCTION

Skilled, effective palpation of bones, fascial [FAY-shul] structures, and muscles provides you with tactile information about their structure and function. This skill in touch and movement is your tool for creating professional, therapeutic treatments for your clients.

In this chapter, you will apply the Four-Step Palpation Protocol to bony landmarks that serve as attachment sites for muscles and associated fascial structures that connect and support bones and muscles.

DID YOU KNOW?

Babies don't have true kneecaps! The patellae are cartilaginous in infancy and ossify, turn into bone, as babies begin to crawl and then to walk.

BONY LANDMARKS

Bone is dynamic, living tissue: it actively responds to stresses placed upon it. While some bony landmarks are present at birth, others, primarily those to which skeletal muscles attach, form in response to stress—the pull of contracting muscle fibers against the tendon where it attaches to bone—and change to adapt to that stress. The relative stress that muscles exert on their bony landmarks creates, to a degree, the relative size and shape of those landmarks.

The consequence to palpation of this dynamic nature of bone is evident each time you palpate a bony landmark. Although every humerus has medial and lateral epicondyles, a medial epicondyle to which muscles that have lifted heavy boxes or played concert piano every day for 30 years attach may feel different in palpation from an epicondyle that has spent those same decades leaning on the arm of an easy chair. Bone health and the condition of bony landmarks may be adversely affected by a sedentary lifestyle, advancing age, and certain diseases. Palpation results must be viewed within the context of all your client's attributes.

Types and Functions Bony Landmarks

Landmarks are found on all bones, as shown in Figures 7–1 and 7–2. Most serve as attachment sites for skeletal muscles that cross synovial, or freely moveable, joints and move the skeleton. Many of these landmarks are **processes** or projections on bones that serve as attachment sites for ligaments and tendons that can be reasonably and comfortably palpated and some are fossae. A **fossa** [FAHS-uh] is a shallow depression in a bone that serves as a surface for muscle attachment. Fossae are not usually easily palpable, because they are filled with muscle tissue.

Table 7–1 lists and defines the types of bony landmarks that are discussed in this chapter. As in many areas of anatomical terminology, some of the terms for bony landmarks may seem arbitrary. Illustrations of individual bony landmarks accompany the following instructions for their palpation.

Process

a projection on a bone that serves as attachment sites for ligaments and tendons.

Fossa

a shallow depression in a bone.

TABLE 7–1

TYPES OF BONY LANDMARKS	
BONY LANDMARK	**DESCRIPTION**
Angle	An abrupt change of direction on the border of a flat bone, such as the superior angle of the scapula.
Border	A long edge on a flat bone, such as the medial border of the scapula.
Condyle [KAHN-dyl]	A large, round protuberance at the end of a long bone, such as the lateral condyle of the tibia.
Crest	A prominent ridge or an elongated projection, such as the iliac crest.
Epicondyle [ep-ih-KAHN-dyl]	A smaller, rounded projection found above a condyle, such as the medial epicondyle of the femur.
Facet [FASS-it]	A flat, smooth articular surface, such as the facets on each vertebra that articulate with other facets on superior and inferior vertebrae.
Foramen [fuh-RAY-mun]	An opening in a bone through which blood vessels, nerves, and ligaments may pass, such as the vertebral foramen, through which the spinal cord passes.
Fossa	A shallow depression in a bone, such as the infraspinous fossa of the scapula.
Head	A rounded articulating projection, supported by the constricted, neck-like portion of a long bone, such as the head of the humerus.
Shaft	The length of a long bone, such as the shaft of the humerus.
Spine	A long, raised ridge, such as the spine of the scapula.
Spinous process	A sharp, slender projection, such as the spinous processes of the vertebrae.
Styloid process	A sharp, pointed projection, such as the styloid process of the ulna.
Trochanter [troh-KANT-ur]	A very large, protruding projection, such as the greater trochanter of the femur.
Tubercle [TOO-bur-kul]	A small, rounded projection, such as the lesser tubercle of the humerus.
Tuberosity [toob-uh-ROSS-ih-tee]	A large, usually roughened projection, such as the gluteal tuberosity of the femur.

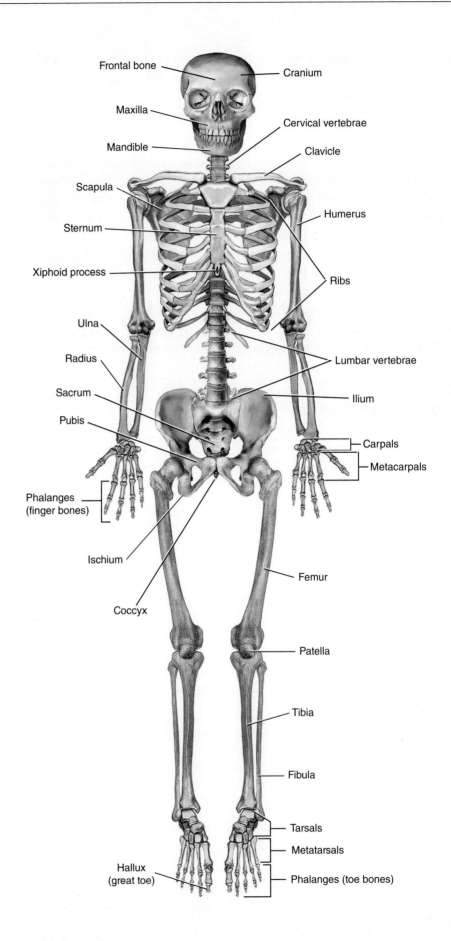

FIGURE 7-1 The skeletal system, anterior view.

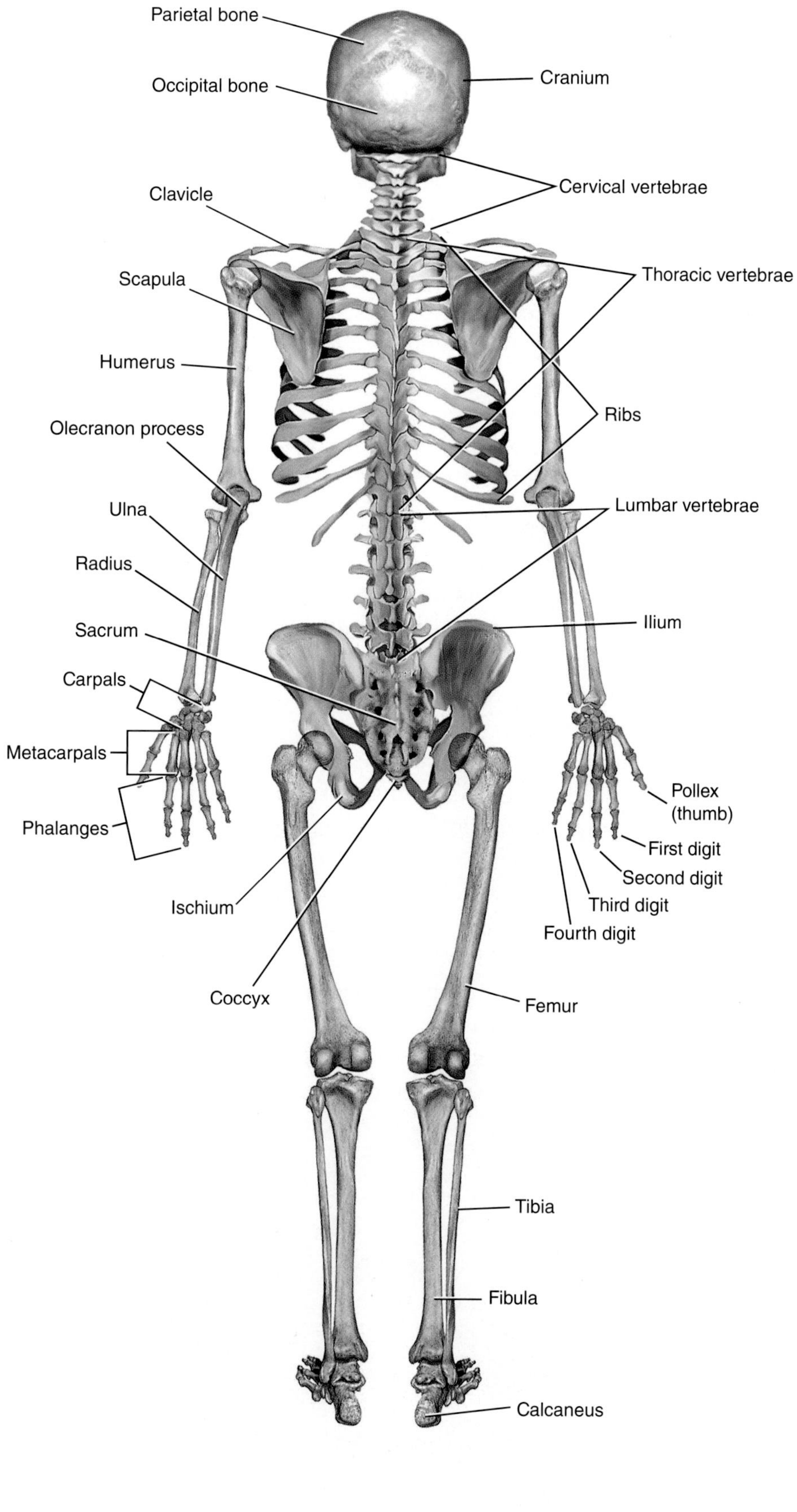

FIGURE 7-2 The skeletal system, posterior view.

Parietal bone

Occipital bone

Clavicle

Scapula

Humerus

Olecranon process

Ulna

Radius

Sacrum

Carpals

Metacarpals

Phalanges

Ischium

Coccyx

Cranium

Cervical vertebrae

Thoracic vertebrae

Ribs

Lumbar vertebrae

Ilium

Pollex (thumb)

First digit

Second digit

Third digit

Fourth digit

Femur

Tibia

Fibula

Calcaneus

FASCIAL STRUCTURES

Connective tissues support and bind together other types of tissue and separate compartments of organs and structures, such as muscles and muscle groups. It is essential to understand the properties and functions of connective tissue because your every massage stroke impacts the levels of connective tissue that lie deep to the skin, whether or not that is your intention.

Connective tissue is composed of a matrix that includes ground substance materials and embedded fibers, along with a few cells. Each type of connective tissue, from solid bone to semisolid fascia to liquid plasma and lymph, has its own composition of matrix and fibers, giving that tissue its functional characteristics.

Types and Functions of Palpable Fascial Structures

Fascia [FAYSH-ah] is connective tissue that surrounds, supports, and separates the structures of the body. Fascia, as seen in the axillary region in Figure 7–3, is a continuous, web-like, layered membrane that extends throughout the body, surrounding and supporting every organ, blood vessel, and nerve and every muscle and muscle group. Fascia also covers and lines each bone and every joint capsule and gives the body its shape around the skeleton.

To understand how fascia connects and supports structures, envision the body as a giant bowl of fruit, containing and wrapped by an immense roll of plastic wrap. Each grape and bunch of grapes, each banana and bunch of bananas, then each orange and every apple, then the bulk of all the fruit together, and, finally, the inner surface of the bowl and the bowl itself is wrapped in the continuous, unending sheet of the plastic wrap.

The properties of fascia include both great tensile strength and pliability. Fascia is so strong that it can endure a certain amount of impact and stretching without injury. Its composition, however, also allows it to "melt" and turn from gel-like to more fluid when a form of energy is applied, such as the heat and mechanical energy of massage. This property is known as **thixotropy**.

Fascia

connective tissue that surrounds, supports, and separates structures.

Thixotropy

the property of fascia that allows it to melt and turn from gel-like to fluid when a form of energy is applied, such as the heat and mechanical energy of massage.

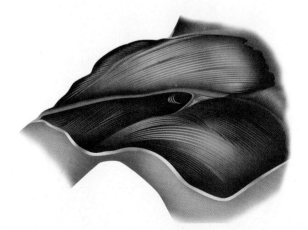

FIGURE 7–3 Superficial and deep fascia, in the axillary region

Two types of fascia are found throughout the body:

- **Superficial fascia** is found just beneath the skin, and is also known as the **hypodermis** [hy-poh-DUR-mis]. Superficial fascia separates the skin from muscles and provides the pathway into muscles for nerves, blood, and lymph vessels.
- **Deep fascia** surrounds and supports organs and body cavities and envelops and permeates skeletal muscles. Deep fascia covers each muscle fiber, each bundle of muscle fibers, each whole muscle, and each entire group of muscles. Extensions of deep fascia connect body structures and form organ compartments. In Figures 7–4 and 7–5, the deep palpable fascial structures are shown in white and are described in detail below.

Extensions of deep fascia form the following connective tissue structures:

- A **tendon** is a cord of connective tissue that attaches muscle to bone. Tendons are extensible and elastic: they can stretch to accommodate the contraction of a muscle and return it to its original shape and length. The Achilles tendon can be seen in Figure 7–5.
- An **aponeurosis** [ap-uh-noo-ROH-sus] is a broad, flat layer of deep fascia that extends to connect muscles or other tendons. Aponeuroses can be found where muscle has no direct bony landmark for attachment, such as in the anterior abdomen and the low back. The abdominal aponeurosis in the anterior trunk can be seen in Figure 7–4.

HERE'S A TIP

In the bowl of fruit described above, superficial fascia would wrap and line the bowl itself, while deep fascia would support and connect individual grapes or bananas and their bunches.

Tendon

a cord of fascial connective tissue that attaches muscles to bone.

Aponeurosis

a broad, flat layer of fascia that extends to connect muscles or other tendons.

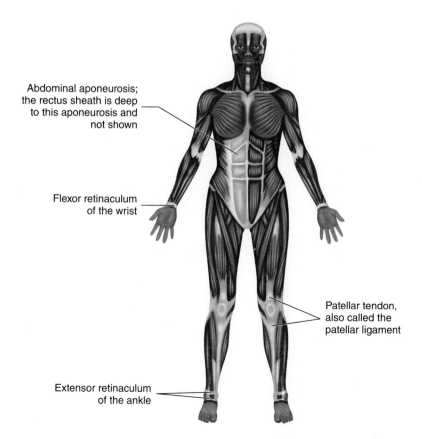

Abdominal aponeurosis; the rectus sheath is deep to this aponeurosis and not shown

Flexor retinaculum of the wrist

Patellar tendon, also called the patellar ligament

Extensor retinaculum of the ankle

FIGURE 7–4 Connective tissue structures on the anterior body.

© Milady, a part of Cengage Learning.

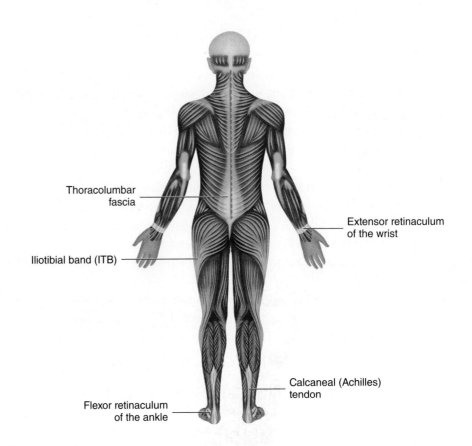

FIGURE 7–5 Connective tissue structures on the posterior body.

Labels in figure:
- Thoracolumbar fascia
- Iliotibial band (ITB)
- Extensor retinaculum of the wrist
- Calcaneal (Achilles) tendon
- Flexor retinaculum of the ankle

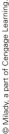

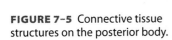

Ligament

a band of fascial connective tissue that unites bones with other bones.

Retinaculum

a fibrous, transverse band of deep fascia that holds body structures in place.

Flexor retinaculum (retinaculum=band)

also called the transverse carpal ligament, a strong fascial band around the anterior aspect of the carpals.

- **Ligaments** unite bones with other bones at joints and maintain the positions of articulating bones during movement. Because its function is to provide stability to a structure during movement, a ligament is distinctly less elastic or extensible than a tendon. The patellar ligament, also called the patellar tendon, can be seen in Figure 7–4.
- A **retinaculum** [ret-in-ACK-yoo-lum] is a fibrous band of deep fascia. Transverse retinacula hold groups of structures together in areas of free movement, such as at the wrist and the ankle, while others provide a connection for soft tissue structures over distances. The **flexor retinaculum** at the ankle can be seen in Figure 7–5.

PALPATION OF BONY LANDMARKS AND FASCIAL STRUCTURES

This chapter applies your knowledge of bones and other connective tissues, along with your knowledge of safe and effective palpation pressure and touch sensitivity, to the palpation of bony landmarks and associated fascial structures, using the Four-Step Palpation Protocol. As described in Chapter 6, The Art of Palpation, the Four-Step Palpation Protocol is a systematic approach to palpation that creates dependable palpation results for treatment planning. The palpations in this chapter are presented using the Four-Step Protocol. For each bony landmark palpation, you will:

1. Position the client and yourself.
2. Locate the bone and palpate the target bony landmark.
3. In some cases, perform a joint action as part of palpation.
4. Evaluate the results of your palpation.

If the target bony landmark has a contralateral counterpart, you will palpate that landmark too and evaluate the results of both palpations for treatment planning. Some structures are simultaneously palpated on both sides of the body.

Although palpation of some of the bony landmarks described below may be performed with the client clothed, standing, or seated, the instructions in this chapter are presented for the client on the massage table, to address positioning and draping concerns. The photographs that accompany individual palpation instructions are intended as guides, not as mandates. Find your own way, taking into account all the factors about the client on your table. Palpation is about *touch*—what you *feel* is more important than what you see.

Whether the target structure is a bony landmark or a muscle, palpation impacts fascia. It is not possible to palpate the body without palpating superficial fascia. Muscle palpation involves palpating the multiple layers of deep fascia that surround muscle fibers, muscles, and muscle groups. As you palpate, lift or roll the skin, you are in contact with superficial fascia.

Fascial tissue can be differentiated from bones or muscles by its distinct palpation feedback:

- Because bone is solid connective tissue, it has no "give" during palpation. Other types of connective tissue are not solid. There is a degree of "give" during palpation of fascia.
- Skeletal muscle is striated, contractile tissue: during active palpation, its bundles of fibers and their contractions may be felt. Fascial fibers do not contract during muscle contractions.

Each type of fascial structure has its own palpation feedback:

- Tendons, because of their extensibility and elasticity, may feel like rubber bands when palpated, depending on their location, their length, and the tone of the muscle they attach to.
- Ligaments, aponeuroses, and retinacula are much less elastic than tendons: their functions of support and stability give them a somewhat strap-like palpation feel.
- The palpation feedback of fascia may vary tremendously, depending on its location and the health of the tissue. Fascia may feel thick or "stuck" or it may feel as if it is resisting or holding on. Fascia may have the feel of bubble wrap and even snap-crackle-and-pop under palpation, or it may feel fluid, gel-like, or yielding.
- Superficial fascia may be quite mobile during palpation. It can be lifted or rolled, or it may be immovable. Extensions of deep fascia, such as the thoracolumbar fascia or the iliotibial band, may have a dense, heavy feel during palpation. Such deep fascial structures will feel less mobile than superficial fascia and may be quite rigid.

HERE'S A TIP

Self-palpation can be helpful to you in learning to palpate bony landmarks. Because there is sometimes little tissue overlaying bony landmarks, persistent palpation in search of a specific landmark can be unpleasant for the client or lab partner on the table. Practice locating the following bony landmarks on your own body, before palpating them on a classmate or client.

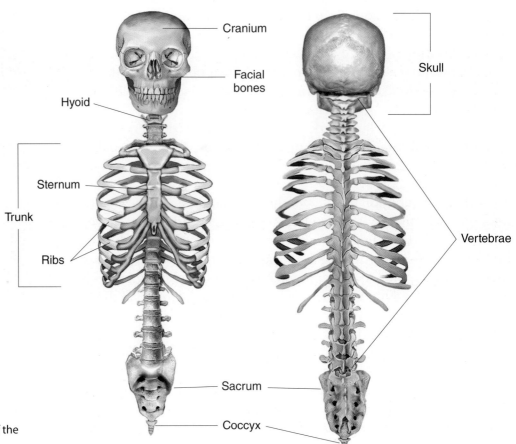

FIGURE 7-6 The bones of the axial skeleton.

Divisions of the Skeleton

The skeleton is divided into two parts:

■ The axial skeleton, seen in Figure 7–6, comprises the head and the torso. It includes the bones of the skull and the face; the bones of the internal ear and the hyoid bone; the sternum and ribs that form the thoracic cage; and the vertebral column, including the sacrum and coccyx; plus all of the associated fascial structures.

■ The appendicular skeleton comprises the extremities or append-ages and the bones that attach them to the axial skeleton. Included in the upper extremity are the clavicle and the scapula; the humerus, radius, and ulna; and the carpals, metacarpals, and phalanges that make up the wrist and hand, plus their associated fascial structures. The lower extremity includes the pelvis, the femur, and the patella; the tibia and the fibula; and the tarsals, metatarsals, and phalanges that make up the ankle and foot; plus associated fascial structures.

PALPATING BONY LANDMARKS AND FASCIAL STRUCTURES ON THE AXIAL SKELETON

Palpating bony landmarks and their associated fascial structures natu-rally includes palpation of the joints where they are found. In the pal-pation instructions that follow, articulations and movements for accompanying joints are described. You are encouraged to explore these articulations and joint movements as you palpate.

The bony landmarks of the axial skeleton described here for palpation include those on several bones of the skull and the face, the hyoid bone, and the sternum, the ribs, and the vertebrae.

The Occiput

The shape of the occiput [AHK-sih-put], shown in Figure 7–7, varies hugely from person to person. It can appear to be bulbous or flat or rounded. Because posterior neck muscles attach to landmarks on the occiput, its shape may have significance for patterns of strain in these muscles. The atlanto-occipital joint connects the spine to the skull and allows you to nod your head "yes."

Palpable landmarks:

- External occipital protuberance: the large, prominent medial bump on the occiput, the most inferior portion of the occiput that is readily palpable.
- Superior nuchal lines: ridges that extend horizontally on either end of the external occipital protuberance.

Articulations:

- The occiput articulates with the parietal and temporal bones of the skull at the lamboidal suture.
- The atlanto-occipital joint: occiput articulates with C1, the atlas, between the superior articular facets of the C1 and the condyles of the occiput.

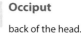

Occiput

back of the head.

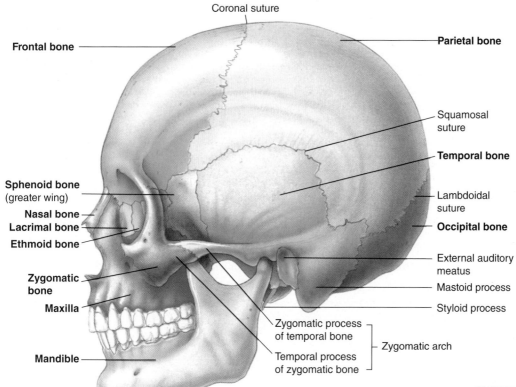

FIGURE 7-7 Cranial and facial bones, lateral view.

© Delmar, Cengage Learning.

Attachments:

- Occipitalis attaches to the occiput.
- Upper Trapezius and Splenius capitis attach to the nuchal lines of the occiput.

Associated structures:

- The nuchal ligament separates the right and left compartments of posterior trunk muscles in the cervical region. Its superficial location over the spinous processes from C7 to the external occipital protuberance interferes with easy palpation of those processes.

Palpating the occipaut:

POSITION:

- Supine client: undrape your client's neck.
- Stand or sit at the head of the table. For palpation of the bony landmarks of the head and face, both hands are considered palpating hands.

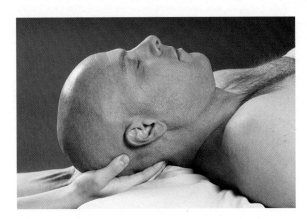

FIGURE 7–8 Palpating the occiput.

LOCATE AND PALPATE:

- With both hands along each side of the spine, palms up, just below the shoulders, palpate the posterior neck with your fingertips, moving toward the skull, as shown in Figure 7–8.
- Gently rotate your client's head into one hand while palpating with the other. Explore the size and shape of the external occipital protuberance, which may vary considerably from person to person.
- Move your fingertips slightly laterally on the occiput to trace the superior nuchal lines. Performing a minimal degree of passive extension of the head may reveal the attachment sites of upper Trapezius along the nuchal lines.

EVALUATE:

- Characterize your findings: is the occiput equally prominent on both sides of the skull? Are the nuchal lines palpable, and palpable on both sides of the skull?
- Compare your findings with palpations of the occiputs on other clients.

OPTION:

- With your client prone: using your mother hand to support the crown of your client's head, place your palpating hand around the cervical spine, with your fingertips and thumb on the inferior occiput.
- Palpate as described above.

Nuchal

neck.

The Nuchal Ligament

The nuchal [NOO-kul] ligament, as shown in Figure 7–9, is a large, flat band of fascia that extends from the external occiput to the spinous

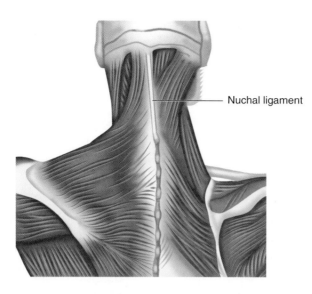

FIGURE 7–9 The nuchal ligament.

process of C7, also called the vertebral prominens [VUR-tuh-brul PRAHM-ih-nenz]. It separates and provides attachment sites for the right and left compartments of posterior neck muscles. Although its location makes palpation of the cervical spinous processes more difficult, the nuchal ligament itself is easily palpated.

Palpating the nuchal ligament:

POSITION:

- Prone client: undrape your client's neck, and adjust the face cradle to create a slight degree of flexion of the neck.
- Stand or sit at the side of the table. Use your mother hand to support your client's head.

LOCATE AND PALPATE:

- Locate the external occipital protuberance, the prominent "bump" on the medial occipital bone.
- Slide your palpating down from your client's occiput to locate the prominent spinous process of C7, the largest and most easily palpable cervical spinous process. The nuchal ligament lies superficial to the spinous processes of C1–C6.
- With the fingers of your palpating hand, strum across the nuchal ligament between these landmarks, as shown in Figure 7–10.

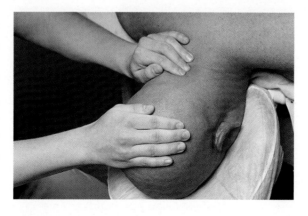

FIGURE 7–10 Palpating the nuchal ligmanet.

DIRECT AND ACTION AND PALPATE:

- To further bring out the nuchal ligament, ask your client to tuck his chin toward his chest and strum across the ligament again.

© Milady, a part of Cengage Learning.

© Milady, a pvart of Cengage Learning. Photography by Yanik Chauvin.

EVALUATE:

- Characterize the mobility of the nuchal ligament: is it freely mobile or is it partially or completely restricted?
- Characterize the tissue quality of the nuchal ligament: does the tissue feel supple or brittle? Does the tissue soften in response to your touch?
- Compare the mobility and tissue quality of the nuchal ligament with your palpation of the nuchal ligament on other clients.

Temporal	*The Temporal Bone*
the temple or side of the skull.	

The temporal bone [TEM-poh-rul BOHN] is visible in Figure 7–7. The temporal bone houses the external opening for the ear, called the external auditory meatus, and articulates with the mandible at the temporomandibular joints. Palpate the temporal bone when assessing possible causes of headache and jaw pain. Temporomandibular joint disorder (TMJD) is described in Chapter 8, Palpating Superficial Muscles of the Axial Skeleton.

Palpable landmarks:
- Mastoid process [MAS-toyd PRAH-ses]: the rounded, superficial process directly posterior to the earlobe.
- Zygomatic process [zy-goh-MAT-ik PRAH-ses]: together with the temporal process of the zygomatic bone, the zygomatic process of the temporal bone forms the zygomatic arch, or cheekbone.

Articulations:
- The temporal bone articulates with the occiput, the parietal bones, the sphenoid, and the zygomatic bones.
- The temporomandibular joints: the mandibular fossae of the temporal bone articulate with the condyles of the mandible.

Attachments:
- Temporalis covers most of the temporal bone.
- The Masseter attaches to the zygomatic arch of the temporal bone.
- Sternocleidomastoid, Splenius capitis, and Longissimus capitis all share attachments on the mastoid process of the temporal bone.

Palpating the temporal bone:

POSITION:
- Supine client: undrape your client's neck.
- Stand or sit at the head of the table. For palpation of the bony landmarks of the head and face with your client supine, both hands are considered palpating hands.

LOCATE AND PALPATE:
- Begin with your palpating fingertips just superior to the ear, as shown in Figure 7–11. Slide your hands around so that they cup the ear: your thumbs will be on the temporal bone, while your fingertips should be curled around the mastoid process of the temporal bone.

- Rotate your hands to slide your fingertips anterior and superior to the ears. Follow the prominent zygomatic process as it widens toward the zygomatic arch.

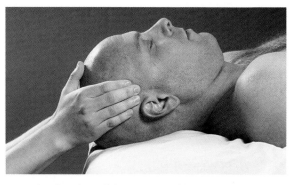

FIGURE 7-11 Palpating the temporal bone.

EVALUATE:

- Characterize your findings: are both sides of the temporal bone the same size and shape? Are the processes equal in angle, shape, and prominence?
- Compare your findings with palpations of the temporal bones on other clients.

The Frontal Bone

Frontal

the front of the skull.

The frontal bone [FRUNT-ul BOHN], visible in Figure 7–7, is superficial to the frontal sinuses and is often assessed and treated on clients with sinus problems.

Palpable landmarks:

- Frontal "ridge": this horizontal ridge begins as part of the orbit, the bony prominence surrounding the eye. The ridge extends, superior to the sphenoid bone, onto the parietal bone.

Articulations:

- The frontal bone articulates with the zygomatic bone and the parietal, sphenoid, maxilla, and nasal bones.

Attachments:

- The anterior portion of Occipitofrontalis [ahk-sip-ih-toh-frun-TAY-lus] covers much of the frontal bone.

Palpating the frontal bone:

POSITION:

- Supine client: undrape your client's neck.
- Stand or sit at the head of the table. For palpation of the bony landmarks of the head and face with your client supine, both hands are considered palpating hands.

LOCATE AND PALPATE:

- Place your thumbs together along the top of your client's skull, fingertips on her eyebrows.
- Slide your fingertips laterally to follow the curve of the orbit around the eye, as in Figure 7–12. Palpate

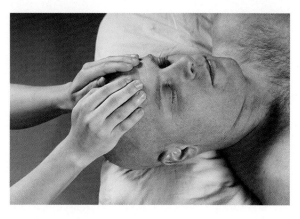

FIGURE 7-12 Palpating the frontal bone.

upward on the lateral frontal bone to feel the frontal ridge. Palpate the ridge to its posterior continuation on the parietal bone.

EVALUATE:

- Characterize your findings: is the ridge of the frontal bone equally prominent on both sides of the skull?
- Compare your findings with palpations of the frontal bone on other clients.

The Parietal Bone

The parietal bone can be seen in Figure 7–7. Although the parietal bone [pur-RY-ate-ul BOHN] curves significantly from the sagittal suture along the top of the skull to the squamous suture, where it articulates with the temporal bone, it is considered a flat bone.

Palpable landmarks:

- Parietal "ridge": this horizontal ridge continues laterally from the frontal bone and curves through the parietal bone to the posterior of the temporal bone, where it terminates in the zygomatic process.

Articulations:

- The parietal bones articulate with the frontal and temporal bones, the occiput and the sphenoid.

Attachments:

- Temporalis and Temporoparietalis attach to the parietal bones.

Palpating the parietal bone:

POSITION:

- Supine client: undrape your client's neck.
- Stand or sit at the head of the table. For palpation of the bony landmarks of the head and face with your client supine, both hands are considered palpating hands.

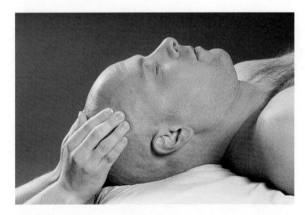

LOCATE AND PALPATE:

- Place your thumbs together along the top of the skull. Your fingers will drape over the parietal bone.
- The ridge will be found as the parietal bone curves toward the temporal bone: explore its anterior-to-posterior orientation. Figure 7–13 illustrates palpation of the parietal bone.

FIGURE 7-13 Palpating the parietal bone.

EVALUATE:

- Characterize your findings: are the parietal bones equally prominent on both sides of the skull? Is the articulation with the zygomatic bone the same size and shape on each side of the face?
- Compare your findings with palpations of the parietal bones on other clients.

The Mandible

The mandible [MAN-duh-bul] is visible in Figure 7–7.
Palpable landmarks:

- Angle: the prominent angle of the mandible is lateral and posterior, superficial, and readily palpable.
- Coronoid process: the coronoid process [KOR-un-noyd PRAH-ses] is the anterior, superior projection. Its superior portion lies deep to the zygomatic arch when the jaw is closed or elevated.
- Condyle: the condyle of the mandible is the posterior, superior projection that articulates with the temporal bone to form the temporomandibular joint.

Articulations:

- The temporomandibular joints: the condyles of the mandible articulate with the fossae of the temporal bone.

Attachments:

- The Masseter and Medial pterygoid muscles attach to the angle of the mandible.
- Temporalis and Masseter attach to the coronoid process, and the Lateral pterygoid muscles attach to the condyle of the mandible.

Mandible

the jaw.

HERE'S A TIP

The angle of the mandible is sometimes obscured by excess adipose tissue and may be positioned posteriorly in someone with an "overbite" or toward the anterior on someone with an "underbite."

Palpating the mandible:

POSITION:

- Supine client: undrape your client's neck.
- Stand or sit at the head of the table. For palpation of the bony landmarks of the head and face with your client supine, both hands are considered palpating hands.

LOCATE AND PALPATE:

- Place your hands along your client's jaw line, so that your fingertips meet at the point of her chin, as shown in Figure 7–14.
- Slide your fingertips around the jaw line to palpate the angle of the mandible, which is superficial and quite prominent on most people.

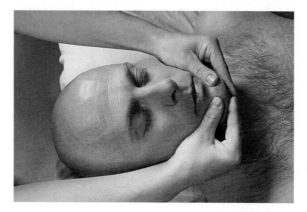

FIGURE 7–14 Palpating the mandible.

■ From the angle of the mandible, sweep your fingertips upward to palpate the condyle.

■ The coronoid process is not as easily palpable because its superior portion lies deep to the zygomatic arch.

DIRECT AN ACTION AND PALPATE:

■ Ask your client to open and close her jaw to palpate the condyle of the mandible during depression and elevation.

■ Ask your client to open her jaw so that you may palpate the coronoid process of the mandible, starting with your fingertips on the zygomatic arch and moving downward onto the coronoid process as it emerges from beneath the arch during depression of the jaw.

EVALUATE:

■ Characterize your findings: is the angle of the mandible equally prominent on both sides of the skull? Are the condyles and coronoid processes equal in size and shape? Do these processes maintain their orientation during elevation and depression of the mandible, or does one process jut laterally?

■ Compare your findings with palpations of the mandible on other clients.

IN THE TREATMENT ROOM

When your client opens and closes her jaw so that you may palpate the condyle of the mandible, any notable prominence of one of the condyles during movement indicates a misalignment at the temporomandibular joint that should point you toward treatment of the muscles of mastication and referral for a dental evaluation.

Hyoid

"U" shaped.

The Hyoid Bone

The hyoid bone [HY-oyd BOHN], seen in Figure 7–15, does not articulate with any other bone. Instead, it is held in place by connective tissue. The hyoid has significance in forensic pathology: in adults, it is fractured during strangulation, aiding determination of cause of death. The hyoid bone stabilizes the hyoid muscles during swallowing.

Palpable landmarks:

■ Body: the large, central portion.
■ Greater cornu: the large, superior bilateral processes.

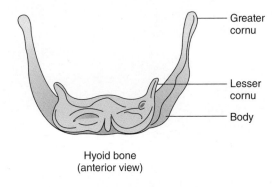

Hyoid bone
(anterior view)

FIGURE 7–15 The hyoid bone.

Articulations:

■ The hyoid is one of the few bones that does not form an articulation with another bone.

Attachments:

■ Eight of the nine Hyoid muscles, excepting Sternothyroid, attach to the mandible.

Palpating the hyoid bone:

POSITION:

■ Supine client: undrape your client's neck and upper chest.

■ Stand or sit at the side of the table. Place your mother hand beneath the neck for support and to discourage head or neck movement.

LOCATE AND PALPATE:

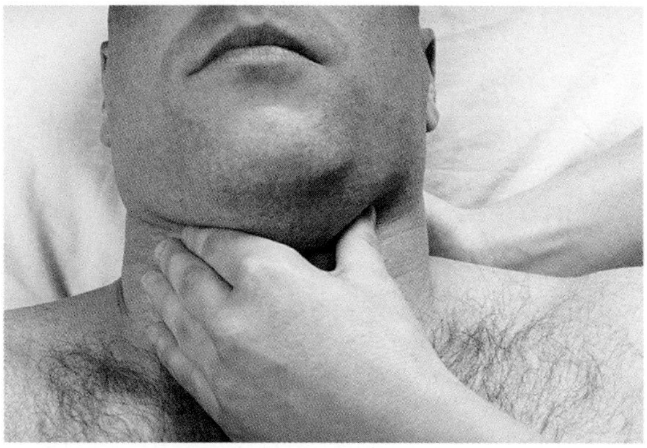

■ Proceed gently and with caution when palpating any structure on the anterior neck. Locate your own hyoid bone before palpating the hyoid on a client.

FIGURE 7-16 Palpating the hyoid bone.

© Milady, a part of Cengage Learning. Photography by Yanik Chauvin.

■ Place your thumb and one or two fingers of your palpating hand on each side of the client's jaw where it meets his neck, just inferior to the angle of the mandible, as in Figure 7–16. Slide your palpating hand inferiorly and medially until you feel bony tissue.

■ Once you have located the body of the hyoid, slide your palpating fingertips laterally and slightly upward to find each greater cornu. Wobbling your fingertips back and forth ever so slightly will let you know you have found them—the hyoid as a whole will move.

■ The central body is readily palpable. Each palpable greater cornu is lateral and superior on the hyoid and especially identifiable during the swallow.

HERE'S A TIP

The hyoid moves significantly during swallowing. Asking your client to swallow as you gently palpate the hyoid lets you know when you've located it.

IN THE TREATMENT ROOM

The anterior neck may be an area of emotional vulnerability for some clients. Be alert to the potential for distress as you palpate structures on the anterior neck: describe the palpation before proceeding and palpate very gently. Palpate during your client's exhalation and check in frequently to be certain your client is comfortable with the technique.

EVALUATE:

■ Characterize your findings: is the hyoid mobile? Is it equally mobile from side to side?

■ Compare your findings with palpations of the hyoid on other clients.

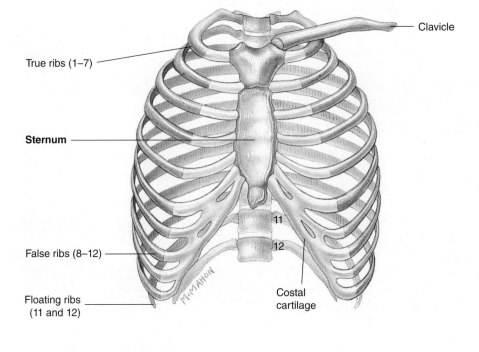

FIGURE 7-17 The sternum and the anterior ribs.

Clavicle

True ribs (1–7)

Sternum

11

12

False ribs (8–12)

Floating ribs (11 and 12)

Costal cartilage

Sternum

the breastbone.

The Sternum

The xiphoid process [ZIFF-oyd PRAH-ses] of the sternum [STUR-num], seen in Figure 7–17 may be absent in some people. It also may be missing because it can break off during forceful or poorly applied chest compressions during CPR and can puncture a lung.

Palpable landmarks:

- Manubrium [muh-NOO-bree-um]: the superior portion of the sternum. The medial notch on the manubrium is called the suprasternal notch.
- Gladiolus [glad-ee-OH-lus] or body: the large, central portion of the sternum.
- Xiphoid process: the inferior, pointed process. Initially cartilaginous, it may become bone over time.

Articulations:

- The sternoclavicular joint: manubrium articulates with the medial clavicle.
- The sternocostal joints: the body of the sternum articulates with the costal cartilage of the ribs.

Attachments:

- An insertion of Sternocleidomastoid, SCM, is on the manubrium.
- Rectus abdominis, the Diaphragm, and the abdominal aponeurosis attach to the xiphoid process.

Palpating the sternum:

POSITION:

- Supine client: you may wish to palpate the sternum through your female client's draped chest.

- Stand or sit at the side of the table.
- Place your mother hand beneath your client's thorax for stability and support.

LOCATE AND PALPATE:

- Because there is little tissue between the skin and the sternum, palpation pressure over the sternum should be very light.
- Place your palpating hand softly over the midline, fingertips at the sterno-clavicular joint. Gently palpate your client's visible and superficial suprasternal notch, as shown in Figure 7–18.
- With your fingertips, gently explore the articulations of the manubrium with the clavicle and the body with the costal cartilage.
- Slide your hand lower on the abdomen to locate the small, somewhat pointy xiphoid process at the inferior end of the sternum. If your client takes in a deep breath, the xiphoid may become more prominent for easier palpation.

EVALUATE:

- Characterize your findings: are the divisions of the sternum palpable?
- Compare your findings with palpations of the sternum on other clients.

OPTION:

- Standing or seated behind your supine client: Slide your mother hand under your client's upper thorax and place your palpating hand over the sternum from above. The heel of your hand will rest lightly on the manubrium as your fingertips palpate the body and xiphoid process of the sternum. This palpation position is easier for longer-armed therapists!

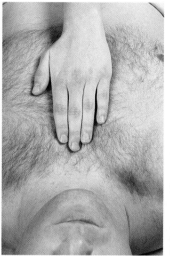

© Milady, a part of Cengage Learning. Photography by Yanik Chauvin.

FIGURE 7–18 Palpating the sternum.

HERE'S A TIP

Be extra mindful of draping when palpating near breast tissue. Always respect your client's individual boundaries and palpate with ongoing consent:

- Your client may be more comfortable if you palpate the sternum over the drape, with the chest remaining covered.
- If your client is large breasted, avoid placing your whole hand over the sternum. Palpate with your fingertips only.
- Alter your position: standing at the side of the table, palpate the sternum with your fingertips only, over the drape from the midline of the body of the sternum, working across the table. Consider palpating from the xiphoid process toward the manubrium of the sternum.
- Your female client may wish to secure her breast tissue with her own hand.

IN THE TREATMENT ROOM

The sternum of a client who has undergone open heart surgery may have been split open and stapled back together during the procedure. The sternum is also easily bruised or cracked by the seatbelt in even a minor car accident, and it may remain painful for many months. Perform palpation of the sternum with complete intake information in mind.

The Ribs

The ribs can be seen in Figure 7–17.

Palpable landmarks:

- Angle: the orientation of each rib as it travels from the anterior of the thorax to the posterior.
- Costal cartilage [KAHS-tul KAR-ti-ledg]: the costal cartilage attaches ribs #2–7 directly to the sternum and ribs #8–10 indirectly. Ribs #11–12 are "floating" ribs, with no sternal articulation.
- Intercostal spaces: between each pair of ribs is an intercostal space filled by the Internal and External intercostal muscles.

Non-palpable landmarks:

- Head: the posterior end of a rib that articulates with the body of a vertebra.
- Tubercle: a posterior projection on a rib that articulates with the transverse process of a vertebra.

Articulations:

- The sternocostal joints: ribs articulate with the manubrium of the sternum via costal cartilage.
- The vertebrocostal joints: heads of ribs and the bodies of thoracic vertebrae articulate with the tubercles of ribs and the transverse processes of thoracic vertebrae.

Attachments:

- Internal and External intercostals attach to each pair of ribs.
- The Diaphragm, Pectoralis major and minor, Rectus abdominis, Serratus anterior, and Transversus abdominis all attach to surfaces of ribs.

Associated structures:

- The abdominal aponeurosis and the rectus sheath.

HERE'S A TIP

Rib #1 is largely deep to the clavicle and is not readily palpable. Ribs #2–10 are palpable for most of their length. Ribs #11–12, the floating ribs, are short, pointy projections just superior to the iliac crest. The floating ribs are only palpable with the client in side-lying or prone position. Palpate them working from medial to lateral only, to avoid causing discomfort to your client.

Palpating the ribs:

Pause as you palpate your client's ribs so that you may experience the movement of ribs at different levels of the thorax during inhalation and exhalation.

POSITION:

- Supine, side-lying, and prone client: drape the breast area for security. Palpate through the drape when indicated.
- Stand or sit at the side of the table. Place your mother hand to support the torso of your side-lying client.

ADDITIONAL NOTES ON POSITIONING:

- With your client in supine position, work from medial to lateral on your client's anterior trunk, seated or standing, working from the opposite side of the table. Place your mother hand beneath the ribcage for stability, or use both hands to palpate.
- With your client in prone position: work from medial to lateral on your client's posterior trunk. Stand, working from the opposite side of the table. Use both hands to palpate.

- Side-lying position is recommended for complete palpation of the ribs on each side of the body and to sense the cage-like, rounded structure of the thorax.
- Palpating both sides of the anterior ribs with the client supine and the posterior ribs with the client prone allows you to compare their structure and angle.

HERE'S A TIP

Breast tissue may interfere with complete palpation of the ribcage in supine or side-lying positions. Drape the area with care, as shown in Figure 7–19a. Your client may prefer that you palpate over the drape. Communicate with your client, asking permission to continue before each repositioning of the palpating hand.

LOCATE AND PALPATE:

WITH YOUR CLIENT SUPINE:

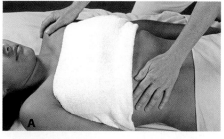

- Starting at the sternocostal joints, where the costal cartilage articulates with the sternum, spread your fingers slightly, as shown in Figure 7–19b, to palpate several ribs at once.
- Note the junction between each rib and its costal cartilage. Explore the web-like structure of the costal cartilage via which ribs #8–10 attach to the sternum.
- Explore the oblique angle of the ribcage as a whole and how this angle changes as you palpate around the thorax.
- Move your fingertips slightly laterally to palpate the intercostal spaces.

WITH YOUR CLIENT PRONE:

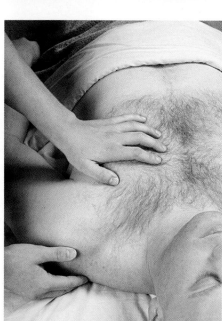

- In the posterior trunk, the ribs are deep to multiple layers of musculature along each side of the spine: the Erector spinae and Transversospinalis groups, plus Latissimus dorsi in the lumbar region and Trapezius in the thoracic region, among others. This musculature may make it difficult to palpate close to the spine.
- The posterior ribs are readily palpable lateral to the Erector spinae and Transversospinalis muscle groups, from T7–T12. From C7–T4, the Rhomboids, which overlie the ribs in the space between the vertebrae and the scapula and the scapula itself, limit palpation. The ribs inferior to T4 are more readily

FIGURE 7–19 (a) Drape your female client's breast area securely and palpate the anterior ribs above and below the drape. (b) Palpating the ribs with your client supine.

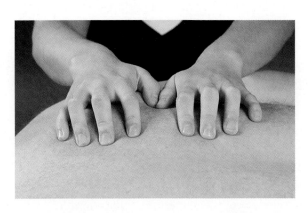

FIGURE 7–20 Palpating the ribs with your client prone.

palpable, as shown in Figure 7–20.

- Note the oblique angle of the ribcage from the posterior aspect. Explore how this angle changes as you palpate around the thorax.
- Move your fingertips slightly laterally to palpate the intercostal spaces.

EVALUATE:

- Characterize your findings: is the size and shape of the ribs equal on each side of the body? Are the intercostal spaces palpable from upper ribs to lower ribs?
- Compare your findings with palpations of ribs on other clients.

OPTION:

- With your client in side-lying position: standing behind your client, place your mother hand, to stabilize her trunk. Palpate the ribcage, following its curve, as in Figure 7–21, taking care to avoid breast tissue. Your client may prefer that you palpate over the drape.

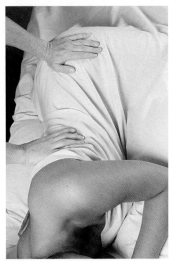

FIGURE 7–21 Palpating the ribs with your client in side-lying position.

IN THE TREATMENT ROOM

Someday you will encounter a client whose ribcage is quite ticklish, making palpation a challenge. Suggest deep breathing and palpate with your whole hand, not your fingertips, on her exhalation. You may also ask your client to place her hand over yours during palpation or give her another task, such as holding the drape in place that may serve as a distraction. Deepening your palpation pressure may also diminish a ticklish response.

Aponeurosis

flat sheet.

Rectus

erect.

The Abdominal Aponeurosis and the Rectus Sheath

The abdominal aponeurosis and the rectus sheath are shown in Figure 7–22. The abdominal aponeurosis is a broad, flat sheet of fascia in

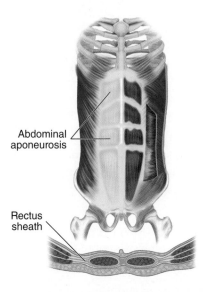

Abdominal aponeurosis

Rectus sheath

FIGURE 7–22 The abdominal aponeurosis and the rectus sheath.

the anterior abdomen that attaches Transversus abdominis, which has no bony attachment, to the abdominal wall. An extension of this deep fascia on the posterior of the aponeurosis forms the rectus sheath, which surrounds the Rectus abdominis muscle and extends from the xiphoid process of the sternum to the crest of the pubic bone.

Palpating the abdominal aponeurosis and the rectus sheath:

POSITION:

- Supine client: undrape the abdomen and cover the breast area, or work over the drape.
- Stand or sit at the side of the table. Use both hands to palpate.

LOCATE AND PALPATE:

- Locate the xiphoid process of the sternum and the pubic crest, the bony anterior prominence of the pelvis described on page 281, as shown in Figure 7–23.
- Palpate the dense fascia that surrounds and supports the muscles in the anterior abdomen between these landmarks, as shown in Figure 7–23. Move your palpating fingertips laterally from each side of the midline to gauge the breadth of the rectus sheath.

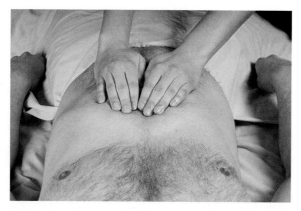

FIGURE 7–23 Palpating the abdominal aponeurosis and the rectus sheath.

© Milady, a part of Cengage Learning. Photography by Yanik Chauvin.

EVALUATE:

- Characterize the mobility of this fascial structure: is it freely mobile or is it partially or completely restricted?
- Characterize the tissue quality of the abdominal aponeurosis and the rectus sheath: does the tissue feel supple or brittle? Does the tissue soften in response to your touch?
- Compare the mobility and tissue quality of the abdominal aponeurosis and the rectus sheath with your palpation of the abdominal aponeurosis and the rectus sheath on other clients.

IN THE TREATMENT ROOM

Your client may be ticklish or feel emotionally vulnerable around the pubic crest area. Discuss and agree to the boundaries of physical touch in this palpation with your client before you begin. Leave the drape in place over the pubic crest and always work within your client's comfort level.

The Vertebrae

The spine, shown in Figure 7–24, typically has 24 vertebrae [VUR-tuh-breye]—seven in the cervical region, 12 in the thoracic region, and five in

Vertebra

to turn.

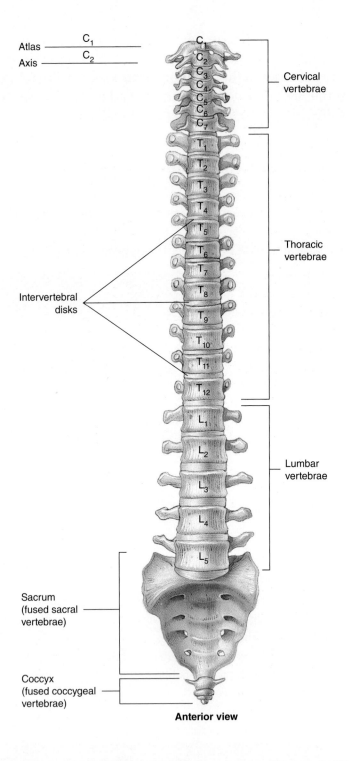

Atlas — C₁
Axis — C₂

C₁
C₂
C₃
C₄
C₅
C₆
C₇

Cervical vertebrae

T₁
T₂
T₃
T₄
T₅
T₆
T₇
T₈
T₉
T₁₀
T₁₁
T₁₂

Intervertebral disks

Thoracic vertebrae

L₁
L₂
L₃
L₄
L₅

Lumbar vertebrae

Sacrum (fused sacral vertebrae)

Coccyx (fused coccygeal vertebrae)

Anterior view

FIGURE 7-24 The vertebral column, anterior view.

the lumbar region. Each typical vertebra, as seen in Figure 7–25, features the same landmarks, which vary in size, shape, and orientation, depending on their region:

- Spinous processes are minimal in C1 and C2, the first and second cervical vertebrae, and are bifurcated or split in C3–5. The spinous process of C7 is visibly longer than other spinous processes.
- Spinous processes in the cervical region point posteriorly. In the thoracic region, they point increasingly to the inferior, while lumbar spinous processes are square-shaped and point posteriorly.

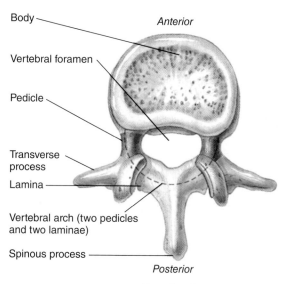

FIGURE 7–25 A typical vertebra.

Superior view

Body

Anterior

Vertebral foramen

Pedicle

Transverse process

Lamina

Vertebral arch (two pedicles and two laminae)

Spinous process

Posterior

© Delmar, Cengage Learning.

- Transverse processes in the cervical region are small and point laterally. In the thoracic region, transverse processes are longer and are angled slightly downward, where they articulate with the ribs. Lumbar transverse processes are broader, shorter, and point more laterally than those in the thoracic region.

Joint range of motion in the spine is also variable. In the thoracic region, the cage-like structure of the ribcage limits the range of motion possible in the cervical and lumbar regions:

- The atlanto-occipital and atlanto-axial allow free movement, but are difficult to access for palpation.
- Intervertebral joints allow freer movement of the spine in the cervical and lumbar regions than in the thoracic region, and although synovial, the vertebrocostal joints allow little movement—only slight gliding—in the thorax, where the cage-like structure of the ribcage limits range of motion.
- The lumbosacral joint supports much of the weight of the torso, and allows for varied movement.

Palpable landmarks on each vertebra:

- Spinous process: the posterior projection.
- Lamina [LAM-uh-nuh]: the surface that lies between the spinous and transverse processes. Sequential laminae create the palpable laminar groove for the attachment of deep paraspinal muscles that run parallel to the spine.
- Transverse processes: the lateral projections.

Non-palpable landmarks:

- Body: the large anterior portion of a vertebra.
- Vertebral arch: arch formed by the laminae of a vertebra and posterior projections called pedicles.
- Vertebral foramen: large, central foramen through which the spinal cord passes.
- Intervertebral foramen: bilateral openings between vertebrae through which spinal nerves pass.

DID YOU KNOW?

The bodies of vertebrae are composed of a superficial layer of hard, compact bone over an inner core of lightweight, spongy bone. Without this mass of lightweight bone, the spine would be too heavy for us to stand upright.

Articulations:

- The atlanto-occipital joint: articular facets of C1, the atlas, articulate with the condyles of the occiput.
- The atlanto-axial joint: the dens, a superior projection on C2, the axis, articulates with the anterior arch of C1, the atlas.
- The lumbosacral joint: the body of the fifth lumbar vertebra articulates with the base of the sacrum.
- The vertebrocostal joints: heads of ribs and the bodies of thoracic vertebrae articulate with the tubercles of the ribs and the transverse processes of thoracic vertebrae.
- The intervertebral joints: the bodies and arches of adjacent vertebrae articulate.

Attachments:

- The Erector spinae and Transversospinalis groups and the Interspinales, Latissimus dorsi, Rhomboids, Serratus posterior superior and inferior, and Trapezius all attach to spinous processes from C7 through the lumbar region.
- The Transversospinalis group attaches along the laminar groove.
- The Erector spinae and Transversospinalis groups, Intertransversarii, Quadratus lumborum, and Psoas major all share attachments on transverse processes.

The spinous processes of cervical and thoracic vertebrae are readily palpable, depending on the degree of the posterior thoracic curvature of your client's spine. Spinous processes in the lumbar region may be more difficult to palpate, depending on the degree of the anterior lumbar curve in your client's spine, and are easiest to palpate with your client standing or seated.

Palpation of the spinous processes of the vertebrae with your client standing, that is, when weight-bearing, is a primary means of postural assessment, and is described in detail in Chapter 6, The Art of Palpation. The palpation of the landmarks of the cervical and thoracic spine described below is described with your client on the massage table and is intended to be a guide to locating the muscles that attach to the vertebrae. Palpation of lumbar spinous processes is described with your client standing or seated.

Palpating the vertebrae:

Palpating cervical and thoracic spinous processes:

POSITION:

- Prone client: undrape your client's neck and back.
- Adjust the face cradle to create slight flexion of your client's head, making the spinous processes in the cervical region more apparent.
- Stand or sit at the side of the table. Place your mother hand on the crown of your client's head or on her shoulder.

LOCATE AND PALPATE:

- Cervical spinous processes: locate the prominent spinous process of C7. Place the fingertips of your palpating hand along the midline. With the fingertips of your palpating hand, palpate through the nuchal ligament toward the occiput, counting the spinous processes toward the head, from C6 to C2, as in Figure 7–26.

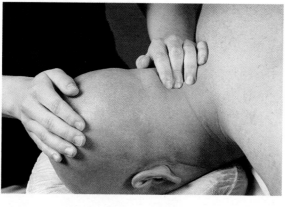

© Milady, a part of Cengage Learning. Photography by Yanik Chauvin.

FIGURE 7-26 Palpation of cervical spinous process.

- Thoracic spinous processes: with the fingertips of your palpating hand, gently palpate the spinous processes down the midline from C7 into the thoracic region, keeping count as you go, T1–T12. The insertion of Trapezius on the spinous process of T12 may be a visual cue.

Palpating lumbar spinous processes:

POSITION:

- Standing or seated client.
- Support your client's standing or seated posture with your mother hand.

LOCATE AND PALPATE:

- Ask your client to lean forward from the waist, as shown in Figure 7–27, until the degree of flexion allows you to palpate the individual spinous processes in the lumbar region without compromising his balance.

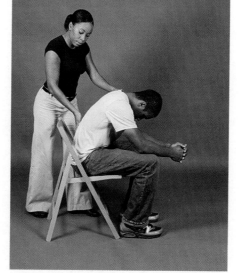

FIGURE 7-27 Palpating lumbar spinous processes on a seated client.

© Milady, a part of Cengage Learning. Photography by Yanik Chauvin.

OPTION:

- With your client prone on the massage table, back draped or undraped, palpate from the lumbar to the cervical region.
- Place your palpating hand along the midline over the lumbar spine. Palpate *up* the spine, toward the head.
- Some therapists find that the direction of movement in this technique allows them to "run into" the spinous processes.

ADDITIONAL OPTION:

- With your client in supine position, slide your mother hand under your client's occiput, to support her head and neck.
- Slide your palpating hand beneath your client's shoulder, with your fingertips at the midline. Locate the prominent spinous process of C7. Palpate upward along the midline, through the nuchal ligament toward the occiput, counting the spinous processes from C6 to C2.

Palpating the laminar groove:

The laminar groove created by the sequential laminae of the vertebral column is deep to layers of bulky paraspinal muscles and may not be readily palpable on all clients.

POSITION:

- ■ Prone client: undrape your client's back.
- ■ Place your mother hand for ease and comfort.

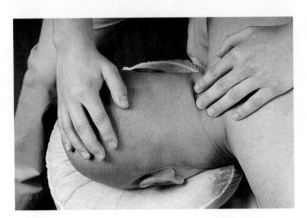

FIGURE 7–28 Palpating the laminae in the laminar groove.

LOCATE AND PALPATE:

- ■ Place your palpating hand along the midline at C7, as in Figure 7–28. Slide the fingers of your palpating hand just lateral to the spinous processes: you will feel the depression that leads toward the laminae and encounter the dense muscle tissue that fills the laminar groove.

Palpating transverse processes:

Transverse processes in the thoracic region of the spine are easier to locate for palpation than in the cervical or lumbar regions. Deviations in the normal spinal curvatures are assessed by palpating the spine following visual assessment.

POSITION:

- ■ Prone client: undrape your client's back.
- ■ Stand or sit at the side of the table. Place your mother hand for ease and comfort.

LOCATE AND PALPATE:

- ■ Cervical transverse processes: the cervical transverse processes are small and difficult to palpate. After palpating the cervical spinous processes as described above, move your fingers laterally to palpate the transverse processes, which are deep to posterior cervical muscles and relatively small, as shown in Figure 7–29.

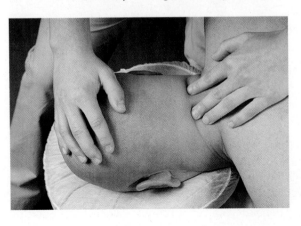

FIGURE 7–29 Palpating the cervical transverse processes of the vertebrae.

- ■ Thoracic transverse processes: locate a thoracic spinous process, as described above. Each transverse process of that thoracic vertebra is about one inch lateral to the spinous process and ever-so-slightly inferior.

- ■ Lumbar transverse processes: the lumbar transverse processes are difficult to locate for palpation, due to the anterior lumbar curve of the spine and the density of the musculature in the lumbar region. You may be able to palpate the lumbar spinous processes as your standing client slowly flexes his trunk to the fullest range.

EVALUATE:

- Characterize your findings: are the size and shape of the vertebral landmarks equal on each side of the body? Are the landmarks palpable throughout each region of the spine?
- Compare your findings with palpations of vertebrae on other clients.

IN THE TREATMENT ROOM

Palpating the curves of your client's spine to assess their relationship to the normal range alerts you to patterns of strain and compensation, as described in Chapter 2, Posture Assessment. Spinal curvatures that are diminished or exaggerated in any region set up patterns of strain in the surrounding musculature and require the body to create compensatory alterations in head and foot positions.

Palpating the curves of the spine:

The spine begins to develop its curves as it responds to bearing the weight of the head and torso when we begin as toddlers to stand and walk. The normal curves of the spine, as shown in Figure 7–30, are:

- To the anterior in the cervical region.
- To the posterior in the thoracic region.

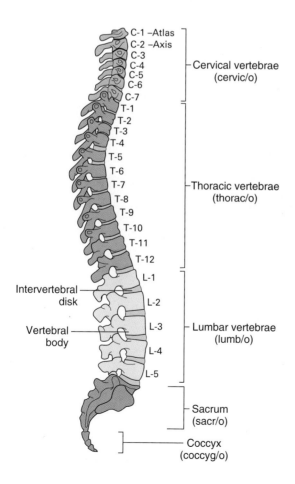

FIGURE 7–30 The normal curves of the spine, lateral view.

- To the anterior in the lumbar region.
- To the posterior over the sacrum.

In addition, the spine may curve laterally and vertebrae may twist or torque, singly or in groups, altering the position of the spine. You will find endless variations on these curvatures in your treatment room. The illustrations of the spine shown in textbooks and the spines of classroom skeletons almost never exist in reality!

POSITIONS:

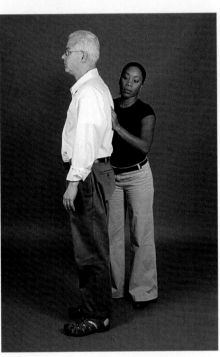

- Standing client: palpate over clothing. Use your mother hand to support your standing client's torso.
- Prone client: undrape the back. Use both hands to palpate your prone client's spine.

LOCATE AND PALPATE:

- With your client standing: support your client's torso, as shown in Figure 7–31. Slowly and gently sweep your palpating hand directly over the spine, from the occiput to the sacrum, noting the length and degree of each of the spinal curves.
- Place your hands on either side of the spine. Beginning at the occiput and palpating toward the sacrum, note any deviance in the spine that may curve it laterally.

FIGURE 7–31 Palpating the curves of the spine on a standing client.

OPTION:

With your client prone, as in Figure 7–32:

- Slowly and gently sweep your palpating hand directly over the spine, noting any variance from the standing—weight bearing—palpation results.

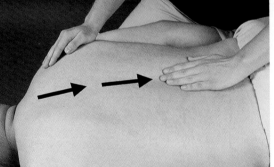

- Place your hands on either side of the spine. Beginning at the occiput and palpating toward the sacrum, note any deviance in the spine that may cause it to curve laterally.

EVALUATE:

- Characterize your findings: are the curvatures of the spine to the proper aspect

FIGURE 7–32 Palpating the curves of the spine on a prone client.

throughout each region of the spine? Does any individual curve feel exaggerated or diminished? Did your palpation find any lateral deviations in the spine?

- Compare your findings with palpations of spinal curvatures on other clients.

The Sacrum

Early in human evolution, the sacrum [SAY-krum] consisted of five separate vertebrae. The sacral tubercles are the remnants of the spinous processes of those vertebrae, while the coccyx, inferior to the sacrum, is the remnant of the tail that once was part of human anatomy. The sacrum is visible in Figure 7–33.

Palpable landmarks:

■ Base of the sacrum: the articulation of the sacrum with the body of L5.
■ Sacral tubercles: remnants of five spinous processes along the midline of the sacrum.

Articulations:

■ The lumbosacral joint: the base of the sacrum articulates with the body of L5.
■ The sacroiliac joint: the sacrum articulates with the ilia of the pelvis.
■ The sacrococcygeal joint: the apex of the sacrum articulates with the coccyx.

Attachments:

■ On the anterior surface: Iliacus, Piriformis.
■ On the posterior surface: Erector spinae and Transversospinalis groups, Gluteus maximus, and Latissimus dorsi.

Associated structures:

■ Thoracolumbar fascia

Sacrum

sacred.

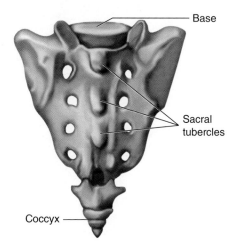

Base

Sacral tubercles

Coccyx

FIGURE 7–33 The sacrum, posterior view.

© Milady, a part of Cengage Learning.

Palpating the sacrum:

POSITION:

- Prone client: for palpation of the sacrum to its articulation with the coccyx, leave the area draped for client comfort and security.
- Stand or sit at the side of the table. Place your mother hand for ease and comfort, and your palpating hand along the midline over the lumbar vertebrae.

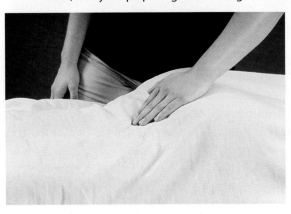

FIGURE 7-34 Palpating the sacrum.

LOCATE AND PALPATE:

- Palpate the midline of the spine, working inferiorly through the anterior lumbar curve until you reach its articulation with the sacrum at L5, the base of the sacrum, as seen in Figure 7–34. The anterior curve will abruptly become posterior over the sacrum.
- The five sacral tubercles are along the midline of the sacrum: laterally on the sacrum, you can palpate the protrusion of the PSIS, the posterior superior iliac spine, as it covers the articulation of the sacrum with the ilia of the pelvis.

EVALUATE:

- Characterize your findings: are all the sacral tubercles palpable? Is the base prominent and palpable?
- Compare your findings with palpations of the sacrum on other clients.

Thoracolumbar Fascia

Thick extensions of deep fascia form palpable structures in the posterior trunk: thoracolumbar [thoh-ruh-koh-LUM-buhr] fascia is found bilaterally in the lower thoracic and lumbar regions and in the upper thoracic region, medial to middle Trapezius. Thoracolumbar fascia is shown in Figure 7–35.

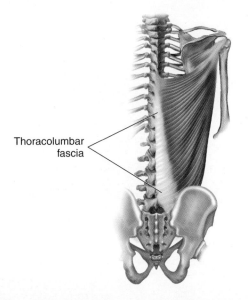

Thoracolumbar fascia

FIGURE 7-35 Thoracolumbar fascia.

Palpating thoracolumbar fascia:

POSITION:

- Prone client: undrape your client's back.
- Stand at the side of the table. Use both hands to palpate.

LOCATE AND PALPATE:

- With one palpating hand, locate the spinous process of C7. With your other palpating hand, locate the base of the sacrum.
- As shown in Figure 7–36, palpate the dense bilateral fascia that overlays the muscles along the spine in the upper thoracic and lower lumbar regions. Explore this tissue with your fingertips. Feel its density begin to "melt" beneath your warm touch.

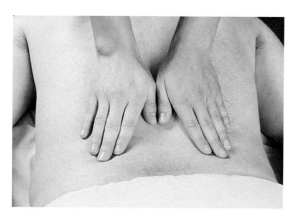

FIGURE 7-36 Palpating thoracolumbar fascia. Palpate using the pads of your finger tips not your thumbs.

© Milady, a part of Cengage Learning. Photography by Yanik Chauvin.

EVALUATE:

- Characterize the mobility of the thoracolumbar fascia: is it freely mobile or is it partially or completely restricted?
- Characterize the tissue quality of this thoracolumbar fascia: does the tissue feel supple or brittle? Does the tissue soften in response to your touch?
- Compare the mobility and tissue quality of this thoracolumbar fascia structure with your palpation of thoracolumbar fascia on other clients.

LEARNING ENHANCEMENT ACTIVITY

Commit to palpating bony landmarks of the axial skeleton at least 10 times in the next 30 days. Note the differences you observe in the prominence of landmarks on the skull, in the movement in the mandible, in the size of the sternum and angles of the ribs, in the prominence of spinous processes, and in the curves of each spine. Record your observations and examine them for any apparent trends: are there differences in gender, age, or physical condition that you note? How can you use this information in treatment planning?

Lab Activity 7–1 on page 299 is designed to develop your palpation skills on bony landmarks and associated structures of the axial skeleton.

PALPATING BONY LANDMARKS AND FASCIAL STRUCTURES ON THE UPPER EXTREMITY

The bony landmarks of the upper extremity described here for palpations include those on the clavicle and the scapula, the humerus, the radius and the ulna, and the carpals, metacarpals, and phalanges of the wrist and hand.

Acromial end

Sternal end

Posterior

Anterior

Curvature

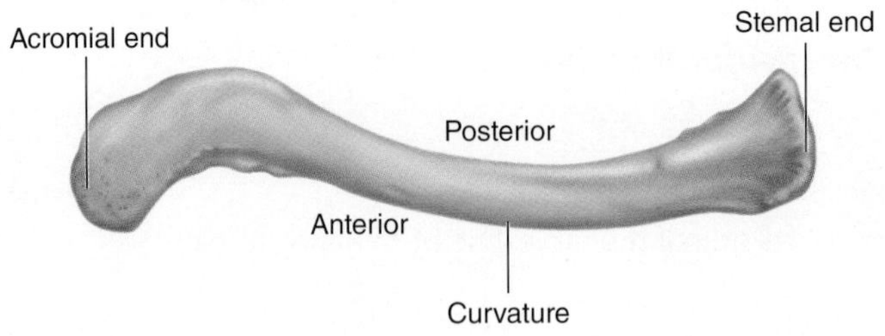

FIGURE 7–37 The clavicle.

Clavicle

key.

The Clavicle

The clavicle [KLAV-ih-kul] is the bone that is broken most often, sometimes on a newborn during birth. A broken clavicle is commonly left untreated and heals on its own. An improperly healed fracture of the clavicle will have consequences for its articulations and for the muscles, which attach to it. The clavicle is shown in Figure 7–37.

Palpable landmarks:

- Sternal end: the medial end of the clavicle.
- Acromial end: the lateral end of the clavicle.
- Curvature of the clavicle: from anterior or convex at the sternal end to posterior or concave at the acromial end.

Articulations:

- The sternoclavicular joint: the sternal end of the clavicle articulates with the manubrium of the sternum.
- The acromioclavicular joint: the acromial end of the clavicle articulates with the acromion of the scapula.

Attachments:

- Anterior Deltoid, Pectoralis major, one head of Sternocleidomastoid (SCM), Subclavian, and Trapezius all attach to surfaces of the clavicle.

Palpating the clavicle:

POSITION:

- Supine client: undrape your client's upper chest.
- Stand or sit at the side of the table. Place your mother hand beneath your client's thorax for stability and support.

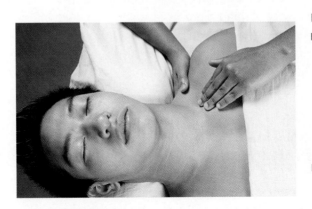

LOCATE AND PALPATE:

- Place your palpating hand softly over the midline, fingertips at the sternoclavicular joint. Gently palpate your client's visible and superficial suprasternal notch.
- Move your palpating hand slightly laterally to locate the sternal end of the

FIGURE 7–38 Palpating the clavicle.

clavicle, as shown in Figure 7–38. Palpate gently. There is little tissue over the clavicle.

- Continue palpating laterally, assessing the convex and concave curve of the clavicle, to the acromial end, where it articulates with the acromion of the scapula.
- Repeat the palpation on the contralateral clavicle. Palpate both clavicles simultaneously, comparing their symmetry.

EVALUATE:

- Characterize your findings. Is the shape of the curve of the clavicle equal on each side of the body? Is one acromial or sternal end more prominent than the other? Is there any indication of a previous break in the clavicle?
- Compare your findings with palpations of clavicles on other clients.

The Scapula

The actions of the scapula [SKAP-yuh-luh], shown in Figure 7–39, occur at the scapulocostal [skap-yuh-loh-KAHS-tul] joints: the articulations of the anterior scapula with posterior thoracic ribs.

Palpable landmarks:

- Angles: superior and inferior.
- Borders: Medial or vertebral and lateral or axillary.
- Spine: extends from the upper third of the medial border on the anterior surface, laterally and superiorly, to become the acromion process.
- Acromion [uh-KROH-mee-un] process: the anterior process that extends from the lateral spine.
- Coracoid [KOR-uh-koyd] process: extends from the anterior surface of the scapula to just below the acromial end of the clavicle.

Scapula

shovel or spade.

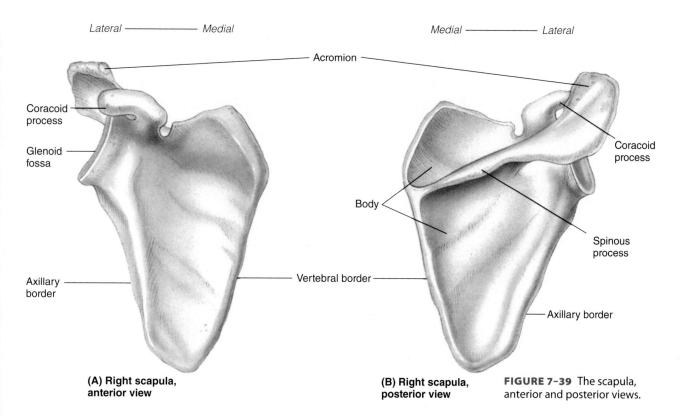

Lateral ——————— Medial   Medial ——————— Lateral

Acromion

Coracoid process

Glenoid fossa

Body

Coracoid process

Spinous process

Axillary border

Vertebral border

Axillary border

(A) Right scapula, anterior view

(B) Right scapula, posterior view

FIGURE 7–39 The scapula, anterior and posterior views.

© Delmar, Cengage Learning.

Non-palpable landmarks:

- Fossae: supraspinous, infraspinous, glenoid, and subscapular.
- Supraglenoid tubercle: tubercle located superior to the glenoid fossa.
- Infraglenoid tubercle: tubercle located inferior to the glenoid fossa.

Articulations:

- The glenohumeral joint: the glenoid fossa of the scapula articulates with the head of the humerus.
- The acromioclavicular joint: the acromion of the scapula articulates with the acromial end of the clavicle.
- The scapulocostal joints: the anterior scapula articulates with posterior thoracic ribs.

Attachments:

- Biceps brachii, Coracobrachialis and Deltoid, Infraspinatus, Levator scapulae and Pectoralis minor, Omohyoid of the Hyoid group, the Rhomboids and Serratus anterior, Subscapularis and Supraspinatus, Teres major and Teres minor, Trapezius and Triceps brachii all have attachments on surfaces of the scapula. Latissimus dorsi sometimes attaches to the scapula as it heads toward the humerus.

Associated structures:

- The **posterior axillary fold** is a mass of tissue created by the junction of Latissimus dorsi and Teres major and a pad of superficial adipose tissue. The size and location of this fold challenges palpation of the lateral border and subscapular surface of the scapula.
- A deep layer of fascia overlays much of the Infraspinatus muscle.

DID YOU KNOW?

Chronic strain in the muscles that attach to the scapula may refer into the axilla, or armpit. A client who reports pain in the axilla, should be evaluated by his primary healthcare provider to eliminate other causes of pain in this region.

Posterior axillary fold

a mass of tissue created by the junction of Latissimus dorsi and Teres major and a pad of adipose tissue.

Palpating the posterior scapula:

HERE'S A TIP

As you palpate, explore the range of movements of the scapula, including the movements of its inferior angle, to differentiate movements of the scapula at the scapulocostal joints from movements of the humerus at the glenohumeral joint.

POSITION:

- Prone client: undrape your client's back.
- Stand or sit at the side of the table. Place your mother hand beneath your client's shoulder joint.

LOCATE AND PALPATE:

- With your mother hand, lift your client's shoulder slightly until the angles and borders of the scapula more apparent.
- Curve your palpating hand around the inferior angle, as in Figure 7–40. Palpate from the inferior angle up the medial or vertebral border to the superior angle. You may need to perform another shoulder lift with your mother hand to locate the superior angle, which is deep to layers of muscle.
- Just below the superior angle on the medial border, locate the origin of the spine. Isolate the spine between your fingertips and thumb, tracing it laterally

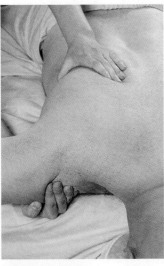

FIGURE 7–40 Palpating the posterior scapula.

to its anterior curve, where it becomes the acromion, the high point of the shoulder.

■ Return your palpating hand to the inferior angle once more. Palpate the lateral border with your thumb or fingertips as far as the superficial tissue will allow, noting the posterior axillary fold and the posterior fibers of Deltoid.

Palpating the anterior scapula:

The acromion process, the coracoid process, and the lateral border of the subscapular fossa are palpable from the anterior.

POSITION:

■ Supine client: support your client's arm in horizontal abduction with your mother hand.

■ Stand at the side of the table.

■ Tuck the drape under your client's arm to ensure security.

LOCATE AND PALPATE:

■ With the fingertips of your palpating hand, palpate the clavicle to its lateral articulation with the acromion—the high point of the shoulder—and the termination of the spine of the scapula.

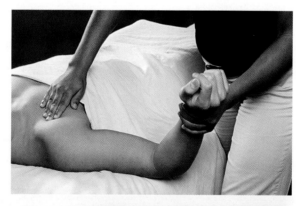

FIGURE 7–41 Palpating the coracoid process.

■ To locate the coracoid process, move your palpating fingertips about 1–1½ inch (2½–3 cm), inferior to the acromion and medial to the head of the humerus, as shown in Figure 7–41. The coracoid process lies beneath the dense fibers of pectoralis major. Proceed gently.

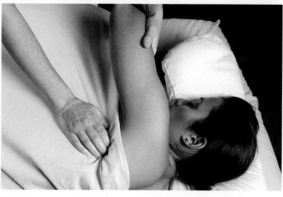

FIGURE 7–42 Palpating the lateral border of the scapula with the client's arm abducted.

■ To palpate the lateral border of the subscapular fossa, support your side-lying client's arm in abduction, as shown in Figure 7–42. Drape your client's breast tissue securely. Slide your palpating fingertips beneath the lateral border of the scapula, following the angle of the ribs.

PERFORM AN ACTION:

■ Gently pull your client's arm forward, applying traction as shown in Figure 7–43, to bring the scapula forward in protraction, increasing your access to the subscapular surface. Palpate during the traction.

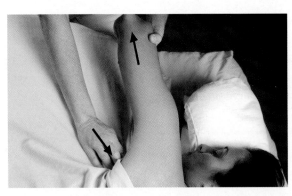

© Milady, a part of Cengage Learning. Photography by Yanik Chauvin.

FIGURE 7–43 Applying traction to the client's arm to facilitate palpation of the lateral border of the scapula.

EVALUATE:

■ Characterize your findings: are the size and shape of the scapular landmarks equal on each side of the body? Are the landmarks equally palpable on each scapula? Does any angle or border protrude unequally?

■ Compare your findings with palpations of the scapulae on other clients.

OPTION:

You can palpate both anterior and posterior landmarks on the scapula with your client in side-lying position:

■ Stand facing your side-lying client, with her arm flexed at her side. Cradling her anterior shoulder with your mother hand, slightly push on the shoulder to retract the scapula, moving it backward, as shown in Figure 7–44. Use the fingertips of your palpating hand to trace the inferior angle and medial border.

■ With additional retraction, you may also be able to palpate the medial border of the subscapular fossa, depending on the degree of free lifting of the scapula away from the posterior ribs allowed by your client's musculature.

■ Slightly elevating the shoulder may make the superior angle of the scapula easier to locate and palpate. Continue palpating to follow the spine of the scapula to its termination on the acromion.

■ Return to the inferior angle once more to palpate the lateral border and subscapular fossa, as described. It is difficult to palpate the coracoid process in side-lying position.

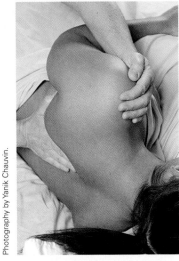

© Milady, a part of Cengage Learning. Photography by Yanik Chauvin.

FIGURE 7–44 Palpating the inferior angle of the scapula with the client in side-lying position.

IN THE TREATMENT ROOM

Manipulating the arm of a large client who is in side-lying position can be a challenge. You may ask the client to support her own arm in abduction, as pictured in Figure 7–45. With the client supporting her abducted arm, you are able to move around the table to palpate the scapula from multiple angles: from the head of the table, from in front of the client, and from behind the client. Note that the degree of access to the subscapular surface, from the medial or vertebral or the lateral or axillary border, will vary considerably, depending on the degree of free movement of the scapula allowed by the surrounding muscles.

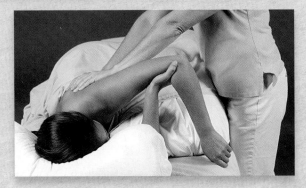

FIGURE 7–45 The client may support her own arm during palpation.

© Milady, a part of Cengage Learning. Photography by Yanik Chauvin.

The Humerus

The head of the humerus [HYOO-muh-rus], as seen in Figure 7–46, may be dislocated by sudden, hard impact to the shoulder from the side, as can happen during football, soccer, or rugby play. Dislocations are excruciatingly painful, but easily treated by putting the head of the humerus back into its socket at the glenoid fossa. Repeated dislocations, however, can result in serious damage to the muscles, tendons, and ligaments that hold the head of the humerus in place.

Palpable landmarks:

- Medial epicondyle: a larger projection at the distal, medial end of the humerus.
- Lateral epicondyle: a smaller, more pointed projection at the distal, lateral end of the humerus.
- Lateral supracondylar ridge: a sharp ridge of bone that extends vertically from the lateral epicondyle.
- Deltoid tuberosity: a roughened, slightly raised prominence midway down the shaft of the humerus.

Humerus

the shoulder.

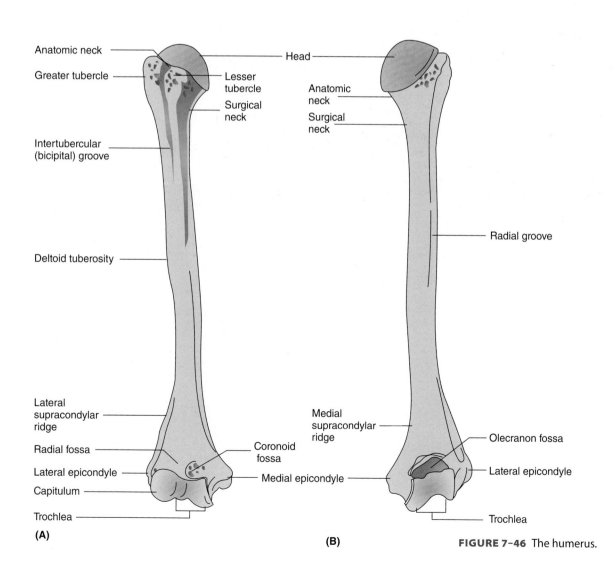

FIGURE 7-46 The humerus.

© Delmar, Cengage Learning.

- Lesser tubercle: a small tubercle at the proximal end or the head of the humerus, located medially and slightly inferior to the greater tubercle.
- Bicipital [by-SIP-ut-ul] or intertubercular [in-tur-too-BUR-kyoo-lur] groove: a deep, vertical groove on the proximal third of the humerus that lies between the greater and lesser tubercles, through which the tendon of the long head of Biceps brachii travels on its way to the scapula.
- Greater tubercle: a large tubercle at the proximal end or the head of the humerus, located laterally and slightly superior to the lesser tubercle.

Non-palpable landmarks:

- Capitulum [kah-PITCH-yuh-lum] and trochlea [TRAHK-lee-uh]: the condyles of the humerus, found at the anterior distal end, around which the processes of the ulna slide in flexion of the forearm.
- Coronoid fossa: the anterior, distal fossa into which slides the coronoid process of the ulna during flexion of the forearm.
- Olecranon fossa: [oh-LEK-ruh-nahn FAHS-uh]: the posterior, distal fossa into which slides the olecranon of the ulna.

Articulations:

- The glenohumeral joint: the head of the humerus articulates with the glenoid fossa of the scapula.
- The humeroulnar joint: the capitulum of the humerus articulates with the head of the radius and the trochlea of the humerus with the trochlear notch of the ulna.

Attachments:

- Anconeus, Biceps brachii and Brachialis, Brachioradialis, Coracobrachialis and Deltoid, extensors and flexors of the forearm, Infraspinatus, Subscapularis and Supraspinatus, Teres major and Teres minor, and Pronator teres and Triceps brachii all share attachments on the humerus.

Palpating the humerus:

POSITION:

- Supine client: undrape your client's arm, securing the drape.
- Stand at the side of the table. Use your mother hand to support the shoulder and humeroulnar joints as you manipulate the humerus.

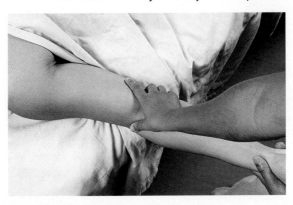

FIGURE 7–47 Palpating the humerus.

© Milady, a part of Cengage Learning. Photography by Yanik Chauvin.

LOCATE AND PALPATE:

- Begin palpation from the distal humerus.
- Slightly rotate your client's arm laterally. Gently grasp the distal humerus between your thumb and fingers, just above the anterior crease at the elbow, as in Figure 7–47.

- As you grasp the distal humerus, either your thumb is palpating the lateral epicondyle and your fingers are palpating the medial epicondyle or vice versa. Each is felt as a sharp protrusion on the distal humerus, though the medial epicondyle is sharper.

- Slide the fingertips of your palpating hand proximally from the lateral epicondyle to palpate the lateral epicondylar ridge, which extends vertically two to three inches on the lateral humerus.

- Slide your palpating hand proximally again on the shaft of the humerus. About one-third of the length down the shaft from the head of the humerus, palpate the deltoid tuberosity. You may feel a hard, tender knot at this site, the insertion of the Deltoid.

- The bicipital groove may be palpated just distal to the acromion of the scapula, deep to the fibers of Deltoid, on the head of the humerus between the greater and lesser tubercles, as shown in Figure 7–48. Take care—deep or persistent palpation of the bicipital groove may cause pain in the tendon of the long head of Biceps brachii, which passes through it.

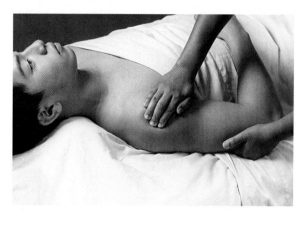

FIGURE 7–48 Palpating the bicipital groove of the humerus.

© Milady, a part of Cengage Learning. Photography by Yanik Chauvin.

- The greater tubercle is lateral to the bicipital groove and superior on the head of the humerus. To make sure you are palpating the head of the humerus and not the acromion, passively flex and extend your client's arm at the glenohumeral joint. The head of the humerus will move, the acromion will not.

- The lesser tubercle is smaller than the greater tubercle and is found medial to the bicipital groove and slightly distal to the greater tubercle. Palpate each tubercle with your fingertips, comparing their relative size and shape.

PERFORM AN ACTION:

- To make sure you are palpating the humerus and not the radius or ulna, passively flex and extend your client's arm at the elbow: the radius and ulna will move, the humerus will not.

EVALUATE:

- Characterize your findings. Are the size and shape of the landmarks on the humerus equal on each side of the body? Are the landmarks equally palpable?

- Compare your findings with palpations of the humerus on other clients.

The Radius and the Ulna

Pronation and supination take place at the proximal and distal radioulnar joints. During these actions, the radius rotates around the ulna, while the ulna remains stable. Palpating the radius and the ulna [UL-nuh] during pronation and supination helps you to experience these complex actions of the radius and the ulna, seen in Figure 7–49.

Radius

rod or spoke of a wheel.

Ulna

elbow.

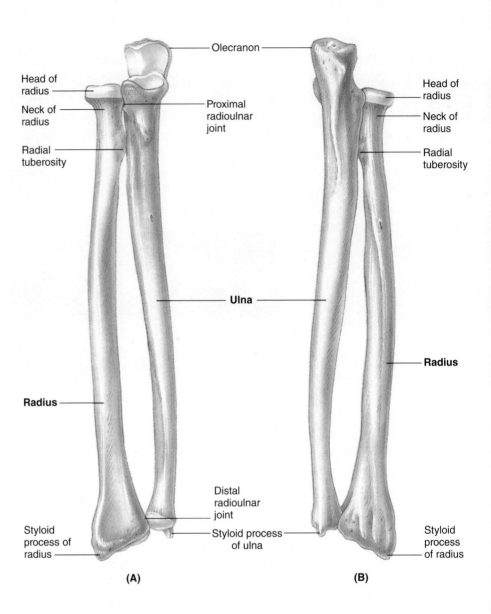

FIGURE 7-49 The radius and the ulna.

(A)   (B)

Palpable landmarks on the radius:
- Styloid process: the distal, lateral projection.
- Shaft: the lateral shaft of the radius is palpable.

Palpable landmarks on the ulna:
- Head and styloid process: the distal, medial projection.
- Shaft: the medial shaft of the ulna is palpable.
- Olecranon: the "elbow," the large, posterior, proximal process.

Non-palpable landmarks on the radius:
- Head: the proximal articular surface.
- Radial tuberosity: roughened area on the medial surface

Non-palpable landmarks on the ulna:
- Coronoid process: proximal, anterior projection.
- Ulnar tuberosity: roughened area distal to the coronoid process.

Articulations:
- The proximal radioulnar joint: the head of the radius articulates with the radial notch of the ulna.

- The distal radioulnar joint: the ulnar notch of the radius articulates with the head of the ulna.
- The humeroulnar joint: the olecranon of the ulna also articulates with the olecranon fossa of the humerus and with the radius and interosseous membrane.

Attachments:

- Anconeus, Brachialis and Brachioradialis, the forearm extensor and flexor groups, Pronator teres, Supinator, and Triceps brachii all share attachments on surfaces of the radius or the ulna.

Palpating the radius and the ulna:

POSITION:

- Supine client: undrape your client's forearm.
- Stand at the side of the table. Use your mother hand to support the wrist as you palpate the supinated radius and ulna and the elbow or the wrist during pronation and supination.

LOCATE AND PALPATE:

- Begin palpation from the distal projections, with your client's forearm comfortably flexed and supinated. You may need to medially or laterally rotate the glenohumeral joint to find the most comfortable position for your supine client, as in Figure 7–50.

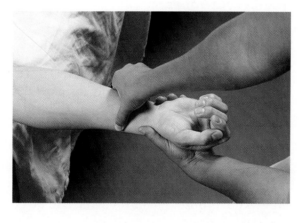

FIGURE 7-50 Palpating the radius and the ulna.

© Milady, a part of Cengage Learning. Photography by Yanik Chauvin.

- Locate and palpate the radius in a proximal direction on the lateral shaft, which becomes more difficult as the fibers of Brachioradialis become denser in the proximal forearm.
- As you palpate the shaft of the radius, pronate and supinate the forearm to feel the radius as it rotates around the stable ulna.
- Locate and palpate the ulna: to palpate proximally on the ulnar shaft, pronate and supinate the forearm to feel that the ulna remains unmoved during the action.
- At the proximal, posterior end of the ulnar shaft, palpate the large, pointed olecranon, also called the olecranon process—the point of the elbow. Palpate the tip of the olecranon as you passively flex and extend the forearm, to experience the movement of the olecranon into the olecranon fossa on the posterior of the humerus. Take care to palpate very lightly: impinging the ulnar nerve here may elicit the "funny bone" response.

PERFORM AN ACTION:

- Slightly adduct and then abduct the wrist to delineate the styloid processes of the radius and the ulna for palpation. The carpals will move, but the radius will not. Note the degree to which the styloid process of the functions to limit adduction and abduction of the wrist.

EVALUATE:

- Characterize your findings: are the size and shape of the landmarks on the radius and ulna equal on each side of the body? Are the landmarks equally palpable?
- Compare your findings with palpations of the radius and ulna on other clients.

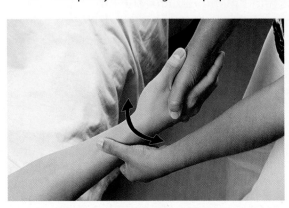

OPTION:

- When pronating and supinating the forearm to palpate the radius and ulna, use your mother hand to "shake hands" with your client, as shown in Figure 7–51, rather than supporting the wrist from below.

FIGURE 7–51 Palpating the radius and ulna with the client's arm in the "handshake" position.

© Milady, a part of Cengage Learning.
Photography by Yanik Chauvin.

The Carpal Bones

The carpals, as seen in Figure 7–52, comprise eight bones, in two rows:

- Proximally, from radial (lateral) to ulnar (medial): scaphoid [SKAF-oyd], lunate [LOO-nayt], triquetrum [try-KWEE-trum], and pisiform [PY-suh-form].
- Distally, from radial to ulnar: trapezium [truh-PEE-zee-um], trapezoid [TRAP-uh-zoyd], capitate [KAP-uh-tayt], and hamate [HAY-mayt].

The pisiform, the most radial carpal in the proximal row, and the scaphoid, the most ulnar carpal in the proximal row, are the most visible and palpable carpals. As the carpal bones glide against one another, a type of circumduction at the wrist can be created.

Articulations:

- The radiocarpal joint: the scaphoid, lunate, and triquetrum carpal bones articulate with the distal radius.
- The carpometacarpal joints: the distal carpal bones articulate with the bases of metacarpals I–V.
- The intercarpal joints: carpals articulate with adjacent carpals.

Attachments:

- Forearm flexors and extensors and the intrinsic muscles of the hand have attachments on carpal bones.
- The tendons of the forearm flexors and extensors travel through the carpal region to insert on the metacarpals and phalanges.

Associated structures:

- The flexor retinaculum, also called the transverse carpal ligament, described next, forms a strong band around the anterior aspect of the carpals.
- The **carpal tunnel** is a narrow passageway through the wrist formed by the flexor retinaculum on the anterior and the carpal bones at its posterior. The median nerve, blood vessels, and tendons of the muscles that flex the hand and fingers pass through this tunnel.

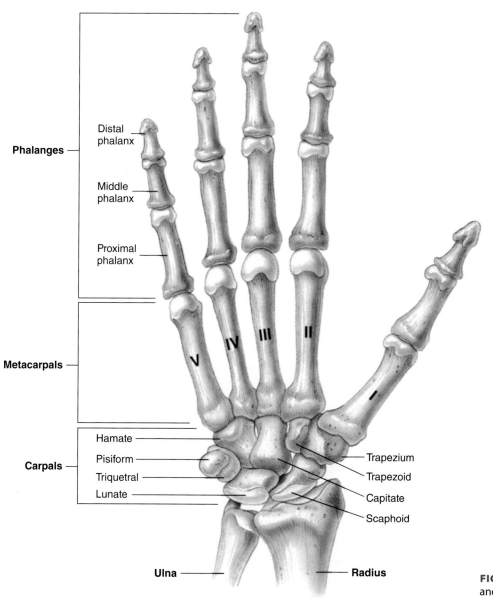

Phalanges

Distal
phalanx

Middle
phalanx

Proximal
phalanx

V   IV   III   II   I

Metacarpals

Carpals

Hamate
Pisiform
Triquetral
Lunate

Trapezium
Trapezoid
Capitate
Scaphoid

Ulna

Radius

FIGURE 7-52 Bones of the wrist
and the hand, dorsal view.

Palpating the carpals:

POSITION:

■ Supine client: undrape your client's forearm.

■ Stand at the side of the table. Use your mother hand to support your client's wrist.

LOCATE AND PALPATE:

■ Place your client's
hand on a cushioned
surface, as shown in
Figure 7–53, or use
both your hands to
support her wrist as
you palpate. With your
client's forearm com-
fortably flexed and

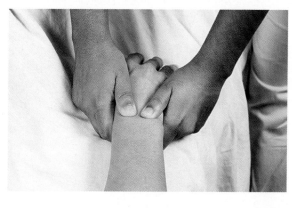

FIGURE 7-53 Palpating the
carpal bones.

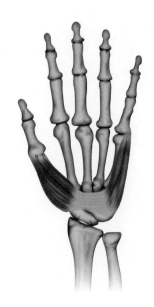

FIGURE 7–54 The flexor retinaculum and the carpal tunnel.

supinated, palpate the anterior wrist. Locate the styloid processes of the radius and the ulna. Slight abduction and adduction of the hand at the wrist will help locate these processes.

- Just distal to the styloid process of the ulna, palpate the prominent, pointed pisiform with your thumb. Ask your client to spread her fingers so that you can feel the muscle insertions on the pisiform bone.
- Just distal to the styloid process of the radius, palpate the prominent tubercle on the scaphoid bone.

With your client's forearm comfortably flexed and pronated, palpate the posterior wrist:

- Place your client's hand on a cushioned surface, or use both your hands to support her wrist as you palpate. Passively flex and extend your client's hand at the wrist to palpate the posterior carpals, which are more evident as her wrist moves through flexion.
- Bring your thumbs together over the posterior carpals and press proximally over the carpals as you flex the wrist, to palpate the extensor retinaculum.

EVALUATE:

- Characterize your findings. Are the size and shape of the landmarks equal on each wrist? Are the landmarks palpable on each wrist?
- Compare your findings with palpations of carpals on other clients.

The Flexor Retinaculum and the Carpal Tunnel

| **Transverse carpal ligament**
| another term for the flexor retinaculum.

| **Carpal tunnel**
| a narrow passageway through the wrist formed by the flexor retinaculum on the anterior and the carpal bones at its posterior.

This strong, dense band of fascia, also called the **transverse carpal ligament**, runs between carpal bones, the pisiform, and the hamate medially and the scaphoid and trapezium laterally. The transverse fibers of this retinaculum, as shown in Figure 7–54, create the **carpal tunnel**, the region through which the median nerve, blood vessels, and the tendons of forearm flexor muscles travel. The flexor retinaculum holds in place the distal tendons of all the forearm flexor muscles except Palmaris longus, whose distal tendon is superficial to the retinaculum and inserts into the palmar aponeurosis. Located on the posterior of the wrist, the extensor retinaculum is less significant, from a therapeutic standpoint.

Palpating the flexor retinaculum and the carpal tunnel:

POSITION:

- Supine client: undrape your client's forearm.
- Stand at the side of the table. Use your mother hand to support your client's wrist.

LOCATE AND PALPATE:

- Locate the pisiform and scaphoid carpals, as described above.
- Using both hands to support and palpate, as in Figure 7–55, place your thumbs on the pisiform and scaphoid carpal bones. Slide your thumbs slightly medially to palpate the fibrous flexor retinaculum. With your fingertips, slightly flex and extend your client's wrist to palpate the transverse borders of the flexor retinaculum.

- Turn your attention to the depression created by the anterior carpals for the carpal tunnel, deep to the flexor retinaculum. Avoid palpating directly over the visible blood vessels in the medial wrist. Use gentle pressure to avoid impinging the median nerve or causing pain in this crowded area.

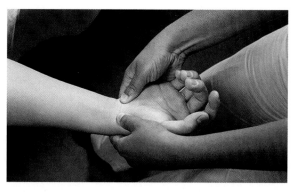

FIGURE 7–55 Palpating the flexor retinaculum and the carpal tunnel.

OPTION:

- On the posterior of the wrist, locate the extensor retinaculum. Palpate gently during passive flexion and extension of the hand at the radiocarpal joint.

EVALUATE:

- Characterize the mobility of the flexor retinaculum: is it freely mobile or is it partially or completely restricted?
- Characterize the tissue quality of this structure: does the tissue feel supple or brittle? Does the tissue soften in response to your touch?
- Compare the mobility and tissue quality of the flexor retinaculum structure with your palpation of the flexor retinaculum on other clients.
- Note any feedback from your client during palpation of the carpal tunnel: did your touch provoke any pain, numbness, or tingling in either hand?

IN THE TREATMENT ROOM

Pain, numbness, or tingling, or weakness in the hand or fingers, specifically, the thumb, first or second fingers, may indicate symptoms of **carpal tunnel syndrome**—compression of the median nerve caused by swelling and irritation of the tissues that travel through the carpal tunnel or by misalignment of one or more of the carpal bones.

Not all hand or finger symptoms indicate carpal tunnel syndrome: pain, tingling, numbness, or weakness that is felt proximal to the wrist is more likely caused by compression of the radial nerve if symptoms are felt on the radial aspect, or of ulnar nerve if symptoms are felt on the ulnar aspect, by a misaligned or herniated vertebral disc or muscle hypertonicity in the cervical or upper thoracic region.

Unfortunately, carpal tunnel syndrome is sometimes a snap diagnosis a physician may make in response to a patient's report of hand pain. Your client's symptoms may not have been fully explored. When a client reports symptoms of dysfunction in her wrist, hand, or fingers, explore all the possibilities in drafting your treatment plan.

Carpal tunnel syndrome (carpal=wrist)

compression of the median nerve caused by swelling and irritation of the tissues that travel through the carpal tunnel or by misalignment of one or more of the carpal bones.

Meta

along with.

Phalanx (-ges)

line of battle.

Metacarpals and Phalanges

Each finger, and the thumb, is called a digit, and each digit is composed of segments called phalanges (the singular is phalanx). The thumb, digit #1, has only a proximal and a distal phalanx. Each remaining digit has three phalanges. Metacarpals [met-uh-KAR-pulz] and phalanges [fun-LAN-jeez] are visible in Figure 7–52.

Metacarpals: usually designated in Roman numerals, I through V, as in Figure 7–52. Metacarpal I articulates with thumb, or the polex, and metacarpal V articulates with the little finger, called digiti minimi.

- Base: the proximal articular prominence.
- Shaft: the length between the base and the head.
- Head: the distal articular prominence.

Phalanges: the fingers and thumb or digits of the hand, designated in Arabic numbers #1–5, with #1 being the thumb and #5 being the little finger.

- Proximal phalanges, on all digits: base, shaft, head.
- Intermediate phalanges, only on digits #2–5: base, shaft, head.
- Distal phalanges, on all digits: base, shaft, head.

Articulations:

- Carpometacarpal (CMC) joints: the distal row of carpals articulates with the bases of metacarpals I–V.
- Metacarpophalangeal (MCP) joints: heads of metacarpals articulate with bases of phalanges.
- Interphalangeal (IP) joints: heads of phalanges articulate with bases of distal phalanges.

Attachments:

- Flexor digitorum superficialis, Flexor digitorum profundus, and Extensor digitorum attach to distal phalanges. The intrinsic muscles of the hand and the muscles of the thenar and hypothenar eminences all have attachments on the metacarpals and phalanges.

Associated structures:

- The palmar aponeurosis covers much of the palmar surface of the hand that overlays the intrinsic muscles of the hand and the tendons of the muscles that flex the fingers. The palmar aponeurosis sits between the thenar and hypothenar eminences of the palm.

Palpating the metacarpals and phalanges:

POSITION:

- Supine client: undrape your client's forearm.
- Stand at the side of the table. Use your mother hand to support the hand and wrist as you palpate the metacarpals.

LOCATE AND PALPATE:

With your client's forearm comfortable flexed and supinated, palpate the palmar aspect:

- Place your client's hand on a cushioned surface, or use both your hands to support her wrist as you palpate, as shown in Figure 7–56.

With your client's forearm comfortable flexed and pronated, palpate the metacarpals from the dorsal aspect:

- The metacarpals are superficial in the posterior hand. Place your palpating thumbs over the posterior carpals. Passively flex and extend your client's wrist: the carpals will move, the metacarpals will not.
- The bases of metacarpals I–V are prominent. As you locate each broad metacarpal base, gently palpate distally through the length of the narrower shaft to the expansion of the head of the metacarpal.
- Repeat this technique on each metacarpal. Compare the very limited range of movement between metacarpals II through V with the range of movement of metacarpal I, the thumb.
- Continue palpating distally with your fingertips, through each MCP joint, onto each phalanx and through each IP joint.

EVALUATE:

- Characterize your findings: are the size and shape of the landmarks equal on each hand? Are the landmarks equally palpable on each hand?
- Compare your findings with palpations of metacarpals and phalanges on other clients.

OPTION:

- You may choose to palpate the phalanges, metacarpals, and carpals working in a proximal direction, beginning with the distal phalanges and palpating toward the carpals.

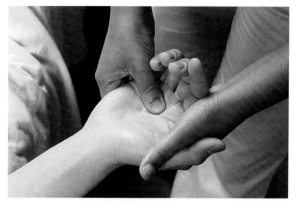

FIGURE 7–56 Palpating the metacarpals and phalanges of the hand with the client's hand supported.

© Milady, a part of Cengage Learning. Photography by Yanik Chauvin.

HERE'S A TIP

It is difficult to palpate the metacarpals on the palmar aspect, because of the dense intrinsic muscles of the hand, though you can easily palpate the palmar aponeurosis, described later in this chapter.

IN THE TREATMENT ROOM

The MCP and IP joints and the bases and heads of metacarpals and phalanges of a client with osteoarthritis in one or both hands or rheumatoid arthritis, or one whose occupation requires repetitive hand movements, may be reddened, gnarled, and tender to touch. Palpate very gently and support the client's joints throughout these palpations and manipulations. You may note significant differences between the bony landmarks of a client's osteoarthritic hand and her unaffected hand.

The Palmar Aponeurosis

The palmar aponeurosis, seen in Figure 7–57, is a thick layer of fascia covering much of the palmar surface of the hand and overlaying both the

Palmar

palm of the hand.

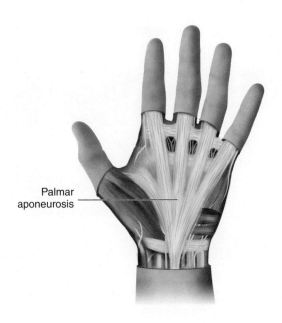

FIGURE 7-57 The palmar aponeurosis.

Palmar aponeurosis

intrinsic muscles of the hand and the tendons of muscles that flex the fingers. Although the hand may be palpated, of course, with your client clothed, palpation is described here as for other structures, with your client disrobed and on the table.

Palpating the palmar aponeurosis

POSITION:

- Supine client: undrape your client's forearm and hand.
- Stand at the side of the table. Use your mother hand to support the hand and wrist as you palpate.

LOCATE AND PALPATE:

- With your client's forearm comfortable flexed and supinated, place her hand on a cushioned surface, or use both your hands to support her wrist as you palpate, as shown in Figure 7–56.
- Using your thumbs, locate the palmar aponeurosis as it flares onto the palmar surface from the Flexor Retinaculum. The aponeurosis lies between the two muscular swellings in the palm, the thenar and hypothenar eminences, described in detail in Chapter 10, Palpating Deeper Muscles and Muscle Groups.
- Palpate the palmar aponeurosis horizontally across your client's palm.

EVALUATE:

- Characterize the mobility of the palmar aponeurosis: is it freely mobile or is it partially or completely restricted?
- Characterize the tissue quality of this structure: does the tissue feel supple or brittle? Does the tissue soften in response to your touch?
- Compare the mobility and tissue quality of the palmar aponeurosis structure with your palpation of the palmar aponeurosis on other clients.

Lab Activity 7–2 on page 300 is designed to develop your palpation skills on bony landmarks and associated structures of the upper extremity.

PALPATING BONY LANDMARKS AND FASCIAL STRUCTURES ON THE LOWER EXTREMITY

The bony landmarks of the lower extremity described here for palpation include those on the pelvis, the femur, and the patella; the tibia and fibula; and the tarsal bones, metatarsals, and phalanges of the foot.

The Pelvis

Pelvis

basin.

The bones of the pelvis, the ilium, ischium, and pubis or pubic bone, are separate at birth, and fuse during early childhood. The fused adult pelvis is shown in Figure 7–58. The male pelvis, as shown in Figure 2–44 in Chapter 2, Posture Assessment, is taller and narrower than the female pelvis. This difference is reflected not only in the placement of its bony landmarks but also the attachment sites of muscles to the pelvis. A woman's femur is also angled more medially, due to the relative width of the female pelvis. You will note distinct differences across gender lines in palpating these structures.

Palpable landmarks on the pelvis:

On the ilium:

- Iliac crest: the entire superior border of the ilium.
- Posterior superior iliac spine (PSIS): the posterior, superior portion of the iliac crest, which overlays the sacroiliac articulation.
- Anterior superior iliac spine (ASIS): the anterior, superior, prominent portion of the iliac spine.
- Anterior inferior iliac spine (AIIS): the anterior, inferior prominence of the iliac spine.

On the ischium:

- Ischial [IS-kee-ul] tuberosity: a rough, thickened tuberosity that is the inferior portion of the ischium.

On the pubis:

- Pubic crest: the anterior border of the body of the pubic bone.

Non-palpable landmarks:

- Acetabulum: deep fossa into which the head of the femur fits.
- External iliac surface or fossa: posterior surface of the ilium.
- Internal iliac surface or fossa: anterior surface of the ilium.
- Obturator foramen: large foramen formed by the ischium through which lower extremity nerve, blood vessels, and tendons travel.

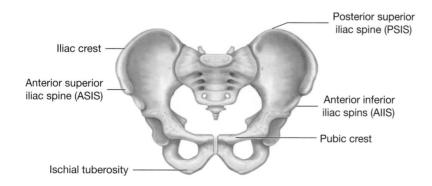

Iliac crest

Anterior superior iliac spine (ASIS)

Ischial tuberosity

Posterior superior iliac spine (PSIS)

Anterior inferior iliac spins (AIIS)

Pubic crest

FIGURE 7-58 The pelvis, anterior view.

Articulations:

- The sacroiliac joint: the posterior ilium articulates with the sacrum.
- The acetabulofemoral joint: the deep acetabulum formed by the ilium, ischium, and pubis articulates with the head of the femur.
- The pubic bones articulate at the pubic symphysis, not a synovial joint.

Attachments:

- The Adductor group and the Abdominal group, deep lateral rotators of the thigh; the Erector spinae and Transversospinalis groups; TFL and the Gluteals, Gracilis, Sartorius, and Pectineus; Iliacus and Psoas major; Quadratus lumborum; and the Quadriceps group all share attachments on the pelvis.

Palpating the ilium, ischium and pubis:

POSITION:

- Side-lying client: for complete palpation of the iliac crest.
- Prone or side-lying client: for palpation of the ischial tuberosity.
- Supine client: for palpation of the pubic crest.
- Drape the abdomen for palpation of the pubic crest. Drape the pelvis for side-lying palpation.
- Stand or sit at the side of the table. Use your mother hand to stabilize your client's trunk in side-lying position. Place for ease and comfort of the prone or supine client.

LOCATE AND PALPATE:

PALPATING THE ILIUM:

- With your client in side-lying position, locate the base of the sacrum with your palpating hand. Move the fingertips of your palpating hand laterally to palpate the PSIS as it forms the iliac crest.

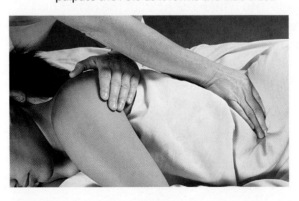

- Palpate the prominence of the iliac crest laterally as it rounds the trunk, as shown in Figure 7–59.
- On the anterior, the ASIS of the iliac crest is prominent and pointed. Palpate medially and inferiorly to locate the much-less-prominent AIIS.

FIGURE 7–59 Palpating the ilium with the client in side-lying position.

PALPATING THE ISCHIUM:

- With your client prone, keep the posterior thigh draped or position it undraped, with the drape secured.

- Locate the popliteal area of the posterior leg. Place your palpating hand as shown in Figure 7–60. Palpate proximally on the posterior thigh, deepening your palpation pressure as you reach the gluteal cleft, the line where the thigh

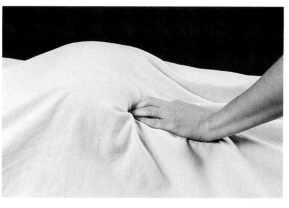

FIGURE 7–60 Palpating the ischium with the client prone.

© Milady, a part of Cengage Learning. Photography by Yanik Chauvin.

joins the buttocks. The ischial tuberosity is large and prominent at the gluteal line.

OPTION:

- You may choose to place your client's leg in the "frogged" position, as shown in Figure 7–61 to palpate the ischial tuberosity, especially if there is a great depth of tissue in the upper thigh and gluteal region.
- Take care to maintain secure draping in the frogged position.
- Clients with limited mobility, especially elders with osteoporosis or who have had hip- or knee-replacement surgery, may not be comfortable in the frogged position. Take care to accommodate the position to the client, not the client to the position.

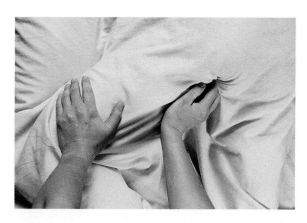

FIGURE 7–61 Palpating the ischial tuberosity with the client's leg "frogged."

© Milady, a part of Cengage Learning. Photography by Yanik Chauvin.

PALPATING THE PUBIC BONE:

- With your client supine, keep the abdomen draped.
- Your palpating hand should be the hand that can rest its ulnar side, not its thumb side, against the pubic crest, shown in Figure 7–62.
- Place your mother hand on your client's shoulder.
- Place your palpating hand over the umbilicus or the navel. Slide your hand to the inferior, deepening your pressure slightly while taking care not to press too deeply over the urinary bladder, until the ulnar aspect of your hand encounters the pubic crest, which is medial in the lower abdomen.

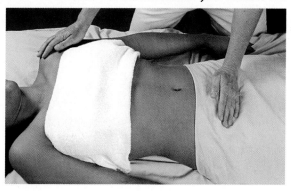

FIGURE 7–62 Palpating the pubic bond with the client in supine position.

© Milady, a part of Cengage Learning. Photography by Yanik Chauvin.

EVALUATE:

- Characterize your findings: are the size and shape of the landmarks equal on each side of the pelvis? Are the landmarks equally palpable on each side of the pelvis?
- Compare your findings with palpations of pelvic landmarks on other clients.

Ilio
the ilium.

Tibial
the tibia.

The Iliotibial Band (ITB)

The Iliotibial [ill-ee-oh-TIB-ee-ul] band, the ITB, shown in Figure 7–63, is prominent in the lateral thigh, extending from the insertion of Tensor fasciae latae, proximal to the greater trochanter of the femur, to the lateral tibia, via the deep fascia that wraps around the tibiofemoral joint. The ITB separates the anterior and posterior compartments of thigh muscles that flex and extend the leg.

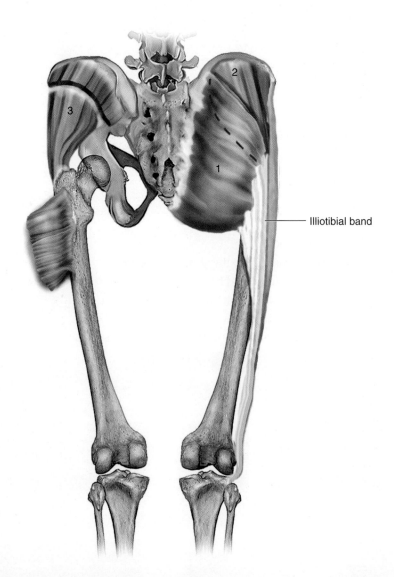

Illiotibial band

FIGURE 7–63 The iliotibial band (ITB).

Palpating the Iliotibial band:

POSITION:

- Side-lying client: place a bolster under your client's knee and foot so that the hip, knee, and ankle are in alignment.
- Stand at the side of the table. Use your mother hand to support your client in side-lying position.

LOCATE AND PALPATE:

- Locate the greater trochanter of the femur and the lateral condyle of the tibia. Palpate the tough, fibrous band of fascia, as shown in Figure 7–64, which attaches at these two land-marks and separates the anterior and posterior compartments of thigh muscles.
- With the fingertips of your palpating hand, strum across the ITB, assessing its tautness and the mobility along its length.

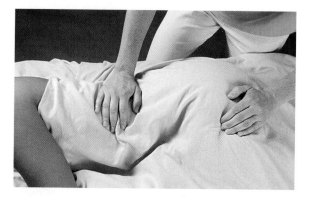

FIGURE 7–64 Palpating the ITB with the client in side-lying position.

EVALUATE:

- Characterize the mobility of the ITB: is it freely mobile or is it partially or completely restricted?
- Characterize the tissue quality of this structure: does the tissue feel supple or brittle? Does the tissue soften in response to your touch?
- Compare the mobility and tissue quality of the ITB with your palpation of the iliotibial band on other clients.

The Femur and the Patella

The angle of the femur [FEE-mur], from its articulation with the pelvis to its articulation with the tibia, is greater on women than on men, due to the wider, deeper female pelvis. This difference in angle has significance for knee-replacement surgery: the size and angle of a woman's knee may make this surgery more complicated and the recovery more difficult. The femur is shown in Figure 7–65.

Palpable landmarks on the femur and patella [puh-TEL-uh]:

On the femur:

- Lateral condyle: the large distal prominence on the lateral femur.
- Medial condyle: the large distal prominence on the medial femur.
- Greater trochanter: the large proximal prominence on lateral femur.
- Lesser trochanter: the smaller proximal prominence on the posterior femur.

On the patella (the patella is not shown in Figure 7–65):

- Apex: the pointed, inferior aspect.
- Base: the broad, superior aspect.

Femur

thigh.

Patella

a pan.

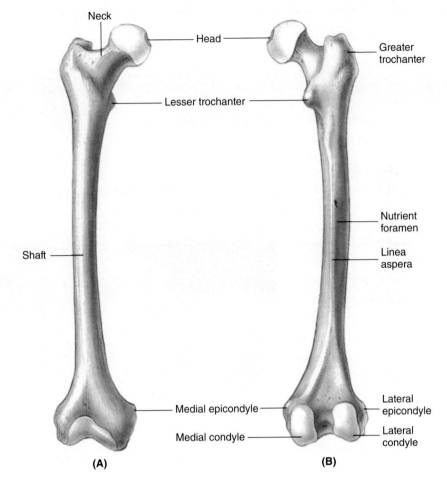

Neck

Head

Greater trochanter

Lesser trochanter

Nutrient foramen

Linea aspera

Shaft

Medial epicondyle

Lateral epicondyle

Medial condyle

Lateral condyle

(A)

(B)

FIGURE 7–65 The femur.

Non-palpable landmarks on the femur:
- Linea aspera: a roughened line on the posterior shaft.
- Intertrochanteric crest: on the posterior between the greater and lesser trochanters.

Articulations:
- The acetabulofemoral joint: the head of the femur articulates with the acetabulum of the pelvis.
- The tibiofemoral joint: the medial condyle of the femur articulates with the medial meniscus and the medial condyle of the tibia, and the lateral condyle of the femur with the lateral meniscus, and the lateral condyle of the tibia.
- The patellofemoral joint: the posterior surface of the patella articulates with the patellar surface of the distal, anterior femur.

Attachments:
- The Adductor group; the deep Lateral rotators; Gastrocnemius and the Hamstrings group; Iliacus and Psoas major; Pectineus and Plantaris; and the Quadriceps group all share attachments on the femur.

Associated structures:
- The iliotibial band (ITB), the patellar tendon, and the pes anserine tendon are fascial structures associated with the femur and the patella.

Palpating the femur and the patella:

POSITION:

- Supine client: thigh slightly flexed and supported at the knee. Undrape your client's thigh and leg.
- Stand at the side of the table. Palpate with both hands, or use your mother hand to support the knee from below.

LOCATE AND PALPATE:

- Palpate the femur: the large medial and lateral condyles are superficial and palpable.
- The medial condyle is deep to the pes anserine tendon and is, usually, a fat pad. It may be less palpable than the lateral condyle.
- At the proximal end of the iliotibial band (ITB), the greater trochanter is a large protuberance on the proximal, lateral femur. Palpate the greater trochanter, as shown in Figure 7–66, to discern its shape and the layers of fascial tissue overlaying it.

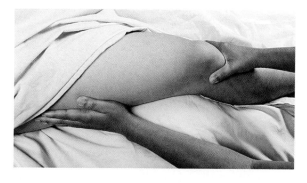

FIGURE 7–66 Palpating the femur with the client in supine position.

© Milady, a part of Cengage Learning. Photography by Yanik Chauvin.

- The lesser trochanter is much less prominent. To palpate the lesser trochanter, move your palpating hand posterior and distal to the greater trochanter. You may or may not be able to palpate the intertrochanteric crest between the two trochanters.
- Palpate the patella: the pointed apex is inferior and fits into the patellar tendon. Follow the ligament distally to its attachment on the tibia. The broad base is superior and receives the quadriceps tendon.

PERFORM AN ACTION:

- To make sure you are palpating on the femur, passively flex and extend your client's leg at the knee. The tibia and fibula move, the femur does not.

EVALUATE:

- Characterize your findings: are the size and shape of the landmarks equal on each femur? Are the landmarks equally palpable on each femur? Are both patellae equal in size, shape, and mobility?
- Compare your findings with palpations of femurs and patellae on other clients.

The Patellar Tendon

The patellar tendon [puh-TEL-uhr TEN-dun], shown with the pes anserine tendon in Figure 7–68 and sometimes called the patellar ligament, is a continuation of the broad tendon of the quadriceps group in the

Patellar

related to the patella.

anterior thigh. The patellar tendon bridges that group attachment onto the anterior surface of the tibia at the tibial tuberosity. The patellar tendon is anterior to the tibiofemoral and patellofemoral joints and is separated from it by a fat pad.

Palpating the patellar tendon:

POSITION:

- Supine client: either elevate your client's foot or remove the bolster beneath her knees to place her leg in passive extension. Undrape your client's thigh and leg.

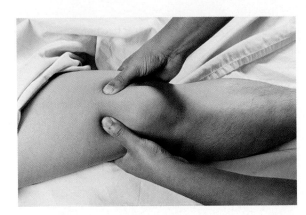

© Milady, a part of Cengage Learning. Photography by Yanik Chauvin.

FIGURE 7-67 Palpating the patellar tendon.

- Stand at the side of the table. Palpate with both hands, or use your mother hand to support the tibiofemoral joint from below.

LOCATE AND PALPATE:

- Circle the patella with your palpating hands, as shown in Figure 7–67. At the superior end of the patella, its base, palpate the broad, fibrous tendon that arises proximal to the patella and inserts onto the tibia at the tibial tuberosity.
- You may compare the mobility of each patellar tendon by palpating it on both legs simultaneously.

EVALUATE:

- Characterize the mobility of the patellar tendon: is it freely mobile or is it partially or completely restricted?
- Characterize the tissue quality of this structure: does the tissue feel supple or brittle? Does the tissue soften in response to your touch?
- Compare the mobility and tissue quality of the patellar tendon structure with your palpation of the patellar tendons on other clients.

Pes anserine

goose's foot.

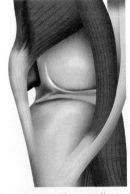

© Milady, a part of Cengage Learning.

FIGURE 7-68 The patellar and pes anserine tendons.

The Pes Anserine Tendon

The pes anserine [PEEZ an-suh-RYNE] is a large tendon in the medial, distal thigh that is shaped like a webbed goose or duck's foot, if the fowl's webs pointed upward from the medial knee. The function of the pes anserine is to receive the distal tendons of Sartorius, Gracilis, and Semitendinosus and attach them to the deep fascia surrounding the tibiofemoral joint. The pes anserine is slightly distal to the large fat pad commonly found in the medial knee, as it inserts onto the medial tibia. The pes anserine tendon is visible in Figure 7–68.

Palpating the pes anserine tendon:

POSITION:

- Supine client: place your client's leg in a "figure 4" position, as in Figure 7–69.
- Stand at the side of the table. Use your mother hand to support your client's leg position.

LOCATE AND PALPATE:

- Locate the medial condyle of the tibia. Palpate through the superficial fat pad to the fibrous pes anserine tendon, which fans out proximally in the distal, medial thigh.

EVALUATE:

- Characterize the mobility of the pes anserine tendon: is it freely mobile or is it partially or completely restricted?
- Characterize the tissue quality of this structure: does the tissue feel supple or brittle? Does the tissue soften in response to your touch?
- Compare the mobility and tissue quality of the pes anserine tendon with your palpation of the pes anserine tendon on other clients.

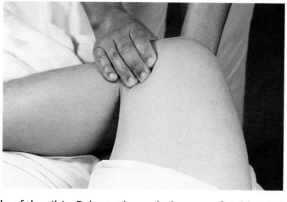

FIGURE 7–69 Palpating the pes anserine tendon.

The Tibia and the Fibula

The tibia [TIB-ee-ah] is the stoutest bone in the body. It receives the entire weight of the head, the torso, and the upper extremities and its distal end creates the medial malleolus [muh-LEE-uh-lus], or "ankle." The fibula [FIB-yuh-luh] is not part of the tibiofemoral joint. Its head is distal to the knee and its distal end creates the lateral malleolus, the other "ankle." The tibia and fibula are shown in Figure 7–70.

Palpable landmarks on the tibia and fibula:

On the tibia:

- Medial malleolus: the distal styloid process.
- Anterior crest: a sharp vertical ridge on the anterior tibia.
- Tibial tuberosity: a prominent projection on the anterior, proximal tibia.
- Medial condyle: the medial, proximal prominence.
- Lateral condyle: the lateral, proximal prominence.

On the fibula:

- Lateral malleolus: the distal styloid process.
- Head: the proximal end of the fibula.

Articulations:

- The tibiofemoral joint: the medial meniscus and medial condyle of the tibia articulate with the medial condyle of the femur, and the lateral meniscus and lateral condyle of the tibia articulate with the lateral condyle of the femur.

Tibia

shinbone.

Fibula

a clasp.

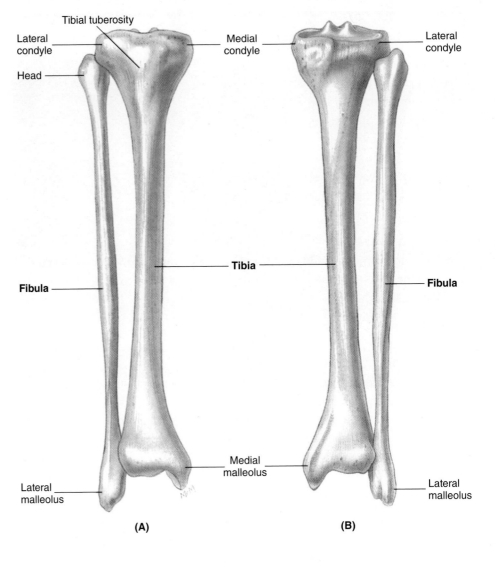

FIGURE 7-70 The tibia and fibula.

(A)   (B)

■ The tibiofibular joint: the lateral condyle of the tibia articulates with the head of the fibula.

■ The talocrural joint: the medial malleolus of the tibia and the lateral malleolus of the fibula articulate with the talus of the tarsal bones.

Attachments:

■ Extensor digitorum longus, Extensor hallucis longus, and Flexor hallucis longus; Gastrocnemius and Soleus; Sartorius and Gracilis; the Hamstrings and Peroneal groups; Plantaris and Popliteus; the Quadriceps group; and Tibialis anterior and Tibialis posterior all share attachments on the tibia or the fibula.

Palpating the tibia and fibula:

POSITION:

■ Supine client: knee slightly flexed and supported. Undrape your client's thigh and leg.

■ Stand at the side of the table. Palpate with both hands, or use your mother hand to support the tibiofemoral joint from beneath.

LOCATE AND PALPATE:

- Begin palpating from the distal end of the leg. Place the fingertips of both hands on the medial malleolus and the lateral malleolus, the "ankles." Note their relative positions: the lateral malleolus on the fibula is more distal than the medial malleolus on the tibia, as shown in Figure 7–71.

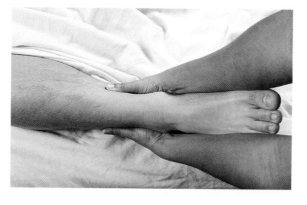

FIGURE 7-71 Palpating the tibia and the fibula.

© Milady, a part of Cengage Learning. Photography by Yanik Chauvin.

- With the fingertips palpating the medial malleolus, continue to palpate proximally on the anterior tibia for the anterior crest, the sharp "shin bone." Lighten your palpation pressure here, because there is very little tissue overlaying the anterior crest of the tibia.

- As you palpate closer to the patellar tendon, find the knobby tibial tuberosity, where the patellar tendon attaches to the proximal tibia.

- Move your palpating fingertips slightly upward and medial and lateral to the tibial-tuberosity, to palpate the large medial and lateral condyles of the tibia. From the lateral condyle of the tibia, drop your palpating fingertips onto the head of the fibula, directly distal to the condyle.

PERFORM AN ACTION:

- To make sure you are not palpating the condyles of the femur, passively flex and extend your client's leg at the knee. The tibia and fibula will move, the femur will not.

EVALUATE:

- Characterize your findings: are the size and shape of the landmarks equal on each leg? Are the landmarks equally palpable on each leg? Are the medial and lateral malleoli equal in size and shape on each leg?

- Compare your findings with palpations of the tibia and fibula on other clients.

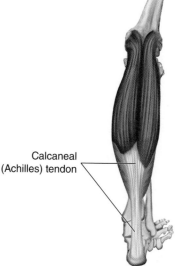

Calcaneal (Achilles) tendon

© Milady, a part of Cengage Learning.

FIGURE 7-72 The calcaneal or Achilles tendon.

The Calcaneal (Achilles) Tendon

Calcaneus

the heel.

In Greek mythology, Achilles [uh-KIL-eez] was a great warrior who died from a wound on his heel. The calcaneal tendon [kal-KAY-nee-ul TEN-dun], also known as the Achilles tendon, is the largest and strongest tendon in the body. The calcaneal tendon inserts both Gastrocnemius and Soleus onto the calcaneus, and is superficial and easily palpable. The calcaneal tendon is shown in Figure 7–72.

Palpating the calcaneal tendon:

POSITION:

- Prone client: undrape the leg.
- Place a bolster under your client's foot, to eliminate plantarflexion.
- Stand at the side of the table. Use your mother hand to stabilize your client's foot.

LOCATE AND PALPATE:

- Locate the calcaneus. Slightly dorsiflex your client's foot to bring out the calcaneal tendon. Follow the tendon to its emergence from the belly of Gastrocnemius, as shown in Figure 7–73.
- You may compare the mobility of the calcaneal tendon by palpating it on both legs simultaneously.

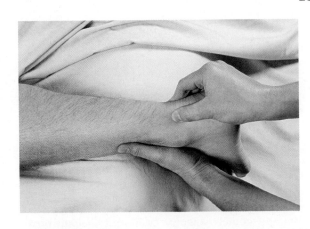

FIGURE 7–73 Palpating the calcaneal (Achilles) tendon.

EVALUATE:

- Characterize the mobility of the calcaneal tendon: is it freely mobile or is it partially or completely restricted?
- Characterize the tissue quality of this structure: does the tissue feel supple or brittle? Does the tissue soften in response to your touch?
- Compare the mobility and tissue quality of the calcaneal tendon with your palpation of the calcaneal tendon on other clients.

Tarsus

flat surface.

The Tarsal Bones

There are seven tarsal [TAR-sul] bones: the talus [TAL-us], the calcaneus [kal-KAY-nee-us], the navicular [nuh-VIK-yuh-lur], the cuboid [KYOO-boyd], and three cuneiform [kyuh-NEE-uh-form] bones. The joints between the tarsal bones allow inversion and eversion of the foot. As the tarsal bones glide against one another, a type of circumduction at the ankle can be created. The bones of the foot are shown in Figure 7–74.

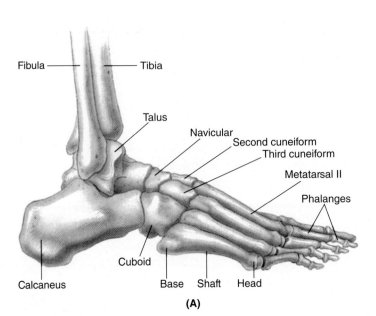

FIGURE 7–74 Bones of the ankle and the foot.

Palpable landmarks:

- Each tarsal bone is palpable, although palpation of the talus is limited by its articulation at the talocrural joint. Palpate as a group.

Articulations:

- The talocrural joint: the medial malleolus of the tibia and the lateral malleolus of the fibula articulate with the talus of the tarsal bones.
- The intertarsal joints: tarsals articulate with other tarsals.
- The tarsometatarsal joints: the three cuneiforms articulate with metatarsals I–V.

Attachments:

- The tendons of the flexors and extensors travel through the tarsal region to insert on the metatarsals and phalanges.

Associated structures:

- The extensor retinaculum forms a strong band around the tarsals on the anterior. The tendons of the extensor muscles of the leg travel deep to this retinaculum.
- The large calcaneal tendon fills the space between the calcaneal tuberosity and the other tarsal bones in the posterior ankle.

Palpating the tarsals:

POSITION:

- Supine client, legs slightly flexed and supported at the knees: undrape the lower leg.
- Stand or sit at the foot of the table. Use your mother hand to support the ankle, or use both hands to palpate.

LOCATE AND PALPATE:

- Place your palpating hands just distal to the medial and lateral malleoli, as shown in Figure 7–75. Palpate the tarsal bones as a group.
- With your thumbs or fingertips, palpate the tarsal bones on the dorsal foot, between the talocrural joint and the tarsometatarsal joints.
- Slide the fingertips of your palpating hand around to the posterior of the tarsal group. Palpate the heel, the calcaneus, noting the prominent calcaneal tendon that attaches to its posterior aspect.

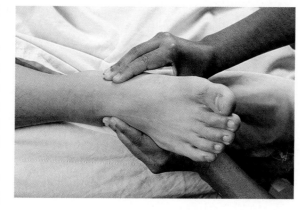

FIGURE 7–75 Palpating the tarsal bones.

© Milady, a part of Cengage Learning. Photography by Yanik Chauvin.

PERFORM AN ACTION:

- To make sure you are on the tarsal bones, invert and evert the foot. The tarsals will move, the tibia and fibula will not.

- Characterize your findings: are the size and shape of the landmarks equal on each ankle and foot? Are the landmarks equally palpable on each ankle?
- Compare your findings with palpations of the tarsal bones on other clients.

Metatarsals and Phalanges

The metatarsals [met-uh-TAR-suls] and phalanges are visible in Figure 7–74. As with the thumb in the hand, the big toe in the foot, digit #1, has only a proximal and a distal phalanx. The metatarsals and phalanges are most easily palpated on the dorsal aspect of the foot.

Metatarsals: usually designated in Roman numerals I–V. Metatarsal I is medial on the foot and articulates with the hallux or big toe, and metatarsal V is lateral on the foot and articulates with digiti minimi pedis, the little toe.

- Base: the proximal articular prominence.
- Shaft: the length between the base and the head.
- Head: the distal articular prominence.

Phalanges: designated in Arabic numbers #1–5, with #1 being the big toe and #5 the little toe.

- Proximal phalanges: base, shaft, head.
- Intermediate phalanges, only on digits #2–5: base, shaft, head.
- Distal phalanges on all digits: base, shaft, head.

Articulations:

- Tarsometatarsal joints: the three cuneiforms articulate with the bases of metatarsals I–V.
- The metatarsophalangeal joints: the heads of metatarsals articulate with the bases of phalanges.
- The interphalangeal (IP) joints: heads of phalanges articulate with bases of distal phalanges.

Attachments:

- The intrinsic muscles of the foot all have attachments on the metatarsals and phalanges.

Associated structures:

- The plantar aponeurosis covers much of the plantar surface of the foot, superficial to the intrinsic muscles of the foot.

Palpating the metatarsals and phalanges:

POSITION:

- Supine client, legs slightly flexed and supported at the knees. Undrape the lower leg.
- Stand or sit at the foot of the table. Use your mother hand to support the ankle, or use both hands to palpate.

LOCATE AND PALPATE:

- With your thumbs on the anterior tarsals, palpate the metatarsals and phalanges, easily palpable on the dorsal aspect of the foot in this position.

- Position yourself comfortably to palpate the plantar aspect of the foot, as shown in Figure 7–76. Carefully palpate the base of Metatarsal I, where Tibialis anterior and Peroneus longus share an insertion. Palpate gently: this insertion is often quite tender.

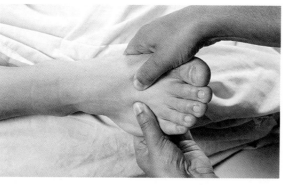

FIGURE 7–76 Palpating the metatarsals and phalanges of the foot.

EVALUATE:

- Characterize your findings: are the size and shape of the landmarks equal on each foot? Are the landmarks equally palpable on each foot?
- Compare your findings with palpations of the metatarsals and phalanges on other clients.

The Extensor Retinaculum

This thick band of deep fascia spans the tarsal bones on the anterior, from the medial malleolus of the tibia to the lateral malleolus of the fibula. With a superior portion that lies over the tarsals and an inferior portion that lies over the metatarsals, as shown in Figure 7–77, the extensor retinaculum holds the tendons of anterior leg muscles, Tibialis anterior, Extensor digitorum longus and Extensor hallucis longus, in place.

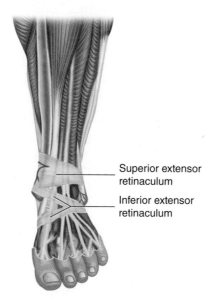

Superior extensor retinaculum

Inferior extensor retinaculum

FIGURE 7–77 The extensor retinaculum.

Palpating the extensor retinaculum:

POSITION:

- Supine client, legs slightly flexed and supported at the knees. Undrape the lower leg.
- Stand or sit at the foot of the table. Use your mother hand to support the ankle, or use both hands to palpate.

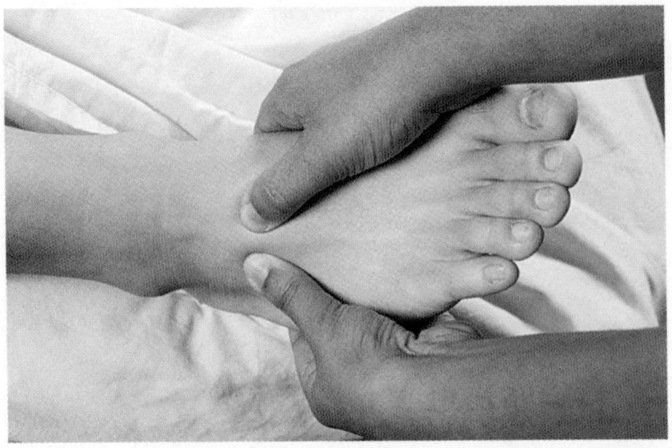

LOCATE AND PALPATE:

- With your fingertips on the medial and lateral malleoli and your thumbs on the plantar surface of your client's foot, as shown in Figure 7–78, slightly dorsiflex your client's foot as you palpate the horizontal superior and inferior segments of the extensor retinaculum.

FIGURE 7–78 Palpating the extensor retinaculum.

- Slightly invert and evert your client's foot, to better palpate the inferior segment of the extensor retinaculum.
- You may compare the mobility of the extensor retinaculum by palpating it on both legs simultaneously.

EVALUATE:

- Characterize the mobility of the extensor retinaculum: is it freely mobile or is it partially or completely restricted?
- Characterize the tissue quality of this structure: does the tissue feel supple or brittle? Does the tissue soften in response to your touch?
- Compare the mobility and tissue quality of the extensor retinaculum with your palpation of the extensor retinaculum on other clients.

Plantar

sole of the foot.

The Arches of the Foot and the Plantar Aponeurosis

The foot contains three distinct arches:

- A medial longitudinal arch, the high arch of the foot, formed by the calcaneus and talus, plus the three cuneiforms and the three medial metatarsals.
- A lateral longitudinal arch, formed by the calcaneus and cuboid bones and the two lateral metatarsals.
- A transverse arch, prominent at the base of the metatarsals, and supported by the distal tendons of Tibialis anterior and Peroneus longus, which insert onto the plantar surface of the base of metatarsal I.

The **plantar aponeurosis**, seen in Figure 7–79, is a tough, thick layer of deep fascia that is superficial to the three layers of intrinsic muscles in the plantar foot. It arises from the plantar aspect of the calcaneus and inserts onto the distal phalanges of each toe.

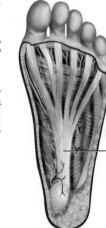

Plantar fascia (aponeurosis)

FIGURE 7–79 The plantar aponeurosis.

Palpating the arches of the foot and the plantar aponeurosis:

POSITION:

- Supine client, legs slightly flexed and supported at the knees. Undrape the lower legs.

- Elevate the feet, if necessary, to raise them to a comfortable working height.
- Stand or sit at the foot of the table. Use both hands to palpate these structures simultaneously on both feet.

LOCATE AND PALPATE:

- On each foot, locate the prominent head of metatarsal I, which lies at the superior end of the medial longitudinal arch. Palpate the medial longitudinal arches from the head of metatarsal I to the plantar aspect of the medial calcaneus.
- On each foot, locate the head of metatarsal V, which lies at the superior end of the lateral longitudinal arch. Palpate the longitudinal arches from the head of metatarsal V to the plantar aspect of the lateral calcaneus.
- Locate the base of metatarsal I, where the distal tendons of Tibialis anterior and Peroneus longus meet and help to maintain the transverse arch. Palpate the transverse arches across the plantar foot to the base of metatarsal V.
- Locate the midline of the plantar aspect of the calcaneus. With the thumbs of your palpating hands, palpate the plantar aponeurosis horizontally across the foot, as shown in Figure 7–80. Follow the aponeurosis toward the distal phalanx on each toe.

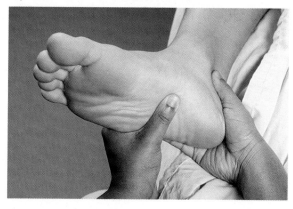

FIGURE 7–80 Palpating the arches of the foot and the plantar aponeurosis.

© Milady, a part of Cengage Learning.

EVALUATE:

- Characterize the mobility of the arches and plantar aponeuroses on each foot: is each aponeurosis freely mobile or is it partially or completely restricted? Are the arches of each foot equally shaped or is any arch on either foot malformed?
- Characterize the tissue quality of these structures: does the tissue feel supple or brittle? Does the tissue soften in response to your touch?
- Compare the mobility and tissue quality of the arches and plantar aponeuroses on each foot with your palpation of the arches and plantar aponeuroses on each foot on other clients.

HERE'S A TIP

Be sure to warm and relax the superficial tissues in the plantar foot before palpating. Palpate gently at first, increasing your pressure slowly, to avoid eliciting a cramp in the foot. If a foot cramp does occur, gently traction the foot to counter the direction of cramp. Avoid wrenching or forcing the foot, which may intensify the cramp or injure the cramping muscles.

Palpate the bony prominences on the plantar foot with care. Sesamoid bones or sharp, painful bone spurs called neophytes may have developed at the bases or heads of the metatarsals or phalanges on one or both feet in response to stress from poorly fitting shoes or an altered gait.

Plantar fasciitis

irritation or inflammation of the plantar aponeurosis.

Heel bone spurs

overgrowths of bone, also called osteophytes, that may develop on the plantar surface of the calcaneus.

IN THE TREATMENT ROOM

Inflammation of the plantar aponeurosis or fascia, shown in Figure 7–81, is called **plantar fasciitis** [PLANT-ur fash-ee-EYE-tis], a painful condition that impacts standing posture and gait and complicates palpation of the plantar foot. Often the result of irritation of the plantar aponeurosis, the symptoms of plantar fasciitis—pain, stiffness, local heat, or swelling—are usually worse first thing in the morning, when the arch of the foot is tight and inflexible, and are made worse by prolonged standing or walking. In about 70 percent of plantar fasciitis cases, the sufferer also has **heel bone spurs,** or osteophytes, shown in Figure 7–82—overgrowths of bone on the calcaneus that can be extremely painful and inhibit normal standing posture and gait.

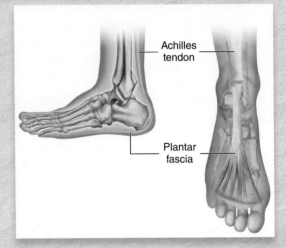

FIGURE 7–81 Plantar fasciitis is a painful condition that impacts standing posture and gait.

Advise a client with persistent plantar foot pain, especially if the pain is made worse by palpation or is accompanied by the hallmarks of inflammation—heat, redness, or swelling—to seek medical evaluation for plantar fasciitis or heel bone spurs, and avoid deep pressure on the plantar foot.

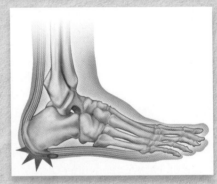

FIGURE 7–82 Heel bone spurs may also painfully alter standing posture and gait.

Lab Activity 7–3 on page 301 is designed to develop your palpation skills on bony landmarks and associated structures of the lower extremity.

SUMMARY

The techniques and procedures outlined in this chapter will help prepare you for palpation of skeletal muscles. They are, however, only a starting place: only through repetition of these techniques and procedures can a massage therapist gain mastery in palpation. The techniques and procedures from this chapter will be utilized in the chapters to come: the remaining chapters describe palpation of individual superficial and deeper skeletal muscles and muscle groups.

LAB ACTIVITIES

LAB ACTIVITY 7–1: PALPATING THE AXIAL SKELETON

1. Working with a partner, palpate the following bony landmarks and associated structures:
   - On the occipital bone: the external occipital protuberance and the superior nuchal lines.
   - On the temporal bone: the mastoid process and the zygomatic process.
   - On the mandible: the angle, the condyle, and the coronoid process.
   - The nuchal ligament.
   - On the hyoid bone: the body and greater cornu.
   - On the sternum: the body, manubrium, and xiphoid process.
   - On the ribs: the angle of the ribs from anterior to posterior, the costal cartilage, and the intercostal spaces.
   - The abdominal aponeurosis and the rectus sheath.
   - On the vertebrae: the spinous and transverse processes and the laminar groove.
   - Spinal curvatures in the cervical, thoracic, and lumbar regions.
   - On the sacrum: the base and sacral tubercles.
   - Thoracolumbar fascia.

2. Decide the order of palpation, the client's position, and the position of your palpating hands—measures for client comfort and security and how you will meet any challenges—then carry out your palpation plan.

3. Palpate the landmarks on the bones and associated structures, using the protocol steps and options listed above—and any more you can devise.

4. Discuss the results of your palpations with your partner:
   - Which bony landmarks were easiest to locate and palpate?
   - Which were more difficult?
   - What made some palpations more difficult?
   - Was palpating the fascial structures difficult?
   - What could have eased this process?

   Discuss what adjustments in positioning or technique might ease the more difficult palpations.

5. How did touch sensitivity enhance the palpation experience?
   - What specific steps did you take during the palpations to increase or focus your touch sensitivity?
   - What differences in touch sensitivity did you note in relation to the palpation pressure used?

6. Switch partners and repeat.

LAB ACTIVITY 7–2: PALPATING BONY LANDMARKS AND ASSOCIATED STRUCTURES OF THE UPPER EXTREMITY

1. Working with a partner, palpate the following bony landmarks and associated structures:
    - On the clavicle: the sternal and acromial ends and the curve of the clavicle.
    - On the scapulae: the acromion and coracoid processes, the angles and borders, and the spine.
    - The lateral and medial epicondyles, the lateral supracondylar ridge, the deltoid tuberosity, the bicipital groove, and the greater and lesser tubercle.
    - On the radius and ulna: the styloid processes and the olecranon of the ulna.
    - The flexor retinaculum, the carpal tunnel, and the palmar aponeurosis.
    - On the radius and ulna: the styloid processes and the olecranon of the ulna.
    - On the wrist: the pisiform and scaphoid carpal bones that border the carpal tunnel and the flexor and extensor retinacula.
    - On the hand: the bases, shafts, and heads of metacarpals I through V and the proximal, intermediate, and distal phalanges of the hand.
    - The flexor retinaculum, the carpal tunnel, and the palmar aponeurosis.

2. Decide the order of palpation, the client's position, and the position of your palpating hands—measures for client comfort and security and how you will meet any challenges—and then carry out your palpation plan.

3. Palpate the landmarks on the bones and associated structures, using the protocol steps and options listed above—and any more you can devise.

4. Discuss the results of your palpations with your partner:
    - Which bony landmarks were easiest to locate and palpate?
    - Which were more difficult?
    - What made some palpations more difficult?
    - Was palpating the fascial structures difficult?
    - What could have eased this process?

    Discuss what adjustments in positioning or technique might ease the more difficult palpations.

5. How did touch sensitivity enhance the palpation experience? What specific steps did you take during the palpations to increase or focus your touch sensitivity? What differences in touch sensitivity did you note in relation to the palpation pressure used?

6. Switch partners and repeat.

LAB ACTIVITY 7–3: PALPATING BONY LANDMARKS AND ASSOCIATED STRUCTURES ON THE LOWER EXTREMITY

1. Working with a partner, palpate the following bony landmarks and associated structures:
   - On the ilium, the PSIS, ASIS, and AIIS along the iliac crest.
   - On the ischium, the ischial tuberosity.
   - On the pubic bone, the pubic crest.
   - The iliotibial band (ITB).
   - The sacroiliac joints.
   - On the femur: the medial and lateral condyles and the greater and lesser trochanters.
   - On the patella: the base and apex.
   - The patellar and pes anserine tendons.
   - On the tibia: the medial malleolus, the anterior crest, the tibial tuberosity, and the condyles.
   - On the fibula: the head and the lateral malleolus.
   - The tarsal bones; the bases, shafts, and heads of metatarsals I through V; and the proximal, intermediate, and distal phalanges of the foot.
   - The extensor retinaculum, the arches of the feet, and the plantar aponeurosis.

2. Decide the order of palpation, the client's position and the position of your palpating hands—measures for client comfort and security and how you will meet any challenges—then carry out your palpation plan.

3. Palpate the landmarks on the bones and associated structures, using the protocol steps and options listed above—and any more you can devise.

4. Discuss the results of your palpations with your partner:
   - Which bony landmarks were easiest to locate and palpate?
   - Which were more difficult?
   - What made some palpations more difficult?
   - Was palpating the fascial structures difficult?
   - What could have eased this process?

   Discuss what adjustments in positioning or technique might ease the more difficult palpations.

5. How did touch sensitivity enhance the palpation experience?
   - What specific steps did you take during the palpations to increase or focus your touch sensitivity?
   - What differences in touch sensitivity did you note in relation to the palpation pressure used?

6. Switch partners and repeat.

CASE PROFILES

Case Profile 1

Tom is a 39-year-old entrepreneur who runs his Internet dating service business from his home, using his laptop as he reclines in his easy chair. He has come for a massage because of persistent headaches and neck pain. When you ask Tom to duplicate his position at his "workstation," you see that he semi-reclines and slumps his head forward. What bony and connective tissue structures would you palpate first in evaluating Tom's presenting complaints? What positions would you place Tom in for palpation?

Case Profile 2

Sandra, 45, drives a delivery truck all day, five days a week. She has pain in her right axilla, or armpit, that has been evaluated by her primary care physician, who found no pathology or disease process that might be causing the pain, which is worse toward the end of the day and the end of the week. Sandra thinks her work has something to do with the pain. What bony structures would you palpate first in evaluating Sandra's presenting problem? What client positions would you use for these palpations?

Case Profile 3

Marie is a 71-year-old woman who recently retired from her work as a ski instructor. After decades on the slopes, Marie has ongoing pain, stiffness, and poor mobility in her hips and knees. What bony and connective tissue structures would you palpate first in evaluating Marie's hips and knees? What changes in position and pressure might be indicated for Marie because of her age and frailty?

STUDY QUESTIONS

1. Name three fascial structures that are palpable on the axial skeleton.
2. What is the difference between superficial and deep fascia?
3. Why is special care recommended in palpating the flexor retinaculum of the wrist?
4. Discuss why you might consider palpating the ITB with your client in side-lying position.
5. Describe how you will drape a client to completely palpate his or her ribcage.
6. Describe complete palpation of the bony landmarks of the mandible.
7. Describe the placement of the mother hand in palpating the bony landmarks of the leg and the foot.
8. Describe your order of palpation of the bony landmarks of the arm and forearm.
9. Describe how you will position your client to palpate all the bony landmarks of the scapula.
10. Describe the challenges of palpating bony landmarks on a client who is obese or elderly.

Palpating Superficial Muscles on the Axial Skeleton

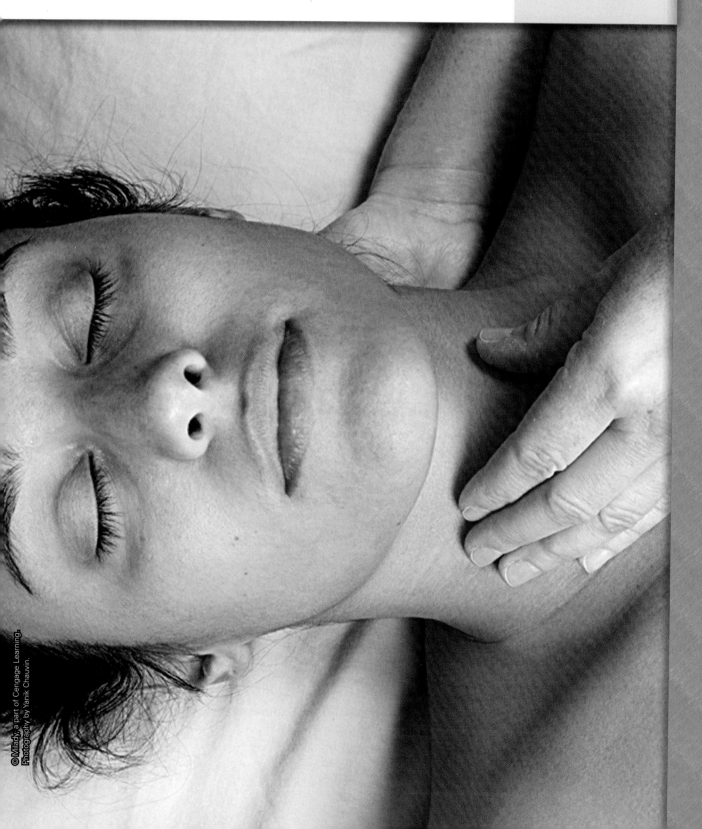

CHAPTER OUTLINE

- **MUSCLES THAT ACT ON THE SCAPULA**
- **MUSCLES THAT ACT ON THE NECK**
- **MUSCLES OF RESPIRATION**
- **MUSCLES THAT ACT ON THE ABDOMEN**
- **MUSCLES OF MASTICATION**

LEARNING OBJECTIVES

- Apply an understanding of the origins, insertions, and actions of specific superficial and intermediate muscles and muscle groups on the axial skeleton to their palpation.

- Apply safe and effective palpation techniques to superficial and intermediate skeletal muscles on the axial skeleton.

- Apply an understanding of client conditions resulting from strain or dysfunction in specific muscles and muscle groups to safe and effective palpation of those muscles and muscle groups.

INTRODUCTION

In this chapter, you will apply the Four-Step Protocol to palpation of superficial muscles on the axial skeleton: those that act on the trunk, the neck, and the head. In keeping with our focus on assessment of a client's body from the core outward, we begin by palpating muscles that attach to the trunk and move the scapula. Palpation of muscles that act on the neck, the chest during respiration, and the abdomen follows. Finally, you will learn how to palpate the muscles of mastication, which attach to the skull and move the mandible.

In the following palpation instructions, the suggestions that are given for directing muscle actions and adding resistance to movement are only a starting place. Develop your own palpation vocabulary as you learn the procedures. Optional positions and muscle actions are also presented for some palpations. Experiment with these options to find procedures that are most effective for you.

Although some of the muscle palpations described in this chapter may be performed with the client clothed, standing or seated, the instructions are presented for the client on the massage table, to address positioning and draping concerns. The photograph that accompanies each palpation is intended as a guide, not as a mandate. With practice and experience, you will find your own way, taking into account all the factors about the client on your table. Palpation is about *touch*—what you feel is more important than what you see.

MUSCLES THAT ACT ON THE SCAPULA

Muscles that act on the scapula shrug shoulders, row boats, reach for the phone, and help us breathe. They surround the scapula on all sides, from posterior to lateral to anterior. Palpable superficial muscles acting on the scapula include Trapezius, the Rhomboids, Levator scapulae and Serratus anterior. Actions of the scapula occur where the anterior scapula articulates with posterior ribs, articulations sometimes called the scapulocostal joints, though they are not true synovial joints.

Trapezius

Trapezius [truh-PEE-zee-us] is a large, flat superficial muscle that covers much of the back, shoulders, and neck. It allows multiple actions on the scapulae and the neck. Trapezius has fibers that run in multiple directions, and for reference is divided into three sections: upper, middle, and lower, visible in Figure 8–1. Trapezius acts primarily on the scapulae, where they articulate with the posterior ribs.

Attachments:

- Origin: the occiput and nuchal ligament and spinous processes of C7–T12.
- Insertion: lateral third of the clavicle, the acromion and the spine of the scapula.

Upper Trapezius actions:

- Elevates and laterally tilts the scapulae at the scapulocostal joints.
- Extends, laterally flexes, and contralaterally rotates the neck at the spinal joints.

Trapezius

trapezoid-shaped.

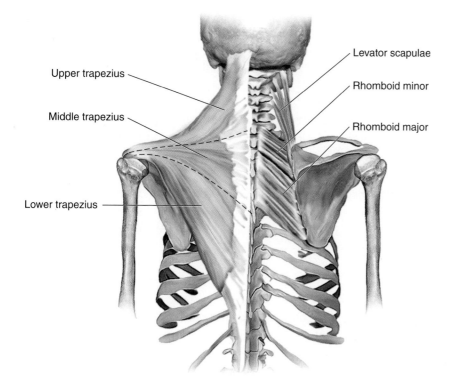

Upper trapezius

Middle trapezius

Lower trapezius

Levator scapulae

Rhomboid minor

Rhomboid major

FIGURE 8-1 Trapezius, the Rhomboids, and Levator scapulae.

Middle Trapezius actions:

■ Retracts the scapulae and pulls them medially, at the scapulocostal joints.

Lower Trapezius actions:

■ Depresses and medially tilts the scapulae at the scapulocostal joints.

Placement:

■ Superficial.

Palpation of Trapezius:

POSITION:

■ Prone client: undrape your client's back.

■ Stand at the side of the table. Use your mother hand to add resistance to movement or use both hands to palpate.

LOCATE AND PALPATE:

■ Locate the occiput and nuchal ligament as it extends to C7. On either side of the nuchal ligament, the fibers of Trapezius are superficial to Splenius capitis and cervicis, and their mass makes upper Trapezius very apparent.

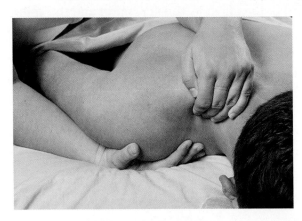

© Milady, a part of Cengage Learning. Photography by Yanik Chauvin.

FIGURE 8-2 Palpating Trapezius with the client in prone position.

■ Locate the lateral clavicle and the acromion. Passively elevate your client's shoulder to make the clavicular insertion more apparent. Palpate the upper fibers of Trapezius in their resting state between these landmarks, as shown in Figure 8–2. Palpate both with and across the grain of muscle fibers.

■ Locate the spinous processes of C7 through T5 and the spine of the scapula. Palpate the middle fibers of Trapezius in their resting state between these landmarks. Note the change in direction of the fibers from inferior-superior to lateral-to-medial. Palpate with and across the grain of muscle fibers.

■ Locate the spinous processes of T5 through T12 and the spine of the scapula. Palpate the lower fibers of Trapezius in their resting state between these landmarks. Note the change in direction of the fibers from lateral-to-medial to a lateral-to-inferior. Palpate with and across the grain of muscle fibers.

DIRECT AN ACTION AND PALPATE:

■ Ask your client to shrug his shoulders: palpate upper Trapezius during elevation of the scapula at the scapulocostal joints. Ask him to slightly lift his head: palpate upper Trapezius during extension of the neck. Palpate with and across the grain of muscle fibers.

- Ask your client to reach behind his back: palpate middle Trapezius during retraction or medial rotation of the scapula at the scapulocostal joints. Palpate with and across the grain of muscle fibers.
- Ask your client to bring his shoulder downward: palpate lower Trapezius during depression of the scapula at the scapulocostal joints. This action is the weakest for palpation.
- Add resistance to movement to any of these actions by placing your mother hand against the direction of movement.

EVALUATE:

- Characterize your palpation feedback from Trapezius: describe the tone, texture, and temperature of the muscle tissue.
- Note the presence of trigger points, tissue adhesions, barriers to palpation, or other findings.
- Compare palpation of both sides of Trapezius, noting how the findings from the second palpation vary.
- Compare with palpations of Trapezius on other clients, noting how the findings from palpation on this client differ.

OPTION:

- With your client supine: ask your client to bend his head toward his shoulder and palpate upper Trapezius during lateral flexion of the head at the neck.
- Ask your client to turn his head away from your palpating hand and palpate upper Trapezius during contralateral rotation of the head at the neck.

DID YOU KNOW?

Trapezius is sometimes called the "starter muscle" in Swedish massage technique: the beginning diamond-shaped effleurage stroke on a client's back perfectly outlines the borders of Trapezius. Because of its size and multiple attachment sites, most massage therapists routinely palpate the contours of Trapezius. Assessment of Trapezius is indicated for a client with postural dysfunctions, especially with rounded shoulders, a kyphotic spinal curvature, or a head-forward posture—linked issues that were discussed in Chapter 2, Posture Assessment—or a client who reports upper back and neck pain or one who works at a computer.

Rhomboids

Although palpated and treated as one muscle, the Rhomboids [RAHM-boyds] are actually two muscles, as shown in Figure 8–1: a superior Rhomboid minor and an inferior, larger Rhomboid major. Their fibers are indistinguishable, and often blend. The Rhomboids retract or bring back the scapulae. They are powerful in reaching and rowing motions and are opposed in those actions by the protraction of Serratus anterior and Pectoralis minor. Rhomboids lie entirely deep to Trapezius, but are palpable.

Rhomboids

rhomboid-shaped.

Attachments:
- Origin: spinous processes of C7–T5.
- Insertion: medial border and root of the spine of the scapula.

Actions:
- Retracts and downwardly rotates the scapulae at the scapulo-costal joints.

Placement:
- Deep to Trapezius.

Palpation of Rhomboids:

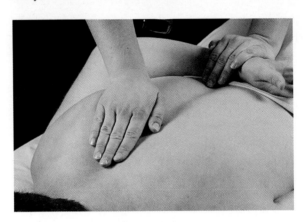

FIGURE 8-3 Palpating the Rhomboids with the client's hand placed in the small of the back.

POSITION:
- Prone client: undrape your client's back and ask him to place the hand on the side of the target muscle in the small of his back, as shown in Figure 8–3.
- Stand at the side of the table. Use your mother hand to support your client's shoulder from beneath.

LOCATE AND PALPATE:
- Locate the spinous processes of C7–T5 and the medial border of the scapula. Place your palpating hand in the area between the scapula and the spine. Palpate the fibers of the Rhomboids between these landmarks in their resting state. Palpate with and across the grain of muscle fibers.

DIRECT AN ACTION AND PALPATE:
- Ask your client to lift his arm from the surface of his back: palpate Rhomboids during retraction of the scapula at the scapulocostal joints, as in Figure 8–3. Palpate with and across the grain of muscle fibers.
- Resistance is not usually necessary when palpating Rhomboids.

EVALUATE:
- Characterize your palpation feedback from the Rhomboids: describe the tone, texture, and temperature of the muscle tissue.
- Note the presence of trigger points, tissue adhesions, barriers to palpation, or other findings.
- Compare palpation of both sides of the Rhomboids, noting how the findings from the second palpation vary.
- Compare with palpations of the Rhomboids on other clients, noting how the findings from palpation on this client differ.

IN THE TREATMENT ROOM

When the Rhomboids are weak, their action of retraction or bringing back of the scapulae is weak and unable to counter the protraction or pulling forward of the scapulae by Serratus anterior or Pectoralis minor (palpation of Pectoralis minor is described in Chapter 10, Palpating Deeper Muscles and Muscle Groups). This scenario is a frequent cause of rounded shoulder. Assessment and palpation of the Rhomboids along with Serratus anterior and Pectoralis minor is always recommended when assessing clients with one or both shoulders rounded to the anterior.

Levator Scapulae

Levator scapulae [lih-VAYT-ur SKAP-yuh-lee] is the dense mass of muscle tissue that extends laterally from the cervical region of the spine to the superior angle of the scapula. Its density is due in part to the twisting of its middle fibers, not truly visible in Figure 8–1. As its name implies, Levator scapulae lifts—elevates—the scapula and shrugs your shoulders. It is a site of frequently discovered trigger points. Levator scapulae lies deep to the upper fibers of Trapezius, but is readily palpable when Trapezius is relaxed.

Attachments:
- Origin: transverse processes of C1–C4.
- Insertion: superior angle and superior third of the medial border of the scapula.

Actions:
- Elevates the scapula at the scapulocostal joints.
- Extends and laterally flexes the neck at the spinal joints.

Placement:
- Deep to Trapezius.

Levator

elevates.

DID YOU KNOW?

Other muscles with twisted fibers include Pectoralis major and Latissimus dorsi. Such twisted fibers add density and bulk in muscles with actions in multiple directions.

Palpation of Levator Scapulae:

POSITION:
- Prone client: undrape your client's neck and upper back.
- Place your client's hand in the small of his back, to relax Trapezius, as in Figure 8–4.
- Stand or sit at the side of the table. Use your mother hand to support your client's hand on his back.

LOCATE AND PALPATE:
- Locate the inverted V-shaped trough in the posterior neck between the upper fibers of Trapezius

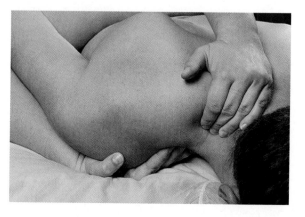

FIGURE 8-4 Palpating Levator scapulae with the client's hand placed in the small of the back.

© Milady, a part of Cengage Learning. Photography by Yanik Chauvin.

and the insertion of SCM on the mastoid process—the palpation site for Splenius capitis, and the superior angle of the scapula.

■ With the fingertips of your palpating hand, palpate Levator scapulae from the trough in the posterior neck to the superior angle of the scapula, in its resting state, as shown in Figure 8–4. Palpate with and across the grain of muscle fibers.

DIRECT AN ACTION AND PALPATE:

■ Ask your client to quickly raise and lower (elevate and depress) his shoulder: palpate Levator scapulae during the elevation of the scapula at the scapulo-costal joints. Palpate with and across the grain of muscle fibers.

■ Adding resistance to the action of Levator scapulae will engage Trapezius, hindering the palpation.

EVALUATE:

■ Characterize your palpation feedback from Levator scapulae: describe the tone, texture, and temperature of the muscle tissue.

■ Note the presence of trigger points, tissue adhesions, barriers to palpation, or other findings.

■ Compare palpation of both sides of Levator scapulae, noting how the findings from the second palpation vary.

■ Compare with palpations of Levator scapulae on other clients, noting how the findings from palpation on this client differ.

IN THE TREATMENT ROOM

Levator scapulae are assessed in a client who reports shoulder pain or when postural analysis shows has one shoulder chronically elevated. Such symptoms or signs may occur if the client typically raises one shoulder to support the weight of a shoulder bag or purse, or sits at a desk chair all day long with one leg tucked under the other, requiring him to raise the opposite shoulder in order to balance the head.

Serratus

serrated edges.

Serratus Anterior

Because of its insertion on the anterior aspect of the scapula, Serratus anterior [ser-RAT-us an-TEER-ee-ur] can hold the scapula against the chest wall. Its name describes its serrated appearance, visible in Figure 8–5. Serratus anterior's action of protraction of the scapula assists Pectoralis minor and opposes the retraction by the Rhomboids, which also attach to the medial border of the scapula. The origins of Serratus anterior are on, not between, ribs #1–8. The External intercostals are in the intercostal spaces between the ribs. Their fibers are perpendicular to the ribs, while the fibers of Serratus anterior are aligned with the ribs.

Attachments:
■ Origin: anterior aspect of ribs #1–8.
■ Insertion: medial border of the scapula, on the anterior aspect.

Actions:
■ Stabilizes, protracts, and upwardly rotates the scapula at the scapulocostal joints.

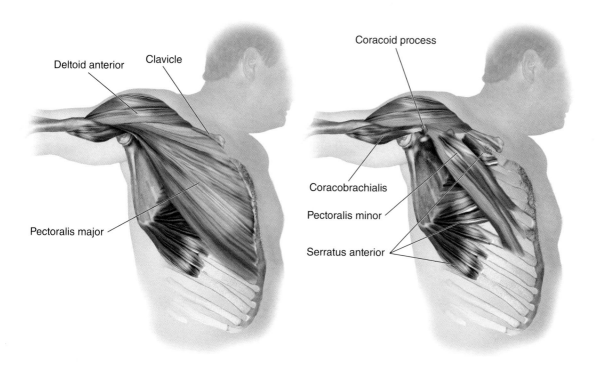

FIGURE 8–5 Serratus anterior wraps around the lateral torso.

Placement:

■ Deep to Latissimus dorsi, Pectoralis major and minor.

Palpation of Serratus Anterior:

POSITION:

■ Side-lying client: palpate through the drape.

■ Flex your client's arm to allow access to the target muscle.

■ Stand at the side of the table, facing your client. Use your mother hand to support your client's flexed arm, as in Figure 8–6.

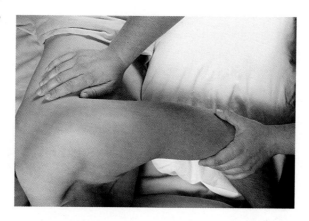

FIGURE 8–6 Palpating Serratus anterior with the client in side-lying position.

LOCATE AND PALPATE:

■ Along the angle of the ribcage, place your palpating hand to follow its curve to locate the origins of Serratus anterior: palpate toward the lateral border of the scapula.

■ Apply slight passive traction on your client's arm to deepen your access beneath the border. Palpate the fibers of Serratus anterior in its resting state between these landmarks. Palpate with and across the grain of muscle fibers.

DIRECT AN ACTION AND PALPATE:

■ Ask your client to push against your mother hand as shown in Figure 8–6 as you resist his movement. Palpate Serratus anterior in resisted protraction of the scapula at the scapulocostal joints. Palpate with and across the grain of muscle fibers.

EVALUATE:

■ Characterize your palpation feedback from Serratus anterior: describe the tone, texture, and temperature of the muscle tissue.

■ Note the presence of trigger points, tissue adhesions, barriers to palpation, or other findings.

■ Compare palpation of both sides of Serratus anterior, noting how the findings from the second palpation vary.

■ Compare with palpations of Serratus anterior on other clients, noting how the findings from palpation on this client differ.

OPTION:

■ With your female client supine: abduct her arm, support it at the elbow with your mother hand, and ask her to hold breast tissue secure with her other hand.

■ Locate the insertions of Serratus anterior on ribs by following the curve of ribs #2–8 laterally on the thorax.

■ Ask your client to push against your resisting mother hand and palpate Serratus anterior during resisted protraction of the scapula.

Lab Activity 8.1 on page 333 is designed to develop your palpation skills on superficial muscles that act on the scapulae.

HERE'S A TIP

A weak Serratus anterior is unable to effectively counter the retraction of Rhomboids, resulting in "winged" scapula, in which the inferior angle of the scapula protrudes from the surface of the ribcage, as shown in Figure 8–7. The relationship between Pectoralis minor, Rhomboids, and Serratus anterior and their actions on the scapulae is one that calls for focused palpation of all three muscles in assessing the range of shoulder problems massage therapists routinely encounter. A winged scapula will be palpable and perhaps visible even through clothing during visual assessment of posture. It also alters the usual position of the coracoid process of the scapula, moving it in a downward, deeper direction. This makes the coracoid process less palpable and in turn alters the position of the attachments of muscles on its surface.

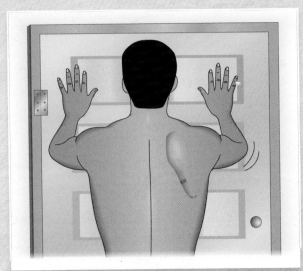

FIGURE 8-7 A "winged" scapula: the inferior angle protrudes from the surface of the ribcage.

MUSCLES THAT ACT ON THE NECK

Muscles in the posterior neck usually extend, laterally flex, ipsilaterally rotate the head and neck, and act on the scapula. Muscles in the anterior neck usually flex, laterally flex, and contralaterally rotate the head and neck. Palpation of the muscles that act on the neck is a skill you will use on a daily basis, throughout your career as a massage therapist!

Sternocleidomastoid (SCM)

Sternocleidomastoid [STUR-noh-KLEE-ih-doh-MAS-toyd], usually, and conveniently, called SCM, has two heads at its origin: one on the sternum and one on the clavicle. The paired SCMs form a "V" in the anterior neck, as seen in Figure 8–8, creating the borders between the endangerment sites of the anterior and posterior triangles of the neck. Because SCM is an anterior neck muscle, it may be difficult to visualize its action as it occurs at spinal joints. Palpate SCM in both its unilateral and bilateral actions, and take care to avoid the anterior triangle of the neck.

> **Sterno**
>
> sternum; cleido = clavicle; mastoid = mastoid process of the temporal bone.

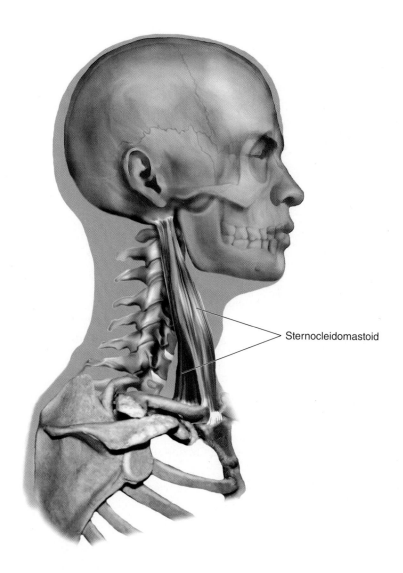

Sternocleidomastoid

FIGURE 8-8
Sternocleidomastoid (SCM).

© Delmar, Cengage Learning.

DID YOU KNOW?

The clavicular head of SCM may attach quite laterally on the clavicle, and may even appear to be a separate structure because it creates a "well" in between the two heads.

Attachments:
- Origin: the superior aspect of the manubrium of the sternum and the medial third of the clavicle.
- Insertion: mastoid process of the temporal bone.

Actions:
- Bilateral: flexes the head at the spinal joints.
- Unilateral: laterally flexes the head at the spinal joints to the same side and contralaterally rotates the head at the spinal joints to the opposite side.

Placement:
- Superficial.

Palpation of SCM:

POSITION:
- Supine client: undrape your client's neck.
- Stand or sit at the head of the table. Use your mother hand to stabilize your client's neck during rotational actions. Use both hands to palpate during flexion and lateral flexion of the head.

LOCATE AND PALPATE:

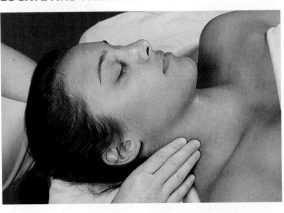

- Locate the mastoid process of the temporal bone, the medial clavicle, and the manubrium of the sternum, just medial to the sternoclavicular joint: gently palpate SCM, in its resting state, between these landmarks, as in Figure 8–9. Palpate with and across the grain of muscle fibers.

FIGURE 8–9 Palpating SCM. Be mindful of the endangerment sites on either side of the muscle belly.

DIRECT AN ACTION AND PALPATE:
- Ask your client to raise her head slightly off the table, making both sides of SCM clearly evident and palpable: palpate SCM during flexion of the head at the spinal joints. *Do not allow your client to keep holding her head off the table! If necessary, ask her to duplicate the action a second time after first releasing and resting the neck.*
- Ask your client to bend her head toward her ear: palpate the same-side SCM during lateral flexion of the head at the spinal joints. Palpate with and across the grain of muscle fibers.
- Ask your client to turn her head away from your palpating hand, to the opposite side of the table: palpate SCM during contralateral rotation of the head at the spinal joints.
- To bring out SCM even more, ask your client to briefly raise her head off the table while it is rotated.
- Do not add resistance to the actions of SCM.

EVALUATE:

- Characterize your palpation feedback from SCM: describe the tone, texture, and temperature of the muscle tissue.
- Note the presence of trigger points, tissue adhesions, barriers to palpation, or other findings.
- Compare palpation of both sides of SCM, noting how the findings from the second palpation vary.
- Compare with palpations of SCM on other clients, noting how the findings from palpation on this client differ.

IN THE TREATMENT ROOM

Trigger points in SCM may refer pain to the sinuses, the teeth, or even to the tongue. Because it flexes the head, SCM is assessed following any whiplash-like strain or injury. **Whiplash** is a sudden, forceful flexion then extension (or vice versa) of the cervical spine, as shown in Figure 8–10. The head snaps back and forth, like the end of a whip, alternately hyperflexing and hyperextending the neck flexor and extensor muscles. Whiplash may occur when someone is struck on the head, runs into a door headfirst, or is hit from behind in a rear-end collision. Symptoms caused by a whiplash injury may include dizziness, headaches, and neck and jaw pain. Muscles assessed in client who has experienced a whiplash-like event include SCM, the Scalene group, described next, and Longus colli, described in Chapter 10, Palpating Deeper Muscles and Muscle Groups. Whiplash may also affect the position of the mandible, straining the muscles of mastication, described later in this chapter, and indicates assessment of the muscles of mastication, described later in this chapter.

There are many reasons to assess SCM: if you note that your client's head is chronically tilted or rotated to one side, for example, recall that SCM laterally flexes to the same side and rotates to the opposite side, and target SCM for palpation.

> **Whiplash**
>
> a sudden, forceful flexion and extension, or vice versa, of the cervical spine, such as that experienced when struck on the head or hit from behind in a rear-end collision.

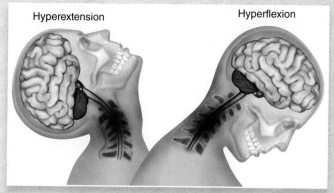

FIGURE 8–10 In a whiplash injury, the head snaps back and forth like the end of whip, alternately hyperflexing and hyperextending the neck flexor and extensor muscles.

Hyperextension　Hyperflexion

© Milady, a part of Cengage Learning.

Scalene Group: Anterior, Middle, Posterior

The anterior, middle, and posterior Scalene [SKAY-leen] muscles originate on cervical transverse processes and insert onto upper ribs, as seen in Figure 8–11. Because of their insertions on ribs #1 and 2, the Scalenes

> **Scalene**
>
> a triangle with three unequal sides.

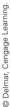

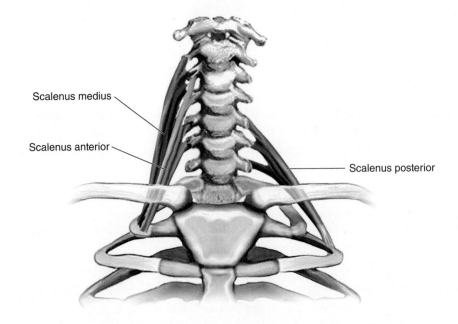

Scalenus medius

Scalenus anterior

Scalenus posterior

FIGURE 8-11 Anterior, middle, and posterior Scalenes.

are considered accessory muscles of respiration: asking your client to take in a deep breath as you palpate will ensure you that you are correctly locating the Scalenes. The Scalenes may be involved in a whiplash-like injury or in thoracic outlet syndrome, described on page 318. Only small sections of the Scalenes are readily palpable.

IN THE TREATMENT ROOM

Recall that the anterior neck region contains two endangerment sites: the anterior and posterior triangles of the neck, described in Chapter 5, the Science of Palpation. Check visually for the exact locations of blood vessels in the anterior neck before palpating these muscles, and avoid any site where pulsing is felt. Make sure you are palpating muscle tissue, not blood vessels or nerves. Keep your palpation pressure superficial in the anterior neck.

Attachments:

Anterior Scalene:

- Origin: anterior tubercles of transverse processes C3–6.
- Insertion: anterior, superior aspect of rib #1.

Medial Scalene:

- Origin: posterior tubercles of transverse processes C2–7.
- Insertion: lateral, anterior aspect of rib #1.

Posterior Scalene:

- Origin: posterior tubercles of transverse processes C5–7.
- Insertion: lateral, anterior aspect of rib #2.

Actions as a Group:

- Bilateral: flexes the neck at the spinal joints and raises ribs #1 and 2 during deep inhalation.
- Unilateral: laterally flexes and assists in contralateral rotation of the neck at the spinal joints.

Placement:

- Superior portions are deep to SCM.

Palpation of the Scalenes group:

POSITION:

- Supine client: undrape your client's neck.
- Stand or sit at the head of the table. Use your mother hand to stabilize your client's neck during rotational actions.

LOCATE AND PALPATE:

- Locate the lateral border of SCM and the insertion of Trapezius on the lateral clavicle by asking your client to elevate her shoulder: this action lifts the clavicle, revealing the posterior triangle where the Scalenes lie.
- Place the fingertips of your palpating hand in the depression between SCM and Trapezius to palpate the Scalenes in their resting state, as in Figure 8–12. Palpate with and across the grain of muscle fibers.

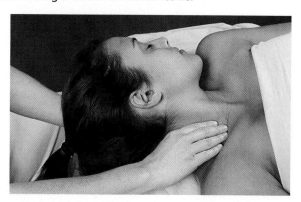

FIGURE 8–12 Gently palpating the Scalenes group in the posterior triangle of the neck.

© Milady, a part of Cengage Learning. Photography by Yanik Chauvin.

DIRECT AN ACTION AND PALPATE:

- Ask your client to lift her slightly off the table. Palpate the Scalenes during flexion of the head at the spinal joints. Do not allow your client to sustain this position. Ask her to repeat the action, if necessary, after resting his neck for a moment.
- With her head resting on the table, ask your client to take a fast, deep breath in: palpate the Scalenes during the deep inhalation.
- Ask your client to bend her head toward his ear. Palpate the same-side Scalenes during lateral flexion of the head at the spinal joints.
- Ask your client to turn her head away from your palpating hand. Palpate the Scalenes during contralateral rotation of the head.
- Do not add resistance to the actions of the Scalenes.

EVALUATE:

- Characterize your palpation feedback from the Scalenes: describe the tone, texture, and temperature of the muscle tissue.
- Note the presence of trigger points, tissue adhesions, barriers to palpation, or other findings.
- Compare palpation of both sides of the Scalenes, noting how the findings from the second palpation vary.
- Compare with palpations of the Scalenes on other clients, noting how the findings from palpation on this client differ.

IN THE TREATMENT ROOM

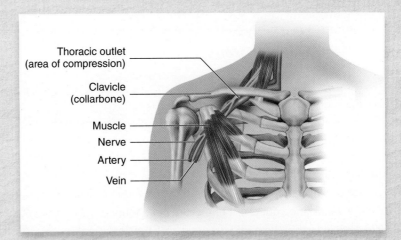

FIGURE 8–13 Thoracic outlet syndrome is characterized by entrapment of nerves in the brachial plexus and/or the blood vessels that supply the arm as they travel between the anterior and middle Scalenes and beneath Pectoralis minor.

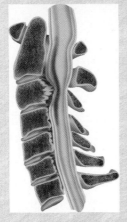

FIGURE 8–14 Bone spurs in the cervical region of the spine may compress delicate structures.

The Scalene muscles, like SCM, are assessed following a whiplash-like strain or injury, and for **thoracic outlet syndrome**, also called TOS: entrapment of nerves in the brachial plexus and/or the blood vessels that supply the arm as they travel between the anterior and middle Scalenes and beneath Pectoralis minor, shown in Figure 8–13. Symptoms of TOS include shooting pains, numbness and weakness, and sometimes discoloration in the affected arm from inadequate blood circulation. Symptoms are progressive and may become serious. Before receiving massage treatment, a client with symptoms of TOS should be medically evaluated to rule out vertebral disc problems, skeletal misalignments, or **bone spurs**, which are overgrowths of bone called osteophytes that can impinge on nearby delicate tissues, shown in Figure 8–14.

Thoracic outlet syndrome

entrapment of nerves in the brachial plexus and/or blood vessels that supply the arm, causing shooting pains, numbness and weakness, and possibly discoloration in the affected arm, due to inadequate circulation.

Bone spur

an overgrowth of bone; also called an osteophyte.

Supra

above or superior

Infra

below or inferior

DID YOU KNOW?

Palpating the Hyoid muscles is an effective means of locating the hyoid bone for treatment with craniosacral therapy.

Hyoids Group: Suprahyoids; Infrahyoids

The eight muscles of the Hyoid group are divided into two subgroups by their location, shown in Figure 8–15: the Suprahyoids [soo-pruh-HY-oyds] lie superior to, attach to, and elevate the hyoid bone. The Infrahyoids [in-fruh-HY-oyds] lie inferior to, attach to, and depress the hyoid bone. As a group, the Hyoids are active during mastication and swallowing. They are easiest to locate during swallowing. Use very superficial pressure when palpating the two Hyoid groups, and communicate with your client to gauge his comfort.

Suprahyoid group attachments:
- Origin: the temporal bone and the mandible.
- Insertion: the superior aspect of the hyoid bone.

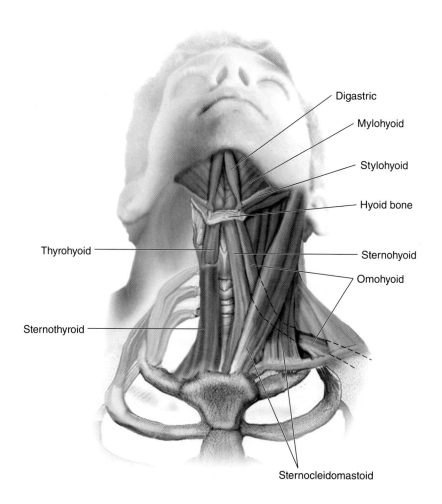

Digastric

Mylohyoid

Stylohyoid

Hyoid bone

Thyrohyoid

Sternohyoid

Omohyoid

Sternothyroid

Sternocleidomastoid

FIGURE 8-15 The Hyoid muscle group.

© Delmar, Cengage Learning.

Infrahyoid group attachments:
- Origin: the sternum, the clavicle, and thyroid cartilage.
- Insertion: the inferior aspect of the hyoid bone.

Actions:
- The Suprahyoids elevate the hyoid bone and the mandible.
- The Infrahyoids depress the hyoid bone and thyroid cartilage.

Placement:
- Superficial, deep only to platysma.

Palpation of the Hyoids group:

POSITION:
- Supine client: undrape your client's neck and upper chest.
- Stand or sit at the side of the table. Use your mother hand to stabilize your client's neck.

LOCATE AND PALPATE:
- Locate the hyoid bone. The Suprahyoids lie superior to the hyoid bone. The Infrahyoids lie inferior to the hyoid bone, medial to SCM, and lateral to the trachea. Place your palpating hand softly around your client's anterior neck: palpate each group in its resting state, as in Figure 8–16.

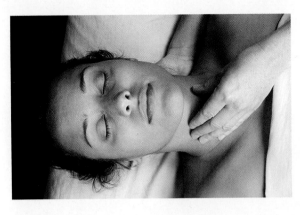

FIGURE 8-16 Gently palpating the Hyoid muscles with the client's neck stabilized.

DIRECT AN ACTION AND PALPATE:

- Ask your client to swallow: place your palpating hand softly over the Suprahyoids during that action. Repeat for the Infrahyoid muscles.

- Do not add resistance to the action of the Hyoids.

EVALUATE:

- Characterize your findings. Compare with palpations of the Hyoids on other clients.

Lab Activity 8–2 on page 333 is designed to develop your palpation skills on superficial muscles that act on the neck.

MUSCLES OF RESPIRATION

Muscles of respiration include the Diaphragm, the External and Internal intercostals, Serratus posterior superior, Serratus posterior inferior, and accessory muscles, such as Pectoralis minor. Of the muscles of respiration, only the superficial External intercostal muscles are readily palpable. Palpation of the deeper Diaphragm, Serratus posterior superior, Serratus posterior inferior, and Pectoralis minor are described in Chapter 10, Palpating Deeper Muscles and Muscle Groups.

External Intercostals

The External intercostal [in-tur-KAHS-tul] muscles, visible in Figure 8–17, elevate the ribs to expand the chest cavity for inhalation. Their fiber

Inter

between; -costal = ribs.

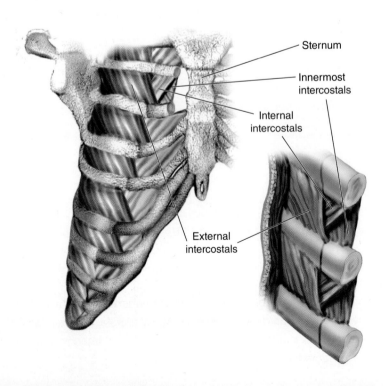

Sternum

Innermost intercostals

Internal intercostals

External intercostals

FIGURE 8-17 The Intercostal muscles.

direction is slightly diagonal, from lateral superiorly to medial interiorly. The deeper Internal intercostals depress the ribs to contract the chest cavity for exhalation, and are not directly palpable.

Attachments:

■ Inferior border of one of ribs #1–11 to the superior border of the next inferior rib.

Actions:

■ Pull the ribs together, which elevates them during inhalation.

Placement:

■ Superficial.

Palpation of the External Intercostals:

POSITION:

■ Supine client: undrape your client's upper chest.

■ Breast tissue may impede palpation of all the External intercostals. You may ask your female client to use her free hand to secure the drape and immobilize breast tissue during this palpation.

■ Stand at the side of the table. Use your mother hand to support your client's torso or palpate with both hands.

LOCATE AND PALPATE:

■ Place the fingertips of your palpating hands along the intercostal spaces between several ribs, as in Figure 8–18, following the angle of the ribcage.

■ The fibers of the External intercostals are angled 45° lateral-to-medial in the intercos-

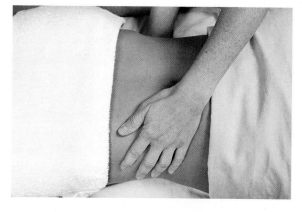

FIGURE 8–18 Palpating the External Intercostal muscles with the client in supine position.

© Milady, a part of Cengage Learning. Photography by Yanik Chauvin.

tal spaces: palpate the fibers of the External intercostals in their resting state, on the inhalation and between breaths. Palpate with and across the grain of muscle fibers.

DIRECT AN ACTION AND PALPATE

■ Ask your client to inhale deeply: palpate the External intercostals during elevation of the ribs.

■ Place your hands around each side of the ribcage to palpate the expansion of the chest cavity.

■ Adding resistance to movement is not useful in palpation of the External intercostals.

EVALUATE:

■ Characterize your palpation feedback from the External intercostals: describe the tone, texture, and temperature of the muscle tissue.

■ Note the presence of trigger points, tissue adhesions, barriers to palpation, or other findings.

■ Compare palpation of both sides of the External intercostals, noting how the findings from the second palpation vary.

■ Compare with palpations of the External intercostals on other clients, noting how the findings from palpation on this client differ.

© Milady, a part of Cengage Learning.

Chronic obstructive pulmonary disease, COPD

a chronic, progressive lung condition that includes chronic bronchitis and emphysema.

IN THE TREATMENT ROOM

The External intercostal muscles are assessed for treatment in clients with ongoing breathing problems, such as asthma or **COPD**, chronic obstructive pulmonary disease, a chronic, progressive lung condition that includes chronic bronchitis and emphysema. A client with emphysema may have a barrel-chested appearance, shown in Figure 8–19, due to "locking" of the Intercostals in an effort to ease breathing.

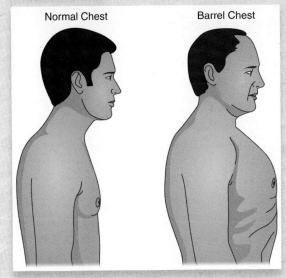

Normal Chest   Barrel Chest

FIGURE 8–19 The labored breathing of a client with COPD results in a "barrel-shaped" chest.

MUSCLES THAT ACT ON THE ABDOMEN

The four Abdominal group muscles, Rectus abdominis, External oblique, Internal oblique, and Transversus abdominis, shown in Figure 8–20, compress the abdominal contents. All except Transversus abdominis, which has no skeletal attachment, also flex and rotate the trunk. Only Rectus abdominis and the External oblique are directly palpable. The actions of the Abdominal group muscles take place at the spinal joints.

IN THE TREATMENT ROOM

Before palpating your client's abdomen, verify that he has no visceral abdominal pain. Recent abdominal medical procedures or unexplained pain contraindicate abdominal pressure.

Rectus = erect

Abdominis = of the abdomen.

Rectus Abdominis

The fibers of Rectus abdominis [REK-tus ab-DAHM-ih-nus] are vertical and contained within the rectus sheath, part of the abdominal

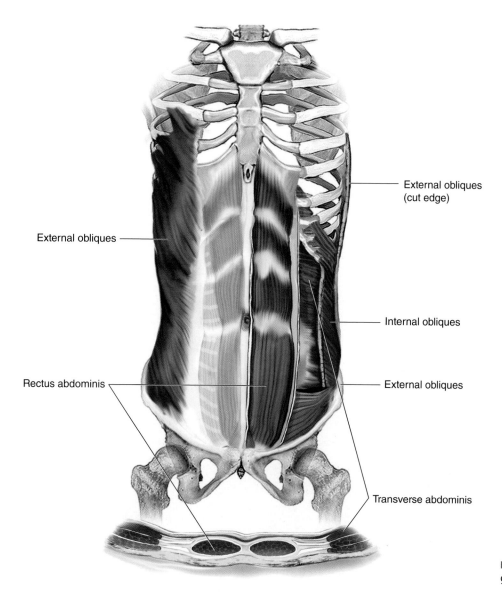

External obliques (cut edge)

External obliques

Internal obliques

Rectus abdominis

External obliques

Transverse abdominis

FIGURE 8-20 The Abdominal group.

© Delmar, Cengage Learning.

aponeurosis. This configuration mirrors the Erector spinae group in the posterior trunk, and Rectus abdominis opposes the Erectors in extension of the trunk. Transverse fibrous bands across Rectus abdominis create the "six-pack" look of a highly toned Rectus abdominis and may be noted during palpation. Rectus abdominis is medial to the other muscles of the abdominal group.

Attachments:
- Origin: pubic crest and symphysis.
- Insertion: xiphoid process of the sternum and costal cartilage of ribs #5–7.

Actions:
- Flexes the trunk at the spinal joints and compresses the abdominal wall.
- Posteriorly tilts the pelvis at the lumbosacral joint.

Placement:
- Superficial.

Palpation of Rectus Abdominis:

POSITION:

- Supine client: place a bolster beneath your client's knees to create passive flexion of the thighs. Palpate through the drape or undrape the abdomen and secure a towel or other covering over the breast area so that it remains in place during directed actions.
- Stand at the side of the table. Place your mother hand beneath your client's shoulder for support during movement.

LOCATE AND PALPATE:

- Place your palpating hand along your client's abdominal midline: locate the origin on the pubic crest and the insertion on the xiphoid process of the sternum.
- Palpate Rectus abdominis in its resting state between these landmarks. Note the transverse fibrous bands that divide Rectus abdominis into sections and palpate with and across the grain of muscle fibers.

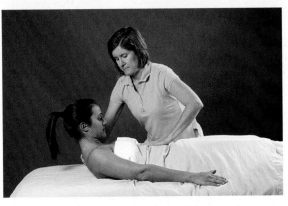

DIRECT AN ACTION AND PALPATE:

- Ask your client to perform a slight curl-up of her trunk. Reinforce the instruction with your mother hand, if appropriate. Palpate Rectus abdominis during flexion of the trunk at the spinal joints, as shown in Figure 8–21.

FIGURE 8–21 Palpating Rectus abdominus with your client flexing the trunk.

- Adding resistance to movement is not useful in palpation of Rectus abdominis.

EVALUATE:

- Characterize your palpation feedback from Rectus abdominis: describe the tone, texture, and temperature of the muscle tissue.
- Note the presence of trigger points, tissue adhesions, barriers to palpation, or other findings.
- Compare with palpations of Rectus abdominis on other clients, noting how the findings from palpation on this client differ.

IN THE TREATMENT ROOM

Avoid exerting palpation pressure over the xiphoid process of the sternum, or palpating too deeply into the abdomen. The abdominal aorta is deep in this region: move away from any area where pulsing is felt.

External Oblique

The External obliques [eks-TUR-nul oh-BLEEKS], seen in Figure 8–20, are superficial and palpable. The fibers of each External oblique are diagonal from lateral-and-superior to medial-and-inferior in the trunk.

Oblique

diagonal.

> ### HERE'S A TIP
>
> To duplicate the fiber orientation of the External obliques, place your hands on your lateral ribcage as if putting them into the side pockets of a short jacket.

Attachments:
- Origin: external surface of the lower eight ribs.
- Insertion: abdominal aponeurosis, the linea alba—a fibrous band at the midline—and the iliac crest.

Actions:
- Bilateral: flexes the trunk at the spinal joints and compresses the abdominal wall.
- Unilateral: laterally flexes and contralaterally rotates the trunk at the spinal joints.

Placement:
- Superficial.

Palpation of External Oblique:

POSITION:
- Supine client: place a bolster beneath your client's knees to create passive flexion of the thighs. Palpate through the drape, if appropriate, or undrape the abdomen and secure a towel or other covering over the breast area so that it remains in place during directed actions.
- Stand at the side of the table. Place your mother hand beneath your client's shoulder for support during movement or use both hands to palpate.

LOCATE AND PALPATE:
- With your palpating hand angled downward and toward the midline, along the ribcage, locate the origin of External oblique on the ribs and the insertion along the anterior iliac crest. The ASIS is a handy landmark, as shown in Figure 8–22.

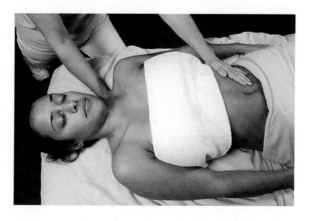

FIGURE 8-22 Palpating the External obliques with your hand placed along the angle of its fibers.

© Milady, a part of Cengage Learning. Photography by Yanik Chauvin.

- Palpate the diagonal fibers of the External obliques in their resting state between these landmarks. Palpate with and across the grain of muscle fibers.

DIRECT AN ACTION AND PALPATE:

■ Ask your client to perform a slight curl-up, again reinforcing the instruction with your mother hand. Palpate External oblique as it flexes the trunk at the spinal joints.

■ Ask your client to twist her torso away from you and palpate External oblique during contralateral rotation of the trunk at the spinal joints. Palpate with and across the grain of muscle fibers.

■ If you place your mother hand on the opposite side of the trunk during contralateral rotation of the target muscle, you may be able to feel the synergistic action of Internal oblique.

■ Adding resistance to the action of External oblique is not recommended.

EVALUATE:

■ Characterize your palpation feedback from the External obliques: describe the tone, texture, and temperature of the muscle tissue.

■ Note the presence of trigger points, tissue adhesions, barriers to palpation, or other findings.

■ Compare palpation of both sides of the External obliques, noting how the findings from the second palpation vary.

■ Compare with palpations of the External obliques on other clients, noting how the findings from palpation on this client differ.

> **Lab Activity 8–3** on page 334 is designed to develop your palpation skills on the superficial abdominal muscles.

MUSCLES OF MASTICATION

The muscles of mastication, or chewing, shown in Figure 8–23, act on the mandible at the temporomandibular joints. Mastication combines five separate movements:

■ Opening and closing the jaw: elevation and depression of the mandible.

■ Moving the jaw forward and backward: protraction and retraction of the mandible.

■ Holding the food in position for chewing and moving the jaw from side to side: lateral deviation of the mandible.

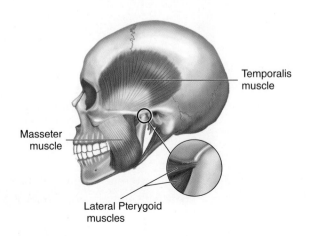

Temporalis muscle

Masseter muscle

Lateral Pterygoid muscles

FIGURE 8–23 The muscles of mastication.

DID YOU KNOW?

Buccinator, a muscle of facial expression, also participates in mastication by compressing food between the cheek and the teeth, though it does not move the mandible and is not significant for palpation.

Temporalis

Temporalis [tem-poh-RAY-lis] is a fan-shaped muscle that lies in a shallow fossa in the temporal bone. The tendinous portion of Temporalis is anterior to the ear, traveling deep to the zygomatic arch toward the coronoid process of the mandible. Temporalis is powerful as it crushes hard-to-chew substances and is most palpable anterior to the top of the external ear.

> **Temporal**
> the temporal bone of the skull.

Attachments:

■ Origin: fossa of the temporal bone.
■ Insertion: coronoid process and ramus of the mandible.

Actions:

■ Elevates and retracts the mandible at the temporomandibular joint.

Placement:

■ Superficial.

HERE'S A TIP

To fully experience the actions of Temporalis, palpate it on yourself as you chew beef jerky or a hard, chewy granola bar—it will be amazingly palpable!

Palpation of Temporalis:

POSITION:

■ Supine client: undrape your client's neck.
■ Stand or sit at the head of the table. Use both hands to palpate.

LOCATE AND PALPATE:

■ Place your hands so that your palpating fingertips lie just anterior to the ear, as in Figure 8–24. Locate and palpate Temporalis in its resting state, from its origin on the temporal bone toward its insertion on the coronoid process of the mandible. The insertion is not directly palpable in the resting state, because it lies beneath the zygomatic arch.

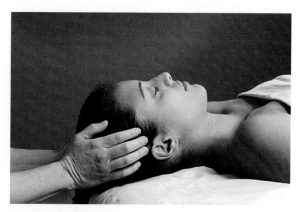

FIGURE 8–24 Bilateral palpation of Temporalis.

© Milady, a part of Cengage Learning. Photography by Yanik Chauvin.

DIRECT AN ACTION AND PALPATE:

■ Ask your client to open and close her jaw: palpate Temporalis during elevation of the mandible at the temporomandibular joint.
■ Do not add resistance to elevation of the mandible.

EVALUATE:

■ Characterize your palpation feedback from Temporalis: describe the tone, texture, and temperature of the muscle tissue.

- Note the presence of trigger points, tissue adhesions, barriers to palpation, or other findings.
- Compare palpation of both sides of Temporalis, noting how the findings from the second palpation vary.
- Compare with palpations of Temporalis on other clients, noting how the findings from palpation on this client differ.

Temporomandibular joint disorder or TMJD

a condition characterized by headaches or dizziness, clicking or popping in the joint, pain, tinnitus, loss of full range of motion, or even locking in the joint. One cause of TMJD may be bruxism (see below). Other causes include osteoarthritis or an injury to the jaw, such as dislocation.

Tinnitus

persistent ringing or noise in the ears.

Bruxism

grinding of the teeth often associated with temporomandibular joint disorder.

IN THE TREATMENT ROOM

The muscles of mastication are assessed in clients who show symptoms of TMJD, **temporomandibular joint disorder**, shown in Figure 8–25. TMJD is characterized by headaches or dizziness, clicking or popping in the joint, pain, ringing in the ears, called **tinnitus** [tih-NYTE-us], and loss of full range of motion or even locking of the joint. One cause of TMJD may be **bruxism** [BRUK-siz-um], or teeth grinding. Other causes include osteoarthritis or an injury to the jaw, such as dislocation or whiplash-type injury. Symptoms are often worse during periods of stress. The lateral displacement of the mandible that can accompany TMJD may result in pain that spreads up into the skull and into the ear itself. Pain may also spread down into the anterior or lateral neck, causing stiffness and hypertonicity in muscles such as Sternocleidomastoid (SCM), the Scalene group, and the lateral cervical fibers of Trapezius. There may be significant tenderness in Temporalis or the lateral occiput on palpation. A client with any of these symptoms should be assessed for TMJD.

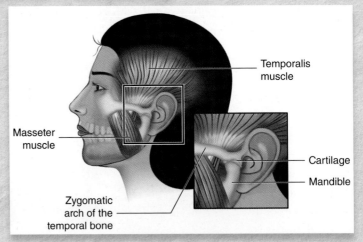

FIGURE 8–25 Temporomandibular joint disorder (TMJD) may cause misalignment or locking of the mandible.

Masseter

means "to chew".

Masseter

The thick Masseter [muh-SEET-ur] has two segments, superficial and deep, and is extremely powerful in elevating the mandible, or closing the mouth. Some sources connect its strength to the need during human evolution to gnaw on raw meat, others to the need to chew rough plant materials. Whatever its evolutionary history is, Masseter is the primary muscle of mastication. The Masseter is often tender in response to trigger points and is prominently involved in TMJD. Simultaneous palpation of both Masseters reveals any misalignment of the mandible. The Masseter is visible in Figure 8–23 and in Figure 8–27.

DID YOU KNOW?

Masseter is often called the strongest muscle in the body.

Attachments:
- Origin: the zygomatic bone and the zygomatic arch.
- Insertion: lateral surface and coronoid process of the mandible.

Actions:
- Elevates the mandible at the temporomandibular joint.

Placement:
- Superficial.

Palpation of Masseter:

POSITION:
- Supine client: undrape your client's neck.
- Stand or sit at the head of the table. Use both hands to palpate.

LOCATE AND PALPATE:
- Place your palpating hands along the zygomatic arch, as shown in Figure 8–26. Locate and palpate Masseter in its resting state, from its origin on the

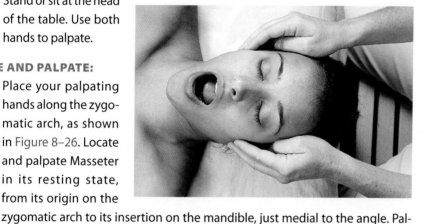

FIGURE 8–26 Palpate Masseter during elevation and depression of the jaw to assess the position of the mandible.

zygomatic arch to its insertion on the mandible, just medial to the angle. Palpate across the grain of the dense fibers of Masseter.

DIRECT AN ACTION AND PALPATE:
- Ask your client to open and close her jaw: palpate Masseter during elevation of the mandible at the temporomandibular joint. Palpate with and across the muscle fibers.
- Do not add resistance to elevation of the mandible.

EVALUATE:
- Characterize your palpation feedback from the Masseter: describe the tone, texture, and temperature of the muscle tissue.
- Note the presence of trigger points, tissue adhesions, barriers to palpation, or other findings.

- Compare palpation of both sides of the Masseter, noting how the findings from the second palpation vary.
- Compare with palpations of the Masseter on other clients, noting how the findings from palpation on this client differ.

IN THE TREATMENT ROOM

Masseter lies just anterior to the parotid gland, a salivary gland shown in Figure 8–27. A hard, swollen, or tender nodule discovered during palpation of the Masseter may be a swollen or inflamed or parotid gland, not a trigger point. Keep the location of the parotid gland in mind, and palpate carefully if your client has pain in this region. Not every tender point is a trigger point!

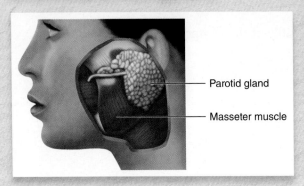

— Parotid gland

— Masseter muscle

FIGURE 8-27 Avoid the parotid gland when palpating the Masseter.

Medial and Lateral Pterygoids

The Pterygoids [TAYR-uh-goyds] can only be palpated intraorally, or from inside the mouth, where Medial pterygoid is the more palpable of the two. As with the other muscles of mastication, the Pterygoids, seen in Figure 8–23, may also be involved in TMJD. Lateral displacement of the mandible will result in stretching of one side of the Pterygoids and shortening of the opposite side. The Medial pterygoid muscle is also called the Internal pterygoid and the Lateral pterygoid is sometimes called the External pterygoid, to indicate their relative positions on the mandible.

HERE'S A TIP

Before you palpate the Pterygoids on a client, practice palpating them on yourself and on willing volunteers until you achieve confidence in the technique.

Attachments:
Medial pterygoid:
- Origin: medial surface of the Pterygoid plate of the sphenoid bone.
- Insertion: medial or internal surface of the mandible.
Lateral pterygoid:
- Origin: lateral surface of the Pterygoid plate of the sphenoid bone.

- Insertion: condyle of the mandible and the Temporomandibular joint capsule.

Actions:

Medial pterygoid:

- Elevates and laterally deviates the mandible at the temporomandibular joint.

Lateral pterygoid:

- Protracts the mandible at the temporomandibular joint.

Placement:

- Deep to Masseter.

Palpation of the Medial and Lateral Pterygoids:

The vertical fibers of Medial pterygoid, seen in Figure 8–28, are palpably distinct from the superior, horizontal fibers of Lateral pterygoid. Change the direction of your palpating fingertips to address the fiber direction of each Pterygoid muscle.

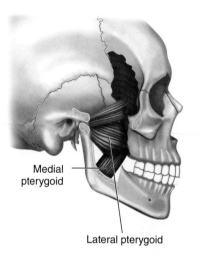

Medial pterygoid

Lateral pterygoid

FIGURE 8-28 Medial and Lateral pterygoids.

© Milady, a part of Cengage Learning.

IN THE TREATMENT ROOM

For intraoral palpation, use the following precautions:

- Wash your hands thoroughly and wear a finger cot or a sterile, disposable exam glove.*
- Describe the palpation procedures for the Pterygoids to your client. Explain why you plan to palpate and potentially treat the Pterygoids.
- Any current dental problem, canker sore, or inflammation in the client's mouth contraindicates intraoral palpation. Ask your client about any contraindicating oral conditions and proceed only with your client's verbal consent and participation.
- The region of the Pterygoids may be tender: adjust your palpation pressure and encourage your client to breathe throughout the palpation.

*Most pharmacies stock single-use, vinyl gloves in various sizes. Avoid the use of latex gloves, to prevent potential problems for anyone who is latex-sensitive.

POSITION:

- Supine client: undrape your client's neck.
- Stand or sit at the head of the table. Use your mother hand to stabilize your client's neck.

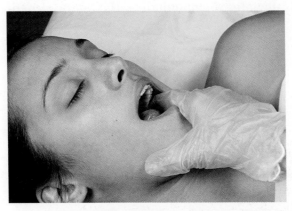

FIGURE 8–29 Discuss intraoral palpation with your client before proceeding to palpate the Pterygoid muscles.

LOCATE AND PALPATE:

- With your client's jaw closed and her mouth relaxed, use your first finger to palpate directly between the cheek and the teeth, as in Figure 8–29, to the back molar on the mandible.
- At the farthest palpable point on the mandible, feel the vertical fibers of the Medial pterygoid. Gently palpate these fibers in the resting state.
- Staying between the cheek and the teeth, move your palpating finger to the farthest palpable point on the maxilla, where the diagonal fibers of Lateral pterygoid are somewhat palpable in their resting state.

DIRECT AN ACTION AND PALPATE:

- To palpate Medial pterygoid in movement, ask your client to open and close her jaw and to move it from side to side: palpate the fibers of Medial pterygoid during elevation and lateral deviation of the mandible the temporomandibular joints.
- To palpate Lateral pterygoid in movement, ask your client to move her jaw forward and backward. You may be able to palpate the fibers of Lateral pterygoid during protraction and retraction of the mandible at the temporomandibular joints.
- Do not add resistance to actions of the mandible.

EVALUATE:

- Characterize your palpation feedback from the Pterygoids: describe the tone, texture, and temperature of the muscle tissue.
- Note the presence of trigger points, tissue adhesions, barriers to palpation, or other findings.
- Compare palpation of both sides of the Pterygoids, noting how the findings from the second palpation vary.
- Compare with palpations of the Pterygoids on other clients, noting how the findings from palpation on this client differ.

> **Lab Activity 8–4** on page 334 is designed to develop your palpation skills on the muscles of mastication.

SUMMARY

As discussed throughout this text, complex movement originates in the core of the body—the axial skeleton—and is carried out in the extremities—the appendicular skeleton. Now that you have successfully palpated the superficial muscles of the axial skeleton, Chapter 9, Palpating Superficial Muscles of the Extremities, will prepare you to palpate muscles in both extremities.

LAB ACTIVITIES

LAB ACTIVITY 8–1: PALPATING SUPERFICIAL MUSCLES THAT ACT ON THE SCAPULA

1. Working with a partner, create a plan for palpating the muscles that act on the scapula:
   - What position will you place your partner in to palpate these muscles?
   - What bony landmarks will you locate?
   - What actions will you direct him to perform?
   - For which palpations is resistance appropriate?
2. Perform palpations of each of the muscles that act on the scapula, using the Four-Step Protocol.
3. What are the antagonist muscles in the actions of your target muscles? Discuss with your partners how palpations of these muscles might be incorporated into your assessment.
4. Evaluate: characterize your palpation findings, as described in the palpation instructions for each muscle:
   - How did touch sensitivity enhance the palpation experience?
   - What specific steps did you take during the palpations to increase or focus your touch sensitivity?
   - What differences in touch sensitivity did you note in relation to the palpation pressure used?
5. Switch partners and repeat. Discuss and compare your experiences.

LAB ACTIVITY 8–2: PALPATING SUPERFICIAL MUSCLES THAT ACT ON THE NECK

1. Working with a partner, create a plan for palpating the muscles that act on the neck:
   - What position will you place your partner in to palpate these muscles?
   - What bony landmarks will you locate?
   - What actions will you direct him to perform?
   - For which palpations is resistance appropriate?
2. Perform palpations of each of the muscles of the neck, using the Four-Step Protocol.
3. What are the antagonist muscles in the actions of your target muscles? Discuss with your partners how palpations of these muscles might be incorporated into your assessment.
4. Evaluate: characterize your palpation findings, as described in the palpation instructions:
   - How did touch sensitivity enhance the palpation experience?
   - What specific steps did you take during the palpations to increase or focus your touch sensitivity?
   - What differences in touch sensitivity did you note in relation to the palpation pressure used?
5. Switch partners and repeat. Discuss and compare your experiences.

LAB ACTIVITY 8–3: PALPATING THE EXTERNAL INTERCOSTALS AND THE SUPERFICIAL ABDOMINAL MUSCLES

1. Working with a partner, create a plan for palpating the External intercostals and the muscles of abdomen:
   - What position will you place your partner in to palpate these muscles?
   - What bony landmarks will you locate?
   - What actions will you direct him to perform?
   - For which palpations is resistance appropriate?
2. Perform palpations of the External intercostals on both sides of the body and Rectus abdominis and the External obliques, using the Four-Step Protocol.
3. What are the antagonist muscles in the actions of your target muscles? Discuss with your partners how palpations of these muscles might be incorporated into your assessment.
4. Evaluate: characterize your palpation findings, as described in the palpation instructions:
   - How did touch sensitivity enhance the palpation experience?
   - What specific steps did you take during the palpations to increase or focus your touch sensitivity?
   - What differences in touch sensitivity did you note in relation to the palpation pressure used?
5. Switch partners and repeat. Discuss and compare your experiences.

LAB ACTIVITY 8–4: PALPATING THE MUSCLES OF MASTICATION

1. Working with a partner, create a plan for palpating the muscles of mastication:
   - What position will you place your partner in to palpate these muscles?
   - What bony landmarks will you locate?
   - What actions will you direct him to perform?
   - For which palpations is resistance appropriate?
2. Perform palpations of each of the muscles of mastication, using the Four-Step Protocol. Follow the precautions described regarding intraoral palpation of the Pterygoids.
3. What are the antagonist muscles in the actions of your target muscles? Discuss with your partners how palpations of these muscles might be incorporated into your assessment.
4. Evaluate: characterize your palpation findings, as described in the palpation instruction.
   - How did touch sensitivity enhance the palpation experience?
   - What specific steps did you take during the palpations to increase or focus your touch sensitivity?
   - What differences in touch sensitivity did you note in relation to the palpation pressure used?
5. Switch partners and repeat. Discuss and compare your experiences.

CASE PROFILES

Case Profile 1

David, 60, is experiencing pain in his neck, mostly on the right side, that runs down from his jaw and up into his head. A lawyer for a telecom company, David has lots of stress in his job and admits he takes the stress home and sometimes wakes up at night in pain because he's clenching his teeth so hard. What muscles will you target for palpation? What other assessments will you perform? Describe any cautions, positioning, or draping considerations for the palpations you plan to perform.

Case Profile 2

Eddie, 27, is a house painter. He works long hours holding a paint sprayer, which is connected to a hose, in his right hand, sweeping it back and forth to apply the paint evenly. After four years at this job, Eddie is experiencing shooting pains and sometimes numbness and tingling down his right arm. By the end of the day, his right arm is so weak that he has to support his right elbow with his left hand. The symptoms are sometimes worst in the morning, after he has slept on his right shoulder. What muscles will you target for palpation? What other assessments will you perform? Describe any cautions, positioning, or draping considerations for the palpations you plan to perform.

Case Profile 3

Maria, 49, was involved in a minor car accident two weeks ago, when her car was hit from behind in a parking lot. She felt okay at first, but now is experiencing some dizziness and headaches, plus pain on the right side of her neck. What muscles will you target for palpation? What other assessments will you perform? Describe any cautions, positioning or draping considerations for the palpations you plan to perform.

STUDY QUESTIONS

1. What precautions for client safety should you take before palpating the Medial and Lateral pterygoids?
2. What type of injury to a client may suggest palpation and assessment of SCM and the Scalene muscles?
3. Which specific endangerment sites are cautions to specific palpations in this chapter?
4. What might be a caution to consider when palpating abdominal muscles?
5. For which muscles in this chapter is applying resistance during palpation not recommended?
6. What are draping concerns and procedures for palpating the Abdominals?

7. Describe the cautions to palpating intraorally, such as for the Pterygoid muscles.
8. Which muscles in this chapter are most effectively palpated on both sides of the client's body simultaneously?
9. Describe how to add resistance to palpation of Serratus anterior.
10. How will you drape a female client to palpate the External intercostal muscles?

Pectoralis Major

Pectoralis major [pek-tor-AL-is MAY-jor] is a thick, layered muscle, divided into clavicular and sternal portions. The lateral fibers of Pectoralis major twist, creating the anterior axillary fold of tissue, just as the twist of lateral fibers in Latissimus dorsi creates the posterior axillary fold. Pectoralis major, as shown in Figure 9–1, is quite powerful and is active in pushing, throwing and punching, particularly in movements that require horizontal adduction of the arm.

During palpation, note the proximity of the anterior fibers of Deltoid, visible in Figure 9–1.

Pectoralis

chest.

> ### HERE'S A TIP
>
> Pectoralis major is most palpable in adduction of the arm in the horizontal plane, especially in the last few degrees of adduction.

Clavicular attachments:
- Origin: medial half and head of the clavicle, the sternum, and costal cartilage of ribs #1–7.
- Insertion: lateral ridge of the bicipital groove of the humerus.

Sternal attachments:
- Origin: sternum and costal cartilage of ribs #1–6.
- Insertion: Lateral ridge of the bicipital groove of the humerus, proximal to the clavicular insertion.

Actions:
- Adducts, horizontally adducts, flexes, and medially rotates the humerus.

Placement:
- Superficial.

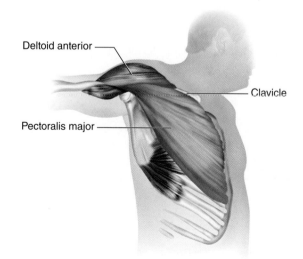

Deltoid anterior

Clavicle

Pectoralis major

FIGURE 9–1 Pectoralis major.

Palpation of Pectoralis Major:

POSITION:

- Supine client. Undrape your client's arm and upper chest. Drape the breast area securely.
- Abduct your client's arm to 90°.
- Stand at the side of the table. Use your mother hand to manipulate your client's arm or to add resistance to movement.
- Breast tissue may impede palpation of the sternal portion of Pectoralis major. Ask your client to use her free hand to secure the drape and immobilize breast tissue during this palpation.

LOCATE AND PALPATE:

- Facing the foot of the table, support your client's passively abducted arm at the elbow. Place your palpating hand just anterior and medial to the anterior axillary fold, taking care to avoid breast tissue, as shown in Figure 9–2.
- On the medial clavicle, locate the origin of the clavicular portion of Pectoralis major. Palpate the muscle fibers to their insertion on the humerus in their resting state between these landmarks. Palpate with and across the grain of muscle fibers.
- The lateral fibers of Pectoralis major are deep to the anterior fibers of Deltoid, which also flexes and medially rotates the humerus. During palpation of lateral Pectoralis major, note that the fibers of anterior Deltoid are more vertical.

DIRECT AN ACTION AND PALPATE:

- Ask your client to reach for her opposite shoulder, horizontal adduction. Palpate Pectoralis major during this action. Contraction of the clavicular portion is strongest and most palpable during the most medial degrees of adduction.
- Ask your client to lift her arm toward her head, flexion. Palpate Pectoralis major during this action. Palpate with and across the grain of muscle fibers.
- With her arm at her side, ask your client to turn her elbow so she can see it. Palpate Pectoralis major in medial rotation of the arm. Palpate with and across the grain of muscle fibers.
- Add resistance to horizontal adduction, flexion, or medial rotation by placing your mother hand on the humerus, distal to the attachment of Pectoralis major, against the direction of movement.

EVALUATE:

- Characterize your palpation feedback from Pectoralis major: describe the tone, texture, and temperature of the muscle tissue.
- Note the presence of trigger points, tissue adhesions, barriers to palpation, or other findings.

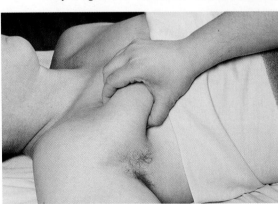

FIGURE 9-2 Palpating Pectoralis major.

- Compare palpation of both sides of Pectoralis major, noting how the findings from the second palpation vary.
- Compare with palpations of Pectoralis major on other clients, noting how the palpation findings on this client differ or are similar.

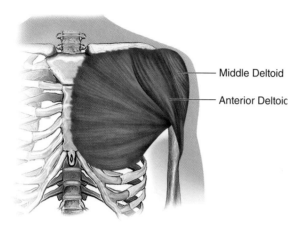

Middle Deltoid

Anterior Deltoic

FIGURE 9–3 Deltoid.

© Milady, a part of Cengage Learning.

Deltoid

Deltoid [DEL-toyd] has three segments—anterior, lateral, and posterior—which allow the full range of motions at the ball-and-socket glenohumeral joint. The large, dense, Deltoid, shown in Figure 9–3, gives the shoulder its shape. Deltoid's origin on the scapula and the clavicle is shared with the insertion of the middle fibers of Trapezius.

Attachments:

Deltoid:

- Origin: lateral third of the clavicle, the acromion, and the lateral spine of the scapula.
- Insertion: deltoid tuberosity of the humerus.

Actions:

- Anterior Deltoid: flexes and medially rotates and horizontally adducts the humerus at the glenohumeral joint.
- Middle Deltoid: abducts the humerus at the glenohumeral joint.
- Posterior Deltoid: extends, laterally rotates, and horizontally abducts the humerus at the glenohumeral joint.

Placement:

- Superficial.

Deltoid

triangular shaped.

HERE'S A TIP

During palpation of anterior and posterior Deltoid, note the degree to which their fibers extend onto the trunk and overlay other muscles, such as Pectoralis major on the anterior and Infraspinatus on the posterior.

Palpation of Deltoid:

POSITION:

- Side-lying client. Undrape your client's arm.
- Stand at the side of the table. Use both hands as palpating hands, or use your mother hand to support your client's elbow during movement or to add resistance to movement.

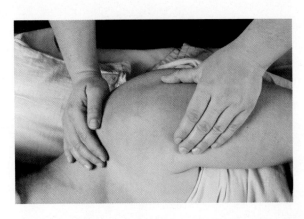

FIGURE 9–4 Palpating Deltoid.

LOCATE AND PALPATE:

- Midway along the length of the lateral humerus, locate the deltoid tuberosity with your thumbs, as in Figure 9–4. *The tuberosity may be quite tender.* Slide your palpating hands proximally on the humerus to locate the acromion of the scapula. Palpate the middle fibers of Deltoid in their resting state between these landmarks. Palpate with and across the grain of muscle fibers.
- Move one palpating hand to the posterior and locate the spine of the scapula. Palpate the posterior fibers in their resting state. Palpate with and across the grain of muscle fibers.
- At the same time, move the other palpating hand to the anterior and locate the lateral clavicle. Palpate the anterior fibers in their resting state. Palpate with and across the grain of muscle fibers.

DIRECT AN ACTION AND PALPATE:

- Ask your client to lift her arm away from her side. Palpate the middle fibers of Deltoid during abduction of the humerus. Palpate with and across the grain of muscle fibers.
- Ask your client to lift her arm toward her face, and then turn her arm so she can see the elbow. Palpate the anterior fibers during flexion and medial rotation of the humerus. Palpate with and across the grain of muscle fibers.
- Ask your client to bring her elbow straight back from her side and then reach behind as if into the backseat of her car. Palpate the posterior fibers during extension and lateral rotation of the humerus. Palpate with and across the grain of muscle fibers.
- Place your mother hand distal to Deltoid on the humerus, against the direction of movement, to add resistance to these actions.

EVALUATE:

- Characterize your palpation feedback from Deltoid: describe the tone, texture, and temperature of the muscle tissue.
- Note the presence of trigger points, tissue adhesions, barriers to palpation, or other findings.
- Compare palpation of Deltoid on both arms, noting how the findings from the second palpation vary.
- Compare with palpations of Deltoid on other clients, noting how the palpation findings on this client differ or are similar.

| Latissimus dorsi |
| wide dorsal surface. |

Latissimus Dorsi

Latissimus dorsi [lah-TIS-ih-mus DOR-see] is a large, flat, posterior trunk muscle. Its superior portion lies deep to lower Trapezius. The "lats" are the only posterior trunk muscle to attach to both the ilium and the arm

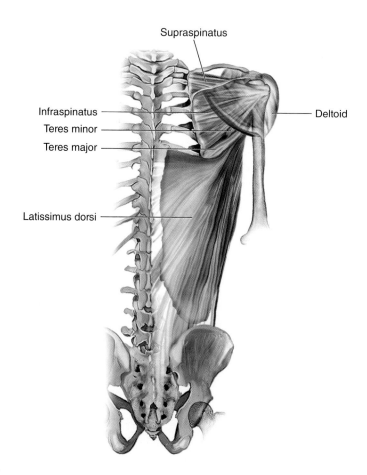

Supraspinatus

Infraspinatus

Teres minor

Teres major

Latissimus dorsi

Deltoid

FIGURE 9–5 Latissimus dorsi, Teres major, Supraspinatus, Infraspinatus, and Teres minor.

© Delmar, Cengage Learning.

and the only one to act on the arm. Latissimus dorsi may seem too large a muscle to act only on the arm, until you consider the action of extension of the arm to push the trunk up from a seated position, which requires considerable muscle power. The lateral fibers of Latissimus dorsi twist as they near their insertion on the humerus, visible in Figure 9–5, creating the posterior axillary fold.

Attachments:

■ Origin: thoracolumbar fascia from T7 to the iliac crest, the lower ribs, and the inferior angle of the scapula.

■ Insertion: medial lip of the bicipital groove of the humerus.

Actions:

■ Extends, adducts, and medially rotates the humerus at the glenohumeral joint.

Placement:

■ Superficial.

> **HERE'S A TIP**
>
> The twisted, lateral fibers of Latissimus dorsi may blend with those of Teres major, making it difficult to palpate their fibers separately.

Palpation of Latissimus Dorsi:

POSITION:

■ Prone client. Undrape your client's back.

■ Passively abduct your client's arm.

■ Stand at the side of the table. Use your mother hand to add resistance to movement or palpate with both hands.

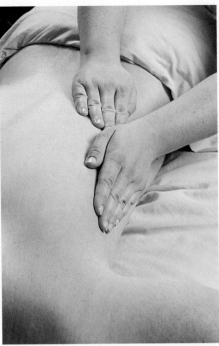

FIGURE 9–6 Palpating Latissimus dorsi.

LOCATE AND PALPATE:

- Locate the PSIS, the posterior superior iliac spine. Palpate laterally and upward on the ribs toward the axilla, palpating along the lateral border of the scapula.
- At the axilla, press the fingertips of your palpating hand toward the medial aspect of the head of the humerus, as shown in Figure 9–6.
- Palpate the expanse of fibers of Latissimus dorsi between these landmarks in their resting state with both hands. Palpate with and across the grain of muscle fibers.

DIRECT AN ACTION AND PALPATE:

- Place your mother hand on the medial aspect of your client's abducted arm. Ask her to bring her arm down to her side as you resist with your mother hand. Palpate Latissimus dorsi during adduction of the humerus. Palpate with and across the grain of muscle fibers.
- With your client's arm by her side, place your mother hand around the olecranon of the ulna. Ask her to push against your hand as you palpate Latissimus dorsi during extension of the humerus. Palpate with and across the grain of muscle fibers.
- With your client's arm by her side, ask her to rotate her arm toward the table as you palpate Latissimus dorsi near its insertion during medial rotation of the humerus. Palpate with and across the grain of muscle fibers.

EVALUATE:

- Characterize your palpation feedback from Latissimus dorsi: describe the tone, texture, and temperature of the muscle tissue.
- Note the presence of trigger points, tissue adhesions, barriers to palpation, or other findings.
- Compare palpation of both sides of Latissimus dorsi, noting how the findings from the second palpation vary.
- Compare with palpations of Latissimus dorsi on other clients, noting how the palpation findings on this client differ or are similar.

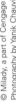

Teres

smooth or cylindrical.

Teres Major

The lateral fibers of Teres major [TAYR-eez MAY-jor] may blend with those of Latissimus dorsi, since they share actions and an attachment on the medial humerus. Teres major is visible in Figure 9–5.

Attachments:

- Origin: lower lateral border and inferior angle of the scapula.
- Insertion: medial ridge of the bicipital groove of the humerus.

Actions:
- Extends, adducts, and medially rotates the humerus at the glenohumeral joint.

Placement:
- Mostly superficial.

DID YOU KNOW?

You can think of Teres major as the cousin who gets ignored at the rotator cuff family reunions: it's a rotator, but is never considered a part of the group, even though Supraspinatus, who never rotates, is! To make matters worse, Teres major is often overshadowed by Latissimus dorsi, the biggest cousin who always does exactly the same things Teres major does—extending, adducting, and medially rotating the humerus—and takes right over, blending its bigger fibers with Teres major without even asking.

HERE'S A TIP

To distinguish the fibers of Teres major from those of Teres minor, place your palpating hand along the muscle tissue attaching to the lateral border of the scapula. Ask your client to medially and then immediately laterally rotate her humerus. The fibers of Teres major, which attach to the inferior portion of the lateral border of the scapula, will contract only during medial rotation. The fibers of Teres minor, which attach to the superior portion of the lateral border of the scapula, will contract only during lateral rotation.

Palpation of Teres Major:

POSITION:
- Prone client. Undrape your client's back.
- Passively abduct your client's arm.
- Stand at the side of the table. Use your mother hand to add resistance to movement or palpate with both hands.

LOCATE AND PALPATE:
- Palpate along the lower lateral border of the scapula. At the axilla, press the fingertips of your palpating hand toward the medial aspect of the head of the humerus, as shown in Figure 9–7. Locate Teres major between the scapula and the medial aspect of the head of the humerus.
- Palpate the fibers of Teres major in their resting state between these landmarks. It will be difficult to

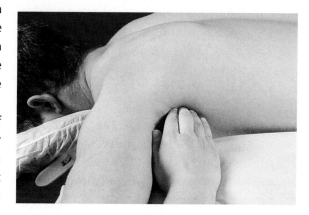

FIGURE 9–7 Palpating Teres major.

distinguish them from Latissimus dorsi. Palpate with and across the grain of muscle fibers.

DIRECT AN ACTION AND PALPATE:

- Place your mother hand on the medial aspect of your client's abducted arm. Ask her to bring her arm down to her side as you resist the movement with your mother hand. Palpate Teres major during adduction of the humerus. Palpate with and across the grain of muscle fibers.
- With your client's arm by her side, place your mother hand around the olecranon of the ulna. Ask her to push against your hand as you palpate Teres major during extension of the humerus. Palpate with and across the grain of muscle fibers.
- With your client's arm by her side, ask her to rotate her arm inwardly as you palpate Teres major near its insertion during medial rotation of the humerus. Palpate with and across the grain of muscle fibers.

EVALUATE:

- Characterize your palpation feedback from Teres major: describe the tone, texture, and temperature of the muscle tissue.
- Note the presence of trigger points, tissue adhesions, barriers to palpation, or other findings.
- Compare palpation of both sides of Teres major, noting how the findings from the second palpation vary.
- Compare with palpations of Teres major on other clients, noting how the palpation findings on this client differ or are similar.

OPTIONS:

All the muscles in the preceding section can be successfully palpated with your client in side-lying position:

- Palpate Pectoralis major from the opposite side of the table, so that you are looking at your client's face.
- Palpate the lower portion of Latissimus dorsi through the drape.

ROTATOR CUFF MUSCLES

The four rotator cuff muscles, Supraspinatus, Infraspinatus, Teres minor, and Subscapularis, originate on the surfaces of the scapula and insert onto the humerus, where their distal tendons form a "cuff" around the head of the humerus. The posterior rotator cuff muscles can be seen in Figure 9–5. Subscapularis attaches to the anterior surface of the scapula. Its palpation is described in Chapter 10, Palpating Deeper Muscles and Muscle Groups. The primary function of the rotator cuff muscles is to stabilize the head of the humerus when the distal humerus is in motion:

- Infraspinatus and Teres minor work together to laterally rotate the arm at the shoulder.
- Subscapularis medially rotates the arm.
- Although called part of the rotator cuff, Supraspinatus does not actually rotate the arm.

The three posterior muscles of the rotator cuff may be palpated as a group, with your client in side-lying position.

Supraspinatus

Supraspinatus [soo-pruh-spy-NAYT-us] works with middle Deltoid in abduction of the arm at the shoulder. It lies deep to middle Trapezius, and with its matching horizontal fiber direction, may be difficult to distinguish in its resting state from Trapezius.

Supraspinatus

above spine.

Attachments:
- Origin: supraspinous fossa of the scapula.
- Insertion: greater tubercle of the humerus.

Actions:
- Abducts the humerus at the glenohumeral joint.

Placement:
- Deep to Trapezius.

Palpation of Supraspinatus:

POSITION:
- Side-lying client. Undrape your client's upper back and arm.
- Stand at the side of the table, facing your client. Use your mother hand to stabilize your client's shoulder and to support her elbow during movement or to add resistance to movement.

LOCATE AND PALPATE:
- With your palpating hand, locate the spine of the scapula. Supraspinatus lies in the fossa superior to the spine. Locate the head of the humerus. Palpate the fibers of Supraspinatus in their resting state between these landmarks, as shown in Figure 9–8. Palpate with and across the grain of muscle fibers.
- Supraspinatus lies deep to the lateral fibers of Trapezius, which does not abduct the humerus and should not interfere with palpation of Supraspinatus.

DIRECT AN ACTION AND PALPATE:
- Ask your client to lift her arm away from her side, abduction at the glenohumeral joint. Palpate the fibers of Supraspinatus during this action. Palpate with and across the grain of muscle fibers.
- Add resistance by placing your mother hand on the humerus, against the direction of movement.

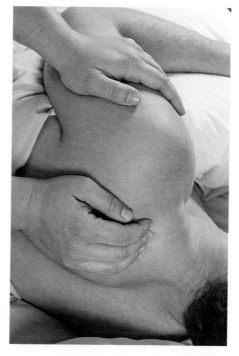

FIGURE 9–8 Palpating Supraspinatus.

EVALUATE:

- Characterize your palpation feedback from Supraspinatus: describe the tone, texture, and temperature of the muscle tissue.
- Note the presence of trigger points, tissue adhesions, barriers to palpation, or other findings.
- Compare palpation of both sides of Supraspinatus, noting how the findings from the second palpation vary.
- Compare with palpations of Supraspinatus on other clients, noting how the palpation findings on this client differ or are similar.

Supraspinatus tendonitis

pain, tenderness to touch, swelling, and local inflammation caused by a strain, tearing, or rupture of the Supraspinatus tendon.

© Milady, a part of Cengage Learning.

IN THE TREATMENT ROOM

When the arm is abducted to a degree that raises it above the shoulder, especially when accompanied by force, such as when throwing a ball, the bursa that lies over its tendon may become entrapped or inflamed, as shown in Figure 9–9, causing symptoms of bursitis, or **Supraspinatus tendonitis**. Symptoms include pain, tenderness to touch, swelling, and local inflammation caused by strain, tearing, or rupture of the Supraspinatus tendon. These injuries to Supraspinatus are common among athletes such as baseball or softball pitchers, especially those who over-train. Weekend warriors in any sport that includes repeated rotations of the shoulder, since circumduction includes abduction, or who neglect to warm up their muscles before activity, are also at risk.

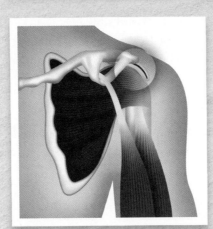

FIGURE 9–9 The inflammation caused by Supraspinatus tendonitis can result in pain and swelling that impinges on nearby nerves.

Infra

inferior or below.

Infraspinatus

Infraspinatus [in-fruh-spy-NAYT-us] fills the infraspinous fossa on the posterior of the scapula, as seen in Figure 9–5, and is largely covered by a thick layer of fascia. Its matching fiber direction and action with Teres minor result in their lateral fibers often blending.

Attachments:
- Origin: infraspinous fossa of the scapula.
- Insertion: greater tubercle of the humerus.

Actions:
- Laterally rotates the humerus at the glenohumeral joint.

Placement:
- Medially, deep to Trapezius and laterally, deep to Deltoid.
- Deep to a layer of thick fascia.

HERE'S A TIP

Wait for the overlying fascia to melt beneath the warmth of your touch before you palpate Infraspinatus' resting fibers.

Palpation of Infraspinatus:

POSITION:

- Side-lying client. Undrape your client's upper back and arm.
- Stand at the side of the table, behind your client. Use your mother hand to stabilize your client's shoulder during movement or to add resistance to movement.

LOCATE AND PALPATE:

- With your palpating hand, locate the spine of the scapula. Infraspinatus lies in the fossa inferior to the spine, as shown in Figure 9–10. Locate the head of the humerus. Palpate the fibers of Infraspinatus in their resting state between these land-marks. Palpate with and across the grain of muscle fibers.

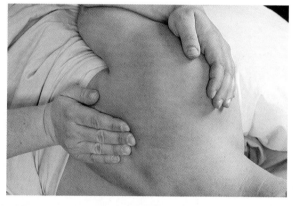

FIGURE 9–10 Palpating Infraspinatus.

- Most of Infraspinatus is covered by a layer of thick fascia, which has its own palpation feedback. The lateral fibers of Trapezius are superficial to Infraspinatus, though Trapezius does not laterally rotate the humerus and so should not interfere with palpation of Infraspinatus.
- The lateral fibers of Infraspinatus are deep to the posterior fibers of Deltoid, which also laterally rotates the humerus. During palpation of lateral Infraspinatus, note that the fibers of Posterior deltoid are more vertical.

DIRECT AN ACTION AND PALPATE:

- Ask your client to reach behind as if into the backseat of a car. Palpate the fibers of Infraspinatus during lateral rotation of the arm. Palpate with and across the grain of muscle fibers.
- Add resistance by placing your mother hand on the posterior humerus, against the direction of movement.

EVALUATE:

- Characterize your palpation feedback from Infraspinatus: describe the tone, textures, and temperature of the muscle tissue.
- Note the presence of trigger points, tissue adhesions, barriers to palpation, or other findings.
- Compare palpation of both sides of Infraspinatus, noting how the findings from the second palpation vary.
- Compare with palpations of Infraspinatus on other clients, noting how the palpation findings on this client differ or are similar.

Teres Minor

As seen in Figure 9–5, Teres minor shares its origin on the lateral border of the scapula with Teres major and a fiber direction and action with Infraspinatus, with which it may blend.

Attachments:
- Origin: upper lateral border of the scapula.
- Insertion: greater tubercle of the humerus.

Actions:
- Laterally rotates the humerus at the glenohumeral joint.

Placement:
- Superficial. Laterally, deep to Deltoid.

Palpation of Teres Minor:

POSITION:
- Side-lying client. Undrape your client's upper back and arm.
- Stand at the side of the table, behind your client. Use your mother hand to stabilize your client's shoulder and to support her elbow during movement or to add resistance to movement.

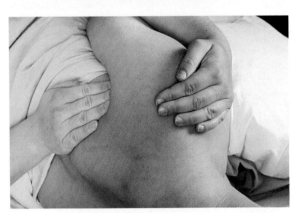

FIGURE 9–11 Palpate Teres minor along with Infraspinatus; their fibers often blend together.

LOCATE AND PALPATE:
- Palpate along the upper lateral border of the scapula. At the axilla, press the fingertips of your palpating hand toward the medial aspect of the head of the humerus, as shown in Figure 9–11. Locate Teres minor between the scapula and the medial aspect of the head of the humerus.
- Palpate the fibers of Teres minor between these landmarks in their resting state. Palpate with and across the grain of muscle fibers.

DIRECT AN ACTION AND PALPATE:
- Ask your client to reach behind as if into the backseat of a car. Palpate the fibers of Teres minor during lateral rotation of the arm. Palpate with and across the grain of muscle.

EVALUATE:
- Characterize your palpation feedback from Teres minor: describe the tone, texture, and temperature of the muscle tissue.
- Note the presence of trigger points, tissue adhesions, barriers to palpation, or other findings.
- Compare palpation of both sides of Teres minor, noting how the findings from the second palpation vary.
- Compare with palpations of Teres minor on other clients, noting how the palpation findings on this client differ or are similar.

IN THE TREATMENT ROOM

Most clients who report shoulder pain on movement should be assessed for problems in the rotator cuff muscles:

- In elder clients, the gradual erosion of bone tissue in the glenohumeral joint, added to the wear and tear of repetitive motions and the progressive loss of tendon elasticity and muscle tissue contributes to inflammation and tears in rotator cuff muscles, as seen in Figure 9–12.
- In clients who spend hours at computers, even the small movements used to type and move a mouse can result in repetitive strain injuries and inflammation in the rotator cuff.

You will note significant variations in the mobility of clients' scapulae when palpating muscles that attach there. Always palpate both sides of the muscles that attach to the scapula, and use scapular mobility as a factor in treatment planning.

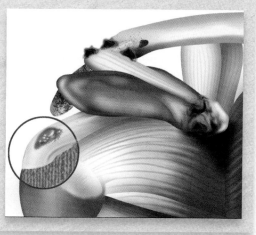

FIGURE 9–12 Wear and tear at the glenohumeral joint can result in inflammation, pain, and tearing of muscle tissue.

Lab Activity 9–1 on page 393 is designed to develop your palpation skills on superficial muscles that act on the arm.

MUSCLES THAT ACT ON THE FOREARM

Palpable muscles that act on the forearm and are superficial or intermediate flex and extend the forearm at the hinge elbow joint. Those described in this chapter include Biceps brachii, Brachialis, Brachioradialis, and Triceps brachii and Anconeus. (Coracobrachialis is described in Chapter 10, Palpating Deeper Muscles and Muscle Groups).

Biceps Brachii

Biceps brachii [By-seps BRAY-kee-ee] has two origins, both on the scapula, and inserts onto the radius. Biceps brachii, therefore, crosses the shoulder and the elbow joint and acts on both. The belly of Biceps brachii, as shown in Figure 9–13, is superficial to the bulkier Brachialis, which also contracts during flexion of the forearm at the humeroulnar joint.

Attachments:
- Short head origin: coracoid process of the scapula.
- Long head origin: supraglenoid tubercle of the glenoid fossa of the scapula.
- Insertion: radial tuberosity.

Actions:
- Flexes the arm at the glenohumeral joint and the forearm at the humeroulnar joint and supinates the forearm at the radioulnar joints.

Placement:
- Superficial.

Biceps

two heads.

Brachius

the arm.

HERE'S A TIP

Near the proximal, tendinous portion of Biceps brachii, the anterior fibers of Deltoid also contract during flexion of the arm at the glenohumeral joint.

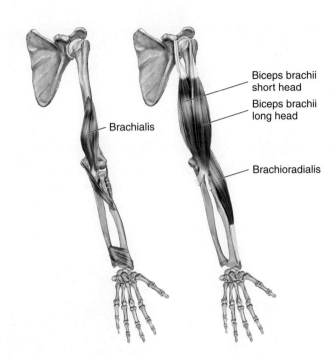

FIGURE 9-13 Biceps brachii, Brachialis, and Brachioradialis.

Palpation of Biceps Brachii:

POSITION:

- Supine client. Undrape your client's arm.
- Stand at the side of the table. Use your mother hand to support the elbow during movement or to add resistance to movement.

LOCATE AND PALPATE:

- Extend your client's arm and supinate her forearm. To locate the radial tuberosity, place your palpating hand on the radius, just distal to the crease of the elbow.
- Locate the long head of Biceps brachii as it travels through the bicipital groove onto the humerus and its short head origin on the coracoid process. Palpate the long, proximal tendinous portions and the fibers of Biceps brachii between these landmarks in their resting state, as shown in Figure 9–14. Palpate with and across the grain of muscle fibers.

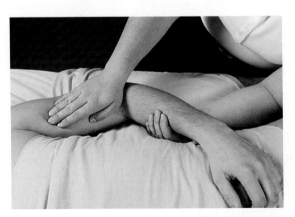

FIGURE 9-14 Palpating Biceps brachii.

DIRECT AN ACTION AND PALPATE:

- Add resistance by placing your mother hand on the proximal forearm, and ask your client to lift her arm straight up from the table, flexion of the arm at the shoulder. Palpate Biceps brachii during this movement. Palpate with and across the grain of muscle fibers.

- Add resistance by placing your mother hand on the distal forearm and ask your client to bend her arm at the elbow, flexion of the forearm at the elbow. Palpate Biceps brachii during this action. Palpate with and across the grain of muscle fibers.
- Ask your client to turn her hand over and then back up again, supination. Palpate Biceps brachii during this action, without resistance. Palpate with and across the grain of muscle fibers.

EVALUATE:

- Characterize your palpation feedback from Biceps brachii: describe the tone, texture, and temperature of the muscle tissue.
- Note the presence of trigger points, tissue adhesions, barriers to palpation, or other findings.
- Compare palpation of both sides of Biceps brachii, noting how the findings from the second palpation vary.
- Compare with palpations of Biceps brachii on other clients, noting how the palpation findings on this client differ or are similar.

Brachialis

Brachialis [bray-kih-AY-lis] is considered a stronger flexor of the forearm than Biceps brachii. Its fibers, as seen in Figure 9–13, are denser, and its origin on the humerus means that its sole action is at the humeroulnar joint. The dense fibers of Brachialis push the slimmer Biceps brachii to the anterior, giving the arm its shape. Brachialis lies deep to Biceps brachii, but is readily palpable because its bulk extends on either side of the belly of Biceps brachii.

Brachialis

of the arm.

DID YOU KNOW?

The configuration of Biceps brachii and Brachialis in the anterior arm is duplicated by Gastrocnemius and Soleus in the posterior leg.

Attachments:
- Origin: distal half of the anterior humerus.
- Insertion: ulnar tuberosity.

Actions:
- Flexes the forearm at the humeroulnar joint.

Placement:
- Deep to Biceps brachii.

Palpation of Brachialis:

POSITION:

- Supine client. Undrape your client's arm.
- Stand at the side of the table. Use your mother hand to support the elbow during movement or to add resistance to movement.

LOCATE AND PALPATE:

- Extend your client's arm and supinate her forearm. To locate the ulnar tuberosity, place your palpating hand on the ulna, just distal to the crease of the elbow.

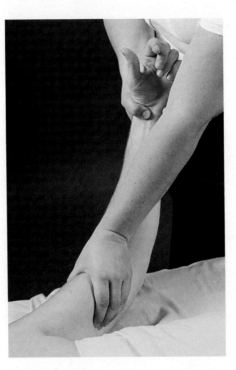

FIGURE 9–15 Palpating Brachialis.

■ Place your palpating hand around the shaft of the humerus, as shown in Figure 9–15, with your thumb and fingertips on either side of Biceps brachii. Palpate the fibers of Brachialis between these landmarks in their resting state. Palpate with and across the grain of muscle fibers.

DIRECT AN ACTION AND PALPATE:

■ Ask your client to bend her arm at the elbow, flexion of the forearm and palpate the fibers of Brachialis during this action. Palpate with and across the grain of muscle fibers.

■ Note that the superficial Biceps brachii prevents complete palpation of the muscle belly of Brachialis. Overcoming this challenge is discussed in the next "In the Treatment Room."

EVALUATE:

■ Characterize your palpation feedback from Brachialis: describe the tone, texture, and temperature of the muscle tissue.

■ Note the presence of trigger points, tissue adhesions, barriers to palpation, or other findings.

■ Compare palpation of both sides of Brachialis, noting how the findings from the second palpation vary.

■ Compare with palpations of Brachialis on other clients, noting how the palpation findings on this client differ or are similar.

IN THE TREATMENT ROOM

When the target muscle lies deep to an adjacent, superficial muscle with which it shares an action, you can inhibit the shared action in the superficial muscle and remove its interference. This differs from the reciprocal inhibition that originates as a reflex in the nervous system and inhibits contraction of an antagonist muscle during contraction of an agonist muscle. For example, Brachialis lies deep to Biceps brachii in the anterior arm. Since both muscles flex for forearm at the humeroulnar joint, directing a client to "bend your arm at the elbow" won't allow you to specifically palpate the fibers of Brachialis, because Biceps brachii is in the way. Here's how inhibiting an action of Biceps brachii assures successful palpation of Brachialis:

■ Remember that Biceps brachii, in addition to flexing the forearm, also supinates the hand. Brachialis' only action is flexion of the forearm at the humeroulnar joint.

- By placing the forearm in pronation, the opposing action to supination, Biceps brachii is weakened and unable to flex the forearm at the humeroulnar joint.
- Brachialis is now the only muscle that will be flexing the forearm and is easily palpated during flexion of the forearm at the humeroulnar joint.

Adding resistance is helpful when inhibiting muscle action during palpation. The resistance must be gentle, however, to prevent the weakened adjacent muscle from trying to rally itself to assist the target muscle. Inhibiting the flexion of Biceps brachii during palpation of Brachialis is shown in Figure 9–16.

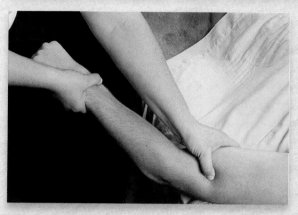

FIGURE 9-16 Inhibiting Biceps brachii to palpate Brachialis.

© Milady, a part of Cengage Learning. Photography by Yanik Chauvin.

Brachioradialis

Brachioradialis [bray-kih-oh-ray-dih-AL-us] is sometimes called the "handshake muscle," because its action of flexion of the forearm at the humeroulnar joint is strongest when the forearm is midway between pronation and supination—the position of the forearm in a handshake. The most prominent muscle in the lateral forearm, visible in Figure 9–13, Brachioradialis is also thought by some sources to participate in pronation and supination of the forearm at the radioulnar joints. Brachioradialis is superficial and readily palpable when the forearm is positioned midway between pronation and supination.

Attachments:
- Origin: lateral supracondylar ridge of the humerus.
- Insertion: styloid process of the radius.

Actions:
- Flexes of the forearm at the humeroulnar joint.

Placement:
- Superficial.

Brachioradialis

the arm; the radius.

DID YOU KNOW?

Brachioradialis is also occasionally described as the "hitchhiking muscle," though this incorrectly promotes the idea that Brachioradialis acts on the thumb—impossible, since it does not cross the wrist onto the hand.

Palpation of Brachioradialis:

POSITION:
- Supine client. Undrape your client's arm.
- Stand at the side of the table. Use your mother hand to support the wrist during movement or to add resistance to movement.

LOCATE AND PALPATE:
- Place your client's arm in neutral, midway between pronation and supination. On the distal radius, locate the styloid process. On the distal lateral humerus, locate

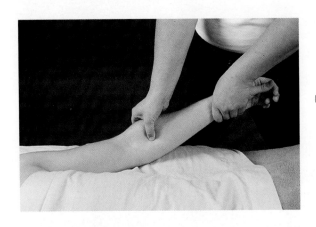

FIGURE 9–17 Palpating Brachioradialis.

the lateral supracondylar ridge. The muscle belly of Brachioradialis lies over the proximal half of the radius.

■ Palpate the fibers of Brachioradialis between these landmarks in their resting state. Palpate with and across the grain of muscle fibers, as shown in Figure 9–17.

DIRECT AN ACTION AND PALPATE:

■ Place your mother hand on the client's hand to provide resistance. Ask your client to bend her arm at the elbow, and palpate Brachioradialis during flexion of the forearm. Palpate with and across the grain of muscle fibers.

EVALUATE:

■ Characterize your palpation feedback from Brachioradialis: describe the tone, texture, and temperature of the muscle tissue.

■ Note the presence of trigger points, tissue adhesions, barriers to palpation, or other findings.

■ Compare palpation of both sides of Brachioradialis, noting how the findings from the second palpation vary.

■ Compare with palpations of Brachioradialis on other clients, noting how the palpation findings on this client differ or are similar.

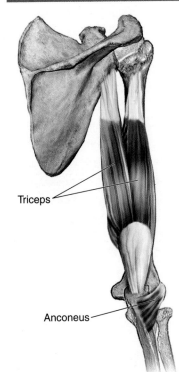

Triceps

Anconeus

FIGURE 9–18 Triceps brachii and Anconeus.

Triceps Brachii

Like Biceps brachii, Triceps brachii [TRY-seps BRAY-kee-ee] attaches to both the scapula and a forearm bone—in this case, the ulna—with more than one head. All three heads of Triceps brachii extend the forearm at the elbow. The long head, with its origin on the scapula, also adducts and extends the arm at the shoulder. Its three heads and crossing of two joints, visible in Figure 9–18, mimic the shape and function of two heads of Biceps brachii and the one head of Brachialis in the anterior arm. Triceps brachii is the sole muscle in the posterior arm and is readily palpable. The long head is the superficial, palpable portion of Triceps brachii.

Attachments:

■ Long head origin: infraglenoid tubercle of the scapula.
■ Lateral head origin: proximal half of the posterior humerus.
■ Medial head origin: distal two-thirds of the posterior humerus.
■ Insertion: olecranon process of the ulna.

Actions:

■ Extends the forearm at the humeroulnar joint.

Placement:

■ Superficial.

Palpation of Triceps Brachii:

POSITION:

- Prone client. Undrape your client's arm.
- Abduct your client's arm off the side of the massage table.
- Stand at the side of the table. Use your mother hand to support the elbow during movement or to add resistance to movement.

LOCATE AND PALPATE:

- With your client's arm passively abducted, as in Figure 9–19, locate the olecranon process of the ulna and the region of the glenoid fossa of the scapula.

The posterior fibers of Deltoid will be superficial here. Palpate the fibers of the long head of Triceps brachii between these landmarks in their resting state. Palpate with and across the grain of muscle fibers.

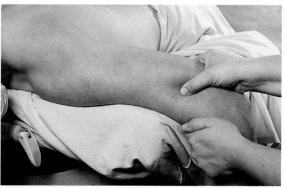

FIGURE 9–19 Palpating Triceps brachii.

© Milady, a part of Cengage Learning. Photography by Yanik Chauvin.

DIRECT AN ACTION AND PALPATE:

- Place your mother hand on your client's proximal ulna. Ask her to push her forearm against your hand and palpate Triceps bachii during resisted extension of the forearm. Palpate with and across the grain of muscle fibers.

EVALUATE:

- Characterize your palpation feedback from Triceps brachii: describe the tone, texture, and temperature of the muscle tissue.
- Note the presence of trigger points, tissue adhesions, barriers to palpation, or other findings.
- Compare palpation of both sides of Triceps brachii, noting how the findings from the second palpation vary.
- Compare with palpations of Triceps brachii on other clients, noting how the palpation findings on this client differ or are similar.

Anconeus

The fibers of the triangular-shaped Anconeus [ayn-KOH-nee-us], visible in Figure 9–18, may blend with Triceps brachii, making it easy to overlook and difficult to palpate separately. Try palpating Anconeus along with Triceps brachii, described above. Both muscles insert on the olecranon process of the ulna. Palpate from this insertion of Anconeus laterally onto the lateral epicondyle of the humerus.

Anconeus

corner of a wall, or a supporting bracket.

DID YOU KNOW?

Anconeus may play a role in lateral epicondylitis, "tennis elbow," described in Chapter 10, Palpating Deeper Muscles and Muscle Groups.

Attachments:

- Origin: lateral epicondyle of the humerus.
- Insertion: olecranon process of the ulna.

Actions:

- Extends the forearm at the humeroulnar joint.

Placement:

- Superficial.

Palpation of Anconeus:

POSITION:

- Prone client. Undrape your client's arm.
- Abduct your client's arm off the side of the massage table.

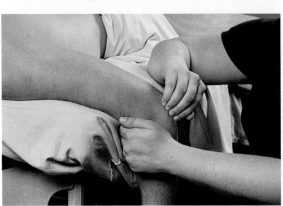

- Stand at the side of the table. Use your mother hand to support the elbow during movement or to add resistance to movement.

LOCATE AND PALPATE:

- With your client's arm passively abducted, as in Figure 9–20, locate the olecranon process of the ulna and lateral epicondyle of the humerus. Palpate the fibers of the fibers of Anconeus between these landmarks in their resting state. Palpate with and across the grain of muscle fibers.

FIGURE 9-20 Palpating Anconeus.

DIRECT AN ACTION AND PALPATE:

- Place your mother hand on your client's proximal ulna. Ask her to push her forearm against your hand and palpate Anconeus during extension of the forearm. Palpate with and across the grain of muscle fibers.

EVALUATE:

- Characterize your palpation feedback from Anconeus: describe the tone, texture, and temperature of the muscle tissue.
- Note the presence of trigger points, tissue adhesions, barriers to palpation, or other findings.
- Compare palpation of both sides of Anconeus, noting how the findings from the second palpation vary.
- Compare with palpations of Anconeus on other clients, noting how the palpation findings on this client differ or are similar.

MUSCLES THAT ACT ON THE HAND

Muscles that act on the hand at the radiocarpal joint include the Forearm flexors and extensors that originate on the humerus and cross the wrist onto the hand. Palpation of the superficial groups of Forearm flexor and extensor muscles, shown in Figures 9–21 and 9–23, is described next. Palpation of individual Forearm flexor and extensor muscles is described in detail in Chapter 10, Palpating Deeper Muscles and Muscle Groups.

Muscles that attach to and act on the hand alone are called the intrinsic muscles of the hand. Their attachments reside within the bones of the hand. Palpation of the intrinsic muscles of the hand is described in detail in Chapter 10, Palpating Deeper Muscles and Muscle Groups.

Forearm Flexor Group

Group attachments:
- Origin: medial epicondyle of the humerus.
- Insertion: carpals, metacarpals, or phalanges.

Actions:
- Flex the wrist, hand, or fingers at the radiocarpal, carpometacarpal, and metacarpophalangeal joints.

Placement:
- Superficial, intermediate, and deep on the anterior forearm.

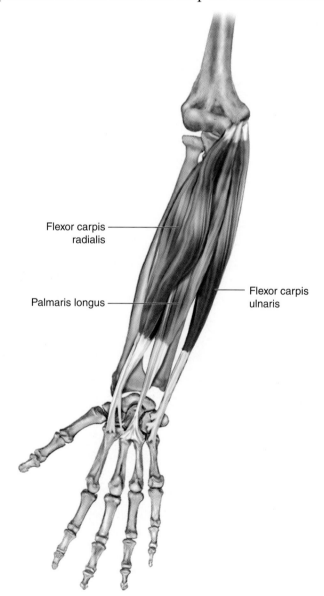

Flexor carpis radialis

Palmaris longus

Flexor carpis ulnaris

FIGURE 9-21 Superficial Forearm flexor muscles.

© Delmar, Cengage Learning.

Palpation of Forearm Flexors:

POSITION:

- Supine client. Undrape your client's arm.
- Place your client's arm in slight lateral rotation, with her forearm supinated at the radioulnar joints.
- Stand at the side of the table. Use your mother hand to support the wrist during movement or to add resistance to movement.

LOCATE AND PALPATE:

- Place your palpating hand around your client's wrist. Palpate the tendons of Forearm flexors that pass through the carpal tunnel and onto the hand, on the radial and ulnar aspects. Locate the prominent medial epicondyle on the distal humerus.

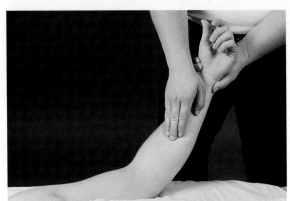

- Palpate the fibers of the Forearm flexor muscle group between these landmarks in their resting state, as shown in Figure 9–22. Palpate with and across the grain of muscle fibers.

FIGURE 9-22 Palpating Forearm flexor muscles as a group.

DIRECT AN ACTION AND PALPATE:

- Ask your client to curl her hand up as you hold it to resist the action. Palpate the Forearm flexor group during flexion of the wrist. Palpate with and across the grain of muscle fibers.

EVALUATE:

- Characterize your palpation feedback from the Forearm flexor muscle group: describe the tone, texture, and temperature of the muscle tissue.
- Note the presence of trigger points, tissue adhesions, barriers to palpation, or other findings.
- Compare palpation of both sides of the Forearm flexor muscle group, noting how the findings from the second palpation vary.
- Compare with palpations of the Forearm flexor muscle group on other clients, noting how the palpation findings on this client differ or are similar.

Forearm Extensor Group

Group attachments:

- Origin: lateral epicondyle of the humerus.
- Insertion: carpals, metacarpals, or phalanges.

Actions:

- Extend the wrist, hand, or fingers at the radiocarpal, carpometacarpal, and metacarpophalangeal joints.

Placement:

- Superficial, intermediate, and deep on the posterior forearm.

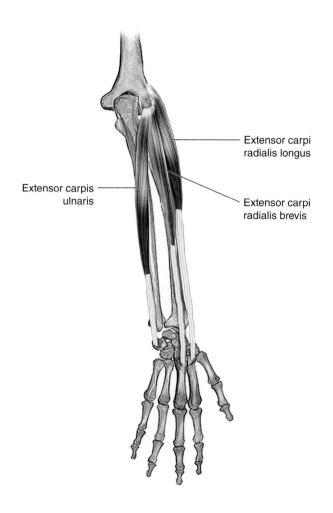

Extensor carpi
radialis longus

Extensor carpis
ulnaris

Extensor carpi
radialis brevis

FIGURE 9–23 Superficial
Forearm extensor muscles.

Palpation of Forearm Extensors:

POSITION:

- Supine client. Undrape your client's arm.
- Place your client's arm in slight medial rotation, with her forearm pronated.
- Stand at the side of the table. Use your mother hand to support the wrist during movement or to add resistance to movement.

LOCATE AND PALPATE:

- Place your palpating hand around your client's wrist. Palpate the tendons of Forearm extensors that pass over the carpals and onto the hand, on the radial and ulnar aspects. Locate the pointed lateral epicondyle on the distal humerus.
- Palpate the fibers of the Forearm extensor muscle group between these landmarks in their resting state, as shown in Figure 9–24. Palpate with and across the grain of muscle fibers.

DIRECT AN ACTION AND PALPATE:

- Ask your client to curl her hand down as you hold it to resist the action. Palpate the Forearm extensor group during extension of the wrist.

EVALUATE:

- Characterize your palpation feedback from the Forearm extensor muscle group: describe the tone, texture, and temperature of the muscle tissue.

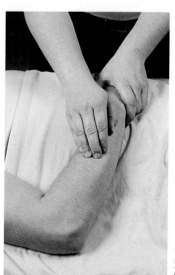

FIGURE 9–24 Palpating Forearm
extensor muscles as a group.

■ Note the presence of trigger points, tissue adhesions, barriers to palpation, or other findings.

■ Compare palpation of both sides of the Forearm extensor muscle group, noting how the findings from the second palpation vary.

■ Compare with palpations of the Forearm extensor muscle group on other clients, noting how the palpation findings on this client differ or are similar.

OPTIONS:

■ If your client has restricted shoulder or elbow mobility, you may choose to palpate the Forearm extensors standing on the opposite side of the table, with her forearm placed across her abdomen. Palpate the Forearm extensors with your client's forearm flexed at 90° to the table.

Lab Activity 9–2 on page 393 is designed to develop your palpation skills on superficial muscles that act on the forearm and hand.

IN THE TREATMENT ROOM

Clients who work with their hands, performing repetitive motions over many hours, or even retirees who spend long hours doing crafts or needlework, may report wrist and hand pain that indicates assessment of the Forearm flexors and extensors. Hand dominance is a factor in Forearm flexor injuries, in a seeming contradiction: although your right-handed client is likely to sustain an overuse injury involving the Forearm flexors on her right side, the Forearm flexors on the left side will be weaker and, potentially, more injury-prone—another reason for palpation of contralateral counterparts.

MUSCLES THAT ACT ON THE THIGH

The ball-and-socket acetabulofemoral joint allows all angular actions: flexion and extension, medial and lateral rotation, frontal and horizontal plane abduction and adduction, and circumduction. The muscles creating these actions attach to the pelvis and the femur, which bear the body's weight when standing and in motion. These muscles, therefore, are large, dense, and targets for injury assessment when a client reports persistent pain or stiffness, especially following exercise. Superficial and intermediate muscles that act on the thigh include Gluteus maximus and Gluteus medius, Tensor fasciae latae (TFL), the Adductor group, and Pectineus, Gracilis, and Sartorius.

Gluteus Maximus

Gluteus

the buttock.

The muscles of the gluteal group—Gluteus maximus [GLOOT-ee-us MAK-sih-mus], medius, and minimus—are large, dense muscles that compose the buttocks and act on the thigh. Gluteus maximus and medius oppose each other in rotation of the thigh at the hip and are shown in Figure 9–25. Gluteus maximus is the largest, most superficial, and most palpable of the Gluteal group. Gluteus maximus is most palpable in extension or hyperextension of the thigh. Gluteus minimus is entirely deep to Gluteus medius and not palpable.

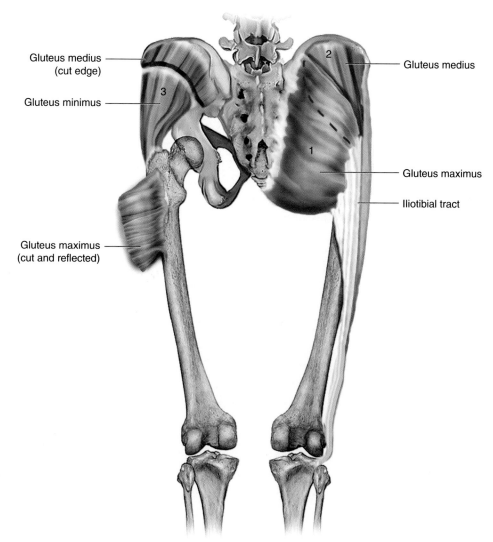

Gluteus medius
(cut edge)

Gluteus minimus

Gluteus maximus
(cut and reflected)

Gluteus medius

Gluteus maximus

Iliotibial tract

© Delmar, Cengage Learning.

FIGURE 9-25 Gluteus maximus, medius, and minimus.

DID YOU KNOW?

The combined actions of Gluteus maximus and Gluteus medius on the thigh at the hip mirror the actions of Deltoid on the arm at the shoulder. Some sources add abduction and adduction to the actions of Gluteus maximus.

Attachments:

- Origin: ilium and iliac crest, posterior inferior sacrum and the lateral coccyx.
- Insertion: iliotibial band (ITB) and the gluteal tuberosity of the femur.

Actions:

- Extends and laterally rotates the thigh at the acetabulofemoral joint.

Placement:

- Superficial.

Palpation of Gluteus Maximus:

POSITION:

- Prone client. Undrape the thigh and hip.
- Stand at the side of the table. Use your mother hand for resistance against movement.

LOCATE AND PALPATE:

- Locate the inferior lateral border of the sacrum and the greater trochanter of the femur. Palpate the fascial tissue at each attachment of Gluteus maximus. Note the direction of the fibers of Gluteus maximus for comparison with the fibers of Gluteus medius.

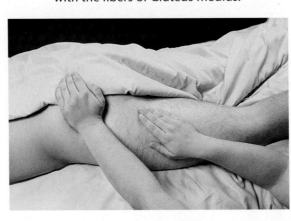

- Palpate the dense fibers of Gluteus maximus between these landmarks in their resting state, as shown in Figure 9–26. Note that the fibers of Gluteus maximus attach only partway along the medial length of the iliac crest. Palpate with and across the grain of muscle fibers.

FIGURE 9-26 Palpating Gluteus maximus.

DIRECT AN ACTION AND PALPATE:

- Ask your client to raise her leg off the surface of the table. Palpate Gluteus maximus during extension of the thigh. Palpate with and across the grain of muscle fibers.

EVALUATE:

- Characterize your palpation feedback from Gluteus maximus: describe the tone, texture, and temperature of the muscle tissue.
- Note the presence of trigger points, tissue adhesions, barriers to palpation, or other findings.
- Compare palpation of both sides of Gluteus maximus, noting how the findings from the second palpation vary.
- Compare with palpations of Gluteus maximus on other clients, noting how the palpation findings on this client differ or are similar.

OPTIONS:

- With your client in side-lying position, palpate through the drape: locate the attachments, as described above. Ask your client to move her thigh backward and palpate during extension of the thigh.
- You can palpate Gluteus maximus, Gluteus medius, and Tensor fasciae latae together in side-lying position.

Gluteus Medius

Gluteus medius acts with Tensor fasciae latae in abducting the thigh at the acetabulofemoral joint, and in opposition to Gluteus maximus in rotation of the thigh at the acetabulofemoral joint. Gluteus medius wraps around the iliac crest, nearly to the anterior superior iliac spine (ASIS), the origin of TFL, tensor fasciae latae. This anterior aspect makes Gluteus medius, visible in Figure 9–25, capable of medial rotation of the thigh at the acetabulofemoral joint. The lower fibers of Gluteus medius are deep to Gluteus maximus and not readily palpable. The upper fibers, however, are superficial and palpable.

Attachments:

- Origin: iliac crest and the external or posterior ilium.
- Insertion: greater trochanter of the femur.

Actions:

- Abducts the thigh. The anterior fibers also medially rotate the thigh at the acetabulofemoral joint.

Placement:

- Posterior portion is deep to Gluteus maximus. The anterior portion is deep to TFL.

> **DID YOU KNOW?**
>
> Gluteus medius is a common intramuscular injection site.

Palpation of Gluteus Medius:

POSITION:

- Side-lying client. Palpate through the drape.
- Stand at the side of the table, behind your client. Use your mother hand to stabilize the hip or to add resistance to movement.

LOCATE AND PALPATE:

- Palpate laterally on the iliac crest from posterior superior iliac spine (PSIS) to ASIS, as in Figure 9–27. The fibers of Gluteus medius are palpable from this portion of the iliac crest to the superior border of Gluteus maximus. The more vertical fibers of Gluteus medius are inactive during extension of the thigh at the acetabulofemoral joint.
- Palpate the fibers of Gluteus medius between these landmarks in their resting state. Palpate with and across the grain of muscle fibers.

DIRECT AN ACTION AND PALPATE:

- Ask your client to lift her thigh up from the table. Palpate the fibers of Gluteus medius during abduction of the thigh. Palpate with and across the grain of muscle fibers.
- Ask your client to turn her knee toward the center of the table and palpate the fibers of Gluteus medius during the medial rotation of the thigh. Palpate with and across the grain of muscle fibers.

EVALUATE:

- Characterize your palpation feedback from Gluteus medius: describe the tone, texture, and temperature of the muscle tissue.
- Note the presence of trigger points, tissue adhesions, barriers to palpation, or other findings.
- Compare palpation of both sides of Gluteus medius, noting how the findings from the second palpation vary.
- Compare with palpations of Gluteus medius on other clients, noting how the palpation findings on this client differ or are similar.

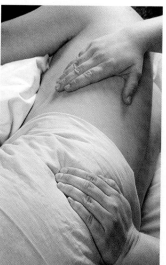

FIGURE 9-27 Palpating Gluteus medius.

© Milady, a part of Cengage Learning. Photography by Yanik Chauvin.

Tensor

stretch.

fasciae

band.

latae

on the side.

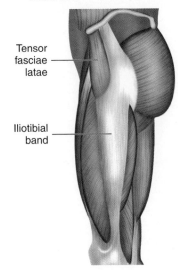

Tensor
fasciae
latae

Iliotibial
band

FIGURE 9-28 Tensor fasciae latae (TFL) and the iliotibial band (ITB).

© Milady, a part of Cengage Learning.

Tensor Fasciae Latae (TFL)

Tensor fasciae latae (TFL) [TEN-sur FASH-ee-ee LAY-tee] can be remembered as the alphabet muscle by using its initials along with those of its attachments: TFL arises from the ASIS and inserts into ITB, the iliotibial band. Seen in Figure 9–28, TFL works with the anterior fibers of Gluteus medius in abduction and medial rotation of the thigh at the acetabulofemoral joint. Tensor fasciae latae is best palpated and treated with the client in side-lying position and is easily palpated along with Gluteus maximus and Gluteus medius.

> **HERE'S A TIP**
>
> A tight TFL can exert pressure along the ITB, making it a common source for lateral knee pain.

Attachments:
- Origin: anterior superior iliac spine and anterior iliac crest.
- Insertion: iliotibial band.

Actions:
- Abducts and medially rotates the thigh at the acetabulofemoral joint.

Placement:
- Superficial.

Palpation of Tensor Fasciae Latae:

POSITION:
- Side-lying client. Palpate through the drape.
- Stand at the side of the table, behind your client. Use your mother hand to stabilize the client's hip or to add resistance to movement.

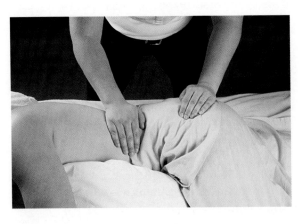

FIGURE 9-29 Palpating Tensor fasciae latae (TFL).

© Milady, a part of Cengage Learning.
Photography by Yanik Chauvin.

LOCATE AND PALPATE:
- Locate the greater trochanter, where the ITB is most easily palpable and where it inserts into TFL. Locate the ASIS. Palpate the fibers of TFL in between these attachments, in its resting state, as shown in Figure 9–29. Palpate with and across the grain of muscle fibers.
- Locate the nearby attachment sites of Gluteus maximus and Gluteus medius.

DIRECT AN ACTION AND PALPATE:
- Ask your client to lift her thigh up from the table and palpate the fibers of TFL and Gluteus medius during the abduction of the thigh. Palpate with and across the grain of muscle fibers.

- Ask your client to turn her knee toward the table and palpate the fibers of TFL and Gluteus medius during the medial rotation of the thigh. Palpate with and across the grain of muscle fibers.
- Ask your client to move her thigh backward and palpate the fibers of Gluteus maximus during the extension of the thigh. Palpate with and across the grain of muscle fibers.
- While palpating Gluteus maximus during extension of the thigh, locate its superior lateral border, where the action of extension is no longer evident. The muscle tissue between this border and the iliac crest is Gluteus medius.

EVALUATE:

- Characterize your palpation feedback from Tensor fasciae latae: describe the tone, texture, and temperature of the muscle tissue.
- Note the presence of trigger points, tissue adhesions, barriers to palpation, or other findings.
- Compare palpation of both sides of Tensor fasciae latae, noting how the findings from the second palpation vary.
- Compare with palpations of Tensor fasciae latae on other clients, noting how the palpation findings on this client differ or are similar.

IN THE TREATMENT ROOM

Muscles that abduct and rotate the femur, such as the Gluteals and TFL, are assessed in clients who report lateral thigh and knee pain: a tight or weak TFL or Gluteus medius can result in strain along the ITB, called **iliotibial syndrome**, following extended exercise, such as running or hiking, shown in Figure 9–28. Clients with iliotibial syndrome may have multiple trigger points in TFL on the affected side, while the ITB may feel as tight as a guitar string.

Iliotibial syndrome

strain along the Iliotibial band in the lateral leg that may refer pain into the knee.

The Adductor Group: Adductor Longus, Adductor Magnus, and Adductor Brevis

Adductor

refers to the action of adduction.

The muscles of the Adductor group in the medial thigh, visible in Figure 9–30, originate on the pubis and insert onto the femur. Adductors longus, magnus, and brevis adduct, flex, and medially rotate the thigh at the acetabulofemoral joint. Adductor magnus alone attaches to the ischial tuberosity, a posterior attachment that allows it to also extend and laterally rotate the thigh at the acetabulofemoral joint, putting it in opposition to segments of itself and to the rest of its group. Of the Adductor group, Adductor longus is the most readily palpable. The proximal tendon of Adductor longus angles laterally from the pubic bone toward the femur and is the most prominent tendon in the groin area. Portions of Adductor magnus are palpable, though much of Adductor magnus is deep to Pectineus and Adductor longus and difficult to distinguish from Adductor longus. Adductor brevis lies between Adductor longus and magnus and its fibers are usually indistinguishable.

DID YOU KNOW?

Pectineus and Gracilis have similar attachments and actions to the adductor group and are sometimes included in it.

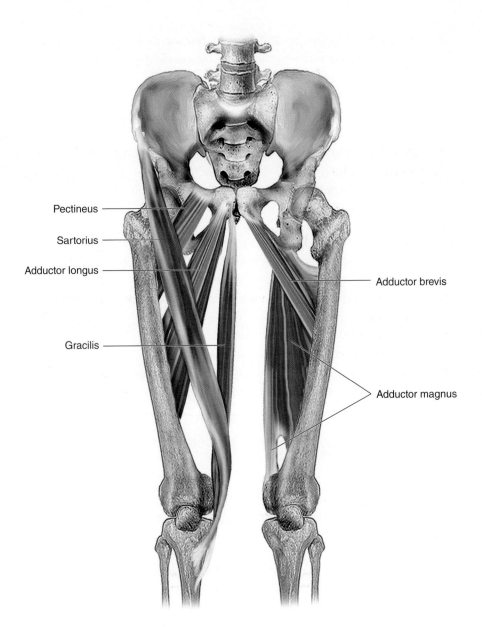

Pectineus

Sartorius

Adductor longus

Adductor brevis

Gracilis

Adductor magnus

FIGURE 9–30 Adductors longus, brevis, and magnus; Pectineus, Sartorius, and Gracilis.

Group attachments:

Adductor longus:

- Origin: pubic crest.
- Insertion: linea aspera of the femur.

Adductor magnus:

- Origin: pubic ramus and the ischial tuberosity.
- Insertion: linea aspera and adductor tubercle of the medial condyle of the femur.

Adductor brevis:

- Origin: pubic ramus.
- Insertion: linea aspera of the femur.

Group actions:

- Adductor longus: adducts, flexes, and medially rotates the thigh at the acetabulofemoral joint.
- Adductor magnus: adducts the thigh at the acetabulofemoral joint. The anterior fibers flex and medially rotate the thigh at the

acetabulofemoral joint and the posterior fibers extend and laterally rotate the thigh at the acetabulofemoral joint.

- Adductor brevis: adducts, flexes, and medially rotates the thigh at
the acetabulofemoral joint.

Placement:

- Adductor longus: mostly superficial.
- Adductor magnus: deep to Pectineus and Adductor longus and
brevis.
- Adductor brevis: deep to Adductor longus and superficial to
Adductor magnus.

Palpation of Adductor Longus and Adductor Magnus:

POSITION:

- Supine client. Place
your client's thigh in
passive abduction at
the acetabulofemoral
joint, as in Figure 9–31.
- Undrape the thigh and
secure the drape as
shown in Figure 9–31.
Encourage your client
to adjust and tighten
the drape to assure her

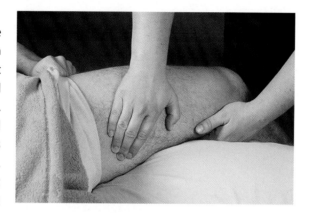

FIGURE 9–31 Palpating the
Adductors.

security while making Adductor longus and magnus available for palpation.
- Stand at the side of the table. Use your mother hand to add resistance to
movement.

LOCATE AND PALPATE:

- With the fingertips of your palpating hand, palpate about one-third down the
medial thigh, where the fibers of Adductor longus become deep to anterior
thigh muscles. Locate the long, prominent tendon of Adductor longus in the
proximal medial thigh.
- Palpate the fibers of Adductor longus between these landmarks in their resting state. Palpate with and across the grain of muscle fibers.
- Medial and distal to Adductor longus are some palpable fibers of Adductor
magnus. Others are medial and posterior to Adductor longus, and may become more apparent during palpation of other muscles, such as Gracilis.

DIRECT AN ACTION AND PALPATE:

- Place your mother hand on the distal medial thigh. Ask your client to bring her
thigh in toward the table and palpate Adductor longus and magnus during the resisted adduction of the femur. Palpate with and across the grain of muscle fibers.

EVALUATE:

- Characterize your palpation feedback from Adductor longus and magnus:
describe the tone, texture, and temperature of the muscle tissue.

- Note the presence of trigger points, tissue adhesions, barriers to palpation, or other findings.
- Compare palpation of both sides of Adductor longus and magnus, noting how the findings from the second palpation vary.
- Compare with palpations of Adductor longus and magnus on other clients, noting how the palpation findings on this client differ or are similar.

IN THE TREATMENT ROOM

Clients who participate in certain sports and activities that include repetitive or sustained adduction of the thigh may report symptoms that indicate assessment of the adductor muscles. Activities such as horseback riding, speed skating, ice hockey, kicking a soccer ball, or other activities that requires fast changes in the direction of movement, as shown in Figure 9–32, may result in inflammation of the adductors or in sudden groin pull. Adductor longus is the muscle most often involved in a groin pull or tear.

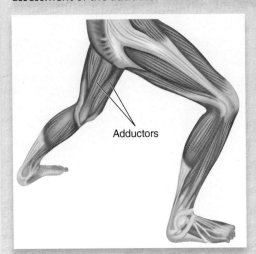

Adductors

FIGURE 9–32 Adductor longus is the muscle most often involved in a groin pull or tear.

Pecten

comb; may refer to the pectineal line of the femur.

HERE'S A TIP

Palpating Pectineus along with Adductor longus and magnus is a good choice, though palpating Pectineus through the drape may be most comfortable for your client. Take care to avoid the femoral nerve and blood vessels in the proximal medial thigh.

Pectineus

Pectineus [pek-TIN-ee-us], shown in Figure 9–30, is sometimes included in the Adductor group. Sources disagree whether Pectineus medially or laterally rotates the thigh at the acetabulofemoral joint (or even whether it rotates the thigh at all). Your assessment of Pectineus may resolve these issues for you on an individual basis.

Attachments:
- Origin: superior anterior pubis.
- Insertion: on the posterior femur, between the lesser trochanter and the linea aspera.

Actions:
- Adducts, flexes, and may medially rotate the thigh at the acetabulofemoral joint.

Placement:
- Superficial, lateral to, and difficult to distinguish from Adductor longus.

Palpation of Pectineus:

POSITION:
- Supine client. Place your client's thigh in passive abduction, as in Figure 9–31.

■ Undrape the thigh and secure the drape as shown in Figure 9–31. Encourage your client to adjust and tighten the drape to assure her security while making Pectineus available for palpation, or palpate through the drape.

■ Stand at the side of the table. Use your mother hand to add resistance to movement.

LOCATE AND PALPATE:

■ Locate the pubic crest, the anterior prominence of the pubic bone, and the proximal diagonal fibers of Adductor longus. The fibers may not be distinguishable from those of Pectineus.

■ Palpate the diagonal fibers of Pectineus in their resting state. Palpate with and across the grain of muscle fibers.

DIRECT AN ACTION AND PALPATE:

■ Place your mother hand on the distal medial thigh. Ask your client to bring her thigh in toward the table. Palpate Pectineus during resisted adduction of the femur. Palpate with and across the grain of muscle fibers.

■ Ask your client to bring her knee toward her head. Palpate Pectineus during flexion of the thigh, as shown in Figure 9–33. Palpate with and across the grain of muscle fibers.

EVALUATE:

■ Characterize your palpation feedback from Pectineus: describe the tone, texture, and temperature of the muscle tissue.

■ Note the presence of trigger points, tissue adhesions, barriers to palpation, or other findings.

■ Compare palpation of both sides of Pectineus, noting how the findings from the second palpation vary.

■ Compare with palpations of Pectineus on other clients, noting how the palpation findings on this client differ or are similar.

FIGURE 9–33 Palpating Pectineus.

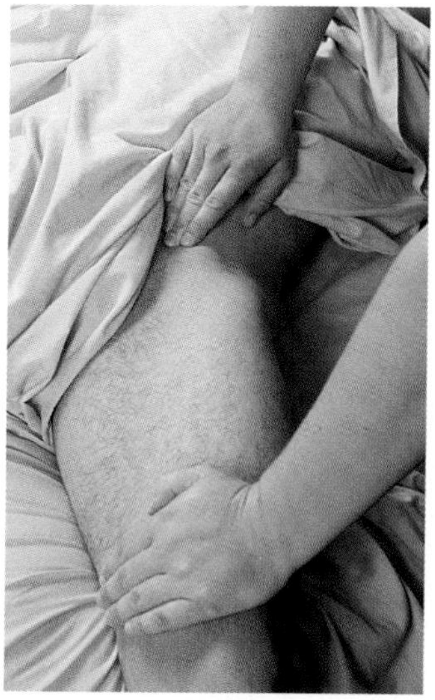

© Milady, a part of Cengage Learning. Photography by Yanik Chauvin.

Gracilis

Gracilis [GRASS-uh-lis] is sometimes called "the fourth Adductor" because it crosses the tibiofemoral joint it acts on the knee, not only on the thigh, as shown in Figure 9–30. Gracilis is a long, slender, superficial muscle in the medial thigh. Its proximal tendon is sometimes confused with the proximal tendon of Adductor longus, and though Gracilis's proximal tendon lacks its diagonal orientation, these tendons may blend. The distal tendon of Gracilis inserts into the pes anserine tendon at the proximal medial tibia.

Attachments:

■ Origin: pubic symphysis and pubic ramus
■ Insertion: pes anserine tendon to the proximal, medial tibia.

Actions:

■ Adducts the thigh at the acetabulofemoral joint and flexes and medially rotates the knee at the tibiofemoral joint.

Placement:

■ Superficial.

Gracilis

slender.

DID YOU KNOW?

The pes anserine tendon, an extension of deep fascia at the medial knee, receives the distal tendons of Gracilis, Sartorius, and Semitendinosus, muscles in the anterior, medial, and posterior thigh. Distinguishing between these muscles is accomplished by palpating from distal to proximal in the thigh.

Palpation of Gracilis:

POSITION:

- Supine client. Place your client's leg in passive abduction, as in Figure 9–31.
- Undrape leg as shown in Figure 9–31. Encourage your client to adjust and tighten the drape to assure her security while making Gracilis available for palpation.
- Stand at the side of the table. Use your mother hand to add resistance to movement.

LOCATE AND PALPATE:

- In the medial knee, locate the pes anserine tendon, usually deep to a pad of adipose tissue. The distal tendon of Gracilis is the middle of the three tendons that insert into the pes anserine, as shown in Figure 9–34. Locate the proximal Gracilis tendon alongside the prominent, diagonal Adductor longus tendon. Their tendons may blend. Palpate the fibers of Gracilis between these landmarks in their resting state. Palpate with and across the grain of muscle fibers.

DIRECT AN ACTION AND PALPATE:

- Place your mother hand just distal to the knee. Ask your client to bring her thigh in toward the table. Palpate the fibers of Gracilis during adduction of the thigh. Gracilis can be distinguished from Semitendinosus in the distal region by its action of adduction. Palpate with and across the grain of muscle fibers.

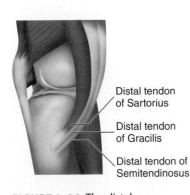

Distal tendon of Sartorius

Distal tendon of Gracilis

Distal tendon of Semitendinosus

FIGURE 9–34 The distal tendon of Sartorius inserts into the pes anserine tendon from the anterior, Gracilis medially, and Semitendinosus from the posterior thigh.

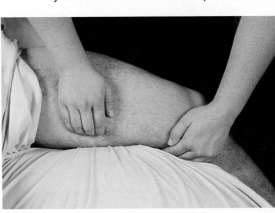

FIGURE 9–35 Palpating Gracilis.

- Bring your client's leg into passive flexion by hanging it off the side of the table, as shown in Figure 9–35. Place your mother hand behind her leg and ask your client to bend her knee; palpate the fibers of Gracilis as you resist flexion of the leg. Palpate with and across the grain of muscle fibers.

- Gracilis can be distinguished from Sartorius by palpating proximally. Gracilis remains in the medial thigh as its fibers lead toward its origin on the pubis, while Sartorius moves laterally toward ASIS.

EVALUATE:

- Characterize your palpation feedback from Gracilis: describe the tone, texture, and temperature of the muscle tissue.
- Note the presence of trigger points, tissue adhesions, barriers to palpation, or other findings.
- Compare palpation of both sides of Gracilis, noting how the findings from the second palpation vary.
- Compare with palpations of Gracilis on other clients, noting how the palpation findings on this client differ or are similar.

Sartorius

Sartorius [sar-TOR-ee-us] is a long, ribbon-like muscle, visible in Figure 9–30, which acts on both the thigh and the leg. The distal tendon of Sartorius is the anterior insertion into the pes anserine. Sartorius is superficial, readily palpable, and sometimes visible.

Sartor

tailor.

DID YOU KNOW?

By laterally rotating the thigh at the acetabulofemoral joint and medially rotating the leg at the tibiofemoral joint, Sartorius allows us to sit cross-legged, giving the muscle its name: Sartor is the Latin word for a tailor—who sits cross-legged as he works. Sartorius is superficial for its entire length and is the longest muscle in the body.

Attachments:
- Origin: anterior superior iliac spine.
- Insertion: pes anserine tendon to the proximal, medial tibia.

Actions:
- Flexes, laterally rotates and abducts the thigh at the acetabulofemoral joint and flexes and medially rotates the leg at the tibiofemoral joint.

Placement:
- Superficial.

Palpation of Sartorius:

POSITION:
- Supine client. Undrape leg as shown in Figure 9–31. Encourage your client to adjust and tighten the drape to ensure her privacy while making Sartorius available for palpation.
- Stand at the side of the table. Use your mother hand to support the knee or to add resistance to movement.

LOCATE AND PALPATE:
- Rest your client's foot on her opposite leg to create passive lateral rotation of the thigh at the acetabulofemoral joint and passive medial rotation of the leg at the tibiofemoral joint, as in Figure 9–36.
- Locate the most anterior of the tendons inserting into the pes anserine. On the anterior pelvis, locate ASIS. Palpate the long, slender fibers of Sartorius between these landmarks in their resting state as they cross over the thigh from medial to lateral. Palpate with and across the grain of muscle fibers.

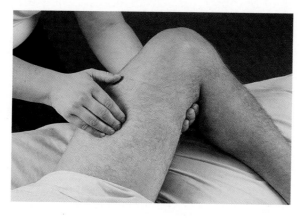

FIGURE 9–36 Palpating Sartorius.

© Milady, a part of Cengage Learning. Photography by Yanik Chauvin.

DIRECT AN ACTION AND PALPATE:

- Ask your client to slide her foot up the leg it rests on. Palpate the fibers of Sartorius during the increased lateral rotation of the thigh at the acetabulofemoral joint, and flexion and medial rotation of the leg at the tibiofemoral joint. Palpate with and across the grain of muscle fibers.

EVALUATE:

- Characterize your palpation feedback from Sartorius: describe the tone, texture, and temperature of the muscle tissue.
- Note the presence of trigger points, tissue adhesions, barriers to palpation, or other findings.
- Compare palpation of both sides of Sartorius, noting how the findings from the second palpation vary.
- Compare with palpations of Sartorius on other clients, noting how the palpation findings on this client differ or are similar.

> Lab Activity 9–3 on page 394 is designed to develop your palpation skills on superficial muscles that act on the thigh.

MUSCLES THAT ACT ON THE LEG

Two powerful muscle groups act on the leg, in opposition to each other: the anterior Quadriceps and the posterior Hamstrings. In each group, there is a long, large, superficial muscle that acts on both the thigh and the leg, and smaller muscles that act only on the leg. These muscle groups are, by and large, flexors or extensors at the hinge joint of the leg at the tibiofemoral joint.

Quadriceps Group: Rectus Femoris, Vastus Lateralis, Vastus Medialis, Vastus Intermedius

Prime extensors of the leg at the knee, the Quadriceps group, [KWAHD-ruh-seps], shown in Figure 9–37, are a great example of reverse action: extension of the leg at the tibiofemoral joint occurs when one rises from a seated position, lifting the entire body into a standing position, or it may occur when one remains seated and simply moves one leg forward. In either instance, extension of the leg at the tibiofemoral joint occurs. The result of the action, however, is quite different. All the quadriceps muscles share an insertion on the tibial tuberosity.

Attachments:

Rectus femoris [REK-tus FEM-uh-rus]:

- Origin: anterior inferior iliac spine.
- Insertion: tibial tuberosity, via the patellar tendon.

Vastus lateralis [VAS-tus lat-uh-RAY-lis]:

- Origin: greater trochanter and linea aspera of the femur.
- Insertion: tibial tuberosity, via the patellar tendon.

Vastus medialis [VAS-tus mee-dee-AY-lis]:

- Origin: medial linea aspera and posterior aspect of the femur.
- Insertion: tibial tuberosity, via the patellar tendon.

Vastus intermedius:

- Origin: anterior proximal femur and the linea aspera.
- Insertion: tibial tuberosity, via the patellar tendon.

HERE'S A TIP

The muscles that act on the leg and foot are readily palpable. Palpating muscles on the legs or feet simultaneously or as groups yields information for assessment and comparison. Simultaneous palpation of both a client's Gastrocnemius, for example, can provide you with information about foot dominance and gait patterns.

Quadriceps

four heads.

Rectus

erect.

Femoris

the thigh.

Vastus

large.

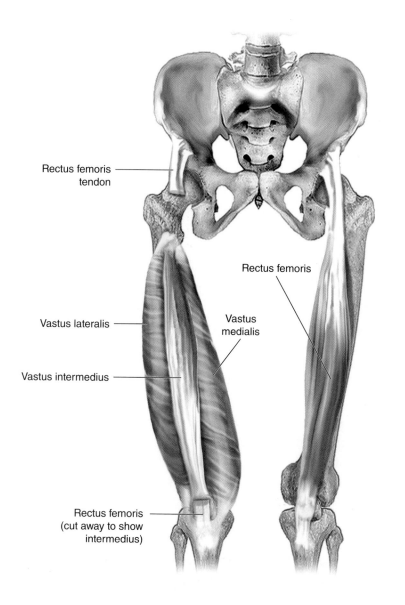

Rectus femoris tendon

Rectus femoris

Vastus lateralis

Vastus medialis

Vastus intermedius

Rectus femoris (cut away to show intermedius)

FIGURE 9–37 The Quadriceps Group: Rectus femoris, Vastus lateralis, Vastus intermedius, and Vastus medialis.

© Delmar, Cengage Learning.

Actions:

- Rectus femoris: flexes the thigh at the acetabulofemoral joint and extends the leg at the tibiofemoral joint.
- Vastus lateralis, medialis, and intermedius: extend the leg at the tibiofemoral joint.

Placement:

- Rectus femoris and Vastus lateralis are superficial.
- Vastus medialis is partially deep to Rectus femoris.
- Vastus intermedius is entirely deep to Rectus femoris.

HERE'S A TIP

Of the four muscles of the Quadriceps group, Vastus intermedius [VAS-tus in-tur-MEE-dee-us] lies entirely deep to Rectus femoris and is not readily palpable.

Palpation of Rectus Femoris:

POSITION:

- Supine client. Undrape the thigh and leg.
- Place a bolster beneath your client's knee to create a degree of passive flexion at the acetabulofemoral and tibiofemoral joints.

■ Stand at the side of the table. Use your mother hand to support the knee or use both hands to palpate.

LOCATE AND PALPATE:

■ Locate the prominent tibial tuberosity, just distal to the patella. Palpate the patellar ligament proximally until it becomes the large, superficial mass of Rectus femoris.

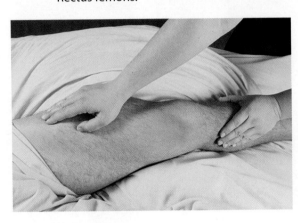

■ Locate the ASIS. Move the fingertips of your palpating hand medially along the anterior ilium to locate the smaller prominence of the AIIS.

■ Palpate the fibers of Rectus femoris between these landmarks in their resting state, as shown in Figure 9–38. Palpate with and across the grain of muscle fibers.

FIGURE 9–38 Palpating Rectus femoris.

DIRECT AN ACTION AND PALPATE:

■ Ask your client to bend her thigh at the hip. Palpate the fibers of Rectus femoris during flexion of the thigh at the acetabulofemoral joint. Palpate with and across the grain of muscle fibers.

■ Ask your client to raise her foot off the table. Palpate the fibers of Rectus femoris during extension of the leg at the tibiofemoral joint. Palpate with and across the grain of muscle fibers.

EVALUATE:

■ Characterize your palpation feedback from Rectus femoris: describe the tone, texture, and temperature of the muscle tissue.

■ Note the presence of trigger points, tissue adhesions, barriers to palpation, or other findings.

■ Compare palpation of both sides of Rectus femoris, noting how the findings from the second palpation vary.

■ Compare with palpations of Rectus femoris on other clients, noting how the palpation findings on this client differ or are similar.

Palpation of Vastus Lateralis and Vastus Medialis:

POSITION:

■ Supine client. Undrape the thigh and leg.

■ Place a bolster beneath your client's knee to create a degree of passive flexion at the acetabulofemoral and tibiofemoral joints.

■ Stand at the side of the table. Use your mother hand to support the knee or use both hands to palpate.

LOCATE AND PALPATE:

■ Locate the prominent tibial tuberosity, just distal to the patella. For Vastus lateralis, locate the greater trochanter of the femur, and for Vastus medialis, locate the border of Sartorius as it crosses over the medial aspect of the femur.

- Place your palpating hands on the medial and lateral aspects of the distal femur, as shown in Figure 9–39. Palpate the fibers of Vastus lateralis and Vastus medialis in their resting state. Palpate with and across the grain of muscle fibers.

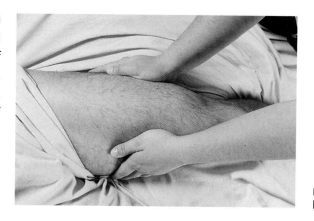

FIGURE 9-39 Palpating Vastus lateralis and Vastus medialis.

© Milady, a part of Cengage Learning. Photography by Yanik Chauvin.

DIRECT AN ACTION AND PALPATE:

- Ask your client to raise her foot off the table. Palpate the fibers of Vastus lateralis and Vastus medialis during extension of the leg. Palpate with and across the grain of muscle fibers.
- Vastus lateralis may be palpated for most of its length, just anterior to the iliotibial band, but where Vastus lateralis is adjacent to the ITB it may be quite tender.
- Vastus medialis is most palpable in its distal aspect, where it forms the pad of flesh medial to the knee.

EVALUATE:

- Characterize your palpation feedback from Vastus lateralis and Vastus medialis: describe the tone, texture, and temperature of the muscle tissue.
- Note the presence of trigger points, tissue adhesions, barriers to palpation, or other findings.
- Compare palpation of both sides of Vastus lateralis and Vastus medialis, noting how the findings from the second palpation vary.
- Compare with palpations of Vastus lateralis and Vastus medialis on other clients, noting how the palpation findings on this client differ or are similar.

IN THE TREATMENT ROOM

A Quadriceps (Quad) strain usually involves Rectus femoris, as shown in Figure 9–40. A Quad strain may be caused by overworking the muscles in any sport that requires bursts of speed, such as soccer or American football, by overstretching of the muscles or by lifting too heavy an object. Pain, stiffness, or signs of inflammation in the anterior thigh are indicators to assess Rectus femoris.

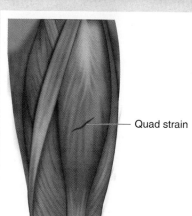

Quad strain

FIGURE 9-40 A quadriceps strain usually involves Rectus femoris.

© Milady, a part of Cengage Learning.

Biceps

two heads.

Femoris

the thigh.

Semi-

partial.

-tendinosus

tendinous.

-membranosus

membranous.

Hamstrings Group: Biceps Femoris, Semitendinosus, Semimembranosus

The three Hamstrings muscles oppose the Quadriceps: they flex the leg at the tibiofemoral joint and extend the thigh at the acetabulofemoral joint. They also assist in rotations of the thigh at the acetabulofemoral joint. Like the Quads, the Hamstrings muscles, seen in Figure 9–41, share a common attachment: their origin on the ischial tuberosity. Biceps femoris [BY-seps FEM-uh-rus] is readily palpable for most of its length. The distal tendon of Semitendinosus [sem-ee-ten-duh-NOH-sus] inserts into the pes anserine tendon from the posterior and is the most prominent tendon in the posterior knee. Semimembranosus [sem-ee-mem-bruh-NOH-sus] is deep on the posterior femur and not readily palpable.

Group attachments:

Biceps femoris:

■ Long head origin: ischial tuberosity.
■ Short head origin: linea aspera of the femur.
■ Insertion: head of the fibula and the lateral condyle of the tibia.

Semitendinosus:

■ Origin: ischial tuberosity.
■ Insertion: pes anserine tendon to the proximal, medial tibia.

Semimembranosus:

■ Origin: ischial tuberosity.
■ Insertion: medial condyle of the tibia.

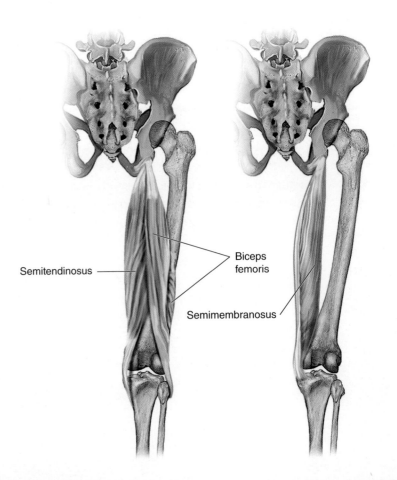

FIGURE 9–41 The Hamstrings Group: Biceps femoris, Semitendinosus, and Semimembranosus.

Group actions:

- Biceps femoris: Long head extends and assists in lateral rotation of the thigh at the acetabulofemoral joint. Both heads flex the leg at the tibiofemoral joint.
- Semitendinosus and Semimembranosus assist in medial rotation of the thigh at the acetabulofemoral joint.
- As a group: extend the thigh at the acetabulofemoral joint and flex the leg at the tibiofemoral joint.

Placement:

- Biceps femoris: superficial.
- Semitendinosus: superficial.
- Semimembranosus: proximally, deep to Semitendinosus and distally, superficial on either side of Semitendinosus.

Palpation of Biceps Femoris:

The four tendons near the posterior knee, from medial to lateral, are those of Sartorius, Gracilis, Semitendinosus, and Biceps femoris. The tendon of Semitendinosus is the largest and most prominent.

POSITION:

- Prone client. Undrape the thigh and the leg.
- Stand at the side of the table. Use your mother hand to add resistance to movement.

LOCATE AND PALPATE:

- In the posterior knee, locate the distal tendon of Biceps femoris, on the lateral aspect. Locate the shared origin on the ischial tuberosity.
- Palpate the fibers of Biceps femoris between these landmarks in their resting state, as shown in Figure 9–42. Palpate with and across the grain of muscle fibers.

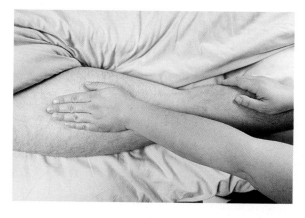

FIGURE 9–42 Palpating Biceps femoris.

© Milady, a part of Cengage Learning. Photography by Yanik Chauvin.

DIRECT AN ACTION AND PALPATE:

- Place your mother hand on the distal, posterior thigh. Ask your client to push her thigh against your hand as you palpate Biceps femoris during extension of the thigh at the acetabulofemoral joint. Palpate with and across the grain of muscle fibers.
- Place your mother hand on the proximal, posterior leg, distal to the knee. Avoid the popliteal area. Ask your client to bend her leg at the knee and palpate the fibers of Biceps femoris during flexion of the leg at the tibiofemoral joint. Palpate with and across the grain of muscle fibers.

EVALUATE:

- Characterize your palpation feedback from Biceps femoris: describe the tone, texture, and temperature of the muscle tissue.

■ Note the presence of trigger points, tissue adhesions, barriers to palpation, or other findings.

■ Compare palpation of both sides of Biceps femoris, noting how the findings from the second palpation vary.

■ Compare with palpations of Biceps femoris on other clients, noting how the palpation findings on this client differ or are similar.

Palpation of Semitendinosus and Semimembranosus:

The distal tendon of Semitendinosus is the most prominent tendon in the posterior medial thigh.

POSITION:

■ Prone client. Undrape the thigh and the leg.

■ Stand at the side of the table. Use your mother hand to add resistance to movement.

LOCATE AND PALPATE:

■ In the posterior knee, locate the large, prominent distal tendon of Semitendinosus, on the medial aspect. Locate the shared origin on the ischial tuberosity.

■ In the posterior knee, locate the distal tendon of Semimembranosus, which lies deep to and is broader than, the distal tendon of Semitendinosus. Locate

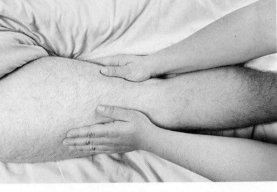

FIGURE 9–43 Palpating Semitendinosus and Semimembranosus.

the shared origin on the ischial tuberosity.

■ Palpate the fibers of Semitendinosus between these landmarks in their resting state, as shown in Figure 9–43. Palpate with and across the grain of muscle fibers.

■ Palpate the fibers of Semimembranosus between these landmarks in their resting state. Its distal belly is deep to and broader than the muscle belly of Semitendinosus. Palpate with and across the grain of muscle fibers.

DIRECT AN ACTION AND PALPATE:

■ Place your mother hand on the proximal, posterior leg, distal to the knee. Avoid the popliteal area. Ask your client to bend her leg at the knee and palpate the long tendon and fibers of Semitendinosus during flexion of the leg. Palpate with and across the grain of muscle fibers.

■ Palpate the fibers of Semimembranosus in their resting state. Its distal belly is deep to and broader than the muscle belly of Semitendinosus. Palpate with and across the grain of muscle fibers.

EVALUATE:

■ Characterize your palpation feedback from Semitendinosus and Semimembranosus: describe the tone, texture, and temperature of the muscle tissue.

- Note the presence of trigger points, tissue adhesions, barriers to palpation, or other finding.
- Compare palpation of both sides of Semitendinosus and Semimembranosus, noting how the findings from the second palpation vary.
- Compare with palpations of Semitendinosus and Semimembranosus on other clients, noting how the palpation findings on this client differ or are similar.

IN THE TREATMENT ROOM

Clients who report pain in the posterior knee, thigh, or hip are assessed for Hamstrings strain. Runners, as in Figure 9–44, and clients who participate in sports that include bursts of speed and sudden changes in the direction of movement are at risk for Hamstrings strain. Those who fail to stretch properly following these activities increase their risk. The Hamstrings muscles are notoriously easy to strain and slow to heal. Your client with a Hamstrings strain may risk re-injury by returning to athletic activity prematurely.

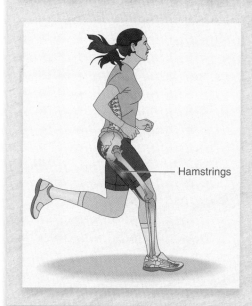

Hamstrings

FIGURE 9–44 The Hamstrings are notoriously easy to strain and slow to heal.

MUSCLES THAT ACT ON THE FOOT

Muscles that act on the foot perform the special movements at the ankle: they dorsiflex and plantarflex the foot at the talocrural joint, invert and evert the foot at the intertarsal joints, and are found in anterior, lateral, and posterior compartments. The superficial and intermediate muscles that act on the foot are visible and readily palpable in their compartments and include Tibialis anterior, Extensor digitorum longus, the Peroneal group, and Gastrocnemius and Soleus.

Tibialis Anterior

The long tendon of Tibialis anterior, shown in Figure 9–45, crosses the tibia from its lateral origin to the medial insertion on the plantar foot, where it meets the distal tendon of Peroneus longus to form a strap-like structure that supports the medial longitudinal arch of the foot. The belly of the muscle is on the lateral tibia.

Tibialis

of the tibia.

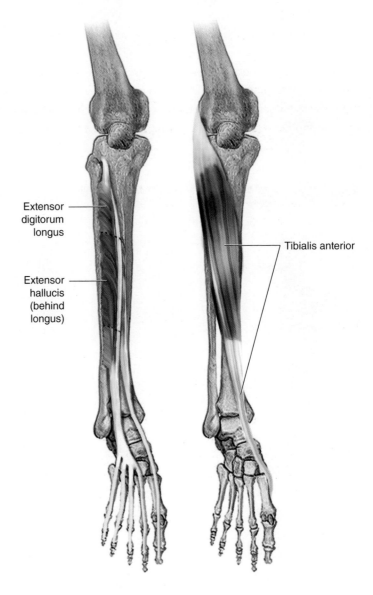

Extensor digitorum longus

Extensor hallucis (behind longus)

Tibialis anterior

FIGURE 9–45 Tibialis anterior and Extensor digitorum longus.

HERE'S A TIP

Palpating Tibialis anterior and Peroneus longus together reveals their strap-like structure around the plantar foot.

Attachments:
- Origin: lateral condyle and proximal half of the anterior tibia.
- Insertion: medial cuneiform and base of metatarsal I.

Actions:
- Dorsiflexes the foot at the talocrural joint and inverts the foot at the intertarsal joints.

Placement:
- Superficial.

Palpation of Tibialis Anterior:

POSITION:
- Supine client. Undrape your client's leg.
- Stand at the foot of the table. Use your mother hand to add resistance to movement.

LOCATE AND PALPATE:
- On the medial foot, locate the base of the first metatarsal, midway on the medial longitudinal arch. This attachment site is often tender.

■ Locate the anterior aspect of the lateral condyle of the tibia. Palpate the long distal tendon as it crosses from its medial insertion to the lateral aspect of the tibia and the fibers of Tibialis anterior between these landmarks in

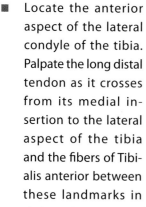
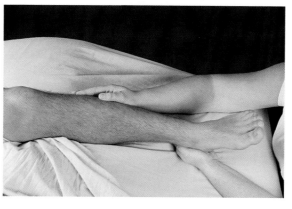

FIGURE 9–46 Palpating Tibialis anterior.

© Milady, a part of Cengage Learning. Photography by Yanik Chauvin.

their resting state, as shown in Figure 9–46. Palpate with and across the grain of muscle fibers.

DIRECT AN ACTION AND PALPATE:

■ Place your mother hand around the dorsal aspect of your client's foot, as in Figure 9–47. Ask your client to push her foot against your hand as you palpate Tibialis anterior during resisted dorsiflexion of the foot at the talocrural joint. Palpate

FIGURE 9–47 Palpating Tibialis against resistance.

© Milady, a part of Cengage Learning. Photography by Yanik Chauvin.

with and across the grain of muscle fibers.

■ Ask your client to turn the sole of her foot in toward the table. Palpate the prominent distal tendon of Tibialis anterior within its tendon sheath during inversion of the foot at the intertarsal joint as it crosses onto the medial aspect of the foot. Palpate with and across the grain of muscle fibers.

EVALUATE:

■ Characterize your palpation feedback from Tibialis anterior: describe the tone, texture, and temperature of the muscle tissue.
■ Note the presence of trigger points, tissue adhesions, barriers to palpation, or other findings.
■ Compare palpation of both sides of Tibialis anterior, noting how the findings from the second palpation vary.
■ Compare with palpations of Tibialis anterior on other clients, noting how the palpation findings on this client differ or are similar.

IN THE TREATMENT ROOM

Anterior or medial leg pain along the tibia indicates an assessment of Tibialis anterior and assessment of possible inflammation due to repetitive stress on the tibia. Clients who are runners, race walkers, and dancers are at risk for

Shin splints

pain along the tibia caused by stress on the connective tissue that attaches Tibialis anterior to the bone.

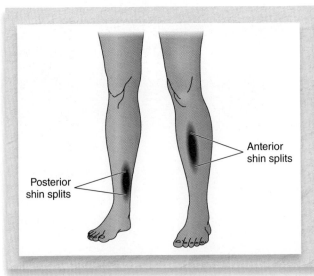

shin splints: pain along the tibia caused by stress on the connective tissue that attaches Tibialis anterior or Tibialis posterior to the bone, as seen in Figure 9–48. Shin splints are slow to heal and reinjury is common.

FIGURE 9–48 Runners, race walkers, and dancers are at risk for shin splints.

Digitorum

the finger or toe.

Extensor Digitorum Longus

The distal tendon of Extensor digitorum longus [eck-STEN-sur DIJ-ih-tor-um LAWNG-gus], visible in Figure 9–45, splits into four segments that travel to the distal phalanges of the toes on the dorsal foot, mirroring the distal tendons of Extensor digitorum in the dorsal hand. Extensor digitorum longus lies between Tibialis anterior and the Peroneal group: its four distal tendons are visible and readily palpable in the dorsal foot.

Attachments:
- Origin: lateral condyle of the tibia and most of the proximal fibula
- Insertion: dorsal surfaces of the intermediate and distal phalanges of toes #2–5.

Actions:
- Extends toes #2–5 at the interphalangeal joints and dorsiflexes the foot at the talocrural joint.

Placement:
- Superficial.

Palpation of Extensor Digitorum Longus:

POSITION:
- Supine client. Undrape your client's leg.
- Stand at the foot of the table. Use your mother hand to add resistance to movement.

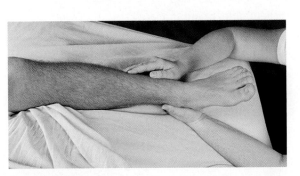

LOCATE AND PALPATE:
- Locate the prominent tendons visible and palpable at the bases of toes #2–5. Palpate the distal Extensor digitorum longus between these landmarks in its resting state, as shown in Figure 9–49.

FIGURE 9–49 Palpating Extensor digitorum longus.

DIRECT AN ACTION AND PALPATE:

- Ask your client to point her toes toward her head. Palpate the tendons of Extensor digitorum longus during extension of toes #2–5 at the interphalangeal joints.

- Place your mother hand around the dorsal aspect of your client's foot, as in Figure 9–47. Ask your client to push her foot against your hand as you palpate Extensor digitorum longus during resisted dorsiflexion of the foot at the talocrural joint.

- The central tendon of Extensor digitorum longus as it crosses the tarsals becomes evident and palpable as your client inverts her foot against slight resistance. Extensor digitorum's tendon is lateral and vertically oriented, while the tendon of Tibialis anterior is medial and angled to the medial foot.

EVALUATE:

- Characterize your palpation feedback from Extensor digitorum longus: describe the tone, texture, and temperature of the muscle tissue.

- Note the presence of trigger points, tissue adhesions, barriers to palpation, or other findings.

- Compare palpation of both sides of Extensor digitorum longus, noting how the findings from the second palpation vary.

- Compare with palpations of Extensor digitorum longus on other clients, noting how the palpation findings on this client differ or are similar.

Peroneal Group

The Peroneals [payr-uh-NEE-uls], sometimes called the Fibulares [fib-yoo-LAYR-eez], are the muscles in the lateral compartment of the leg, shown in Figure 9–50. Peroneus longus is visible and readily palpable

Peroneus

pin of a clasp or brooch.

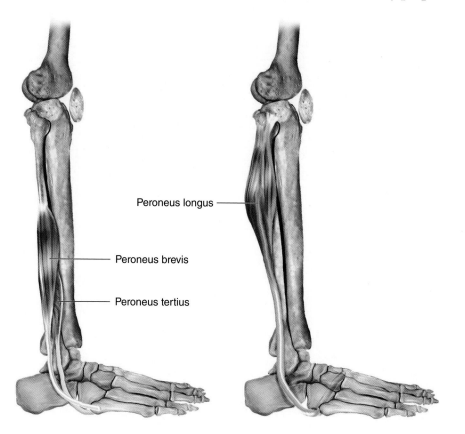

Peroneus longus

Peroneus brevis

Peroneus tertius

FIGURE 9–50 Peroneus longus, brevis, and tertius.

in the lateral leg. Peroneus brevis lies mostly deep to Peroneus longus and shares its action, making it difficult to differentiate. Only the distal tendon of Peroneus tertius is palpable.

DID YOU KNOW?

The distal tendon of Peroneus longus, the most superficial muscle in the group, takes an abrupt 90° turn just below the lateral malleolus, into the deep muscle layers of the plantar foot, and meets the distal tendon of Tibialis anterior at the base of metatarsal #1. Together, these distal tendons help to form the medial longitudinal arch of the foot and create a strap-like support beneath the foot.

Attachments:
Peroneus longus:
- Origin: head and proximal length of the fibula and the lateral condyle of the tibia.
- Insertion: medial cuneiform and base of metatarsal I.

Peroneus brevis:
- Origin: distal two-thirds of the fibula.
- Insertion: lateral on the base of metatarsal V.

Peroneus tertius:
- Origin: distal third of the fibula.
- Insertion: base of metatarsal V.

Actions:
- Peroneus longus and brevis: plantarflex the foot at the talocrural joint and evert the foot at the intertarsal joints.
- Peroneus Tertius: dorsiflexes the foot at the talocrural joint and everts the foot at the intertarsal joints.

Placement:
- Peroneus longus is superficial. Peroneus brevis is mostly deep to Peroneus longus.
- Peroneus tertius is superficial in the lateral, dorsal foot.

Palpation of the Peroneal Group:

POSITION:
- Supine client. Undrape your client's leg.
- Stand at the foot of the table. Use your mother hand to add resistance to movement.

LOCATE AND PALPATE:
- Just posterior to the lateral malleolus, locate the distal tendons of Peroneus longus and brevis as they enter into the deep muscular layers of the plantar foot.
- Locate the base of the first metatarsal, the shared insertion site of Tibialis anterior and Peroneus longus.

- On the proximal lateral leg, locate the lateral condyle of the tibia and, just distal, the head and proximal fibula.

- Palpate the fibers of Peroneus longus and brevis between these landmarks in their resting state, as shown in Figure 9–51. Palpate with and across the grain of muscle fibers.

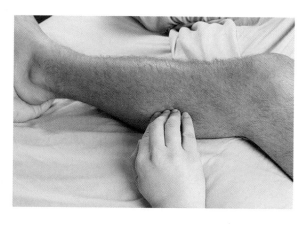

FIGURE 9–51 Palpating Peroneus longus and brevis.

© Milady, a part of Cengage Learning. Photography by Yanik Chauvin.

- Locate the distal tendons of Extensor digitorum longus and Tibialis anterior as they cross over the tarsals. The distal tendon of Peroneus tertius is found between them. Palpate the distal Peroneus tertius in its resting state. Palpate with and across the grain of muscle fibers.

DIRECT AN ACTION AND PALPATE:

- Place your mother hand around the dorsal aspect of your client's foot, as in Figure 9–47. Ask your client to turn the sole of her foot away from the center of the table, and palpate Peroneus longus and brevis during resisted eversion of the foot at the intertarsal joints.

- Repeat the palpation during resisted dorsiflexion of the foot at the talocrural joint by Peroneus longus and brevis. Palpate with and across the grain of muscle fibers.

- Ask your client to again evert her foot at the intertarsal joints without resistance, as you simultaneously palpate the insertion of the Peroneus longus tendon into the deep muscular layer of the plantar foot at its lateral aspect and its ultimate insertion onto the base of the first metatarsal.

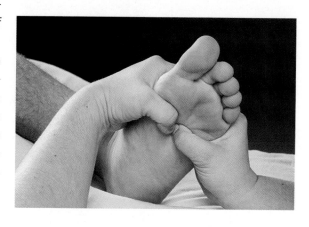

FIGURE 9–52 Palpating the strap-like structure of the distal tendons of Tibialis anterior and Peroneus longus.

© Milady, a part of Cengage Learning. Photography by Yanik Chauvin.

- Ask your client to turn the sole of her foot toward and away from the center of the table as you palpate the strap-like structure created around the plantar foot by the tendons of Tibialis anterior and Peroneus longus during inversion and eversion of the foot at the intertarsal joints, as in Figure 9–52.

- Place your mother hand around the plantar aspect of your client's foot. Ask her to push her foot toward the foot of the table as you palpate the distal fibers of Peroneus tertius during resisted plantar flexion of the foot at the talocrural joint.

EVALUATE:

- Characterize your palpation feedback from the Peroneals: describe the tone, texture, and temperature of the muscle tissue.
- Note the presence of trigger points, tissue adhesions, barriers to palpation, or other findings.
- Compare palpation of both sides of the Peroneals, noting how the findings from the second palpation vary.
- Compare with palpations of the Peroneals on other clients, noting how the palpation findings on this client differ or are similar.

IN THE TREATMENT ROOM

The distal tendons of Tibialis anterior and Peroneus longus are assessed when a client reports arch pain or muscle cramps in her foot. In addition, an inversion sprain of the ankle may tear or rupture tendons of the Peroneal muscles. Finally, sports that include side-to-side movements, especially fast side-to-side starts and stops, such as tennis players must do, can strain the Peroneals.

The most common ankle sprains are inversion sprains, shown in Figure 9–53, in which the ankle is forcefully inverted, such as when your foot suddenly slides off a curb. The distal tendons of the Peroneal muscles are pulled and strained during an inversion sprain.

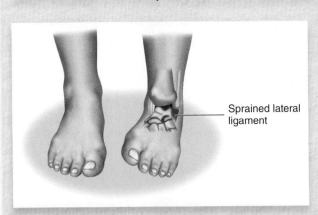

Sprained lateral ligament

FIGURE 9–53 An inversion sprain is the most common type; it may stretch or tear the tendon of Peroneus longus.

gasterkneme

belly leg.

Gastrocnemius

Gastrocnemius [gas-trok-NEEM-e-us] is the prominent posterior leg muscle that gives the leg its shape. Gastrocnemius and Soleus share an insertion on the calcaneus via the Achilles, or calcaneal, tendon. Together, Gastrocnemius and Soleus are sometimes called Triceps surae, acknowledging the three heads and common insertion, shown in Figure 9–54. Both heads of Gastrocnemius are superficial, visible, and readily palpable in the posterior leg, as is the huge Achilles tendon.

DID YOU KNOW?

The two heads of Gastrocnemius, which cross two joints, and its superficial placement over the deeper and more dense Soleus, mirror the relationship of Biceps brachii to Brachialis in the arm.

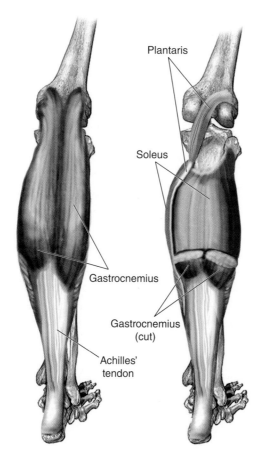

FIGURE 9–54 Gastrocnemius and Soleus, or Triceps surae.

Attachments:

Medial head:

- Origin: posterior surface of the medial condyle of the femur.
- Insertion: posterior calcaneus via the calcaneal or Achilles tendon.

Lateral head:

- Origin: posterior surface of the lateral condyle of the femur.
- Insertion: posterior calcaneus via the calcaneal or Achilles tendon.

Actions:

- Plantarflexes the foot at the talocrural joint and assists in flexing the leg at the tibiofemoral joint.

Placement:

- Superficial.

Palpation of Gastrocnemius:

POSITION:

- Prone client. Undrape the lower leg.
- Place a bolster beneath your client's ankle to create slight dorsiflexion of the foot.
- Stand at the foot of the table. Use your mother hand to add resistance to movement.

LOCATE AND PALPATE:

- On the calcaneus, locate the broad attachment of the Achilles tendon. Locate the medial and lateral condyles of the femur. Palpate the fibers of the two

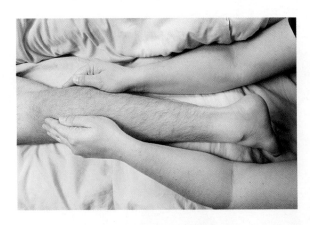

FIGURE 9–55 Palpating Gastrocnemius.

heads of Gastrocnemius between these landmarks in their resting state, avoiding the popliteal area, as shown in Figure 9–55. Palpate with and across the grain of muscle fibers.

DIRECT AN ACTION AND PALPATE:

- Ask your client to point her toes. Palpate the fibers of Gastrocnemius during plantarflexion of the foot at the talocrural joint. Palpate with and across the grain of muscle fibers.
- Place your mother hand on your client's plantar foot. Ask her to bend her knee as you palpate Gastrocnemius during resisted flexion of the leg at the tibiofemoral joint. Palpate with and across the grain of muscle fibers.

EVALUATE:

- Characterize your palpation feedback: describe the tone, texture, and temperature of the muscle tissue.
- Note the presence of trigger points, tissue adhesions, barriers to palpation, or other findings.
- Compare palpation of both sides of Gastrocnemius, noting how the findings from the second palpation vary.
- Compare with palpations of Gastrocnemius on other clients, noting how the palpation findings on this client differ or are similar.

IN THE TREATMENT ROOM

Gastrocnemius is prone to painful spasms and cramps during exertion, during sleep, or even on the massage table:

- During exertion, Gastrocnemius may cramp or spasm due to overuse or an electrolyte imbalance caused by loss of fluids through perspiration.
- During sleep, Gastrocnemius may cramp or spasm because leg movement is restricted by bedding or due to a chronic deficiency in blood levels of calcium, potassium, or magnesium. If this is the cause, it is likely that both legs will cramp.
- On the massage table, a client's Gastrocnemius may spasm or cramp for several additional reasons: the bolster beneath her ankle may be creating strain or this client may have chronically shortened Gastrocnemius from wearing high heels, to the degree that the slight dorsiflexion created by the bolster triggers a spasm or cramp, as shown in Figure 9-56. If this is

the case, removing the bolster and repositioning the leg may alleviate the cramp.

- Diagnosing an electrolyte imbalance or vitamin deficiency is clearly outside the scope of practice of massage therapy. Suggesting and demonstrating stretches for Gastrocnemius, and perhaps advising alternate footwear, is within your scope of practice.

- Assessing Gastrocnemius is indicated whenever your client reports pain, spasms, or cramps in her posterior leg. If your client also complains of intense heel pain, the Achilles tendon may be injured, indicating assessment by her primary healthcare practitioner.

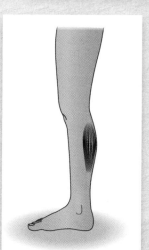

FIGURE 9–56 Positioning the client's leg to prevent cramping of Gastrocnemius or Soleus.

Soleus

The fibers of Soleus [SOH-lee-us] are denser than those of the two-headed Gastrocnemius, and its dense belly pushes Gastrocnemius outward, creating the shape of the calf, as seen in Figure 9–55.

Soleus

flat sandal.

HERE'S A TIP

Gastrocnemius and Soleus may be easily palpated together. Remember that Soleus acts solely on the foot.

Soleus lies deep to Gastrocnemius for most of its length. Because its distal bulk is medial and lateral to Gastrocnemius, it is palpable distally, medial to the Achilles tendon.

Attachments:

- Origin: head and proximal third of the fibula and the posterior tibia.
- Insertion: posterior calcaneus via the calcaneal or Achilles tendon.

Actions:

- Plantarflexes the foot at the talocrural joint.

Placement:

- Mostly deep to Gastrocnemius, superficial medially.

Palpation of Soleus:

POSITION:

- Prone client. Undrape the lower leg.
- Place a bolster beneath your client's ankle to create slight dorsiflexion of the foot. at the talocrural joint.
- Stand at the foot of the table. Use your mother hand to add resistance to movement or use both hands to palpate.

LOCATE AND PALPATE:

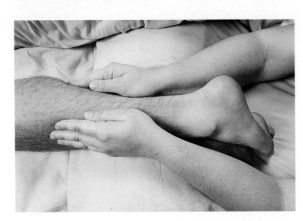

FIGURE 9-57 Palpating Soleus.

© Milady, a part of Cengage Learning.
Photography by Yanik Chauvin.

- On the calcaneus, locate the broad attachment of the Achilles tendon. Move the fingertips of your palpating hands medial and lateral to the Achilles tendon, as in Figure 9–57. Palpate the fibers of Soleus between these landmarks in their resting state. Palpate with and across the grain of muscle fibers.

DIRECT AN ACTION AND PALPATE:

- Ask your client to point her toes. Palpate the fibers of Soleus during plantarflexion of the foot. Use your mother hand to add resistance, if necessary. Palpate with and across the grain of muscle fibers.

EVALUATE:

- Characterize your palpation feedback from Soleus: describe the tone, texture, and temperature of the muscle tissue.
- Note the presence of trigger points, tissue adhesions, barriers to palpation, or other findings.
- Compare palpation of both sides of Soleus, noting how the findings from the second palpation vary.
- Compare with palpations of Soleus on other clients, noting how the palpation findings on this client differ or are similar.

Lab Activity 9–4 on page 394 is designed to develop your palpation skills on superficial muscles that act on the leg and foot.

SUMMARY

With the completion of the palpations described in this chapter, you have successfully palpated the superficial muscles of the body in their entirety. In Chapter 10, Palpating Deeper Muscles and Muscle Groups, you are challenged to utilize your palpation skills for assessment of deeper structures.

LAB ACTIVITIES

LAB ACTIVITY 9-1: PALPATING SUPERFICIAL MUSCLES THAT ACT ON THE ARM

1. Working with a partner, create a plan for palpating the following muscles: what position will you place your partner in to palpate these muscles? What bony landmarks will you locate? What actions will you direct her to perform? For which palpations is resistance appropriate?
   - Pectoralis major
   - Latissimus dorsi
   - Teres major
   - Supraspinatus
   - Infraspinatus
   - Teres minor
2. Perform palpations of each of the muscles, using the Four-Step Protocol.
3. What are the antagonist muscles in the actions of your target muscles? Discuss with your partner how palpations of these muscles might be incorporated into your assessment.
4. Evaluate: characterize your palpation findings, as described in the palpation instructions.
5. How did touch sensitivity enhance the palpation experience? What specific steps did you take during the palpations to increase or focus your touch sensitivity? What differences in touch sensitivity did you note in relation to the palpation pressure used?
6. Switch partners and repeat. Discuss and compare your experiences.

LAB ACTIVITY 9-2: PALPATING SUPERFICIAL MUSCLES THAT ACT ON THE FOREARM AND HAND

1. Working with a partner, create a plan for palpating the muscles listed below: what position will you place your partner in to palpate these muscles? What bony landmarks will you locate? What actions will you direct her to perform? For which palpations is resistance appropriate?
   - Biceps brachii
   - Brachialis
   - Brachioradialis
   - Triceps brachii
   - Anconeus
   - Forearm flexor group
   - Forearm extensor group
2. Perform palpations of these two muscle groups, using the Four-Step Protocol.
3. What are the antagonist muscles in the actions of your target muscles? Discuss with your partners how palpations of these muscles might be incorporated into your assessment.

4. Evaluate: characterize your palpation findings, as described in the palpation instructions.

5. How did touch sensitivity enhance the palpation experience? What specific steps did you take during the palpations to increase or focus your touch sensitivity? What differences in touch sensitivity did you note in relation to the palpation pressure used?

6. Switch partners and repeat. Discuss and compare your experiences.

LAB ACTIVITY 9–3: PALPATING SUPERFICIAL MUSCLES THAT ACT ON THE THIGH

1. Working with a partner, create a plan for palpating the muscles listed below: what position will you place your partner in to palpate these muscles? What bony landmarks will you locate? What actions will you direct her to perform? For which palpations is resistance appropriate?
   - Gluteus maximus
   - Gluteus medius
   - Tensor fasciae latae
   - The Adductor group
   - Pectineus
   - Gracilis
   - Sartorius

2. Perform palpations of these muscles together, using the Four-Step Protocol.

3. What are the antagonist muscles in the actions of your target muscles? Discuss with your partners how palpations of these muscles might be incorporated into your assessment.

4. Evaluate: characterize your palpation findings, as described in the palpation instructions.

5. How did touch sensitivity enhance the palpation experience? What specific steps did you take during the palpations to increase or focus your touch sensitivity? What differences in touch sensitivity did you note in relation to the palpation pressure used?

6. Switch partners and repeat. Discuss and compare your experiences.

LAB ACTIVITY 9–4: PALPATING SUPERFICIAL MUSCLES THAT ACT ON THE LEG AND FOOT

1. Working with a partner, create a plan for palpating the muscles listed below: what position will you place your partner in to palpate these muscles? What bony landmarks will you locate? What actions will you direct her to perform? For which palpations is resistance appropriate?
   - Quadriceps group
   - Hamstrings group
   - Tibialis anterior

- Extensor digitorum longus
- Peroneal group
- Gastrocnemius
- Soleus

2. Perform palpations of these muscles together, using the Four-Step Protocol.
3. What are the antagonist muscles in the actions of your target muscles? Discuss with your partners how palpations of these muscles might be incorporated into your assessment.
4. Evaluate: characterize your palpation findings, as described in the palpation instructions.
5. How did touch sensitivity enhance the palpation experience? What specific steps did you take during the palpations to increase or focus your touch sensitivity? What differences in touch sensitivity did you note in relation to the palpation pressure used?
6. Switch partners and repeat. Discuss and compare your experiences.

CASE PROFILES

Case Profile 1

Myla, 29, works as a sales consultant for an interior design firm. Myla carries a large, heavy portfolio of fabric samples with her to her sales calls, over her left shoulder. She also pitches in a softball league on weekends. Myla has persistent pain and stiffness in both shoulders and pain in her upper-right back. What muscles or muscle groups will you target for palpation on Myla? What client positions and draping will you use for these palpations?

Case Profile 2

Oscar, 45, plays soccer three evenings a week and coaches a soccer team on the weekends. He complains of burning pain down the back and close to the groin on the inside of his right thigh. The pain down the back of his thigh doesn't get better, even when he works out harder before and after soccer. What muscles or muscle groups will you target for Oscar? What client positions and draping will you use for these palpations?

Case Profile 3

Stephanie is a 22-year-old graduate student, majoring in dance. In addition to her dance classes and rehearsals, Stephanie teaches aerobics every weekend at a community center, on a hard concrete floor, to help pay for her tuition. Stephanie has pain in her right lateral knee and hip and experiences sharper pain in her left shin. What muscles or muscle groups will you target for palpation on Stephanie? What client positions and draping will you use for these palpations?

STUDY QUESTIONS

1. Describe palpation of the Posterior rotator cuff muscles: positioning, draping, actions to direct to your client, and using resistance.

2. How can you distinguish the actions of Teres major and Teres minor during palpation?

3. How can you effectively palpate Brachialis and distinguish it from Biceps brachii during flexion of the forearm at the humeroulnar joint?

4. What are some common causes of rotator cuff injuries?

5. What muscle or fascial structure will you target for palpation in your client who reports pain in the lateral knee?

6. In what way is your client's hand dominance a factor in assessing palpation results of your her forearm flexor and extensor muscles?

7. Describe the recommended positioning and draping for palpating the Adductor muscles.

8. How would you position your client to palpate Biceps femoris during extension of the thigh?

9. What is the function of the pes anserine in the medial knee?

10. Which muscles in this chapter might be best palpated with your client in side-lying position? Why?

Palpating Deeper Muscles and Muscle Groups

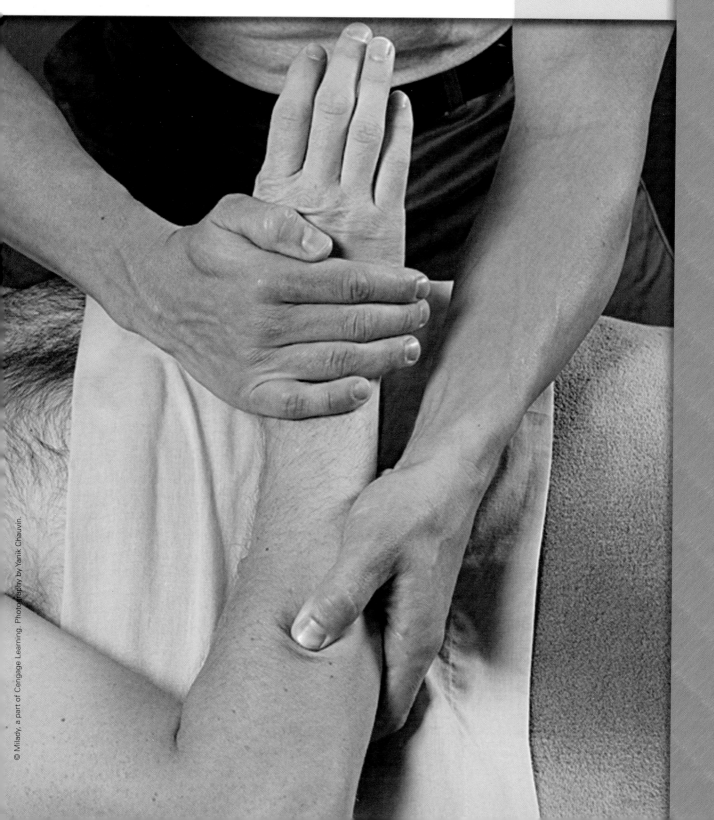

CHAPTER OUTLINE

- **CONSIDERATIONS IN PALPATION OF DEEPER MUSCLES**
- **DEEPER MUSCLES THAT ACT ON THE HEAD AND NECK**
- **DEEPER MUSCLES OF RESPIRATION**
- **DEEPER MUSCLES THAT ACT ON THE SPINE**
- **DEEPER MUSCLES THAT ACT ON THE SCAPULA**
- **DEEPER MUSCLES THAT ACT ON THE ARM AND FOREARM**
- **DEEPER MUSCLES THAT ACT ON THE WRIST AND HAND**
- **INTRINSIC MUSCLES OF THE HAND**
- **DEEPER MUSCLES THAT ACT ON THE THIGH**
- **DEEPER MUSCLES THAT ACT ON THE FOOT**
- **INTRINSIC MUSCLES OF THE FOOT**

LEARNING OBJECTIVES

- Apply safe and effective palpation techniques to deeper skeletal muscles and muscles of selected groups.

- Apply an understanding of client conditions resulting from strain or dysfunction in specific muscles and muscle groups to safe and effective palpation of those muscles and muscle groups.

CONSIDERATIONS IN PALPATION OF DEEPER MUSCLES

Palpation of deeper muscles may be indicated for a variety of reasons:

- When the symptoms of muscle pain or stiffness that a client reports are not supported by your findings from palpation of the superficial or intermediate muscles at the site of pain.
- When palpation of the specific agonist and antagonist muscles in the action that caused the pain does not result in enough information to form an assessment.
- Whenever palpation of superficial or intermediate muscles fails to provide the information you are looking for, deeper muscles are assessed.

Palpation of deeper muscles is obviously less direct than palpation of more superficial muscles, yet it can be a valuable assessment tool. Deeper palpation requires heightened touch sensitivity and, often, great patience. You must wait for the client's superficial tissue to "melt" beneath your palpating hands in order to access the deeper musculature. The client's sense of security and comfort during palpation of deeper muscles comes from your ease with the technique. In turn, your ease springs from your familiarity with the anatomy of the target structures. Confident palpation allows your client to feel secure. Practice these techniques until your touch is masterful.

> **HERE'S A TIP**
>
> During palpation of deeper muscles, you experience how the layering of muscles and the variance in fiber directions produces precise movements in groups of muscles.

Meet the Challenge of Deeper Palpation

Make these adjustments in the Four-Step Palpation Protocol:

- Palpate deeper muscles during a directed action, adding resistance whenever necessary. Palpation of the fibers of deeper muscles in their resting state is difficult.
- Palpate the muscle *only* in its resting state, however, if there is a chance that performing or resisting the directed action will elicit cramping or pain in the muscle.
- Move on to another assessment technique if palpation of a particular deep muscle on a particular client is not producing useful feedback or if it may cause painful compression of superficial tissues.

Maintain Client Safety and Comfort

Palpating deeper muscles is not always a comfortable process for the client. These steps will help to soften your client's palpation experience:

- Avoid palpating over the sites of delicate structures, such as nerves and blood vessels.
- Describe your intentions to your client. Demonstrate palpation on the non-injured target muscle and the action you wish your client to perform.
- Pay attention to the palpation feedback from superficial tissue. Avoid injuring superficial tissue in the effort to palpate deeper tissue.
- Resist the temptation to increase palpation pressure. Instead, work with your client's breath: synchronize your breathing to his, and slowly increase the depth of your palpatory touch on his exhalation.

Enlist the Body's Help

If you pay close attention, your client's body will help you in the process of deeper palpation:

- Superficial muscles "glide" over deeper muscles. The muscle that is gliding under your touch is not the target of deeper palpation. Direct your palpation attention toward the muscle *beneath* the muscle that glides beneath your touch.
- Remember that fascia turns from "gel-like to fluid" with the application of energy in the form of heat from your hands. Pay attention to the melting of fascia and the relaxation of superficial muscles that will make deeper target muscles more accessible for palpation.
- It's unlikely that the direction of all the fibers in the target muscle is identical to that of the superficial muscle. Use your knowledge of the fiber direction of the target muscle to assess the accuracy of your palpation.

DEEPER MUSCLES THAT ACT ON THE HEAD AND NECK

The deeper muscles included in this section are Rectus capitis major and minor and Obliquus capitis superior and inferior of the Suboccipital group in the posterior neck, along with Longus colli in the anterior neck. Posterior neck muscles usually extend the head at spinal joints. Anterior neck muscles usually flex the head at spinal joints.

Suboccipital Group

Deep in the posterior neck, the Suboccipital group [sub-ahk-SIP-ut-ul], shown in Figure 10–1 originates on C1, the Atlas, and C2, the Axis, and largely inserts onto the occiput along the nuchal lines. The fiber direction of the Suboccipital muscles described below is either vertical, *Rectus* [REK-tus], which means "erect," or diagonal, *Oblique* [oh-BLEEK], which means "at an angle," creating their actions of extension and ipsilateral rotation.

Sub-occipital

under occiput.

> ### DID YOU KNOW?
>
> In appearance, the shape and orientation of the Suboccipitals mirror the Hyoids, in the anterior neck.

IN THE TREATMENT ROOM

The Suboccipital muscles are assessed when a client reports upper-neck stiffness or bilateral headache pain that may spread from the occiput to the temporal region. Because the Suboccipitals lie deep to layers of tissue in the posterior neck, palpation is challenging.

Rectus

erect.

Capitis

head.

Attachments:
Rectus capitis posterior major
- Origin: spinous process of C2.
- Insertion: lateral on the inferior nuchal line of the occiput.

Rectus capitis posterior minor
- Origin: posterior arch of C1 and spinous process of C2.

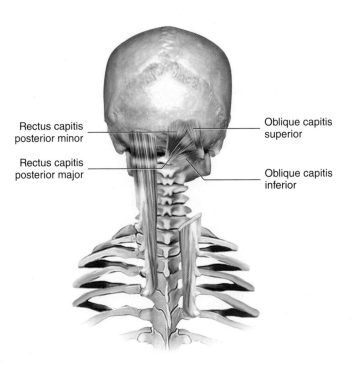

Rectus capitis posterior minor

Rectus capitis posterior major

Oblique capitis superior

Oblique capitis inferior

FIGURE 10–1 Suboccipital group.

■ Insertion: medial on the inferior nuchal line of the occiput.

Obliquus capitis superior

■ Origin: Transverse process of C1.

■ Insertion: between the inferior and superior nuchal lines of the occiput.

Obliquus capitis inferior

■ Origin: spinous process of C2.

■ Insertion: posterior on the transverse process of C1.

Actions:

Rectus capitis posterior major

■ Extends and laterally flexes the head and neck at the spinal joints.

Rectus capitis posterior minor

■ Extends the head and the neck at the spinal joints.

Obliquus capitis superior

■ Extends and ipsilaterally rotates the head at the spinal joints.

Obliquus capitis inferior

■ Ipsilaterally rotates the head at the spinal joints.

Placement:

■ Deep to Trapezius, Sternocleidomastoid (SCM), Splenius capitis, and Semispinalis of the Transversospinalis group and posterior to the spine.

Obliquus

oblique or diagonal fibers.

Palpation of the Suboccipital group:

POSITION:

■ Supine client. Undrape your client's neck.

■ Sit at the head of the table. Use both hands to palpate.

LOCATE AND PALPATE:

■ Warm the superficial muscles and tissues thoroughly, by massaging the area or applying a warm pack.

■ Place your hands beneath your client's occiput, as in Figure 10–2. To facilitate relaxation, encourage your client to breathe deeply and let his jaw drop slightly open.

■ Locate insertions of the Suboccipital muscles on the nuchal lines of the occiput, deep to thick layers of superficial muscle and fascia.

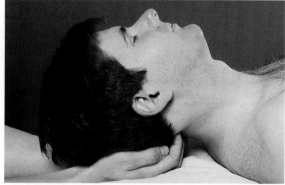

FIGURE 10–2 Palpating the Suboccipitals.

© Milady, a part of Cengage Learning. Photography by Yanik Chauvin.

■ Move the fingertips of your palpating hands medially and to the inferior on the occiput, toward the Suboccipital origins on C1 and C2. Allow time for the superficial tissues to relax and melt beneath your hands.

■ Palpate the Rectus capitis and Obliquus capitis muscles in their resting state. Palpate with and across the grain of muscle fibers.

INITIATE AN ACTION AND PALPATE:

- With one hand, gently rotate your client's head ipsilaterally, while continuing to palpate the same-side Suboccipitals during passive ipsilateral rotation.
- With both hands, gently allow an increase in the degree of extension of your client's head. Palpate the Suboccipitals during passive extension.

EVALUATE:

- Characterize your palpation feedback from the Suboccipitals: describe the tone, texture, and temperature of the muscle tissue.
- Note the presence of trigger points, tissue adhesions, barriers to palpation, or other findings.
- Compare palpation of both sides of the Suboccipitals, noting how the findings from the second palpation vary.
- Compare with palpations of the Suboccipitals on other clients, noting how the findings from palpation on this client differ or are similar.

Splenius

patch.

Splenius Capitis

Together, Splenius capitis [SPLEE-nee-us KAP-uh-tis] and the deeper Splenius cervicis [SPLEE-nee-us SUR-vuh-sis], shown in Figure 10–3, form a "V" in the posterior neck, just as Sternocleidomastoid (SCM), forms a "V" in the anterior neck. Splenius capitis is somewhat palpable for part of its length, though it lies deep to both Trapezius and the Rhomboids. Splenius cervicis is not palpable.

Attachments:

- Origin: inferior nuchal ligament and the spinous processes of C7–T4.

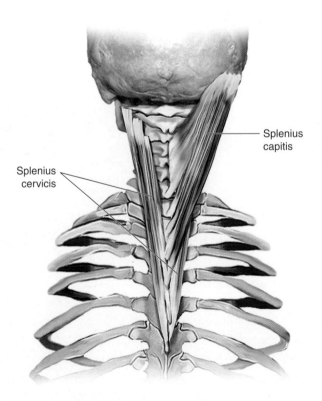

Splenius
capitis

Splenius
cervicis

FIGURE 10-3 Splenius capitis is superficial to Splenius cervicis, and more palpable.

- Insertion: mastoid process of the temporal bone and the lateral occiput.

Actions:

- Bilateral: extends the head and the neck at the spinal joints.
- Unilateral: ipsilaterally rotates the head at the spinal joints.

Placement:

- Splenius capitis is deep to Trapezius and SCM.
- Splenius cervicis is deep to Splenius capitis.

Palpation of Splenius Capitis:

POSITION:

- Prone client: undrape your client's neck and upper back.
- Stand or sit at the side of the table. Use your mother hand to support your client's head.

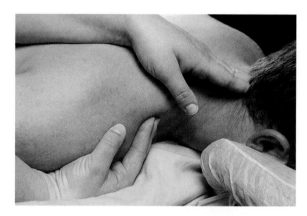

FIGURE 10–4 Palpating Splenius capitis with the client in prone position.

© Milady, a part of Cengage Learning. Photography by Yanik Chauvin.

LOCATE AND PALPATE:

- Locate the lateral border of the upper fibers of Trapezius, the largest mass of superficial muscle tissue in the posterior neck, and the mastoid process of the temporal bone, as shown in Figure 10–4. You may notice the proximal attachment of SCM on the mastoid process.
- Palpate the fibers of Splenius capitis in their resting state between these landmarks, with the fingertips of your palpating hand in the inverted V-shaped trough between upper Trapezius and SCM. Palpate with and across the grain of muscle fibers.

DIRECT AN ACTION AND PALPATE:

- Ask your client to lift his head slightly from the face cradle: palpate Splenius capitis during extension of the head.
- Ask your client to turn his head slightly. Palpate Splenius capitis on the same side during ipsilateral rotation of the head. Palpate with and across the grain of muscle fibers.

EVALUATE:

- Characterize your palpation feedback from Splenius capitis: describe the tone, texture, and temperature of the muscle tissue.
- Note the presence of trigger points, tissue adhesions, barriers to palpation, or other findings.
- Compare palpation of both sides of Splenius capitis, noting how the findings from the second palpation vary.
- Compare with palpations of Splenius capitis on other clients, noting how the findings from palpation on this client differ or are similar.

HERE'S A TIP

Do not add resistance to the actions of Splenius capitis. To do so may cause injury to your client.

Colli

neck.

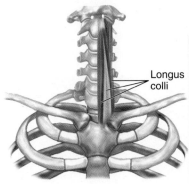

FIGURE 10-5 Longus colli.

Longus Colli

Longus colli [LONG-us KAHL-eye] is located on the anterior surface of the cervical spine. Longus colli, shown in Figure 10–5, is one of the muscles most often injured in a whiplash-type injury: as the head is snapped backward, Longus colli is forcefully stretched beyond its normal range of motion.

IN THE TREATMENT ROOM

Because Longus colli lies very deep in the anterior neck, its palpation requires gently moving aside anterior neck structures such as the trachea and SCM, to gain access to the anterior cervical spine. Encourage your client to relax his neck and to let his head get "heavy." Palpate as he exhales. Note that the common carotid artery is nearby. Move your hand immediately away from any area where pulsing is felt. In order to follow the roundedness of the anterior neck with the natural curve of your palpating hand, work across the table, as shown in Figure 10–6.

Attachments:
- Origin: anterior tubercles of transverse processes of C3–6.
- Insertion: anterior surface of bodies of C4 and anterior tubercles of C5–6.

Actions:
- Flexes, laterally flexes, and ipsilaterally rotates the head at the spinal joints.

Placement:
- Deep to the Hyoids, the trachea, and the esophagus in the anterior cervical region, and anterior to the spine.

Palpation of Longus Colli:

HERE'S A TIP

Palpating deeply into the anterior neck can be scary for both you and the client. Review the placement of nearby blood vessels and nerves to build your confidence in this palpation.

POSITION:
- Supine client. Undrape your client's neck.

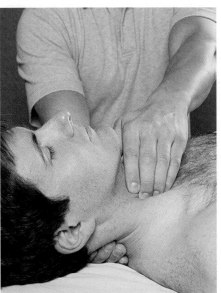

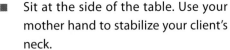

- Sit at the side of the table. Use your mother hand to stabilize your client's neck.

LOCATE AND PALPATE:
- Working across the table, locate the medial border of the opposite SCM with the fingertips of your palpating hand. Take care to avoid resting your hand on your client's throat. To facilitate location of the medial border of SCM, ask your client to turn his head toward your palpating hand.
- Gently work your fingertips in between the medial border of SCM and the trachea, just inferior to the hyoid bone, as shown in Figure 10–6.

FIGURE 10-6 Palpating Longus colli.

- Check in with your client, to be sure he is comfortable with this palpation.
- Continue to press gently but firmly toward the lateral aspect of the anterior cervical spine. Locate and palpate the vertical fibers of Longus colli in their resting state.

DIRECT AN ACTION AND PALPATE:

- Ask your client to lift his head slightly up from the table. Palpate Longus colli during flexion of the head.
- Ask your client to bend his head toward his shoulder and palpate Longus colli during lateral flexion of the head.
- Ask your client to turn his head away from your palpating hand and palpate Longus colli during ipsilateral rotation of the head.

EVALUATE:

- Characterize your palpation feedback from Longus colli: describe the tone, texture, and temperature of the muscle tissue.
- Note the presence of trigger points, tissue adhesions, barriers to palpation, or other findings.
- Compare palpation of both sides of Longus colli, noting how the findings from the second palpation vary.
- Compare with palpations of Longus colli on other clients, noting how the findings from palpation on this client differ or are similar.
- Do not add resistance to the actions of Longus colli.

IN THE TREATMENT ROOM

SCM also flexes and laterally flexes the neck. It may interfere with palpation of the inferior fibers of Longus colli during these actions.

DEEPER MUSCLES OF RESPIRATION

Deeper muscles that participate in respiration include the Diaphragm, Serratus posterior superior, and Serratus posterior inferior.

The Diaphragm

The Diaphragm [DY-uh-fram] is the main muscle of respiration. It is one of the rare skeletal muscles whose control is both involuntary and voluntary. Normal, quiet respiration is involuntary, but when the body needs oxygen, the respiratory centers in the brain send nerve impulses to exert voluntary control over the Diaphragm to increase the volume of air taken in. As seen in Figure 10–7, the Diaphragm has no bony insertion. Instead, it inserts into a large central tendon that attaches to the connective tissue surrounding the lungs.

Only a small anterior segment of the Diaphragm is palpable. Accurate palpation is more likely during the client's exhalation as the Diaphragm ascends into the chest cavity. Suggest some slow, deep breaths to your

Diaphragm

midriff or partition.

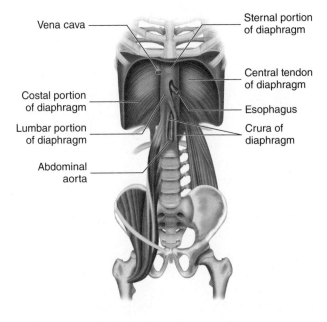

FIGURE 10-7 The Diaphragm and associated structures.

client to engage voluntary control of respiration, before you palpate his Diaphragm.

Attachments:

- Origin: the xiphoid process, lower six ribs and their costal cartilage, and ligaments, bodies, and transverse processes of upper lumbar vertebrae.
- Insertion: a central tendon into connective tissue surrounding the lungs.

Actions:

- Contraction or descending of the Diaphragm increases the volume of the thoracic cavity during inhalation, while relaxation or ascending of the Diaphragm decreases the volume of the thoracic cavity during exhalation.

Placement:

- Transverse in the thoracic cavity, deep to the ribs and external and internal Intercostal muscles, and separates the thoracic cavity from the abdominal cavity.

IN THE TREATMENT ROOM

Palpation of the Diaphragm may be hampered by upper-belly fat in some clients. Placing your client in side-lying position may ease access for this palpation.

HERE'S A TIP

It may be helpful to ask your client to cough once as you sink your fingertips into the abdomen to palpate the Diaphragm. This brief contraction of the abdominal muscles demonstrates to your client that he is in control of the depth of your palpation in this region.

Palpation of the Diaphragm:

POSITION:

- Supine client. Place a bolster beneath his knees to slacken the abdomen.
- Palpate through the drape or undrape the abdomen and cover your female client's breast area with a towel.
- Sit or stand at the side of the table. Use your mother hand to stabilize the ribcage, or palpate with both hands.

LOCATE AND PALPATE:

- Work across your client's body, as shown in Figure 10–8. Place the fingertips of your palpating hand or the thumbs of both hands beneath the costal cartilage of the inferior ribs, lateral to the xiphoid process. Avoid exerting pressure over the xiphoid process.

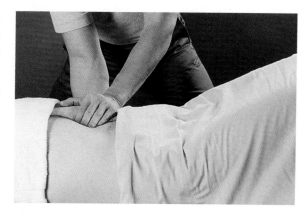

FIGURE 10–8 Palpating the Diaphragm.

© Milady, a part of Cengage Learning. Photography by Yanik Chauvin.

DIRECT AN ACTION AND PALPATE:

- Ask your client to take in a slow, deep breath.
- As your client begins to exhale, palpate beneath the inferior ribs as the Diaphragm ascends in the thoracic cavity.

EVALUATE:

- Characterize your palpation of the Diaphragm: describe the position that worked best for this palpation and how much of the Diaphragm was palpable.
- Note the presence of trigger points, tissue adhesions, barriers to palpation, or other findings.
- Compare with palpations of the Diaphragm on other clients, noting how the findings from palpation on this client differ or are similar.

Serratus Posterior Superior (SPS)

Serratus [ser-RAT-us] posterior superior, SPS, elevates the upper ribs on the posterior during deep inhalation, expanding the capacity of the thoracic cavity, just as Pectoralis minor elevates the same ribs on the anterior (Figure 10–9).

Attachments:
- Origin: spinous processes of C7–T2 and the nuchal ligament.
- Insertion: posterior surfaces of ribs #2–5.

Actions:
- Elevates ribs #2–5 during deep inhalation at the scapulocostal joints.

Serratus

serrated or notched like the edge of a saw.

HERE'S A TIP

Serratus posterior superior lies deep in the upper back. It may be best palpated during the initial stage of deep inhalation, provided the overlying muscles have been relaxed.

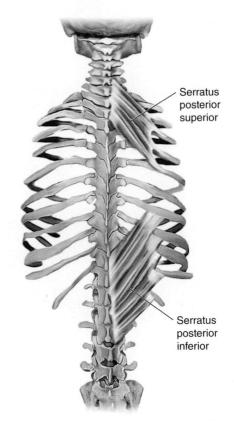

FIGURE 10-9 Serratus posterior superior and inferior.

Placement:

■ Deep to Trapezius and Rhomboids, superficial to the Erector spinae and Transversospinalis muscles in the thoracic region.

Palpation of Serratus Posterior Superior:

POSITION:

■ Prone client. Undrape your client's back and abduct his arm, allowing it to drape off the table.

■ Stand at the head of the table. Use both hands for palpation.

LOCATE AND PALPATE:

■ Warm the superficial muscles and tissues thoroughly, by massaging the area or applying a warm pack.

■ Place your palpating hands along each side of the spine, between the spine and the medial border of the scapula. Allow your hands to slowly relax and melt through the superficial tissues overlying both sides of SPS, as shown in Figure 10–10.

■ Focus your attention on the serrated shape of SPS as it inserts onto ribs #2–5.

■ Synchronize your breathing with your client's, encouraging slow, rhythmic breaths.

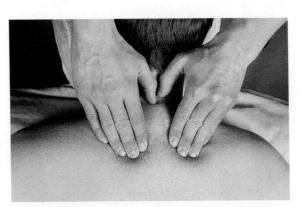

FIGURE 10-10 Palpating Serratus posterior.

DIRECT AN ACTION AND PALPATE:

- Ask your client to inhale deeply and palpate the diagonal fibers and serrated insertions of SPS during elevation of ribs #2–5.

EVALUATE:

- Characterize your palpation feedback from Serratus posterior superior: describe the tone, texture, and temperature of the muscle tissue.
- Note the presence of trigger points, tissue adhesions, barriers to palpation, or other findings.
- Compare palpation of SPS on both sides of the trunk, noting how the findings from the second palpation vary.
- Compare with palpations of SPS on other clients, noting how the findings from palpation on this client differ or are similar.

Serratus Posterior Inferior (SPI)

Both Serratus posterior inferior, SPI, and SPS originate on spinous processes of the spine and insert onto ribs. With their fibers oriented diagonally to one another, they act together in deep, forceful inhalation: as SPS lifts upper ribs to expand the chest cavity for deeper inhalation, SPS stabilizes or holds in place the lower ribs.

SPI lies deep to Latissimus dorsi and superficial to the Erector spinae group in the low back. It is best palpated when Latissimus dorsi is relaxed, although if SPI is also relaxed, Latissimus dorsi may be difficult to locate. Serratus posterior inferior is visible in Figure 10–9.

IN THE TREATMENT ROOM

Its action of stabilization of ribs, instead of movement of ribs, makes palpation of Serratus posterior inferior difficult during a directed action.

Attachments:
- Origin: spinous processes of T11–12.
- Insertion: inferior borders of ribs #9–12.

Actions:
- Stabilizes or depresses ribs #9–12 at the vertebrocostal joints during deep inhalation.

Placement:
- Deep to Latissimus dorsi and superficial to the Erector spinae and Transversospinalis muscles in the lower thoracic and lumbar regions.

Palpation of Serratus Posterior Inferior:

POSITION:

- Prone client. Undrape your client's back.
- Stand at the side of the table. Use both hands for palpation.

LOCATE AND PALPATE:

- Warm the superficial muscles and tissues thoroughly, by massaging the area or applying a warm pack.

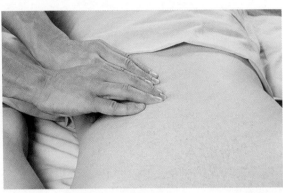

FIGURE 10–11 Palpating Serratus posterior inferior.

- Place your palpating hands along each side of the spine, in the lumbar region. Allow your hands to slowly relax and melt through the superficial tissues overlying both sides of Serratus posterior inferior, as shown in Figure 10–11.

- Focus your attention on the serrated shape of Serratus posterior inferior as it inserts onto ribs #9–12.

- Synchronize your breathing with your client's, encouraging slow, rhythmic breaths.

DIRECT AN ACTION AND PALPATE:

- Ask your client to breathe deeply and on his inhalation palpate the diagonal fibers and serrated insertions of SPI as they stabilize ribs #9–12.

EVALUATE:

- Characterize your palpation feedback from Serratus posterior inferior: describe the tone, texture, and temperature of the muscle tissue.

- Note the presence of trigger points, tissue adhesions, barriers to palpation, or other findings.

- Compare palpation of both sides of SPI, noting how the findings from the second palpation vary.

- Compare with palpations of SPI on other clients, noting how the findings from palpation on this client differ or are similar.

DEEPER MUSCLES THAT ACT ON THE SPINE

Deeper muscles included in this section include the Erector spinae and Transversospinalis groups and Quadratus lumborum, which lies between these two groups in the lumbar region.

Erector Spinae Group: Spinalis, Iliocostalis, and Longissimus

The Erector spinae group [ih-REK-tur SPY-nuh], sometimes called the paraspinals, forms the prominent bulge along each side of the spine, as shown in Figure 10–12. Spinalis [spy-NAY-lis], Iliocostalis [ih-lee-oh-kahs-TAY-lis], and Longissimus [lahn-JISS-ih-mus] share common origins on the sacrum and the pelvis, are contained within a sheath arising from the thoracolumbar fascia, and insert onto the posterior trunk at multiple sites from the lumbar region to the occiput. As prime extensors of the spine, the Erector spinae muscles support the posture of the torso by holding the torso erect.

The Erector spinae muscles lie deep in the posterior trunk, but their bulk on each side of the lumbar spine, especially in clients with

Erector

holds upright.

Spinae

spine.

Spinalis

"of the spine."

Ilio

of the ilium.

Costal

the ribs.

Longissiumus

"long".

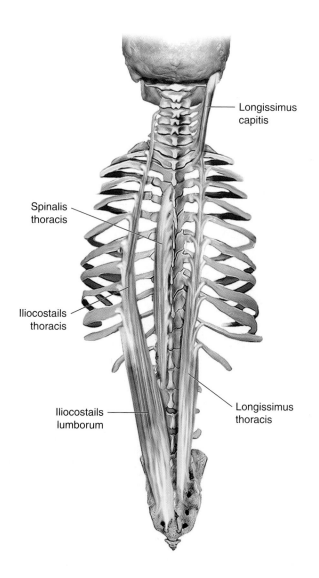

Longissimus
capitis

Spinalis
thoracis

Iliocostails
thoracis

Iliocostails
lumborum

Longissimus
thoracis

FIGURE 10-12 The Erector
spinae muscle group: Spinalis,
Iliocostalis, and Longissimus.

© Delmar, Cengage Learning.

well-developed muscles, renders them palpable. The Erectors are
most easily palpated as a group, in three regions: lumbar, thoracic, and
cervical.

Group attachments:

- Origins: the posterior medial iliac crest and the sacrum; transverse processes of vertebrae and ribs.

- Insertions: superior transverse and spinous processes of vertebrae, superior ribs and the occiput, and the mastoid process of
the temporal bone.

Group actions:

- Unilateral: laterally flexes and ipsilaterally rotates the trunk and
the head at the spinal joints and anteriorly tilts the pelvis at the
sacrolumbar joint.

- Bilateral: extends the trunk and the head at the spinal joints.

Group placement:

- Deep to Latissimus dorsi in the lumbar region, deep to Serratus
posterior superior and inferior, Trapezius, the Rhomboids, and

Splenius capitis in the thoracic and cervical regions. Superficial to the Suboccipital muscles in the cervical region and to the Transversospinalis muscles in the lumbar, thoracic, and cervical regions.

Palpation of Spinalis, Iliocostalis, and Longissimus:

POSITION:

- Prone client. Undrape your client's back.
- Stand at the side of the table. Use your mother hand to add resistance to movement or use both hands to palpate.

LOCATE AND PALPATE:

- Warm the superficial muscles and tissues thoroughly, by massaging the area or applying a warm pack.

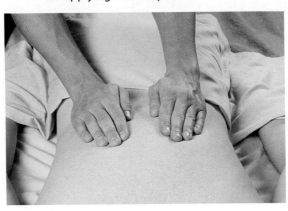

FIGURE 10–13 Palpation of the Erector spinae muscle group.

- Place one hand along each side of your client's lumbar spine, as in Figure 10–13, where the Erector spinae muscles are most prominent. Move each hand slightly laterally to palpate the breadth of the muscle group in the lumbar region. Palpate with and across the grain of muscle fibers.

- The thoracic and cervical segments of the Erector spinae muscles are less prominent and are much more difficult to palpate in their resting state.

DIRECT AN ACTION AND PALPATE:

- Ask your client to raise his head and upper trunk off the surface of the table. Add gentle resistance with your mother hand, if necessary, and palpate each side of the lumbar Erector spinae muscles individually during extension of the trunk.
- If resistance is not added, palpate both sides of the lumbar Erector spinae muscles simultaneously during extension of the trunk.
- Repeat the procedure in the thoracic and cervical regions of the Erector spinae group.

EVALUATE:

- Characterize your palpation feedback from the Erectors: describe the tone, texture, and temperature of the muscle tissue.
- Note the presence of trigger points, tissue adhesions, barriers to palpation, or other findings.
- Compare palpation of both sides of the Erectors, noting how the findings from the second palpation vary.
- Compare with palpations of the Erectors on other clients, noting how the findings from palpation on this client differ or are similar.

OPTION:

For palpation during lateral flexion of the trunk at the spinal joints:

- With your client in side-lying position, un-drape his back, tucking the drape securely.
- Stand facing your client, as in Figure 10–14. Use your mother hand to add resistance to movement.
- Place your mother hand on your client's shoulder. Ask your client to lift his torso off the table as you resist the movement. Palpate the Erector spinae muscles during lateral flexion of the trunk.

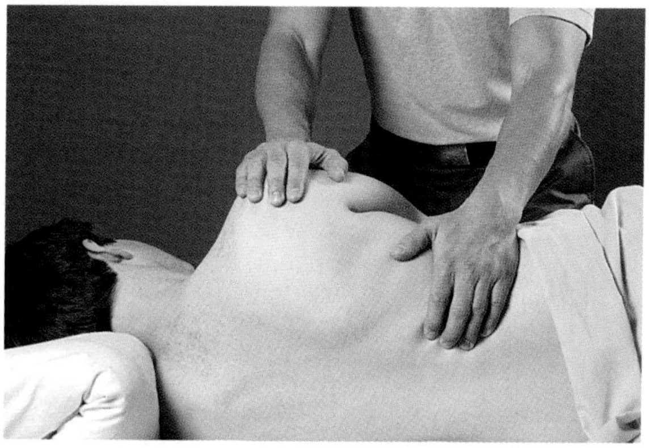

FIGURE 10–14 Side-lying palpation of the Erectors during their unilateral actions.

© Milady, a part of Cengage Learning. Photography by Yanik Chauvin.

HERE'S A TIP

To palpate during both lateral flexion and ipsilateral rotation at the spinal joints, ask your client to remain clothed and seated. Stand behind your client, direct the appropriate actions, and palpate through his clothing.

IN THE TREATMENT ROOM

The ease or difficulty of palpating the Erector spinae muscles is created in part by the nature of your client's spinal curvatures: the muscles in this group will be deeper or more superficial, depending on the region and degree of deviation from normal. In a client with an exaggerated thoracic curve, kyphosis or hyperkyphosis, the thoracic-level Erectors will be more superficial. The lumbar Erectors may be deeper in a client whose lumbar curve results in lordosis or hyperlordosis, a lumbar curve that is exaggerated to the anterior.

In a client with an "S" or "C" shaped scoliosis curve in the lumbar region, the Erector spinae muscles in one side of the spine will be chronically lengthened, while those on the other side of the spine will be "jammed" or shortened, as seen in Figure 10–15. Either finding will be palpable.

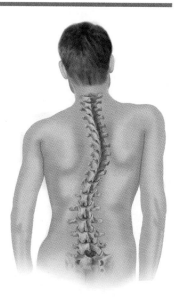

FIGURE 10–15 In a client with scoliosis, the Erector spinae muscles in one side of the spine will be chronically lengthened, while those on the other side of the spine will be "jammed" or shortened.

© Milady, a part of Cengage Learning.

Transverso

transverse processes.

Spinalis

refers to spinous processes.

Multi

many.

Rotatores

rotational.

Transversospinalis Group: Semispinalis, Multifidus, and Rotatores

The Transversospinalis group [tranz-vur-soh-spy-NAY-lis] lies deep to the Erector spinae muscles and also extends in segments from the pelvis to the head, as seen in Figure 10–16. The segments of Rotatores spinae [roh-tuh-TOHR-ees] extend from one vertebra to the vertebra directly above; segments of Multifidus [mul-TIF-ih-dus] span two to four vertebrae, while Semispinalis [sem-ee-spy-NAY-lis] extends in three regions, from T12 to the occiput.

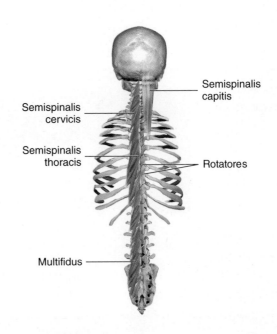

Semispinalis
capitis

Semispinalis
cervicis

Semispinalis
thoracis

Rotatores

Multifidus

FIGURE 10–16 The Transversospinalis muscle group: Semispinalis, Multifidus, and Rotatores.

HERE'S A TIP

Of the muscles in this group, Multifidus may be palpable in the lumbar and lower thoracic region and Semispinalis may be palpable in the cervical region. The Rotatores are too deep to be palpated.

It is quite difficult to distinguish the Transversospinalis muscles from the Erector spinae muscles, but it is worth trying!

Group attachments:
- Origins: posterior sacrum and PSIS; transverse processes of vertebrae.
- Insertions: spinous processes and laminae of vertebrae, to the occiput.

Group actions:
- Unilateral: lateral flexion and contralateral rotation of the trunk and head at the spinal joints.
- Bilateral: extension of the trunk and head at the spinal joints and anterior tilt of the pelvis at the lumbosacral joint.

Placement:
- Deep to Latissimus dorsi in the lumbar region; deep to Trapezius, SCM, the Rhomboids, and Splenius capitis in the thoracic and cervical regions; deep to the Erector spinae muscles in the lumbar, thoracic, and cervical regions. Superficial to the Suboccipital muscles in the cervical region.

Palpation of Multifidus and Semispinalis:

POSITION:
- Prone client. Undrape your client's back.
- Stand at the side of the table. Use your mother hand to add resistance to movement or use both hands to palpate.

LOCATE AND PALPATE:

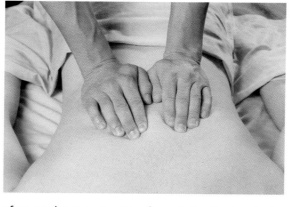

© Milady, a part of Cengage Learning. Photography by Yanik Chauvin.

- Warm the superficial muscles and tissues thoroughly, by massaging the area or applying a warm pack.
- Place one hand along each side of your client's lumbar spine, as in Figure 10–17, where Multifidus may be most palpable. Direct the focus of your palpatory attention through the Erectors to the deepest layer of muscles. Palpate with and across the grain of muscle fibers.
- The cervical segments of Semispinalis are much more difficult to palpate in their resting state.

FIGURE 10–17 Palpating Semispinalis and Multifidus.

DIRECT AN ACTION AND PALPATE:

- Ask your client to raise his head and upper trunk off the surface of the table. Add gentle resistance with your mother hand, if necessary, and palpate each side of the lumbar region of Multifidus individually during extension of the trunk.
- Repeat your instruction and resistance while palpating Semispinalis in the cervical region during extension of the trunk.

EVALUATE:

- Characterize your palpation feedback from the Transversospinalis muscles: were you able to palpate them and distinguish them from the Erectors?
- If you can, describe the tone, texture, and temperature of the muscle tissue.
- Note the presence of trigger points, tissue adhesions, barriers to palpation, or other findings.
- Compare palpation of both sides of the Transversospinalis muscles, noting how the findings from the second palpation vary.
- Compare with palpations of the Transversospinalis muscles on other clients, noting how the findings from palpation on this client differ or are similar.

OPTION:

For palpation during lateral flexion of the trunk:

- With your client in side-lying position, undrape his back, tucking the drape securely.
- Stand facing your client, as in Figure 10–14. Use your mother hand to add resistance to movement.
- Place your mother hand on your client's shoulder. Ask your client to lift his torso off the table as you resist the movement. Palpate the Transversospinalis muscles during lateral flexion of the trunk.

Quadratus Lumborum

Known as "QL," Quadratus lumborum [kwah-DRA-tus lum-BOHR-um] is considered a primary muscle to assess and treat in clients with persistent, urgent low-back pain. Visible in Figure 10–18, QL is both a mover, in lateral flexion of the spine and elevation of the pelvis, and a stabilizer,

Quadratus

square.

Lumborum

of the lumbar spine.

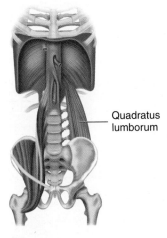

Quadratus
lumborum

FIGURE 10–18 Quadratus
lumborum.

because it attaches to the 12th rib and stabilizes it during respiration. Some sources consider QL an accessory muscle of respiration. Quadratus lumborum is a major source of low-back pain, because it participates in many compound movements of the trunk and hip—walking, stepping up stairs, getting out of a car, and so on.

HERE'S A TIP

In clients with deviations in the normal spinal curvature, which includes nearly everyone, Quadratus lumborum may be significantly impacted and therefore, vulnerable to injury: one side may be chronically shortened or "jammed," while the other side is chronically lengthened. Quadratus lumborum should be assessed and palpated on any client with low-back pain.

IN THE TREATMENT ROOM

The square-shaped Quadratus lumborum lies deep to the lumbar Erectors and may be difficult to palpate on clients whose lumbar Erectors are well developed. QL's vertical fibers can best be palpated by hooking your fingertips beneath the lateral border of the lumbar Erectors, as shown in Figure 10–19, to palpate the lateral fibers of QL unilaterally.

Attachments:
- Origin: posterior iliac crest.
- Insertion: transverse processes of L1–4 and the 12th rib.

Actions:
- Unilateral: laterally flexes the trunk at the spinal joints and elevates the pelvis at the lumbosacral joint.
- Bilateral: extends the trunk at the spinal joints.

Placement:
- Deep to the Erector spinae group.

Palpation of Quadratus Lumborum:

POSITION:
- Prone client. Undrape your client's back.
- Stand at the side of the table. Use your mother hand to add resistance to movement or use both hands to palpate.

LOCATE AND PALPATE:
- Warm the superficial muscles and tissues thoroughly, by massaging the area or applying a warm pack.
- Locate the posterior iliac crest and the 12th rib. Hook the fingertips of your palpating hand beneath the bulk of the lumber Erectors in this area, as shown in Figure 10–19, and palpate medially to reach the lateral edge of the vertical fibers of Quadratus lumborum in their resting state.

DIRECT AN ACTION AND PALPATE:

- Place your mother hand along the superior border of the posterior iliac crest to provide resistance. Ask your client to push his hip against your mother hand and palpate one side of Quadratus lumborum during unilateral elevation of the pelvis.

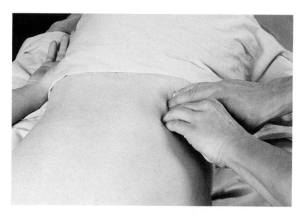

FIGURE 10-19 Palpating Quadratus lumborum with your client prone.

© Milady, a part of Cengage Learning. Photography by Yanik Chauvin.

EVALUATE:

- Characterize your palpation feedback from Quadratus lumborum: describe the tone, texture, and temperature of the muscle tissue.
- Note the presence of trigger points, tissue adhesions, barriers to palpation, or other findings.
- Compare palpation of both sides of Quadratus lumborum, noting how the findings from the second palpation vary: is one side jammed or stretched?
- Compare with palpations of Quadratus lumborum on other clients, noting how the findings from palpation on this client differ or are similar.

OPTION:

For palpation during lateral flexion of the trunk:

- With your client in side-lying position, undrape his back, tucking the drape securely.
- Stand facing your client and work across the table, as shown in Figure 10–20. Use your mother hand to add resistance to movement.
- Place your mother hand on your client's shoulder. Ask your client to lift his torso off the table as you resist the movement. Palpate Quadratus lumborum during lateral flexion of the trunk at the spinal joints.

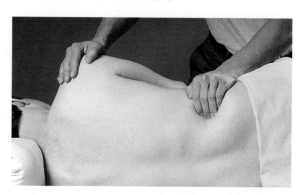

FIGURE 10-20 Palpating Quadratus lumborum with your client in side-lying position.

© Milady, a part of Cengage Learning. Photography by Yanik Chauvin.

DEEPER MUSCLES THAT ACT ON THE SCAPULA

The deeper muscle in this group is Pectoralis minor.

Pectoralis Minor

Pectoralis minor lies deep to Pectoralis major in the anterior chest, as shown in Figure 10–21. Its attachment on the coracoid process of the scapula is shared with Coracobrachialis and the short head of Biceps

Pectoralis

chest or breast.

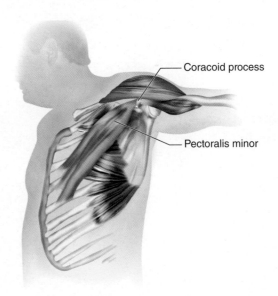

Coracoid process

Pectoralis minor

FIGURE 10–21 Pectoralis minor.

© Milady, a part of Cengage Learning.

brachii. Because it elevates ribs to expand the chest cavity, Pectoralis minor is considered an accessory muscle of respiration.

HERE'S A TIP

Palpation of Pectoralis minor may be uncomfortable for some clients. Proceed slowly and with care. Work with your client's breath and check on his comfort level during the palpation.

Attachments:
- Origin: anterior ribs #3–5.
- Insertion: coracoid process of the scapula.

Actions:
- Protracts and depresses the scapula at the scapulocostal joints.
- Elevates ribs #3–5 during forceful inhalation.

Placement:
- Deep to Pectoralis major.

Palpation of Pectoralis Minor:

POSITION:
- Supine client. Undrape your client's arm and upper chest. Take care to drape the breast area securely. Your female client may prefer to hold the drape with her hand and immobilize breast tissue during this palpation.
- Abduct your client's arm to 90°.
- Stand at the side of the table. Use your mother hand to manipulate your client's arm.

LOCATE AND PALPATE:
- Warm the superficial muscles and tissues thoroughly, by massaging the area or applying a warm pack.

- Standing beside your client, support your client's passively abducted arm at the elbow. Place the fingertips of your palpating hand beneath the anterior axillary fold, as shown in Figure 10–22 taking care to avoid the breast tissue of a female client.

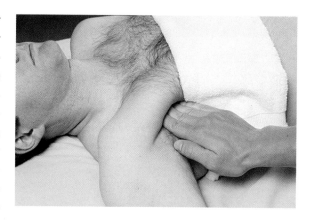

FIGURE 10–22 Palpating Pectoralis minor on a supine client.

© Milady, a part of Cengage Learning. Photography by Yanik Chauvin.

- Palpate medially, deep to Pectoralis major, along the curve of the upper ribcage. Slightly adduct your client's arm horizontally to move Pectoralis major out of the way.

- The fibers of Pectoralis minor are perpendicular to the ribs. Palpate Pectoralis minor in its resting state between these landmarks. Palpate gently. Pectoralis minor may be quite tender. Palpate with and across the grain of muscle fibers.

DIRECT AN ACTION AND PALPATE:

- Ask your client to take in a quick, deep breath. Palpate Pectoralis minor during inhalation. Palpate with and across the grain of muscle fibers.

- Adding resistance to movement is not appropriate in palpation of Pectoralis minor.

EVALUATE:

- Characterize your palpation feedback from Pectoralis minor: describe the tone, texture, and temperature of the muscle tissue.

- Note the presence of trigger points, tissue adhesions, barriers to palpation, or other findings.

- Compare palpation of Pectoralis minor on both sides of the anterior trunk, noting how the findings from the second palpation vary.

- Compare with palpations of Pectoralis minor on other clients, noting how the findings from palpation on this client differ or are similar.

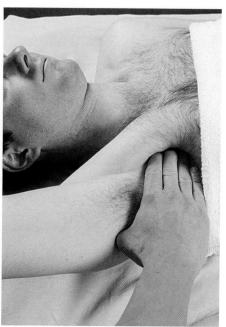

OPTIONS:

Place your client in side-lying position to alter the position of breast tissue, or leave your client in the supine position and change the direction of your palpating hand, as shown in Figure 10–23:

- Stand behind your client. Use your mother hand to support his arm in slight extension.

FIGURE 10–23 Alternate position for palpating Pectoralis minor.

© Milady, a part of Cengage Learning. Photography by Yanik Chauvin.

- Proceed with palpation of Pectoralis minor as described above.

Pectoralis minor syndrome

one type of Thoracic outlet syndrome in which Pectoralis minor entraps nearby structures: the shoulders are rounded to the anterior when protraction of the scapula is sustained by a tight Pectoralis minor and are not counterbalanced due to weakness in Serratus anterior.

Lab Activity 10–1 on page 455 is designed to develop your palpation skills on deeper muscles that act on the axial skeleton.

IN THE TREATMENT ROOM

Pectoralis minor is assessed when postural assessment reveals shoulders that are rounded to the anterior. When protraction of the scapula is sustained by a tight Pectoralis minor and is not counterbalanced due to weakness in Serratus anterior, the result is a chronically rounded shoulder. Pectoralis minor is also assessed for **Pectoralis minor syndrome**, one type of Thoracic outlet syndrome (TOS), in which a chronically tight Pectoralis minor may entrap nearby nerves, ligaments, and blood vessels, as shown in Figure 10–24. Sometimes caused by a whiplash injury or repetitive strain of Pectoralis minor or Serratus anterior, symptoms of Pectoralis minor syndrome occur on the same side of the body as the injury, and may include numbness and tingling in the hand and fingers; pain in the upper anterior chest, shoulder, and arm; and weakness in the arm and hand. The client may be unable to grasp and hold an object without dropping it. In a client with Pectoralis minor syndrome, the muscle itself may also be very tender to the touch.

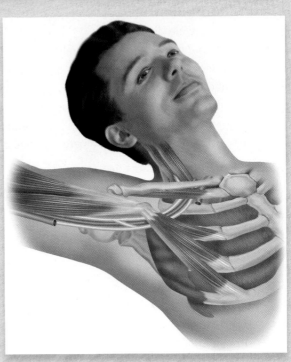

FIGURE 10–24 Pectoralis minor syndrome is one form of TOS.

DEEPER MUSCLES THAT ACT ON THE ARM AND FOREARM

Muscles described in this section include Subscapularis, the anterior Rotator cuff muscle; Coracobrachialis, which is deep to Biceps brachii; and Pronator teres and Supinator, which oppose each other in the proximal forearm. Muscles in this section flex, adduct, and medially rotate the arm at the shoulder, and pronate and supinate the forearm at the proximal radioulnar joint.

HERE'S A TIP

When describing joint and muscle actions, note the following:

- "Arm" refers to the upper extremity from the shoulder joint to the elbow joint.
- "Forearm" refers to the upper extremity from the elbow joint to the wrist joint.
- "Thigh" refers to the lower extremity from the hip joint to the knee joint.
- "Leg" refers to the lower extremity from the knee joint to the ankle joint.

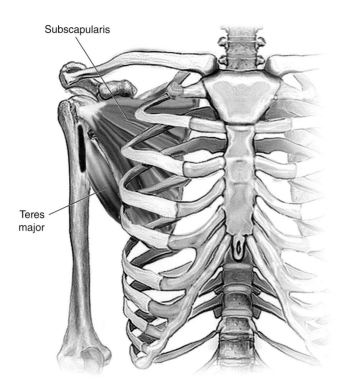

Subscapularis

Teres
major

© Milady, a part of Cengage Learning.

FIGURE 10–25 Subscapularis, anterior view.

Subscapularis

Because Subscapularis [sub-skap-yuh-LAYR-us] originates on the anterior scapula, as seen in Figure 10–25, and inserts onto the medial aspect of the humerus, it works with Latissimus dorsi and Teres major to medially rotate the humerus in opposition to Infraspinatus and Teres minor. Note in Figure 10–25 the proximity of the fibers of Latissimus dorsi and Teres major to those of Subscapularis.

Sub

under or beneath.

Scapularis

of the scapula.

HERE'S A TIP

Subscapularis cannot be palpated in its entirety, but its lateral fibers can be palpated on the anterior aspect of the lateral border of the scapula. Palpation of Subscapularis may be more challenging on clients with limited or restricted scapular movement, though this also indicates assessment and treatment of Subscapularis.

Be sure your palpation is *deep to* the lateral border of the scapula. Teres major, another medial rotator of the arm, attaches to the inferior lateral border of the scapula. You might confuse Teres major with the lateral fibers of Subscapularis.

Attachments:
- Origin: anterior surface, the subscapular fossa, of the scapula.
- Insertion: lesser tubercle of the humerus.

Actions:
- Medially rotates the humerus at the glenohumeral joint.

Placement:
- On the anterior surface of the scapula.

Palpation of Subscapularis:

POSITION:

- Side-lying client. Undrape your client's upper back and arm.
- Support your client's arm in passive flexion to 90°.
- Stand at the side of the table, facing your client. Use your mother hand to stabilize your client's shoulder during movement or to add resistance to movement during palpation.

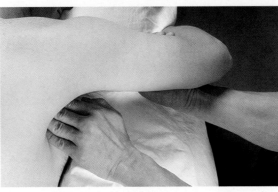

© Milady, a part of Cengage Learning.
Photography by Yanik Chauvin.

FIGURE 10–26 Palpate Subscapularis with your client in side-lying position.

LOCATE AND PALPATE:

- Holding your client's arm in passive flexion, as in Figure 10–26, locate the lateral or axillary border of the scapula with your palpating hand. Slide your fingertips or your thumb toward the medial aspect of the head of the humerus.
- Add slight traction to your client's arm as you palpate beneath the scapula, on its anterior surface. The lateral fibers of Subscapularis are slightly palpable.
- Palpate the lateral fibers of Subscapularis in their resting state.

DIRECT AN ACTION AND PALPATE:

- Ask your client to turn his arm so that he can see his elbow. Palpate the lateral portion of Subscapularis during medial rotation of the humerus.

EVALUATE:

- Characterize your palpation feedback from Subscapularis: describe the tone, texture, and temperature of the muscle tissue.
- Note the presence of trigger points, tissue adhesions, barriers to palpation, or other findings.
- Compare palpation of both sides of Subscapularis, noting how the findings from the second palpation vary.
- Compare with palpations of Subscapularis on other clients, noting how the findings from palpation on this client differ or are similar.

OPTION:

With your client supine:

- Abduct your client's arm. Proceed as for palpation of Serratus anterior, described in Chapter 8, Palpating Superficial Muscles of the Axial Skeleton, turning your attention to the lateral portion of the anterior scapula and directing your client to medially rotate his arm as an action.

| **Coraco** |
| of the coracoid process of the scapula. |

| **Brachialis** |
| of the arm. |

Coracobrachialis

Coracobrachialis [kor-uh-koh-bray-kih-AY-lis] shares its proximal attachment on the coracoid process of the scapula with Pectoralis minor and the short head of Biceps brachii. In fact, its proximal fibers may blend with those of Biceps. Coracobrachialis assists Biceps brachii in flexion of the arm

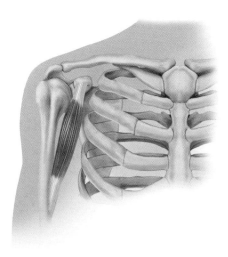

FIGURE 10-27 Coracobrachialis.

at the shoulder. Since they share that action and their fibers may blend, Coracobrachialis is most easily palpable during adduction of the arm at the glenohumeral joint. Coracobrachialis is shown in Figure 10–27.

Attachments:

- Origin: coracoid process of the scapula.
- Insertion: medial shaft of the humerus.

Actions:

- Flexes and adducts the humerus at the glenohumeral joint.

Placement:

- Deep to Deltoid, Pectoralis major, and the short head of Biceps brachii.

Palpation of Coracobrachialis:

POSITION:

- Supine client. Undrape your client's arm and upper chest. Take care to drape the breast area securely.
- Abduct your client's arm to about 45°.
- Stand at the side of the table. Use your mother hand to support the elbow and provide resistance to movement.
- You may ask your female client to use her free hand to secure breast tissue during this palpation.

LOCATE AND PALPATE:

- Warm the superficial muscles and tissues thoroughly, by massaging the area or applying a warm pack.
- Locate the insertion of Coracobrachialis on the medial humerus, about one-third down its length, between the bellies of Brachialis and Triceps brachii, as shown in Figure 10–28.
- Locate the coracoid process of the scapula.

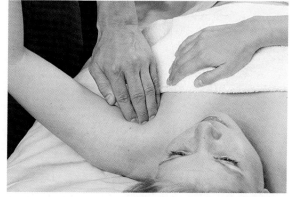

FIGURE 10-28 Palpating Coracobrachialis.

HERE'S A TIP

The more horizontal direction of Coracobrachialis' fibers should help you discern it from Pectoralis minor and the short head of Biceps brachii at the attachment site on the coracoid process of the scapula.

Palpate the vertical fibers of Coracobrachialis between its attachments, in their resting state. Palpate with and across the grain of muscle fibers.

DIRECT AN ACTION AND PALPATE:

- Place your mother hand along your client's distal medial arm. Ask him to push against your hand as you palpate Coracobrachialis during adduction of the arm. Palpate with and across the grain of muscle fibers.

EVALUATE:

- Characterize your palpation feedback from Coracobrachialis: describe the tone, texture, and temperature of the muscle tissue.
- Note the presence of trigger points, tissue adhesions, barriers to palpation, or other findings.
- Compare palpation of both sides of Coracobrachialis, noting how the findings from the second palpation vary.
- Compare with palpations of Coracobrachialis on other clients, noting how the findings from palpation on this client differ or are similar.

Pronator teres

refers to its action of pronation round.

Supinator

refers to its action of supination.

FIGURE 10-29 Pronator teres, Supinator, and Pronator quadratus.

Pronator Teres; Supinator

Pronator teres [proh-NAY-tohr TIHR-ees] works with the distal and deeper Pronator quadratus to pronate the forearm. Supinator [SOO-puh-nayt-ur] lies deep in the proximal, posterior forearm, is assisted in supination of the forearm by Biceps brachii, and opposes Pronator teres. It is easiest to palpate Pronator teres and Supinator at the same time, as described next, during the unresisted actions of pronation and supination. Both Pronator teres and Supinator are visible in Figure 10–29.

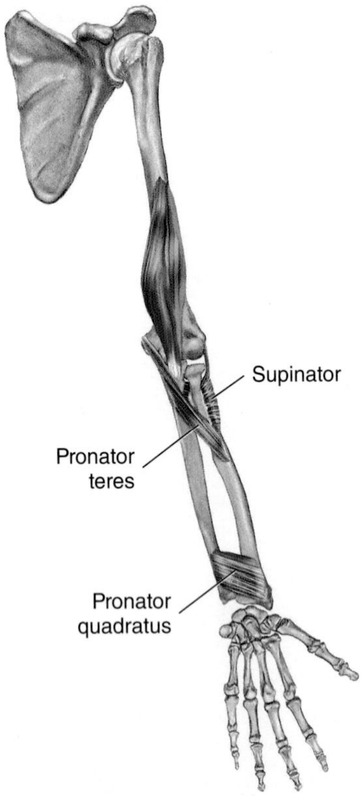

DID YOU KNOW?

Palpation of Pronator quadratus is not advisable. Its depth in the distal anterior wrist would make palpation in this area painful.

Pronator teres attachments:
- Origin: medial epicondyle of the humerus, via the common flexor tendon shared with Forearm flexor muscles.
- Insertion: mid-lateral surface of the radius.

Actions:
- Pronates the forearm at the radioulnar joints and assists in flexion of the forearm at the elbow.

Placement:
- Proximally, superficial. Distally, deep to Brachioradialis.

Supinator attachments:
- Origin: lateral epicondyle and the ulna, below the radial notch.
- Insertion: lateral surface of the proximal radius.

Actions:
- Supinates the forearm at the proximal radioulnar joint.

Placement:
- Deep to Forearm flexors.

Palpation of Pronator Teres and Supinator:

POSITION:

- Supine client. Undrape your client's arm.
- Stand or sit at the side of the table. Use your mother hand to support your client's forearm or to add resistance.

LOCATE AND PALPATE:

- Place your client's hand in the handshake position, midway between pronation and supination. Grasp his forearm with your palpating hand, as shown in Figure 10–30, with your thumb and fingertips placed just

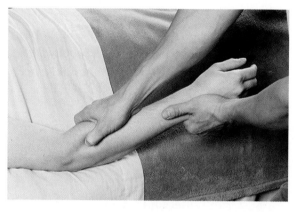

FIGURE 10-30 Palpating Pronator teres and Supinator simultaneously.

© Milady, a part of Cengage Learning. Photography by Yanik Chauvin.

distal to the elbow joint, anterior and posterior to Brachioradialis. Your thumb will palpate one of the target muscles as your fingertips palpate the other.

- Palpate between the superficial layers of forearm flexor and extensor muscles to reach the horizontal fibers of Pronator teres on the anterior and Supinator on the posterior. Palpate both muscles in their resting state. Palpate with and across the grain of muscle fibers.

DIRECT AN ACTION AND PALPATE:

- Ask your client to turn his palm toward the floor and then back up again, as you resist the action with your mother hand. Palpate Pronator teres and Supinator during pronation and supination of the forearm at the radioulnar joints. Palpate with and across the grain of muscle fibers.

EVALUATE:

- Characterize your palpation feedback from Pronator teres and Supinator: describe the tone, texture, and temperature of the muscle tissue.
- Note the presence of trigger points, tissue adhesions, barriers to palpation, or other findings.
- Compare palpation of both sides of Pronator teres and Supinator, noting how the findings from the second palpation vary.
- Compare with palpations of Pronator teres and Supinator on other clients, noting how the findings from palpation on this client differ or are similar.

DEEPER MUSCLES THAT ACT ON THE WRIST AND HAND

Palpation of the deep Forearm flexors and extensors, described in this section, is challenging. Client comfort must be maintained, and the individual muscles can be difficult to distinguish from one another.

Forearm Flexors

Muscles that flex the hand at the wrist share a common origin on the medial epicondyle of the humerus but have varying insertions, depending on whether or not they also act on the fingers of the hand. Among the palpable muscles of the Forearm flexor group, the tendons of Palmaris longus and Flexor carpi radialis are the longest. The tendons of Flexor carpi ulnaris and Flexor digitorum superficialis arise more distally. In the palpations described below, the Flexors are palpated as a group, from the radial aspect to the ulnar aspect of the anterior forearm. *Refer to the Table 1–7, Muscle Name Components, to help you locate each forearm muscle according to the clues in its name.*

Flexor Carpi Radialis

Flexor carpi radialis [FLEK-sur KAR-pih ray-dee-AY-lis] is visible in Figure 10–31.
    Attachments:
    ■   Origin: medial epicondyle of the humerus.
    ■   Insertion: base of metacarpals II and III.
    Actions:
    ■   Flexion and radial deviation of the hand at the radiocarpal joint.
    Placement:
    ■   Superficial in the anterior forearm.

Palmaris Longus

Palmaris longus [pahl-MAYR-is LONG-us] is also visible in Figure 10–31.
    Attachments:
    ■   Origin: medial epicondyle of the humerus.
    ■   Insertion: palmar aponeurosis.
    Actions:
    ■   Flexes the hand at the radiocarpal joint.
    Placement:
    ■   Superficial in the anterior forearm.

Fslexor Digitorum Superficialis

Flexor digitorum superficialis [FLEK-sur dij-ih-TOR-um soo-pur-fish-ee-AY-lis] is visible in Figure 10–32.
    Attachments:
    ■   Origin: medial epicondyle of the humerus and the coronoid process of the ulna.
    ■   Insertion: anterior surfaces of middle phalanges of digits #2–5, via its four tendons.

HERE'S A TIP

Working accurately and confidently helps to maintain client comfort during the repeated requests for resisted movement.

Radialis

the radius.

Palmaris

the palmar surface of the hand.

Digitorum

the digits.

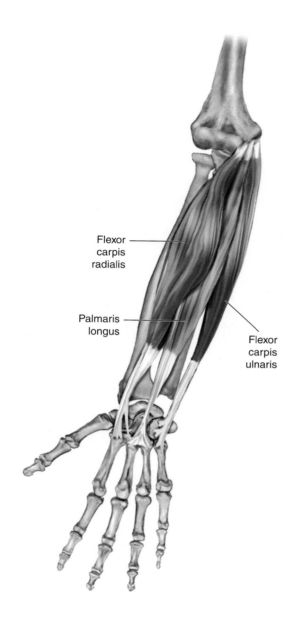

FIGURE 10-31 Flexor carpi radialis, Flexor carpi ulnaris, and Palmaris longus.

Actions:

■ Flexes digits #2–5 at the MCP and IP joints.

Placement:

■ Superficial in the anterior forearm.

Flexor Carpi Ulnaris

Flexor carpi ulnaris [FLEK-sur KAR-pih ul-NAYR-is] is visible along with Flexor carpi radialis and Palmaris longus in Figure 10–31.

Attachments:

■ Origin: medial epicondyle of the humerus.
■ Insertion: carpals and base of metatarsal V.

Actions:

■ Flexion and ulnar deviation of the hand at the radiocarpal joint.

Placement:

■ Superficial on the ulnar aspect of the anterior forearm.

Carpi ulnaris

wrist of the ulna.

HERE'S A TIP

When palpating the Forearm flexor muscles, work carefully in the distal aspect to avoid exerting pressure over the median, radial, and ulnar nerves, as well as the blood vessels that travel through the carpal tunnel.

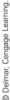

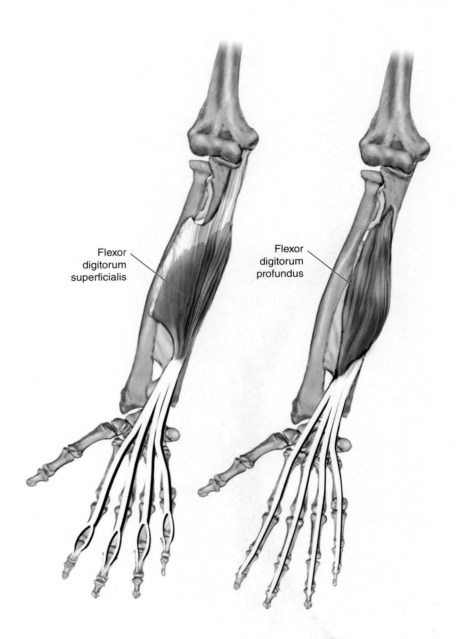

Flexor digitorum superficialis

Flexor digitorum profundus

FIGURE 10-32 Flexor digitorum superficialis.

Palpation of Flexor Carpi Radialis, Palmaris Longus, Flexor Digitorum Superficialis, and Flexor Carpi Ulnaris:

POSITION:

- Supine client. Undrape your client's arm.
- Stand or sit at the side of the table. Use your mother hand to add resistance.

LOCATE AND PALPATE:

- Locate the distal tendon of Flexor carpi radialis, which is prominent in the anterior forearm, just medial to Brachioradialis.
- Locate the distal tendon of Palmaris longus, which is superficial to the Flexor retinaculum as it inserts into the Palmar aponeurosis.
- Locate the distal tendon of Flexor digitorum superficialis, which splits into four segments distal to the Flexor retinaculum and inserts onto digits #2–5.

- Locate the Flexor retinaculum over the anterior wrist. Locate the distal tendon of Flexor carpi ulnaris just distal to the retinaculum, on the ulnar aspect of the carpals.
- Locate the shared proximal attachment on the medial epicondyle of the humerus, as pictured in Figure 10–33, and palpate the common flexor tendon.

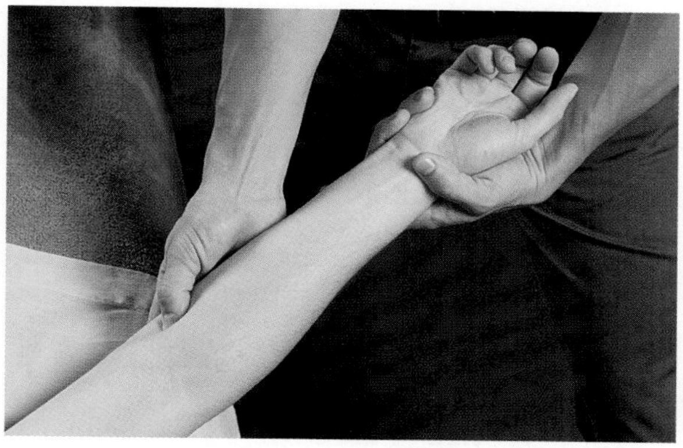

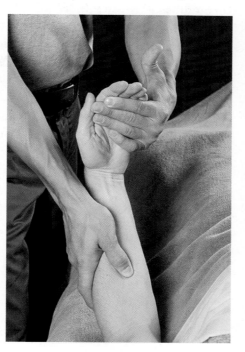

FIGURE 10–33 Palpating the Forearm flexors.

© Milady, a part of Cengage Learning. Photography by Yanik Chauvin.

- Palpate the lengthy tendon and vertical fibers of each Forearm flexor, toward the belly of its muscle. Palpate the fibers in their resting state, with and across the grain.
- In addition, palpate the four tendons of Flexor digitorum superficialis in the proximal direction, from the anterior surfaces of the digits through palmar aponeurosis and the Flexor retinaculum to the broad intermediate tendon, deep to the thin, distal tendon of Palmaris longus, toward the belly of its muscle. Palpate the fibers in their resting state, with and across the grain.

DIRECT AN ACTION AND PALPATE:

- Hold your client's hand securely with your mother hand, as shown in Figure 10–34. Ask him to push his hand against yours while you palpate the fibers of Flexor carpi radialis, Palmaris longus, and Flexor digitorum superficialis in flexion of the hand.
- Ask your client to turn his wrist away from the table as you palpate the fibers of Flexor carpi radialis during abduction of the hand.
- Ask your client to turn his wrist toward the table as you palpate the fibers of Flexor carpi ulnaris during adduction of the hand.
- Do not allow your client to maintain an isometric contraction. Ask him to perform an action once and relax before performing it again, or to push against your hand, then relax before pushing again.

FIGURE 10–34 Palpating the Forearm flexors against resistance.

© Milady, a part of Cengage Learning. Photography by Yanik Chauvin.

EVALUATE:

- Characterize your palpation feedback from the Forearm flexor muscles: describe the tone, texture, and temperature of the muscle tissue.
- Note the presence of trigger points, tissue adhesions, barriers to palpation, or other findings.

■ Compare palpation of both sides of the Forearm flexor muscles, noting how the findings from the second palpation vary.

■ Compare with palpations of the Forearm flexor muscles on other clients, noting how the findings from palpation on this client differ or are similar.

IN THE TREATMENT ROOM

Cautions apply when palpating the Forearm flexors and extensors. Blood vessels travel through toward the hand, and client comfort must be maintained. Look for blood vessels and avoid any area where pulsing is felt.

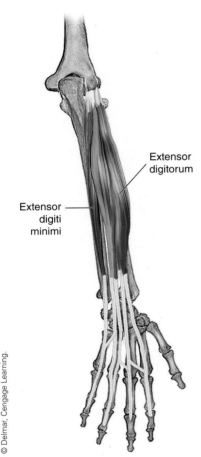

Extensor digitorum

Extensor digiti minimi

© Delmar, Cengage Learning.

FIGURE 10–35 Extensor digitorum and Extensor digiti minimi.

Forearm Extensors

Muscles that extend the hand at the wrist share a common origin on the lateral epicondyle of the humerus but varying insertions, depending on whether or not they also act on the fingers of the hand. The tendinous portions of the forearm extensors arise more distally than those of the flexors, with that of Extensor carpi radialis longus extending most proximally in the lateral posterior forearm. The Extensors are palpated as a group, working both medially and laterally from the prominent and intermediate Extensor digitorum.

Extensor Digitorum

Extensor digitorum [ik-STEN-sur dij-ih-TOHR-um] is shown in Figure 10–35.

Attachments:

■ Origin: lateral epicondyle of the humerus.

■ Insertion: posterior surfaces of digits #2–5.

Actions:

■ Extends digits #2–5 at the MCP and IP joints.

Placement:

■ Superficial in the posterior forearm.

Extensor Carpi Radialis Brevis

Extensor carpi radialis brevis [ik-STEN-sur KAR-pih ray-dee-AY-lis BREH-vis] is seen in Figure 10–36.

Attachments:

■ Origin: lateral epicondyle of the humerus.

■ Insertion: dorsal surface of the base of metacarpal III.

Actions:

■ Extends the hand at the radiocarpal joint.

Placement:

■ Mostly superficial in the posterior forearm on the radial side.

Extensor Carpi Radialis Longus

Extensor carpi radialis longus [ik-STEN-sur KAR-pih ray-dee-AY-lis LONG-us] is also visible in Figure 10–36.

Attachments:

- Origin: lateral supracondylar ridge of the humerus.
- Insertion: dorsal surface of metacarpal II.

Actions:

- Extends and abducts the hand at the radiocarpal joint.

Placement:

- Superficial in the posterior forearm.

Extensor Digiti Minimi

Extensor digiti minimi [ik-STEN-sur DIJ-ih-ty MIN-ih-mee] is visible along with Extensor digitorum in Figure 10–35.

Attachments:

- Origin: lateral epicondyle of the humerus.
- Insertion: digit #5, the "little" finger.

Actions:

- Extends the little finger at the MCP and IP joints.

Placement:

- Superficial in the posterior forearm.

Extensor Carpi Ulnaris

Extensor carpi ulnaris [ik-STEN-sur KAR-pih ul-NAYR-us] is visible along with Extensor carpi radialis longus and Extensor radialis brevis in Figure 10–36.

Attachments:

- Origin: lateral epicondyle of the humerus.
- Insertion: dorsal surface of the base of metacarpal III.

Actions:

- Extends and adducts the hand at the radiocarpal joint.

Placement:

- Extensor carpi ulnaris is superficial in the posterior forearm.

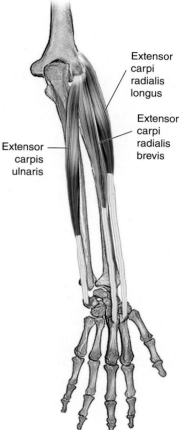

Digiti minimi

little finger, digit #5.

Extensor carpi radialis longus

Extensor carpi radialis brevis

Extensor carpis ulnaris

© Delmar, Cengage Learning.

FIGURE 10–36 Extensor carpi radialis longus and brevis; Extensor carpi ulnaris.

Palpation of Extensor Digitorum, Extensor Carpi Radialis Brevis, Extensor Carpi Radialis Longus, Extensor Digiti Minimi, and Extensor Carpi Ulnaris:

POSITION:

- Supine client. Undrape your client's arm and drape it across his abdomen.
- Stand or sit at the side of the table. Use your mother hand to add resistance.

LOCATE AND PALPATE:

- Locate the common extensor tendon and the lateral supracondylar ridge of the humerus.
- Locate and palpate the Extensor retinaculum over the posterior wrist, as pictured in Figure 10–37.
- Locate the distal tendon of Extensor digitorum, which splits into four visible segments distal to the Extensor retinaculum and inserts onto digits #2–5. Its tendon is broad and intermediate as it travels beneath the Extensor retinaculum in the posterior forearm. Its distal tendons are readily palpable on the dorsal hand and

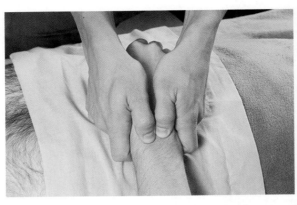

FIGURE 10–37 Palpating the Extensor Retinaculum.

- on the dorsal surfaces of digits #2–5. Extensor digitorum has the most prominent muscle belly in the posterior forearm.
- Locate the vertical fibers of Extensor carpi radialis brevis, toward the radial aspect. Its distal tendon is deep to muscles that act on the thumb.
- Locate the distal tendon of Extensor carpi radialis longus on the radial aspect of the posterior forearm. At the wrist, it also lies deep to muscles that act on the thumb. Locate it proximal to these muscles.
- Locate the distal tendon of Extensor digiti minimi, toward the ulnar aspect from Extensor digitorum, palpable on the dorsal surface of digit #5, the little finger.
- Locate the distal tendon of Extensor carpi ulnaris, on the ulnar aspect of the posterior forearm, just posterior to the belly of Flexor carpi ulnaris. Its distal tendon does not extend onto the dorsal surface of the hand.
- Palpate the vertical fibers of the prominent tendons of Extensor digitorum, from their insertion on the posterior surface of the digits through the dorsal hand toward the muscle belly in the intermediate posterior forearm. Palpate the muscle belly fibers in their resting state, with and across the grain of fibers.
- Palpate the tendons and vertical fibers of each other Forearm extensor muscle, in their resting state. Palpate with and against the grain of fibers.

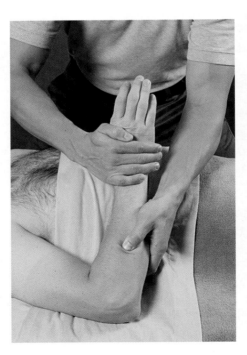

FIGURE 10–38 Palpating the deep Forearm extensors against resistance.

DIRECT AN ACTION AND PALPATE:

- Support your client's hand in your mother hand. Ask him to bend his fingers backward, as you palpate Extensor digitorum during extension of fingers #2–5 at the MCP and IP joints.
- Hold your client's hand securely with your mother hand, as shown in Figure 10–38. Ask his to push his hand against yours as you palpate the fibers of the remaining extensor muscles during extension of the hand.
- Ask your client to turn his hand toward his thumb and palpate Extensor carpi radialis longus during abduction of the hand.
- Ask your client to turn his hand toward his little finger and palpate Extensor carpi ulnaris during adduction of the hand.

EVALUATE:

- Characterize your palpation feedback from the Forearm extensor muscles: describe the tone, texture, and temperature of the muscle tissue.

- Note the presence of trigger points, tissue adhesions, barriers to palpation, or other findings.
- Compare palpation of both sides of the Forearm extensor muscles, noting how the findings from the second palpation vary.
- Compare with palpations of the Forearm extensor muscles on other clients, noting how the findings from palpation on this client differ or are similar.

IN THE TREATMENT ROOM

Lateral epicondylitis, also called tennis elbow, and **Medial epicondylitis**, also called golfer's elbow, are common causes of elbow pain and inflammation, due to overuse of the Forearm flexor and extensors muscles and/or Anconeus, that attach to the medial and lateral epicondyle of the humerus. Symptoms of Lateral epicondylitis, shown in Figure 10–39—misnamed, because the cause is more likely to involve gripping or lifting than playing tennis—include pain and tenderness in response to touch on the lateral elbow. Pain may radiate down the arm and worsens during extension of the forearm. Symptoms of Medial epicondylitis, shown in Figure 10–40, are similar, on the medial aspect of the elbow, with the same radiation of pain, but with worsening during flexion of the forearm. Symptoms of bursitis in the elbow, a similar inflammation, typically are felt on the posterior and do not usually radiate down the arm. Because symptoms of these conditions include inflammation, palpate carefully. Avoid sites of heat, swelling, or redness.

Lateral epicondylitis

also called tennis elbow, a condition including pain, inflammation, and tenderness to touch at or near the lateral epicondyle of the humerus; often follows intensive lifting or gripping.

Medial epicondylitis

also called golfer's elbow, a condition including pain, inflammation, and tenderness to touch at or near the lateral epicondyle of the humerus; common in golfers.

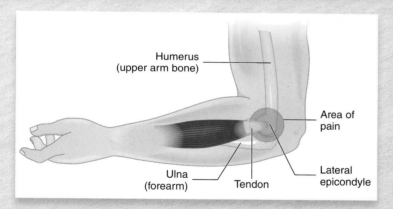

FIGURE 10–39 Lateral epicondylitis, or "tennis elbow."

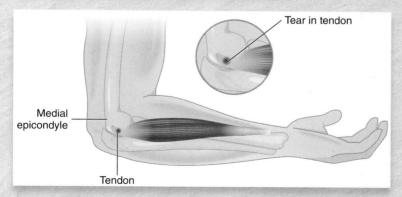

FIGURE 10–40 Medial epicondylitis, or "golfer's elbow."

INTRINSIC MUSCLES OF THE HAND

The intrinsic muscles of the hand have their origins and insertion within the hand. These muscles do not cross the radiocarpal joint. They act only on the digits of the hand, the thumb, and fingers.

The intrinsic muscles described below for palpation include those of the thenar and hypothenar eminences of the hand and the Palmar and Dorsal interossei.

Muscles of the Thenar and Hypothenar Eminence of the Hand

The thenar eminence [THEE-nar EM-uh-nents] is a large, fleshy mound at the base of the thumb, on the palmar surface of the hand, shown in Figure 10–41, which comprises three muscles that abduct, flex, and oppose the thumb. All share origins on the flexor retinaculum and various carpal bones. These three muscles, Abductor pollicis brevis, Flexor pollicis brevis, and Opponens pollicis, are often assessed in habitual computer users and electronic game players, who routinely overuse their thumbs. The muscle fibers are quite dense and when bruised, may be slow to heal.

The hypothenar eminence [hy-PAHTH-uh-nahr EM-uh-nents] is a somewhat smaller, fleshy mound on the ulnar side of the palmar surface of the hand, also visible in Figure 10–40, comprising three muscles that act on the little finger. These muscles, too, share origins on the carpal bones and the flexor retinaculum and their actions mirror those of the muscles of the thenar eminence. The muscles of the hypothenar eminence, Abductor digiti minimi manus, Flexor digiti minimi manus, and Opponens digiti minimi manus, abduct, flex, and oppose the little finger and are palpable on the ulnar side of the palmar surface.

Abductor Pollicis Brevis

Abductor pollicis brevis [ab-DUK-tur PAHL-ih-sus BREH-vis] is visible in Figure 10–42.

Attachments:
- Origin: trapezium and scaphoid carpal bones and the flexor retinaculum.
- Insertion: radial aspect of the proximal phalanx of the thumb.

Thenar

the hand.

Pollicis

the thumb.

Hypo

smaller.

HERE'S A TIP

The palpation instructions that follow are for palpation of your client supine on the table. You may, of course, palpate the intrinsic muscles of the hand on a clothed and seated client. You may also choose to palpate the muscles of both eminences simultaneously.

DID YOU KNOW?

Massage therapists who work with poor hand positioning may strain the muscles of the thenar eminence by overworking their thumbs.

FIGURE 10–41 The thenar and hypothenar eminences of the hand.

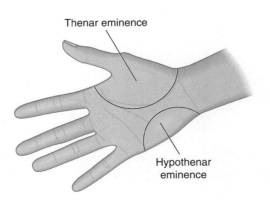

Thenar eminence

Hypothenar eminence

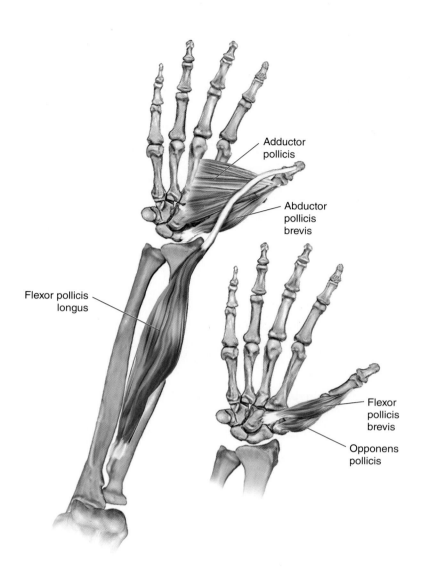

Adductor
pollicis

Abductor
pollicis
brevis

Flexor pollicis
longus

Flexor
pollicis
brevis

Opponens
pollicis

FIGURE 10–42 Muscles of the thenar eminence: Flexor pollicis brevis, Abductor pollicis brevis, and Opponens pollicis.

© Delmar, Cengage Learning.

Actions:

■ Abducts the thumb (digit #1) at the first carpometacarpal joint.

Placement:

■ The superficial muscle of the thenar eminence.

Flexor Pollicis Brevis

Flexor pollicis brevis [FLEK-sur PAHL-ih-sus BREH-vis] is also visible in Figure 10–42.

Attachments:

■ Origin: trapezium, trapezoid, and capitate carpal bones and the flexor retinaculum.

■ Insertion: radial aspect of the proximal phalanx of the thumb.

Actions:

■ Flexes the proximal phalanx of the thumb and assists in opposition of the thumb at the first carpometacarpal joint.

Placement:

■ The intermediate level muscle of the thenar eminence.

Opponens

refers to the action of opposition.

Opponens Pollicis

Opponens pollicis [uh-POH-nenz PAHL-ih-sus] is visible along with Abductor pollicis brevis and Flexor pollicis brevis in Figure 10–42.

Attachments:
- Origin: trapezium and the flexor retinaculum.
- Insertion: radial aspect of the first metacarpal, metacarpal I.

Actions:
- Opposes the thumb at the first carpometacarpal joint.

Placement:
- The deepest muscle of the thenar eminence.

Manus

the hand.

Abductor Digiti Minimi

Abductor digiti minimi [ab-DUK-tur DIJ-ih-ty MIN-ih-mee] is shown in Figure 10–43.

Attachments:
- Origin: pisiform carpal bone and the tendon of Flexor carpi ulnaris.
- Insertion: ulnar side of the proximal phalanx of metacarpal V, the little finger.

Actions:
- Abducts the little finger at the MCP joint.

Placement:
- The superficial muscle of the hypothenar eminence.

Flexor Digiti Minimi or Flexor Digiti Minimi Manus

Flexor digiti minimi [FLEK-sur DIJ-ih-ty MIN-ih-mee] is shown in Figure 10–43.

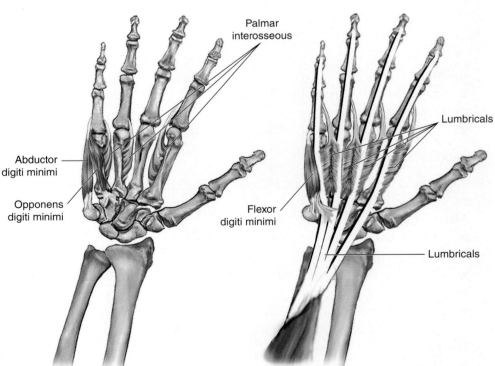

FIGURE 10–43 Muscles of the hypothenar eminence: Abductor digiti minimi, Flexor digiti minimi, and Opponens digiti minimi.

Attachments:

- Origin: the hamate carpal bone and the flexor retinaculum.
- Insertion: base of the proximal phalanx of metacarpal V, the little finger.

Actions:

- Flexes the little finger at the MCP joint.

Placement:

- The intermediate level muscle of the hypothenar eminence.

Opponens Digiti Minimi or Opponens Digiti Minimi Manus

Opponens Digiti Minimi [uh-POH-nenz DIJ-ih-ty MIN-ih-mee] can be seen in Figure 10–43, along with Abductor digiti minimi and Flexor digiti minimi.

Attachments:

- Origin: the hamate carpal bone and the flexor retinaculum.
- Insertion: ulnar border of metacarpal V, the little finger.

Actions:

- Opposes the little finger toward the thumb at the MCP joint.

Placement:

- This is the deepest muscle of the hypothenar eminence.

Palpation of Abductor, Flexor and Opponens Pollicis, and Abductor, Flexor, and Opponens Digiti Minimi:

> **HERE'S A TIP**
>
> Abductor pollicis brevis is the most superficial of the thenar eminence muscles and palpable along its length. Flexor pollicis brevis is intermediate and palpable proximally. Opponens pollicis is deepest and likely not palpable.
>
> Abductor digiti minimi manus is the most superficial of the hypothenar muscles and palpable along its length. Flexor digiti minimi manus is intermediate and palpable along its length. Opponens digiti minimi is deepest and likely not palpable.

POSITION:

- Supine client. Undrape your client's arm and supinate his hand.
- Stand or sit at the side of the table. Use your mother hand to support your client's hand or to add resistance.

LOCATE AND PALPATE:

For muscles of the thenar eminence:

- Locate the lateral aspect of the flexor retinaculum. Locate the radial aspect of the proximal phalanx of the thumb, just distal to the first joint.
- Palpate the prominent, dense bellies of the muscles of the thenar eminence in their resting state between these attachments, as shown in Figure 10–44. The muscle bellies may be difficult to distinguish from one another. Palpate with and against the grain of muscle fibers.

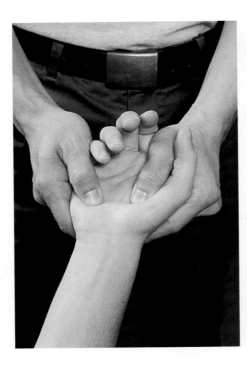

FIGURE 10-44 Palpating the muscles of the thenar and hypothenar eminences simultaneously.

For muscles of the hypothenar eminence:

- Locate the ulnar aspect of the flexor retinaculum. Locate the base of the proximal phalanx of the little finger, just distal to the fifth MCP joint, as shown in Figure 10–43.

- Palpate the prominent bellies of the muscles of the hypothenar eminence in their resting state between these attachments. The muscle bellies may be difficult to distinguish from one another. Palpate with and against the grain of muscle fibers.

DIRECT AN ACTION AND PALPATE:

For muscles of the thenar eminence:

- Ask your client to bend his thumb sideways, away from his hand, and palpate Abductor pollicis brevis during abduction of the thumb.

- Ask your client to bend his thumb toward his wrist and palpate Flexor pollicis brevis during flexion of the thumb.

- Ask your client to bend his thumb toward his little finger and attempt to palpate Opponens pollicis during opposition of the thumb.

For muscles of the hypothenar eminence:

- Ask your client to bend his little finger sideways, away from his hand, and palpate Abductor digiti minimi manus during abduction of the little finger.

- Ask your client to bend his thumb toward his wrist and palpate Flexor digiti minimi manus during flexion of the little finger.

- Ask your client to bend his thumb toward his little finger and attempt to palpate Opponens digiti minimi during opposition of the little finger.

- Add gentle resistance, if necessary.

EVALUATE:

- Characterize your palpation feedback from the muscles of the thenar and hypothenar eminence: describe the tone, texture, and temperature of the muscle tissue.

- Note the presence of trigger points, tissue adhesions, barriers to palpation, or other findings.

- Compare palpation of both sides of the muscles of the thenar and hypothenar eminence, noting how the findings from the second palpation vary.

- Compare with palpations of the muscles of the thenar and hypothenar eminence on other clients, noting how the findings from palpation on this client differ or are similar.

DID YOU KNOW?

In traditional Chinese medicine, the thenar eminence is known as the "big fish," while the hypothenar eminence is called the "little fish."

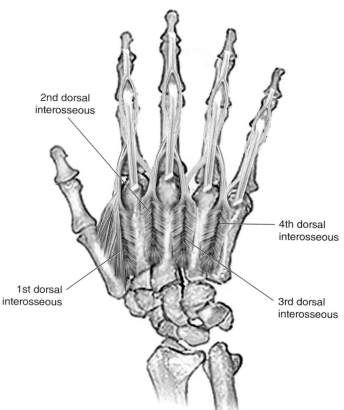

2nd dorsal interosseous

4th dorsal interosseous

1st dorsal interosseous

3rd dorsal interosseous

FIGURE 10-45 The Dorsal interossei muscles.

Palmar and Dorsal Interossei

The Interossei [in-tur-AHS-ee-eye] lie between the metacarpals of the hand. Their diagonal fibers abduct and adduct the fingers. Since the third finger is intermediate on the hand, it does not move during abduction and adduction. The more easily palpable Dorsal interossei are shown in Figure 10–45.

Attachments:

Palmar interossei:

- Origins: bases of metacarpals II, IV, and V on the palmar aspect.
- Insertions: proximal phalanges of digits #2, 4, and 5 on the palmar aspect.

Dorsal interossei:

- Origins: shafts of metacarpals I–V on the dorsal aspect.
- Insertions: proximal phalanges of digits #2, 3, and 4 on the dorsal aspect.

Actions:

Palmar interossei:

- Adduct digits #2, 4, and 5 at the MCP joints.

Dorsal interossei:

- Abduct digits #2, 3, and 4 at the MCP joints.

Placement:

- The Palmar interossei are deep to other intrinsic hand muscles on the palmar aspect.
- The Dorsal interossei are superficial on the dorsal aspect of the hand.

Dorsal

situated at the back.

Interosseous

between bones.

IN THE TREATMENT ROOM

The Palmar and Dorsal interossei may be strained by picking up an object that is too large for one's hand or by grabbing for an object being dropped.

HERE'S A TIP

Both the Palmar and Dorsal interossei muscles can be palpated along with the other intrinsic hand muscles, although the Palmar aponeurosis and thickened palmar skin make palpation of the Palmar interossei more difficult. If your client has osteoarthritis in either or both hands, adjust palpation pressure around swollen joints and avoid sites of local inflammation.

Palpation of the Palmar and Dorsal Interossei:

POSITION:

- Supine client. Undrape your client's arm. You may palpate the Palmar and Dorsal interossei simultaneously.
- Stand or sit at the side of the table. Use both hands to palpate.

LOCATE AND PALPATE:

For the Palmar interossei:

- Using your fingertips, gently palpate in between metacarpals II, III, IV, and V on the palmar aspect a shown in Figure 10–46, moving distally on the hand toward the proximal phalanges of digits #2, 4, and 5.
- Palpate the diagonal fibers of the Palmar interossei in their resting state.

For the Dorsal interossei:

- Using your thumbs, gently palpate in between metacarpals I to V on the dorsal aspect, moving distally on the hand toward the proximal phalanges of digits #2, 3, and 4, as shown in Figure 10–46.
- Palpate the diagonal fibers of the Dorsal interossei in their resting state.

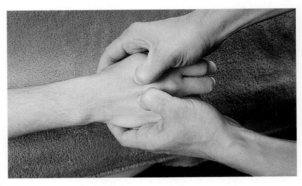

FIGURE 10–46 Palpating the Palmar and Dorsal interossei of the hand simultaneously.

DIRECT AN ACTION AND PALPATE:

For the Palmar interossei:

- Ask your client to spread his fingers, then bring them back together. Palpate the fibers of the Palmar interossei between digits #2, 4, and 5 during adduction of #2, 4, and 5.

For the Dorsal interossei:

- Ask your client to spread his fingers, and palpate the fibers of the Dorsal interossei during abduction of digits #2, 3, and 4.

EVALUATE:

- Characterize your palpation feedback from the Palmar and Dorsal interossei: describe the tone, texture, and temperature of the muscle tissue.
- Note the presence of trigger points, tissue adhesions, barriers to palpation, or other findings.
- Compare palpation of the Palmar and Dorsal interossei on both hands, noting how the findings from the second palpation vary.
- Compare with palpations of the Palmar and Dorsal interossei on other clients, noting how the findings from palpation on this client differ or are similar.

Lab Activity 10–2 on page 456 is designed to develop your palpation skills on deeper muscles that act on the arm, forearm, and hand.

DEEPER MUSCLES THAT ACT ON THE THIGH

These deeper palpable muscles flex, laterally rotate, and adduct the thigh. They include Iliopsoas and the Lateral rotator group.

Psoas Major and Iliacus (iliopsoas)

Iliacus [ih-LYE-uh-kus] and Psoas major [SOH-us MAY-jor] together are called Iliopsoas [ih-lee-oh-SOH-us], because they share attachments and actions. Their fibers may blend distally. Around 40 percent of the population also has a Psoas minor, which is a smaller muscle. Shown in Figure 10–47, Psoas major and Iliacus create the most powerful hip flexion of all the hip flexors and are active in walking, stepping, running, and jumping. Although Psoas major originates on the lumbar vertebrae and Iliacus originates on the anterior surface of the ilium, they each share an insertion on the lesser trochanter. Actions may be unilateral or bilateral and vary, depending on whether the origin or the insertion is fixed, an example of reverse action. The palpations described are for Psoas major and Iliacus together.

   Attachments:

   ■   Origin of Psoas major: transverse processes and bodies of lumbar
        vertebrae.

Ilio

the ilium.

Psoas

the loin or groin.

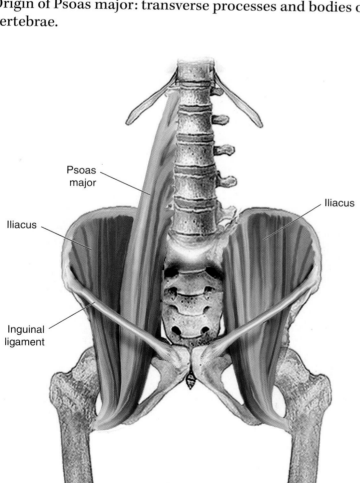

Psoas major

Iliacus

Iliacus

Inguinal ligament

FIGURE 10–47 Psoas major and Iliacus.

© Delmar, Cengage Learning.

- Origin of Iliacus: anterior iliac fossa.
- Insertion of Psoas major and Iliacus: lesser trochanter of the femur.

Actions:

- Unilateral: both muscles flex and laterally rotate the thigh at the acetabulofemoral joint.
- Bilateral: Psoas major flexes and laterally flexes the trunk at the spinal joints. Both muscles anteriorly tilt the pelvis at the lumbosacral joint.

Placement:

- Deep against the posterior wall in the abdominal cavity, just superior to the inguinal crease, the junction between the flexed thigh and the torso.

HERE'S A TIP

Although deep to the viscera in the abdominal cavity, Psoas major and Iliacus are palpated from the anterior. Placing your client in a semi-side-lying position allows the abdominal organs to shift away from the pelvis, easing access for palpation. To create a semi-side-lying position, shown in Figure 10–48:

- Start with your client in supine position.
- Place a wedge or pillow beneath your client's pelvis on the side to be palpated, to elevate the pelvis and allow gravity to move the abdominal organs away from the pelvis.

Palpate slowly, working gently but firmly through the superficial layers of tissue. Because distal fibers of Psoas major and minor may blend with those of iliacus as they near the lesser trochanter, the palpation feedback may seem to come from a single muscle. *Caution: when moving medially in the abdomen to locate the belly of Psoas, you are near the abdominal aorta. Immediately move away from any area where pulsing is felt.*

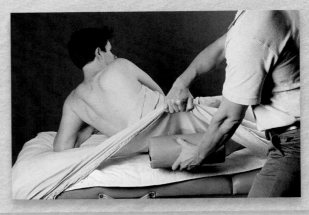

FIGURE 10-48 Place a wedge beneath your client's pelvis to create a semi-side-lying position.

Palpation of Psoas Major and Iliacus (Iliopsoas):

Note the location of the inguinal ligament, seen in Figure 10–47. Avoid exerting pressure on the inguinal ligament, especially during flexion of the thigh at the acetabulofemoral joint.

POSITION:

- Semi-side-lying client. Undrape the abdomen, covering the chest area securely, or work through the drape.
- Place your client's thigh in passive flexion, with his leg supported by a bolster at the knee.
- Stand at the side of the table, facing your client. Use your mother hand to stabilize your client's torso and to provide resistance to movement.

LOCATE AND PALPATE:

- Locate the anterior iliac crest and the inguinal crease, made visible by your client's flexed thigh. To locate the belly of Psoas major, move your palpating hand medial to the ASIS toward the umbilicus, about one-third of the distance.
- Palpating on your client's exhalation, sink the fingertips of your palpating hands into the well created by the shape of the anterior ilium, as shown in Figure 10–49. The vertical fibers of Iliopsoas will seem to line the ilium and become denser as they approach the inguinal crease. Palpate the fibers of Psoas major in their resting state.

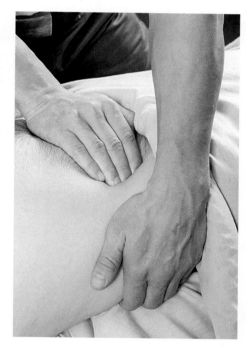

FIGURE 10–49 Palpating Psoas major and Iliacus with your client in semi-side-lying position.

- The fibers of Iliacus lie against the anterior wall of the ilium. You may only be able to distinguish its fibers from those of Psoas major on a client with very little adipose abdominal tissue.

DIRECT AN ACTION AND PALPATE:

- Ask your client to bring his knee toward his chest as you palpate Psoas major and Iliacus. The strong fibers may literally eject your palpating hand, ensuring that your palpation is accurate. Palpate Psoas major and Iliacus during flexion of the thigh.
- Alter the angle of the fingertips of your palpating hand and ask your client to repeat his thigh flexion. Palpate the fibers in their length. If you are able to isolate the fibers of Iliacus, they may blend with Psoas major distally.
- Place your mother hand against your client's anterior thigh to resist flexion and palpate Psoas major and Iliacus during resisted flexion of the thigh.

EVALUATE:

- Characterize your palpation feedback from Psoas major and Iliacus: describe the tone, texture, and temperature of the muscle tissue.
- Note the presence of trigger points, tissue adhesions, barriers to palpation, or other findings.
- Compare palpation of Psoas major and Iliacus on both sides, noting how the findings from the second palpation vary.

■ Compare with palpations of Psoas major and Iliacus on other clients, noting how the findings from palpation on this client differ or are similar.

OPTION:

With your client in supine position: place a bolster under your client's knees to create passive flexion of the thigh, as described in the above palpation.

■ Work from the opposite side of the table, so that you can curl your fingertips into the anterior ilium.

■ Proceed with the palpation as described.

IN THE TREATMENT ROOM

Iliopsoas syndrome

also called Iliopsoas tendonitis, an inflammation of the distal fibers of Iliopsoas, aggravated by forceful or repeated thigh flexion.

Psoas major and Iliacus are assessed in clients who report groin or low-back pain. Clients who report groin pain when climbing stairs or running on an inclined surface may be experiencing **Iliopsoas syndrome**, shown in Figure 10–50, also called Iliopsoas tendonitis, an inflammation of the distal fibers of Iliopsoas, aggravated by forceful or repeated thigh flexion. Dancers, hikers, runners, and other track athletes who report groin pain should be assessed for Iliopsoas syndrome, especially if the pain increases with hyperextension of the thigh. Iliopsoas is also active just before stepping off one foot and onto the other while walking. Assess Iliopsoas in clients who report pain during this phase of gait.

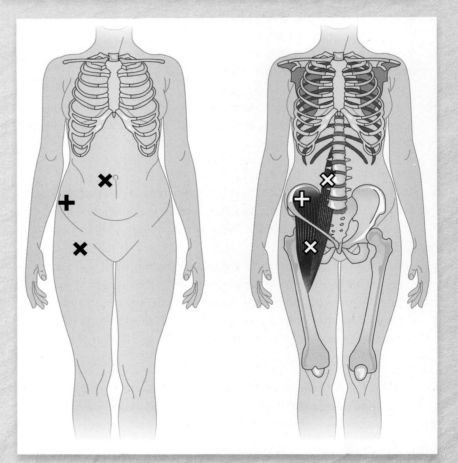

FIGURE 10–50 Iliopsoas syndrome may create trigger points in the predictable pattern shown here.

Deep Lateral Rotators Group

The deep lateral rotators, shown in Figure 10–51, include six horizontal muscles that originate on the sacrum or the pelvis and insert onto the greater trochanter of the femur, with horizontal fibers. Deep to Gluteus maximus, the lateral rotators are on the same plane as Gluteus medius. The Lateral rotators are active in abduction and lateral thigh rotation. They are listed here in their relative positions on the pelvis, from superior to inferior.

Piriformis

Piriformis is superficial and superior in the group and the most palpable Lateral rotator. Piriformis [peer-ih-FOR-mis] is visible in Figure 10–51.
Attachments:
- Origin: anterior sacrum, greater sciatic notch, and the anterior surface of the sacrotuberous ligament.
- Insertion: superior on the greater trochanter of the femur.

Superior Gemellus

Superior gemellus is just inferior to piriformis and their insertions on the greater trochanter are adjacent. Superior gemellus [soo-PEER-ee-ur jih-MEL-us] is visible in Figure 10–51.
Attachments:
- Origin: outer surface of the ischial spine.
- Insertion: medial on the greater trochanter of the femur.

Obturator Internus

The lateral tendons of Superior gemellus, Obturator internus, and Inferior gemellus may blend as they near their insertion on the greater trochanter. Obturator internus [AHB-tuh-rayt-ur in-TUR-nus] is visible in Figure 10–51.

> ### DID YOU KNOW?
>
> The Lateral rotators can also contralaterally rotate the pelvis in a reverse action, if the thigh is fixed. To experience this action, plant your foot firmly on the ground, and then twist your hips in the opposite direction. This "plant and cut" movement is common in field sports, such as football and soccer.

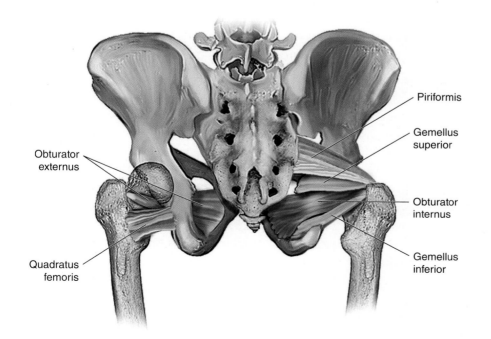

Piriformis

Gemellus superior

Obturator internus

Gemellus inferior

Obturator externus

Quadratus femoris

Piriformis

"pear-shaped."

Superior gemellus

"twin."

Obturator internus

refers to the obturator foramen.

FIGURE 10–51 The deep Lateral rotators of the thigh, posterior view.

© Delmar, Cengage Learning.

Attachments:
- Origin: internal pelvis, surrounding the obturator foramen.
- Insertion: posterior on the greater trochanter of the femur.

Inferior Gemellus

Inferior gemellus is located between Obturator internus and Obturator externus in the deep Lateral rotator group. Inferior gemellus [in-FEER-ee-ur jih-MEL-us] is visible in Figure 10–51.
Attachments:
- Origin: ischial tuberosity.
- Insertion: posterior on the greater trochanter of the femur.

Obturator Externus

Obturator externus is quite deep in its group, and not individually palpable. Obturator externus [AHB-tuh-rayt-ur eks-TUR-nus] is visible in Figure 10–51.
Attachments:
- Origin: pubis and the ischium, medial to the obturator foramen.
- Insertion: trochanteric fossa of the femur between the greater and lesser trochanters.

Quadratus femoris [kwah-DRA-tus FEM-uh-rus] is visible in Figure 10–51.
Attachments:
- Origin: ischial tuberosity.
- Insertion: intertrochanteric crest of the femur between the greater and lesser trochanters.

Actions:
- As a group: lateral rotation and abduction of the thigh at the acetabulofemoral joint and contralateral rotation of the pelvis at the spinal joints if the thigh is fixed. Piriformis can also medially rotate the thigh at the acetabulofemoral joint when the thigh is flexed at the acetabulofemoral joint.

Placement:
- The Lateral rotators are deep to Gluteus maximus and either deep to or on the same plane as Gluteus medius.

HERE'S A TIP

The dense fibers of Gluteus maximus make palpating the lateral rotators challenging. Because of their shared fiber direction, they are best palpated as a group. Palpating the group with your client in side-lying position allows him to fully medially or laterally rotate the thigh unimpeded by the table. In addition, assessing hip or groin pain often involves palpating both Psoas major and the Lateral rotators, a task made easier for the client if he can remain in one position for both palpations and subsequent treatment, making side-lying rather than prone the position of choice for palpating both groups. The sciatic nerve, which serves the entire lower extremity and may be as big around as your index finger at its root, is situated in between piriformis and superior gemellus. Take care to avoid impinging the sciatic nerve during palpation.

Palpation of Deep Lateral Rotators:

POSITION:

- Side-lying client. Work through the drape.
- Place your client's thigh in passive flexion, with his knee supported by a bolster.
- Stand at the side of the table, behind your client. Use your mother hand to provide resistance to movement.

LOCATE AND PALPATE:

- Warm the superficial muscles and tissues thoroughly, by massaging the area or applying a warm pack.
- Locate the lateral border of the sacrum and the greater trochanter.
- Palpate the horizontal fibers of the Lateral rotators between

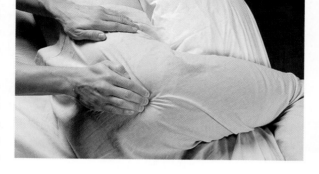

these landmarks in their resting state, as shown in Figure 10–52. Palpate with and against the grain of the fibers.

- It will be difficult to distinguish individual muscles within the group in their resting state.

© Milady, a part of Cengage Learning. Photography by Yanik Chauvin.

FIGURE 10–52 Palpating the deep Lateral rotators with your client in side-lying position.

DIRECT AN ACTION AND PALPATE:

- Ask your client to turn his knee toward the ceiling, which laterally rotates the thigh at the acetabulofemoral joint. Palpate the fibers of the lateral rotators during lateral rotation of the thigh.

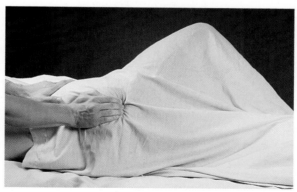

FIGURE 10–53 Isolating Piriformis for palpation may help you to assess Piriformis syndrome.

© Milady, a part of Cengage Learning. Photography by Yanik Chauvin.

- To isolate Piriformis, ask your client to turn his knee toward the ceiling, laterally rotating the thigh, and then immediately toward the table surface, medially rotating the thigh as shown in Figure 10–53. Since Piriformis is the only muscle in this group that can both laterally and medially rotate the thigh, it is evident during this action.
- Adding resistance to rotational actions may result in a cramp or spasm in Piriformis.

EVALUATE:

- Characterize your palpation feedback from the Lateral rotators: describe the tone, texture, and temperature of the muscle tissue.
- Note the presence of trigger points, tissue adhesions, barriers to palpation, or other findings.

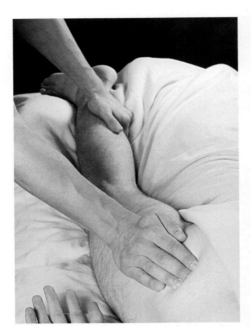

FIGURE 10-54 Palpating the deep Lateral rotators with your client prone.

- Compare palpation of both sides of the Lateral rotators, noting how the findings from the second palpation vary.
- Compare with palpations of the Lateral rotators on other clients, noting how the findings from palpation on this client differ or are similar.

OPTION:

With your client in prone position:

- Place your client's leg in passive flexion at the tibiofemoral joint. Ask him to push his leg against your resisting mother hand, shown in Figure 10-54, which laterally flexes the thigh at the acetabulofemoral joint.

IN THE TREATMENT ROOM

Symptoms of **Piriformis syndrome** occur when Piriformis of the deep lateral rotators creates pressure or irritation on the sciatic nerve as it travels between Piriformis and Superior gemellus, causing pain, numbness, or tingling in the gluteal region, or referring symptoms down the posterior leg or even into the groin. The pain from Piriformis syndrome is deep and made worse by walking, stepping up stairs, or squatting. Piriformis is pierced by either the sciatic or peroneal nerve, visible in Figure 10-55, in 10-15 percent of the population.

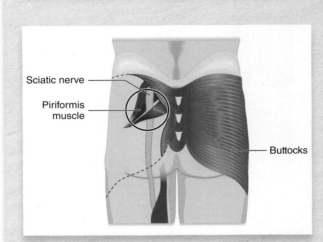

FIGURE 10-55 Piriformis syndrome is usually caused by pressure or irritation on the sciatic nerve as it travels between Piriformis and Superior gemellus.

To assess your client for Piriformis syndrome, *gently* point his knee, with his thigh and leg flexed, toward his shoulder on the unaffected side of his body, as shown in Figure 10-56.

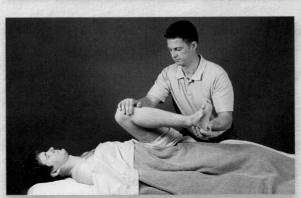

FIGURE 10-56 *Gently* point your supine client's knee, with his thigh and leg flexed, toward his shoulder on the unaffected side of his body, to assess for Piriformis syndrome.

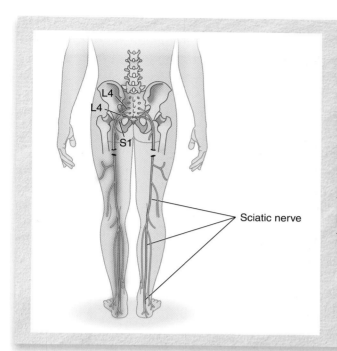

Symptoms of Piriformis syndrome may be indistinguishable from those of **sciatica**, a condition that can be caused by compression of the sciatic nerve root, shown in Figure 10–57, or by a disc herniation or vertebral misalignment in the lumbar region of the spine.

Sciatica

pain, tingling, or numbness in the hip or groin caused by compression of the sciatic nerve root, usually by a disc herniation in the lumbar region.

FIGURE 10–57 Sciatica is usually caused by compression on the sciatic nerve in the lumbar region of the spine.

DEEPER MUSCLES THAT ACT ON THE FOOT

Three deep flexors of the foot in the posterior leg oppose Tibialis anterior and Extensor digitorum in the anterior leg.

Deep Flexors of the Foot

Tibialis Posterior

Tibialis posterior [tib-ih-AL-is poh-STEER-ee-ur], shown in Figure 10–58, is the primary inverter of the foot at the intertarsal joints.

  Attachments:

- Origin: proximal posterior tibia and fibula and the interosseous membrane.
- Insertion: tarsal bones, except the talus, and plantar surfaces of metatarsals II–IV.

  Actions:

- Plantarflexes the foot at the talocrural joint and inverts the foot at the intertarsal joints.

  Placement:

- Deep to Soleus, deepest of the deep flexors of the foot.

Flexor Digitorum Longus

Flexor digitorum longus [FLEK-sur dij-uh-TOR-um LONG-us] is seen in Figure 10–58. The long belly of Flexor digitorum longus is medial in this group.

  Attachments:

- Origin: middle posterior tibia.
- Insertion: plantar surface of distal toes #2–5.

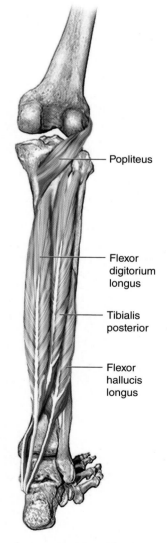

Popliteus

Flexor digitorium longus

Tibialis posterior

Flexor hallucis longus

FIGURE 10–58 The deep Flexors of the foot: Tibialis posterior, Flexor digitorum longus, and Flexor hallucis longus.

Actions:
- Flexes toes #2–5 at the metatarsophalangeal (MTP) and interphalangeal (IP) joints and plantarflexes the foot at the talocrural joint and inverts the foot at the intertarsal joints.

Placement:
- Deep to Soleus.

Hallucis

big toe.

Flexor Hallucis Longus

Flexor hallucis longus [FLEK-sur HAL-yuh-sis LONG-us] is visible along with Tibialis posterior and Flexor digitorum longus in Figure 10–58. The belly of Flexor hallucis longus is lateral in this group.

Attachments:
- Origin: distal two-thirds of the fibula.
- Insertion: plantar surface of the big toe, digit #1.

Actions:
- Flexes the big toe, plantar flexes the foot at the talocrural joint, and inverts the foot at the intertarsal joints.

Placement:
- Deep to Soleus.

HERE'S A TIP

Sometimes known as **T**om, **D**ick, and **H**arry, **T**ibialis posterior, Flexor **d**igitorum longus, and Flexor **h**allucis longus are palpable at their distal tendons, especially in the strong action of flexion of the toes. The distal tendons of individual muscles in this group are difficult to discern. Palpate them as a group. Take care to avoid the tibial artery and nerve, which travel alongside these deep flexors of the leg.

Palpation of Tibialis Posterior, Flexor Digitorum Longus, and Flexor Hallucis Longus:

POSITION:
- Supine client. Undrape your client's leg. Use your mother hand to support the foot.
- Stand or sit at the opposite side of the table, facing your client's medial leg and foot.

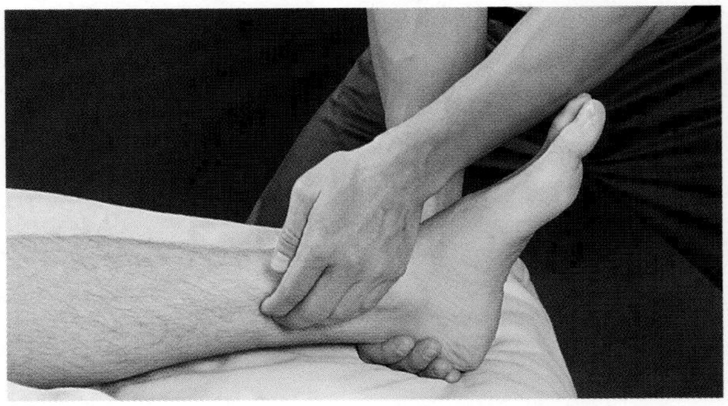

FIGURE 10–59 Palpating the distal tendons of Tibialis posterior, Flexor digitorum longus, and Flexor hallucis longus.

LOCATE AND PALPATE:
- Warm the superficial muscles and tissues thoroughly, by massaging the area.
- Locate the calcaneal tendon and the medial malleolus, as shown in Figure 10–59.

■ Palpate the distal tendons of Tibialis posterior, Flexor digitorum longus, and Flexor hallucis longus as they round the posterior of the medial malleolus and travel toward the deep muscular layers on the plantar surface of the foot.

DIRECT AN ACTION AND PALPATE:

■ Ask your client to point his toes. Palpate the distal tendons during plantar-flexion of the foot at the talocrural joint.

■ Ask your client to wiggle his toes. Palpate the distal tendons during flexion of the toes at the MTP and IP joints.

■ Ask your client to turn the bottom of his foot toward you. Palpate the distal tendons during inversion of the foot at the intertarsal joints.

EVALUATE:

■ Characterize your palpation feedback from Tibialis posterior, Flexor digitorum longus, and Flexor hallucis longus: describe the tone, texture, and temperature of the muscle tissue.

■ Note the presence of trigger points, tissue adhesions, barriers to palpation, or other findings.

■ Compare palpation of Tibialis posterior, Flexor digitorum longus, and Flexor hallucis longus on both feet, noting how the findings from the second palpation vary.

■ Compare with palpations of Tibialis posterior, Flexor digitorum longus, and Flexor hallucis longus on other clients, noting how the findings from palpation on this client differ or are similar.

INTRINSIC MUSCLES OF THE FOOT

The Intrinsic Muscles of the Foot

The intrinsic muscles of the foot move the toes and are critical in gait, because they flex and extend the toes and stabilize side-to-side balance and the arches of the foot. Those on the plantar aspect of the foot are found in layers, deep to the tough plantar aponeurosis. Abductor hallucis [ab-DUK-tur HAL-yuh-sis], Abductor digiti minimi pedis [ab-DUK-tur dij-it-ty MIN-eh-mee], and Flexor digitorum brevis [FLEK-sur dij-ih-TOR-um BREH-vis], shown in Figure 10–60 lie in the superficial plantar layer

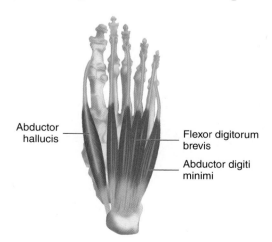

Abductor hallucis

Flexor digitorum brevis

Abductor digiti minimi

FIGURE 10–60 The palpable Plantar intrinsic muscles of the foot.

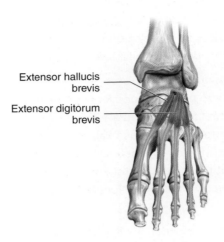

Extensor hallucis brevis

Extensor digitorum brevis

FIGURE 10–61 The palpable Dorsal intrinsic muscles of the foot.

and share an origin on the calcaneus. The origins of Extensor digitorum brevis [ik-STEN-sur dij-ih-TOR-um BREH-vis] and Extensor hallucis brevis on the dorsal aspect of the foot, seen in Figure 10–61, are also on the calcaneus, but on the dorsal aspect. These superficial intrinsic muscles are readily palpable and can be palpated as a group.

Abductor Hallucis

Abductor hallucis is a long muscle on the medial aspect of the plantar foot. It cramps easily, so palpate with care.

Attachments:
- Origin: plantar surface of the calcaneus.
- Insertion: medial on the proximal phalanx of toe #1, the big toe.

Actions:
- Abducts and flexes toe #1 at the MTP joint.

Placement:
- In the superficial muscle layer on the plantar aspect, medial to the plantar aponeurosis.

Abductor Digiti Minimi Pedis

The term "pedis" is added to the name of this muscle to distinguish it from the Abductor digiti minimi of the hand. Abductor digiti minimi pedis may be weak, and the digit itself may be quite tender, if the little toe has been sprained or broken, even long in the past. Palpate this site with care.

Attachments:
- Origin: plantar surface of the calcaneus.
- Insertion: lateral on the proximal phalanx of toe #5, little toe.

Actions:
- Abducts and flexes toe #5 at the MTP joint.

Placement:
- In the superficial muscle layer on the plantar aspect, lateral to the plantar aponeurosis.

Flexor Digitorum Brevis

This strong flexor may also cramp easily. Warm the plantar surface of the foot thoroughly before palpating.

Attachments:

- Origin: plantar surface of the calcaneus.
- Insertion: middle phalanges of toes #2–5.

Actions:

- Flexes toes #2–5 at the MTP and IP joints.

Placement:

- In the superficial muscle layer on the plantar aspect, lateral to Abductor hallucis, medial to Abductor digiti minimi pedis, and deep to the plantar aponeurosis.

Extensor Digitorum Brevis

Extensor digitorum brevis is deep to the distal tendons of Extensor digitorum longus, and its tendons are located in between those of Extensor digitorum longus. Note that it does not act on digiti minimi, the little toe.

Attachments:

- Origin: dorsal surface of the calcaneus.
- Insertion: middle phalanges of toes #2–5.

Actions:

- Extends toes #2–5 at the MTP and proximal IP joints.

Placement:

- The split muscle bellies are partly superficial, deep to the distal tendons of Extensor digitorum longus.

Extensor Hallucis Brevis

Extensor hallucis brevis is the big toe's equivalent of Extensor digitorum brevis.

Attachments:

- Origin: dorsal surface of the calcaneus.
- Insertion: dorsal surface of toe #1, the big toe.

Actions:

- Extends toe #1 at the MTP joint and IP joints.

Placement:

- Mostly superficial; medial to Extensor digitorum brevis.

Palpation of Abductor Hallucis, Abductor Digiti Minimi Pedis, Flexor Digitorum Brevis, and Extensor Digitorum Brevis and Extensor Hallucis Brevis:

Warming the superficial tissue on the plantar aspect before palpating these muscles will help to discourage painful cramping in the client's foot.

POSITION:

- Supine client. Undrape your client's leg and foot.
- Use your mother hand to provide resistance. Palpate the palmar and dorsal foot simultaneously, using both hands.
- Stand or sit at the foot of the table.

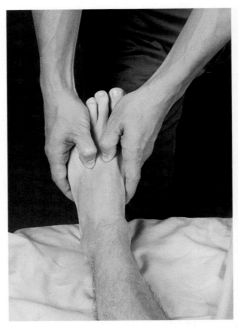

FIGURE 10–62 Palpating the Plantar and Dorsal intrinsic muscles of the foot simultaneously.

LOCATE AND PALPATE:

■ Warm the superficial muscles and tissues thoroughly, by massaging the area.

■ Locate the calcaneus and the proximal phalanges of each of the toes. With your fingertips, locate the fascial plantar aponeurosis that lies intermediate in the plantar foot and extends onto each toe, as shown in Figure 10–62.

■ For Abductor hallucis and Abductor digiti minimi pedis: palpate the muscle bellies that are medial and lateral to the plantar aponeurosis. Palpate the longitudinal fibers in their resting state, with and against the grain.

■ For Flexor digitorum brevis: palpate the dense muscle belly that lies directly deep to the intermediate plantar aponeurosis. Palpate the longitudinal fibers in their resting state, with and against the grain.

■ For Extensor digitorum brevis: locate the muscle belly that lies just deep and lateral to the tendons of Extensor digitorum longus with your thumbs, traveling toward the phalanges of toes #2–5, in the proximal dorsal foot, as shown in Figure 10–61. Palpate the fibers in their resting state, with and against the grain.

■ For Extensor hallucis brevis: locate the muscle belly that lies medial to the belly of Extensor digitorum brevis, traveling toward the phalanges of toe #1, in the proximal dorsal foot, also shown in Figure 10–60. Palpate the fibers in their resting state, with and against the grain.

DIRECT AN ACTION AND PALPATE:

■ For Abductor hallucis and Abductor digiti minimi pedis: ask your client to spread his toes. Palpate the fibers of Abductor hallucis and Abductor digiti minimi pedis during abduction of toes #1 and #5.

■ For Flexor digitorum brevis: ask your client to wiggle his toes. Palpate the fibers of Flexor digitorum brevis during flexion of toes #2–5.

■ For Extensor digitorum brevis: ask your client to wiggle his toes. Palpate the fibers of Extensor digitorum brevis during extension of toes #2–5.

■ For Extensor hallucis brevis: ask your client to wiggle his big toe. Palpate the fibers of Extensor hallucis brevis during extension of toe #1.

EVALUATE:

■ Characterize your palpation feedback from the Intrinsic muscles of the foot: describe the tone, texture, and temperature of the muscle tissue.

■ Note the presence of trigger points, tissue adhesions, barriers to palpation, or other findings.

■ Compare palpation of both sides of the Intrinsic muscles of the foot, noting how the findings from the second palpation vary.

■ Compare with palpations of the Intrinsic muscles of the foot on other clients, noting how the findings from palpation on this client differ or are similar.

Lab Activity 10–3 on page 456 is designed to develop your palpation skills on deeper muscles that act on the thigh, leg, and foot.

SUMMARY

Palpating deeper muscles can be a challenging but ultimately rewarding process. Focused palpation of deeper muscles and specific muscle groups enhances your tactile and assessment skills. The feedback from each deeper palpation is grounded in your previous assessments of your client's posture and gait and palpation of his bones, fascial structures, and superficial muscles. Together, these assessment techniques yield valuable treatment-planning information and create your unique therapeutic skills.

LAB ACTIVITIES

LAB ACTIVITY 10–1: PALPATING DEEPER MUSCLES THAT ACT ON THE AXIAL SKELETON

1. Working in a group of three, palpate the deeper muscles listed below: what position will you place your partner in to palpate these muscles? What bony landmarks will you locate? What actions will you direct him to perform? For which palpations is resistance appropriate?
   - Suboccipital group
   - Longus colli
   - The Thoracic diaphragm
   - Serratus posterior superior and Serratus posterior inferior
   - Erector spinae group
   - Transversospinalis group
   - Quadratus lumborum
   - Pectoralis minor

2. Perform palpations of each of the muscles in this group, using the Four-Step Protocol, on each member of the group.

3. What are the antagonist muscles in the actions of your target muscles? Discuss with your partners how palpation of these muscles can be incorporated into your assessment.

4. Switch partners and repeat the palpations until all group members have palpated all the muscles and have been palpated.

5. Evaluate: characterize your palpation findings, as suggested in the palpation guide above, and compare them with those of the group. Discuss which muscles were easier to palpate on some members of the group and which were more difficult and what differences in the palpation experience were evident to each group member.

6. How did touch sensitivity enhance the palpation experience? What specific steps did you take during the palpations to increase or focus your touch sensitivity? What differences in touch sensitivity did you note in relation to the palpation pressure used?

LAB ACTIVITY 10–2: PALPATING DEEPER MUSCLES THAT ACT ON THE ARM, FOREARM, AND HAND

1. Working in a group of three, palpate the muscles listed below: what position will you place your partner in to palpate these muscles? What bony landmarks will you locate? What actions will you direct him to perform? For which palpations is resistance appropriate?
   - Subscapularis
   - Coracobrachialis
   - Pronator teres and Supinator
   - Deep Forearm flexors
   - Deep Forearm extensors
   - Intrinsic muscles of the hand

2. Perform palpations of each of the muscles in this group, using the Four-Step Protocol, on each member of the group.

3. What are the antagonist muscles in the actions of your target muscles? Discuss with your partners how palpation of these muscles can be incorporated into your assessment.

4. Switch partners and repeat the palpations until all group members have palpated all the muscles and have been palpated.

5. Evaluate: characterize your palpation findings, as suggested in the palpation guide above, and compare them with those of the group. Discuss which muscles were more palpable on some members of the group and which were more difficult, and what differences in the palpation experience were evident to each group member?

6. How did touch sensitivity enhance the palpation experience? What specific steps did you take during the palpations to increase or focus your touch sensitivity? What differences in touch sensitivity did you note in relation to the palpation pressure used?

LAB ACTIVITY 10–3: PALPATING DEEPER MUSCLES THAT ACT ON THE THIGH, LEG, AND FOOT

1. Working in a group of three, palpate the muscles listed below: what position will you place your partner in to palpate these muscles? What bony landmarks will you locate? What actions will you direct him to perform? For which palpations is resistance appropriate?
   - Iliopsoas
   - Deep Lateral rotators group
   - Tibialis posterior, Flexor digitorum longus, and Flexor hallucis longus
   - Intrinsic muscles of the foot

2. Perform palpations of each of the muscles in this group, using the Four-Step Protocol, on each member of the group.

3. What are the antagonist muscles in the actions of your target muscles? Discuss with your partners how palpation of these muscles can be incorporated into your assessment.

4. Switch partners and repeat the palpations until all group members have palpated all the muscles and have been palpated.

5. Evaluate: characterize your palpation findings, as suggested in the palpation guide above, and compare them with those of the group. Discuss which muscles were more palpable on some members of the group and which were more difficult, and what differences in the palpation experience were evident to each group member?

6. How did touch sensitivity enhance the palpation experience? What specific steps did you take during the palpations to increase or focus your touch sensitivity? What differences in touch sensitivity did you note in relation to the palpation pressure used?

CASE PROFILES

Case Profile 1

Andre, 32, is afraid he's developing heart disease: he has pain and tenderness in his upper chest and weakness in his left arm. His symptoms have developed since he was in a car accident six months ago, when he was hit from behind, and his stress level has been high ever since. He's not sleeping well and often wakes up at night with his left shoulder hurting and tingling. What muscles or muscle groups will you target for palpation on Andre? What client positions and draping will you use for these palpations? Which antagonist muscles will you also palpate? Will you refer Andre to his doctor for an evaluation, and if so, why?

Case Profile 2

Katie, 19, a student, has chronic pain and stiffness on the right side of her low back and hip. The pain is always worse after she walks several miles to campus each day, carrying her two-year-old daughter to campus day care. Once in class, the pain can get even worse: at 6 feet (183 cm) tall, Katie is uncomfortable in the cramped chairs in her crowded classroom. What muscles or muscle groups will you target for palpation on Katie? What client positions and draping will you use for these palpations? Which antagonist muscles will you also palpate?

Case Profile 3

Jim, 24, lost 50 pounds in the last year and is training hard for his first marathon, after years without exercising. After the first few miles, Jim begins to suffer intense pain in his right buttock, which soon spreads to his groin. The pain worsens when he runs in the desert, where he has to make frequent, sudden turns to avoid low-lying cactus. Sometimes, the pain is accompanied by tingling and "pins and needles" down his right leg. What muscles or muscle groups will you target for palpation on Jim? What client positions and draping will you use for these palpations? Which antagonist muscles will you also palpate?

STUDY QUESTIONS

1. What adjustments to the Four-Step Palpation Protocol may have to be made for palpation of deeper muscles?
2. What steps will you take to ensure client safety and comfort during palpation of deeper muscles?
3. Describe the steps for locating Longus colli for palpation, including which nearby structures might be impacted.
4. Characterize any postural deviations observed during palpations of the Erector spinae or Quadratus lumborum muscles: what is the impact of these deviations on the muscles in specific regions of the Erectors, or on the position of the pelvis?
5. Characterize your experience in palpating Pectoralis minor: did palpation of either side of Pectoralis minor reflect any difference in the forward protraction of one shoulder?
6. Characterize the palpation findings from the forearm flexors and extensors: how different was the tone and texture of each muscle group on the dominant versus non-dominant hand? How different was the palpation feedback from one partner to another?
7. Describe the steps for locating and palpating Psoas major. What adjustments in positioning were necessary for success? How did coordinating your client's breath with an action contribute to your palpation success?
8. What caution is necessary when palpating the deep lateral rotator muscles? What symptoms and potential conditions indicate palpating this muscle group?
9. Compare and contrast Piriformis syndrome and Sciatica.
10. Which muscles described in Chapter 9, Palpating Superficial Muscles of the Extremities, have distal tendons that help form the arch of the foot? Which palpations described in this chapter will at the same time palpate those distal tendons?

STUDY QUESTION ANSWERS

CHAPTER 1 STUDY QUESTIONS

1. Which part of the skeleton, axial, or appendicular, has more planar joints? How does this predominance of planar joints affect range of motion in the axial skeleton?
   - **Answer:** planar joints are mostly found in the axial skeleton, including the acromioclavicular and sternoclavicular joints and the vertebrocostal joints. Because planar joints allow only a minimum of gliding action, the range of motion at a planar joint is slight. This limited range of motion in the planar joints of the axial skeleton contributes to the stability of the trunk.

2. Which types of synovial joints allow circumduction? What other joints can allow movements that seem to duplicate circumduction?
   - **Answer:** ball-and-socket synovial joints, found at the glenohumeral joint of the shoulder and the acetabulofemoral joint of the hip, allow true circumduction. The gliding actions found in the intercarpal joints of the wrist and the intertarsal joints of the ankle can create a type of circumduction and some sources conclude that circumduction can also occur at the metacarpophalangeal (MCP) and metatarsophalangeal (MTP) joints.

3. At which joints does true rotation—rotation of a bone around a single axis—occur? What other joints allow movement that may be considered a type of rotation?
   - **Answer:** true rotation occurs at the spinal joints, allowing rotation of the trunk and the head. In this action, the spine itself is the axis around which the trunk or the head rotates. Pronation and supination, during which the radius "rotates" around the immobile ulna at the proximal and distal radioulnar joints, is considered a type of rotation.

4. In what planes can abduction of the arm take place? Describe how the abduction of the arm differs in these planes.
   - **Answer:** abduction of the arm at the glenohumeral joint can occur in both the frontal and horizontal planes. In abduction of the arm at the glenohumeral joint in the frontal plane, the arm is raised from its anatomical position away from the midline of the body. In abduction of the arm at the glenohumeral joint in the horizontal plane, the arm is first flexed in the frontal plane and then moved away from the midline of the body while in a flexed position.

5. List the factors that create joint fit.
   - **Answer:** joint fit is created by the overall structure of the joint, the angle at which the ends of the bones articulate, and the tautness of the ligaments that support the joint.

6. Name the layers of connective tissue that wrap around the layers of a skeletal muscle, from superficial to deep.
   - **Answer:** epimysium, the most superficial; perimysium, the middle; and endomysium, the deepest layer of connective tissue wrapping in muscle tissue.

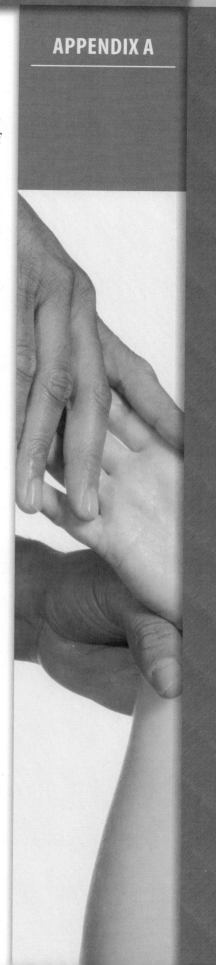

7. How does the direction of fibers in a skeletal muscle create the line of pull of that muscle?
   - **Answer:** during concentric contraction, muscle fibers are pulled toward the center of the muscle, the muscle belly. If the fibers are oriented vertically, the line of pull of the muscle will probably flex or extend the bone being acted on. If the fiber direction is horizontal, the line of pull of the muscle will probably abduct or adduct the bone being acted on.

8. Contrast isotonic and isometric muscle contractions. Which causes a muscle to fatigue more quickly?
   - **Answer:** during an isotonic muscle contraction, muscle length changes. The muscle may shorten, as during a concentric isotonic contraction, or lengthen, as during an eccentric isotonic contraction. During an isometric muscle contraction, the muscle length does not change, though the degree of contraction is sustained. Isometric contractions result in rapid muscle fatigue, because the sustained contraction requires greater energy use.

9. Contrast the functions of phasic and postural muscles. Give an example of each type of muscle.
   - **Answer:** phasic muscles move the skeleton. Postural muscles stabilize and support the posture of the body. Examples of phasic muscles include the Scalenes, the Rhomboids, and Deltoid. Examples of postural muscles include SCM and the Erector spinae and Transversospinalis groups.

10. Contrast Type I and Type II muscle fibers. Which fiber type contracts faster? Which fatigues most quickly?
    - **Answer:** Type I muscle fibers, also called "slow twitch," are the smallest muscle fibers. They are slow to fatigue, have a rich blood supply, and the velocity of their contractions is slow. Type IIB muscle fibers, also called "fast twitch," are the largest fibers. They are the quickest to fatigue; their blood supply is low and the velocity of their contractions is fast.

CHAPTER 2 STUDY QUESTIONS

1. Why do postural compensations develop?
   - **Answer:** postural compensations often develop to allow the body to maintain equilibrium despite postural deviations.

2. Describe the postural landmarks you look for in an initial, 60-second visual assessment of your client's posture.
   - **Answer:** check her head position in relation to her spine; the angle of her chin in relation to her suprasternal notch; and the position of her hands. Are her thumbnails visible or do you see the back of one or both hands? Are her fingertips at an even level as her arms hang alongside her thighs?

3. Describe two potential postural compensations that may result from scoliosis.
   - **Answer:** functional short leg or unilateral elevation of one side of the pelvis and unilateral elevation of one shoulder.

4. What is one potential lifestyle habit that may result in functional kyphosis?
   - **Answer:** habitual slumping of the trunk, common among clients who spend long hours at a poorly designed computer workstation, may cause a kyphotic thoracic curve.

5. Describe two pathological conditions that may impact posture.
   - **Answers:** ankylosing spondylitis, osteoporosis, Parkinson's disease, and rheumatoid arthritis, among others.

6. Describe the three arches of the foot and the impact of flat feet on the lower extremity.
   - **Answer:** the arches of the foot include a lateral longitudinal arch, a medial longitudinal arch, and a transverse arch. In a client with flat feet, weight transfers to the medial longitudinal arch of the foot and the deep muscles of the leg. Flattening of the foot lengthens it, slightly and persistently contracting the distal tendons of flexor and extensor muscles that attach to the distal phalanges of the toes. The toes may buckle upward, called claw toe, or they may buckle upward proximally and then downward distally, called hammertoe.

7. How do you assess a client for swayback when he is seated or supine on your table?
   - **Answer:** with your client seated, slide your fist laterally between his lumbar spine and the chair. If your fist can pass easily and unimpeded between the chair and your client's spine, the lumbar curve may be exaggerated. With your client supine, slide your hands laterally beneath both the cervical and lumbar regions of the spine. If your hands can pass easily and unimpeded across the spine in either region, the cervical and lumbar curves may be exaggerated

8. Contrast AROM and PROM.
   - **Answer:** AROM is active range of motion: the client demonstrates the range of motion at a joint, unassisted. PROM is passive range of motion: a massage therapist moves a client's joint through its range of motion without the client's participation.

9. Name two possible causes for an elevated shoulder.
   - **Answer:** as compensation for unilateral elevation of a hip, on either side of the body, or as the result of continuously carrying a heavy bag or purse on that shoulder.

10. Describe the appropriate scope of practice for a massage therapist in performing posture assessments.
    - **Answer:** visual observation of the elements of posture, including the relative positions of joints and bony structures; manual

assessment of the movement of structures during range of joint motion; and recording of objective and subjective findings of assessments in written form, for the purposes of identifying treatment goals and procedures.

CHAPTER 3 STUDY QUESTIONS

1. How does arm swing or lack of arm swing impact gait?
   - **Answer:** normal arm swing is synchronized with step and contributes to balanced, even gait. If arm swing is limited or impeded, step length shortens and the cadence of gait increases in order to maintain equilibrium.
2. During which stage of the stance phase of gait does the pelvis tilt anteriorly and during which stage does it tilt posteriorly?
   - **Answer:** The pelvis tilts anteriorly on the opposite side during the heel-strike stage of stance and tilts posteriorly during the heel-off stage.
3. What muscle dysfunctions may disturb these actions of pelvic tilt?
   - **Answer:** Hypotonicity or hypertonicity in muscles that tilt or elevate the pelvis, such as the Erector spinae group or Quadratus lumborum.
4. Describe two pathological conditions that may impact gait.
   - **Answer:** fibromyalgia, myasthenia gravis, osteoarthritis, osteoporosis, rheumatoid arthritis, Alzheimer's disease, amyotrophic lateral sclerosis (ALS), dystonia, multiple sclerosis, Parkinson's disease, and stroke are some of the conditions that may alter gait. *Review the chapter information on these conditions to describe them thoroughly.*
5. Describe two postural deviations that may impact gait and what that gait might look like.
   - **Answer:** the gait of a client with lordosis may be altered—the transition from heel strike, when the pelvis is tilted to the anterior, through foot flat to midstance, when the pelvis posteriorly tilts, may be stiff and incomplete. The gait of a client with excessive inversion may be altered—the inversion of the foot increases the risk for an inversion sprain of the ankle during normal gait on even a slightly inclined surface.
6. Describe the relationship between heel strike and short-leg syndrome.
   - **Answer:** the heel strike of a client with a functionally short leg may be significantly harder on the long-leg side of her body.
7. How does walking on a treadmill alter someone's gait?
   - **Answer:** the strip of moveable tread in which the walker must remain may inhibit normal step width, as does the intrusion of side support bars. Treadmill gait also inhibits normal step length because most people hold the support bars with both hands, eliminating any natural arm swing from their gait. Normal cadence may also be disrupted by the enforced pace of the treadmill.

8. Contrast the time spent in non-support during walking gait and running gait.
   - **Answer:** during normal walking gait, there is no period of non-support because one foot is always on the ground. During running gait, there are periods of non-support, when both feet are off the ground. When either foot hits the ground and bears the full weight of the body, there is increased impact on weight-bearing joints. During non-support, there is no impact on weight-bearing joints.

9. Describe the most effective way to assess unilateral hip elevation during gait.
   - **Answer:** ask your client to place her hands on her hips as she walks toward you.

10. Foot slap may be caused by weakness in what muscles?
    - **Answer:** weak or hypotonic plantarflexors of the foot, such as Gastrocnemius or Soleus.

CHAPTER 4 STUDY QUESTIONS

1. Contrast complex movement and simple movement. What makes a movement complex? Give an example of a simple movement and a complex movement.
   - **Answer:** a complex movement is one that involves multiple joint and muscle actions in both the axial and appendicular skeleton. One example of a complex movement is walking, which involves joint and muscle actions throughout the body. A simple movement does not involve multiple joint and muscle actions in both the axial and appendicular skeleton; for example, bending the head forward or backward, which involves only cervical spinal joints and muscles that flex the head at spinal joints.

2. Describe why turning the pages of this textbook may be considered a complex movement.
   - **Answer:** multiple joint and muscle actions are involved in turning the page of a book. The arm may medially and laterally rotate at the glenohumeral joint, for example, utilizing muscles that perform those actions, such as Anterior and Posterior deltoid, Infraspinatus, and Teres minor. Other actions may include pronation and supination at the radioulnar joints and actions at the radiocarpal, intercarpal, metacarpophalangeal (MCP), and interphalangeal (IP) joints.

3. Describe how the initiation and transition stages of a complex movement may resemble one another.
   - **Answer:** each stage may last only a second or two and may involve postural muscles more than phasic muscles.

4. How do you identify one joint action from another on a structure during a complex movement?
   - **Answer:** by duplicating the actions of the joint during palpation of the muscles that act on it.

5. Why is it important to identify antagonist muscles in complex movements?
   - **Answer:** antagonist muscles are vulnerable to injury during complex movements because, among other things, they both allow and limit the movement.

6. Describe the role of postural deviations in deconstructing complex movements. Do they cause or result from performing complex movements?
   - **Answer:** functional postural deviations may result from strains created by incorrectly performing a complex movement or from injurious repetition of a complex movement. Existing functional or structural postural deviations may force an unnatural performance of a complex movement that places strain on joints and soft tissue structures.

7. Describe the role of gait in deconstructing complex movements. Do alterations or disruptions in gait cause or result from performing complex movements?
   - **Answer:** many complex movements include a measure of gait, including the transfer of weight from one limb to the other during complex movements. Weight transfer during complex movement may be one opportunity for dysfunction or injury. Alterations or disruptions in gait, as with postural deviations, can both cause or result from performing complex movements.

8. How does recreating a complex movement contribute to deconstructing it?
   - **Answer:** by allowing you to experience within your own body the breadth and variety of joint and muscle actions contained with the specific complex movement.

9. How does deconstructing a complex movement contribute to selecting target structures for palpation?
   - **Answer:** once you have recreated the complex movement with your own body, you are able to identify the joint actions and muscle actions contained within it and can target those agonist and antagonist muscles for palpation.

10. How does deconstructing a complex movement contribute to planning subsequent assessments and creating a treatment plan?
   - **Answer:** once you grasp the elements of a complex action, you understand its potential for the dysfunction or strain that brought your client in for treatment. You are able to form an effective treatment plan that may include suggesting alterations to complex movements that will prevent reinjury or referring your client to appropriate practitioners, such as physical or occupational therapists, who can help him restructure his movements.

CHAPTER 5 STUDY QUESTIONS

1. How does the rate of perception of sensation affect palpation, both from the standpoint of the client and the therapist?
   - **Answer:** a client or massage therapist's perception of pressure, temperature, or pain may be disrupted by injury, a medical condition, or by certain medications.
2. How does adaptation to sensation affect palpation, both from the standpoint of the client and the therapist?
   - **Answer:** the longer that palpatory touch is perceived by either the client or the therapist, the more likely it is that adaptation to the sensations of pressure, temperature, or pain may result in inaccurate palpation feedback.
3. How does limb dominance affect palpation findings?
   - **Answer:** structures on the client's dominant limb may be slightly larger and the muscle fibers stronger than on the non-dominant limb. Structures on the client's non-dominant limb may be weaker and slightly more injury-prone.
4. What are three or more conditions that may alter perception of sensation? How might each condition impact the experience of palpation from the standpoint of the client and the therapist?
   - **Answer:** cancer, carpal tunnel syndrome (CTS,) chronic pain syndrome, circulatory disorders, diabetic neuropathy, fibromyalgia, multiple sclerosis (MS), nerve entrapment, spinal cord injury, and stroke are among the conditions which may affect perception of sensation. The effects may be directly connected to the condition itself or may arise as a result of treatment for the condition, such as medication side effects. *Review the chapter information on these conditions to describe how each may impact the palpation experience.*
5. Describe the location of endangerment sites on the head and neck.
   - **Answer:** inferior to the ear, the anterior triangle of the neck, and the posterior triangle of the neck.
6. Name three sites on the body that are potential areas of injury due to fragile skin on an elder client.
   - **Answer:** on the head, the back of the head and the ears. On the trunk, the angles of the scapula, the spinous processes of the vertebrae, the sacrum, the ischial tuberosity, and the ribs. On the upper extremity, the elbow. On the lower extremity, the greater trochanter, the condyles of the tibia, the malleoli, and the heels.
7. What are two recommendations for safe palpation on a client who is obese?
   - **Answer:** avoid the urge to use deeper pressure, and position your client so that her joints are supported.

8. What do you need to know about the medications and dosages taken by a client with a chronic illness?
   - **Answer:** what medications is she taking, how much, and how often? A client with a chronic illness may be taking multiple medications, which may require frequent dosage changes and may result in intensification of side effects. Some medication side effects may preclude certain massage or palpation techniques.

9. Name two or more skin conditions that may be systemic contraindications to palpation or massage.
   - **Answer:** if widespread, these skin conditions contraindicate massage: boils, burns, and blisters; fungal infections; herpes zoster, impetigo, rashes, or scaly spots; squamous cell carcinoma or melanoma; and tumors, warts, or unhealed flesh wounds.

10. Contrast acute and chronic pain; suggest words a client may use to describe each type of pain.
   - **Answer:** acute pain is pain of less than six months' duration and is often described as breathtaking, sharp, intense, or prickling. Chronic pain may have begun as acute pain but has persisted for more than six months and may be described as deep, aching, throbbing, or burning pain.

CHAPTER 6 STUDY QUESTIONS

1. Why might you use less pressure when palpating a bony landmark than when palpating a muscle?
   - **Answer:** because there is often less tissue between the skin and the bony landmark. Pressure is reduced to maintain client comfort.

2. Name two strategies for working through tissue barriers.
   - **Answer:** focus on slowly sinking or melting into tissue, working with the tissue rather than forcing through it. Work within the client's current range of motion; work with the client's breath, and introduce gentle rocking or stabilized shaking.

3. Why is touch sensitivity important to effective palpation? Name three strategies for enhancing touch sensitivity.
   - **Answer:** enhanced touch sensitivity replaces the need for deeper pressure during palpation. *Review the chapter information to select your strategies for enhancing touch sensitivities.*

4. Describe the role of the mother hand during palpation. How does using the mother hand contribute to good body mechanics?
   - **Answer:** the mother hand, or the non-palpating hand, is placed on the client's body to stabilize both the client and therapist's position and to add to the client's sense of security and comfort. Working with both hands on the client's body contributes to the therapist's equilibrium during palpation.

5. Contrast poor and preferred hand positions. What are the benefits of maintaining good hand positions during palpation?
   - ■ **Answer:** poor hand positions include palpating only with the fingertips, raising most of the hand off the client's body, hyperextending the wrist or the fingers, positioning the palpating hand counter to the curve of a structure, tightening the hand to maintain fingertips-only touch or maintaining touch with only one hand; and not using the mother hand. Preferred hand positions for palpation include palpating with the whole hand, resting the palpating hand on the client's body, keeping the wrist in "neutral" and the fingers only slightly flexed, positioning the palpating hand along the curve of a structure, relaxing the hand to increase sensory input and reassure the client, and maintaining touch with both hands, using the mother hand. Using good hand positions during palpation ensures greater relaxation and comfort for both the client and the therapist and provides better palpation results.

6. Name three structures that are more easily palpated with the client in side-lying position, and describe two challenges for the massage therapist when working with a side-lying client.
   - ■ **Answer:** palpation with the client in side-lying position facilitates palpation of some otherwise hard-to-access muscles, such as Subscapularis, and allows easy, full range of motion assessment of the ball-and-socket joint at the shoulder. It also eases palpation of structures on the lateral aspect, such as Serratus anterior, Tensor fasciae latae, the iliotibial band (ITB), and the Peroneal muscles. Challenges for the therapist include altering body mechanics to avoid bending her trunk laterally; maintaining outward, not downward, pressure; and raising the table one or two notches to accommodate good body mechanics when working on a side-lying client.

7. Why is using lay terminology for directing client muscle actions important? Name four lay terms you have developed to replace anatomically correct terms for muscle actions.
   - ■ **Answer:** using lay terminology ensures clarity of communication with the client, prevents misunderstanding, and prevents the building of barriers between massage therapist and client. *Review the chapter information to devise the lay terms you will utilize.*

8. What are two cautions to remember when applying resistance to movement during palpation?
   - ■ **Answer:** resistance during palpation should never cause discomfort. If adding resistance causes pain, it should be stopped immediately. Resistance should not be applied to a muscle that is already strained.

9. When is adding resistance to movement beneficial during palpation? Where is the mother hand placed when adding resistance?
   - ■ **Answer:** adding gentle resistance requires the muscle to strengthen the force of contraction, easing palpation of the

muscle fibers during muscle action. The resistance to increased movement places an additional, controlled stress on the muscle, and the stronger contraction in response to that stress makes the muscle fibers more apparent for palpation. The mother hand is placed to counter the direction of movement of the structure.

10. Contrast hypotonic and hypertonic muscle tone. List and describe three self-defined terms you plan to use in evaluating palpation results for treatment planning.

   - **Answer:** a hypotonic muscle is one with decreased or lost tone. A hypertonic muscle is one with increased, perhaps even rigid, tone. *Review the chapter information to define the terms you will utilize in evaluating palpation results.*

CHAPTER 7 STUDY QUESTIONS

1. Name the three fascial structures that are palpable on the axial skeleton.
   - **Answer:** the nuchal ligament, the abdominal aponeurosis, and thoracolumbar fascia.
2. What is the difference between superficial and deep fascia?
   - **Answer:** superficial fascia is found just beneath the skin. It separates the skin from muscles and provides the pathway into muscles for the nerves and the blood and lymph vessels. Deep fascia surrounds and supports organs and body cavities and envelops and permeates skeletal muscles. Deep fascia covers each muscle fiber, each bundle of muscle fibers, each whole muscle, and each entire group of muscles. Extensions of deep fascia connect body structures and form organ compartments.
3. Why is special care recommended in palpating the flexor retinaculum of the wrist?
   - **Answer:** the flexor retinaculum is superficial to the carpal tunnel, through which travel tendons, delicate blood vessels, and nerves.
4. Discuss why you might consider palpating the ITB with your client in side-lying position.
   - **Answer:** side-lying palpation of the ITB to give complete access to the length of the ITB without straining the body mechanics of the therapist. Side-lying palpation of the ITB also allows full access to the adjacent musculature of the client.
5. Describe how you will drape a client to completely palpate his or her ribcage.
   - **Answer:** begin with the client supine or side-lying and palpate over the sheet or place a towel or folded pillowcase over the breast area. With the client prone, no special draping is required.
6. Describe complete palpation of the bony landmarks of the mandible.
   - **Answer:** place your hands along your client's jawline, so that your fingertips meet at the point of her chin. Slide your fingertips around the jaw line to palpate the angle of the mandible. From the angle of the mandible, sweep your fingertips upward to palpate the condyle. Ask your client to open and close her jaw to

palpate the condyle of the mandible during depression and elevation. Ask your client to open her jaw so that you may palpate the coronoid process of the mandible, starting with your fingertips on the zygomatic arch and moving downward onto the coronoid process as it emerges from beneath the arch during depression of the jaw.

7. Describe the placement of the mother hand in palpating the bony landmarks of the leg and the foot.
   - **Answer:** during palpation of the tibia and fibula, you palpate with both hands or use your mother hand to support the tibiofemoral joint from beneath. During palpation of the tarsals and associated structures, use your mother hand to stabilize your client's foot. During palpation of the malleoli and actions at the talocrural and intertarsal joints, use your mother hand to support the ankle, or use both hands to palpate. To palpate structures on the foot, use both hands to palpate simultaneously on both feet.

8. Describe your order of palpation of the bony landmarks of the arm and forearm.
   - **Answer:** begin palpation with the clavicle and the scapula. Next, palpate the humerus, the radius, and the ulna; and then the carpals, metacarpals, and phalanges, working from distal to proximal on each structure.

9. Describe how you will position your client to palpate all the bony landmarks of the scapula.
   - **Answer:** begin with a prone client to palpate the posterior scapula only and a supine client to palpate the anterior scapula only. With your client in side-lying position, you can palpate both anterior and posterior landmarks on the scapula.

10. Describe the challenges of palpating bony landmarks on a client who is obese or elderly.
    - **Answer:** on a client who is obese, there may be an excess of tissue between the skin and bony landmarks, which is a challenge to effective palpation. Focus and touch sensitivity may help the massage therapist in these palpations. On an elderly client, there may be very little tissue between the skin and bony landmarks, so that palpation pressure must be very light. In addition, elder skin may be very fragile over bony landmarks, adding to the challenge of palpation on this client.

CHAPTER 8 STUDY QUESTIONS

1. What precautions for client safety should you take before palpating the Medial and Lateral pterygoids?
   - **Answer:** wash your hands thoroughly and wear a finger cot or a sterile, disposable exam glove.

2. What type of injury to a client may suggest palpation and assessment of SCM and the Scalene muscles?
   - **Answer:** a whiplash-type injury, in which the head is hyperflexed and hyperextended at the cervical spinal joints.

3. Which specific endangerment sites are cautions to specific palpations in this chapter?
   - **Answer:** the area inferior to the ear, the anterior and posterior triangles of the neck, the xiphoid process of the sternum, and the abdomen.
4. What might be a caution to consider when palpating abdominal muscles?
   - **Answer:** avoid the xiphoid process of the sternum and avoid applying pressure over the area of the abdominal aorta. Before palpating your client's abdomen, verify that he has no visceral abdominal pain. Recent abdominal medical procedures or unexplained pain contraindicate abdominal pressure.
5. For which muscles in this chapter is applying resistance during palpation not recommended?
   - **Answer:** applying resistance to movement during palpation of Splenius capitis, SCM, the Scalenes, and the Hyoids; Rectus abdominis and the External obliques; and Masseter and Temporalis is not recommended.
6. What are draping concerns and procedures for palpating the Abdominals?
   - **Answer:** palpate over the drape, or undrape the abdomen and place a towel or pillowcase securely over the breast area so that it will remain in place during directed actions.
7. Describe the cautions to palpating intraorally, such as for the Pterygoid muscles.
   - **Answer:** current dental problems, a canker sore, or inflammation in the client's mouth contraindicate intraoral palpation. Proceed only with your client's verbal consent and participation. The region of the Pterygoids may be tender. Adjust palpation pressure and encourage the client to breathe evenly throughout the palpation.
8. Which muscles in this chapter are most effectively palpated on both sides of the client's body simultaneously?
   - **Answer:** Temporalis and Masseter.
9. Describe how to add resistance to palpation of Serratus anterior.
   - **Answer:** ask your client to push against your mother hand as you resist protraction of the scapula at the scapulocostal joints.
10. How will you drape a female client to palpate the external Intercostal muscles?
    - **Answer:** undrape your client's upper chest only. You may ask your female client to use her free hand to secure the drape and immobilize her breast tissue during this palpation.

CHAPTER 9 STUDY QUESTIONS

1. Describe palpation of the posterior rotator cuff muscles: positioning, draping, actions to direct your client, and resistance.
   - **Answer:** begin with the client in side-lying position, stand at the side of the table. Use your mother hand to stabilize your client's

shoulder and to support her elbow during movement or to add resistance to movement. Add resistance by placing your mother hand on the humerus, against the direction of movement. Ask your client to lift her arm away from her side and palpate the fibers of Supraspinatus during abduction of the arm at the glenohumeral joint. Ask your client to reach behind as if into the backseat of a car and palpate the fibers of Infraspinatus during lateral rotation of the arm at the glenohumeral joint. Ask your client to reach behind as if into the backseat of a car and palpate the fibers of Teres minor during lateral rotation of the arm at the glenohumeral joint.

2. How can you contrast the actions of Teres major and Teres minor during palpation?

   ■ **Answer:** ask the client to first medially and then laterally rotate her arm at the glenohumeral joint. The fibers of Teres minor will be palpable during lateral rotation, while the fibers of Teres major will be palpable during medial rotation of the arm at the glenohumeral joint.

3. How can you effectively palpate Brachialis and delineate it from Biceps brachii during flexion of the forearm at the humeroulnar joint?

   ■ **Answer:** by placing the forearm in pronation, Biceps brachii is weakened and unable to flex the forearm at the humeroulnar joint. Brachialis is now the only muscle that will be flexing the forearm and is easily palpated during flexion of the forearm at the humeroulnar joint.

4. What are common causes of rotator cuff injuries?

   ■ **Answer:** when the arm is abducted to a degree that raises it above the shoulder, especially when accompanied by force, such as when throwing a ball, the rotator cuff muscles may be injured. "Weekend warriors" in any sport that includes repeated rotations of the shoulder, since circumduction includes abduction, or who neglect to warm up their muscles before activity, are also at risk. In elder clients, the gradual erosion of bone tissue in the glenohumeral joint, added to the wear and tear of repetitive motions and the progressive loss of tendon elasticity and muscle tissue, contributes to inflammation and tears in rotator cuff muscles. In clients who spend hours at computers, even the small movements used to type and move a mouse can result in repetitive strain injuries and inflammation in the rotator cuff.

5. What muscle or fascial structure will you target for palpation in your client who reports pain in the lateral knee?

   ■ **Answer:** Tensor fasciae latae (TFL) and the ITB.

6. In what way is your client's hand dominance a factor in assessing palpation results of your client's Forearm flexor and extensor muscles?

   ■ **Answer:** the Forearm flexor and extensor muscles on the client's dominant side may be larger and stronger. The Forearm flexor and extensor muscles on the client's non-dominant side may be smaller, weaker, and more injury-prone.

7. Describe the recommended positioning and draping for palpating the Adductor muscles.
   - **Answer:** begin with the client supine and place your client's thigh in passive abduction at the acetabulofemoral joint. Undrape the thigh and secure the drape. Encourage your female client to adjust and tighten the drape to ensure her security while making Adductor longus and magnus available for palpation.

8. How would you position your client to palpate Biceps femoris during extension of the thigh?
   - **Answer:** begin with your client prone and undrape the thigh and the leg.

9. What is the function of the pes anserine in the medial knee?
   - **Answer:** the pes anserine tendon facilitates the insertion of the distal tendons of artorius, Gracilis, and Semitendinosus onto the medial tibia.

10. Which muscles in this chapter might be best palpated in side-lying position? Why?
    - **Answer:** Deltoid, Supraspinatus, Infraspinatus, Teres minor, Gluteus medius, and TFL are best palpated with the client in side-lying position because access to the muscles is unimpeded and full range of motion is best achieved.

CHAPTER 10 STUDY QUESTIONS

1. What adjustments to the Four-Step Protocol may have to be made for palpation of deeper muscles?
   - **Answer:** palpate deeper muscles during a directed action, adding resistance whenever necessary. Palpation of the fibers of deeper muscles in their resting state is difficult. Palpate the muscle only in its resting state, however, if there is a chance that performing or resisting the directed action will elicit cramping or pain in the client. Move on to another assessment technique if palpation of a particular deep muscle on a particular client is not producing useful feedback or if it may cause painful compression of superficial tissues.

2. What steps will you take to ensure client safety and comfort during palpation of deeper muscles?
   - **Answer:** avoid palpating over the sites of delicate structures, such as nerves and blood vessels. Describe your intentions to your client. Demonstrate palpation on a non-injured target muscle and the action you wish your client to perform. Pay attention to the palpation feedback from superficial tissue. Avoid injuring superficial tissue in the effort to palpate deeper tissue. Resist the temptation to increase palpation pressure. Instead, work with your client's breath: synchronize your breathing to his, and slowly increase the depth of your palpatory touch on his exhalation.

3. Describe the steps for locating Longus colli for palpation, including what nearby structures might be impacted.
   - **Answer:** working across the table, locate the medial border of the opposite SCM with the fingertips of your palpating hand. Take care to avoid resting your hand on your client's throat. To facilitate locating the medial border of SCM, ask your client to turn his head toward your palpating hand. Gently work your fingertips in between the medial border of SCM and the trachea, just inferior to the hyoid bone. Check in with your client, to be sure he is comfortable with this palpation. Continue to press gently but firmly toward the lateral aspect of the anterior cervical spine. Locate and palpate the vertical fibers of longus colli in their resting state. Avoid impacting nearby structures such as the trachea, nerves, and blood vessels.

4. Characterize any postural deviations observed during palpations of the Erector spinae or Quadratus lumborum muscles. What is the impact of these deviations on the muscles in specific regions of the Erectors or on the position of the pelvis?
   - **Answer:** postural deviations in the spine may force muscles on one side of the spine to lengthen and shorten on the opposite side of the spine. The pelvis may be tilted to the anterior or unilaterally elevated if one side of the muscles alongside the spine is chronically shortened.

5. Characterize your experience in palpating Pectoralis minor. Did palpation of either side of the muscle reflect any difference in the forward protraction of one shoulder?
   - **Hint:** refer to the information regarding pectoralis minor syndrome, and investigate the type of injury that may impact Pectoralis minor.

6. Characterize the palpation findings from the Forearm flexors and extensors: how different was the tone and texture of each muscle group on the dominant versus the non-dominant hand? How different was the palpation feedback from one partner to another?
   - **Hint:** refer to the information about dominance in Chapter 5, The Science of Palpation.

7. Describe the steps for locating and palpating Psoas major. What adjustments in positioning were necessary for success? How did directing your client's breath and an action contribute to your palpation success?
   - **Hint:** Psoas major palpation may require positioning your client more than once.

8. What caution is necessary when palpating the deep lateral rotator muscles? What symptoms and potential conditions indicate palpating this muscle group?
   - **Answer:** take care to avoid impinging the large sciatic nerve that travels deep to Piriformis. Symptoms of Piriformis syndrome may include pain, numbness, or tingling in the gluteal region or referring symptoms down the posterior leg or even into the groin.

9. Contrast Piriformis syndrome and sciatica.
   - **Answer:** the symptoms for both Piriformis syndrome and sciatica may be identical, though the causes vary. Piriformis syndrome is usually caused by compression of the sciatic nerve as it passes between Superior gemellus and Piriformis, in the deep lateral rotator group. In some instances, the sciatic nerve pierces Piriformis, causing the symptoms. Sciatica is usually caused by compression of the sciatic nerve root as it exits the lumbar spine, perhaps by a herniated disc or a misalignment of the lumbar vertebrae.

10. Which muscles described in Chapter 9, Palpating Superficial Muscles of the Extremities, have distal tendons that help form the arch of the foot? Which palpations described in this chapter will at the same time palpate those distal tendons?
    - **Answer:** the distal tendons of Tibialis anterior and Peroneus longus help form the transverse arch of the foot. Palpation of the intrinsic muscles of the plantar foot will also palpate these distal tendons at their insertion on the base of the first metatarsal.

CASE PROFILES

Each client is individual. Although her anatomy is the same as all other human beings, the expression and the experience of her anatomy is hers alone. With that in mind, you can be aware that there are no "right" or "wrong" answers to the case profiles presented in *Touch & Movement: Palpation and Kinesiology for Massage Therapists*. As massage therapists, we assess the client in front of us on a given day, not a textbook profile. In reading and discussing the case profiles presented here, use your instincts, knowledge, and judgment, along with those of your classmates and the professionals who are available to guide you. The discussion points presented are a starting point for group discussion, which is strongly recommended. Some of the discussion points refer you to subsequent chapters in the text. Although you may form an initial plan for a client based upon the material presented in that case profile's chapter, taking another look at each case once you have learned all the assessment information presented in *Touch & Movement: Palpation and Kinesiology for Massage Therapists* allows you to fully utilize your assessment skills.

CHAPTER 1 CASE PROFILES

Case #1

Matt is a first-time client. When he made his appointment, he mentioned low-back pain after standing for more than 20 minutes or so. Will you assess Matt's standing or seated posture or both? What other assessments might you perform? What questions will you ask Matt?

- **Discussion points:** because Matt is a first-time client, it is important to perform "baseline" assessments of his standing and seated posture and his gait. Additional assessments may include asking Matt to demonstrate the standing posture that usually brings on his pain. Questions for Matt may center on the duration of his back pain and its specific location, any history of back injuries or surgeries, his usual level of physical activity, and how he has been treating his pain.

Case #2

Courtney, 21, is an avid skateboarder. She complains of pain in her right hip and knee. Will you assess Courtney's standing or seated posture or both? Will you assess her gait? What other assessments might you perform? What questions will you ask Courtney?

- **Discussion points:** assessing Courtney's standing posture and her gait is a starting point. It will also be important to assess her skating posture, utilizing information presented later in this Appendix. Duplicating Courtney's skating movements by deconstructing the complex movement of skateboarding, presented in Chapter 4, Deconstructing Complex Movements, will help you to target joints, muscles, and muscle groups for assessment. Additional questions for Courtney may focus on the frequency and duration of her skating

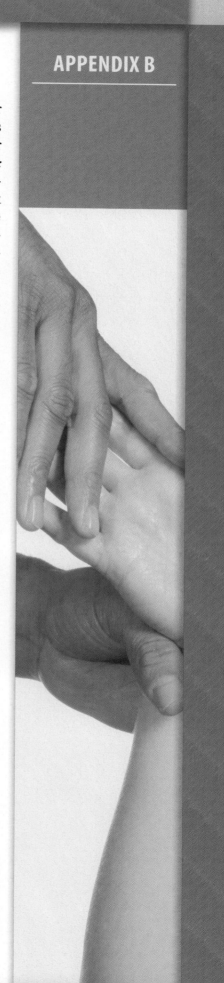

sessions, any past injuries she has experienced, pain in any other areas of her body, and what she has been doing to treat her pain and how it has worked for her.

Case #3

Clem, 72, walks for three miles every morning. Recently, he has been suffering from a very sore right shoulder after his morning walk. Will you assess Clem's standing or sitting posture or both? Will you assess his gait? What structures might you palpate? What questions will you ask Clem?

- **Discussion points:** assessing Clem's standing posture and his gait are important in creating a treatment plan. Asking Clem to duplicate the gait he uses during his morning walk will be helpful: people often adopt a different gait during exercise than they use during normal walking. Because his pain is centered in his right shoulder, utilize the information about arm swing in Chapter 3, Gait Assessment, to examine how he swings his right arm during his morning walk. Your assessment of his posture and gait will help you to select target structures for palpation, although the muscles that act on the arm are likely targets. An important question for Clem will be whether he holds a walking stick or cane in his right hand when he walks or whether he is accompanied on his walk by a dog, who may strain Clem's shoulder by pulling on his lead. Additional questions may concern how he treats his shoulder pain and what other health conditions he is being treated for and whether his walking shoes are comfortable and replaced often.

CHAPTER 2 CASE PROFILES

Case #1

Megan is a healthy, 36-year-old stay-at-home mom who complains of constant soreness in her right lumbar area, especially after a long walk. Her left shoulder and neck are also often sore. Your initial visual assessment shows that the hem of Megan's T-shirt is hiked up on the right and that her head is slightly tilted toward her left shoulder. What postural assessments will you perform next? What do you suspect is the source of Megan's neck, shoulder, and low-back pain?

- **Discussion points:** subsequent postural assessments would include examining the symmetry of Megan's shoulders and hips, any anterior or posterior tilt of her pelvis, and the curvature of her spine. Candidates as sources for Megan's shoulder and low-back pain may include structural or functional short-leg syndrome, lordosis or swayback, or kyphosis accompanied by a compensatory swayback.

Case #2

Sid, 27, is the editor of an online e-mag. He says his neck, shoulders, and upper back give him constant pain. In his downtime, Sid plays video poker while talking on his phone. What postural assessments will you perform on Sid? What do you immediately expect to find? What work habits may be contributing to Sid's back and neck problems?

- **Discussion points:** assessing Sid's seated posture at the computer may reveal the source of his pain. Ask Sid to demonstrate his customary work-station posture. Assess the position of his lumbar spine in relation to the back of his chair and the compensations it creates. Ask Sid to show you how he manages to use his phone at his work station: he may be straining muscles by holding it in between his neck and his shoulder. Ask Sid how many hours a day he spends at his computer work station and whether or not he schedules regular breaks to move around the room. Sid's work station may be poorly set up, adding to his pain.

Case #3

Janice, 47, is otherwise in great shape but complains of an aching pain in her left thigh and hip after standing all day at her job in a rare-book store. In visually assessing Janice's posture, you notice that her right leg remains slightly bent as she stands. What postural assessments will you perform next? What do you suspect is the source of Janice's left thigh and hip pain?

- **Discussion points:** Janice's thigh and hip pain be may caused by a structurally or functionally shortened left leg. She unconsciously levels her hips to maintain equilibrium by chronically flexing her right thigh at the hip, an action that throws all her body weight onto her left leg. Assess Janice for short-leg syndrome.

CHAPTER 3 CASE PROFILES

Case #1

Bethany, 31, is a flight attendant who works long shifts on intercontinental flights. She reports to you that she is experiencing pain and sometimes even numbness down the outside of both her thighs. What alteration of Bethany's gait may be resulting in this pain? What could be the cause of the alteration in gait?

- **Discussion points:** Bethany's gait may be altered for several reasons. She may wear high heels while she works, causing her to shorten her step length, or she may have to rotate her torso and narrow her step width to negotiate the narrow airplane aisles. Bethany's pain may be the result of iliotibial band syndrome.

Case #2

Joe, 38, just bought a new treadmill and has been walking on it for five miles each day. Dissatisfied with the weight loss he's had in the past month, he has raised the angle of his treadmill to increase the difficulty of his workout. Now, Joe tells you he is having pain, stiffness, and some cramping in the muscles in the back of his legs and in his hips. What alteration of Joe's gait may be resulting in Joe's symptoms? What could be the cause of the alteration in gait?

- **Discussion points:** Joe's gait on his new treadmill may not be normal. Joe may have narrowed his step width and limited or eliminated his natural arm swing. Either alteration in gait may be contributing to his hip pain. In addition, by creating an incline in his walking surface, Joe has altered the angle of his foot during the stance phase of his gait, potentially straining the muscles and associated structures on his posterior leg.

Case #3

Jeanette, 63, has osteoporosis. She tells you that sometimes her right foot catches on the ground while she's walking, and she's very afraid she might fall. What postural and/or gait assessments will you perform on Jeanette? What postural deviations and muscle dysfunctions may account for her walking problem?

- **Discussion points:** because of Jeanette's age and her osteoporosis, the risk of fracturing her femur during a fall is high. A structurally or functionally shortened leg may contribute to the appearance of foot drop on her longer-leg side. Assessment of Jeanette's standing posture and her gait are recommended. An additional question for Jeanette may include asking about the use of area rugs, on which she might trip. Examining Jeanette's shoes for wear patterns may reveal foot problems that suggest a referral to her health-care provider.

CHAPTER 4 CASE PROFILES

Case #1

CJ, 24, reports that he's had pain in his left lower back ever since he had to stow his heavy backpack in the overhead compartment of the plane on his trip home last week. During which stage of this complex movement might CJ have strained his left lower back? During which joint actions? Which agonist and antagonist muscles may have been involved? Could any postural deviations have contributed to his injury? What assessments and palpations do you plan to perform?

- **Discussion points:** CJ may have strained his lumbar Erector spinae or Transversospinalis group muscles or his Quadratus lumborum during the active stage of lifting a heavy object above his head. The actions of those agonist muscles would have been opposed by Transversus abdominis and the Abdominal obliques. Joint actions may have included hyperextension of his trunk in the lumbar region spinal joints. Several postural deviations may have played a role: increased anterior pelvic tilt, head-forward posture, unilaterally elevated hip, or iliotibial band syndrome.

Case #2

Sara, a 36-year old waitress, had to miss her last massage appointment to work an extra shift. She is tired and tense today. Sara takes most of the session to relax, but toward the end seems to deeply relax and may even be asleep when you leave the room. When Sara comes out of your treatment room, she's limping and rubbing her right hip and tells you she hurt herself getting up from the table. During which stage of this complex movement might Sara have strained her right hip? During which joint actions? Which agonist and antagonist muscles may have been involved? Could any postural deviations or gait patterns contributed to her injury? What assessments and palpations do you plan to perform?

- **Discussion points:** Sara may have strained her low back and hip during the initiation or action stages of getting off the massage table. In those stages, joint actions may include flexion, extension, lateral flexion, and rotation of the trunk at the lumbar spinal joints and flexion, extension, medial, and lateral rotation the thigh at the acetabulofemoral joint. Muscles acting as agonists and antagonists in those actions include the Gluteals, Psoas major, Tensor fasciae latae, the Lumbar erector spinae and Transversospinalis groups, and Quadratus lumborum, among others. Postural deviations such as unilateral elevation of either hip or increased pelvic tilt may be contributing factors. Assessment of all the structures and muscles listed above, plus the associated structures such as her iliotibial band (ITB) and thoracolumbar fascia is recommended. Sara's fatigue and deep relaxation during the massage may have contributed to the strain by causing her to move too quickly—before her muscles were ready to move—and without her normal awareness of balance. It is always a good idea to caution clients to take their time getting off the table, moving slowly and making sure they are alert and in equilibrium.

Case #3

Jennifer, 39, is a busy single mom and massage therapist who has recently started working out at a health club. Jenn has pain in her mid-back and posterior cervical muscles. How do you assess the potential causes of Jenn's pain? What complex movements might you ask her to perform? What posture deviations or gait dysfunctions might you look for, and how will you assess them?

- **Discussion points:** assessment of Jennifer's pain might begin by asking her to demonstrate some massage strokes, working at her usual table height, and the exercises she is doing at the health club. Postural assessment would focus on examining Jennifer's spinal curvatures for a head-forward posture, rounded shoulders, kyphosis, or swayback.

CHAPTER 5 CASE PROFILES

Case #1

Juan, 45, is a new client who has never had a massage before. For months, he has had pain that travels from his right hip into his lateral leg. He says the pain is deep and aching. Sometimes taking an over-the-counter pain pill helps, but the pain now tends to return quickly, even after taking his usual dosage. Looking at Table 5.2, how would you characterize Juan's pain? In listening to the words Juan uses to describe his pain, is it likely to be acute, chronic, or breakthrough pain or a combination of these?

■ **Discussion points:** Juan is experiencing somatic pain that has become chronic, but seems to become acute when he experiences breakthrough pain.

Case #2

Emily, 27, is a nursing assistant in an assisted living facility where she cares for elder patients, sometimes helping them into and out of their wheelchairs. She tells you she has pain, tingling, and numbness in her right hip and sometimes in her right low back. Looking at Table 5.4, what condition could be causing Emily's symptoms? How might this condition impact Emily's perception of touch during palpation?

■ **Discussion points:** Emily seems to be experiencing nerve entrapment, possibly due to Piriformis syndrome or sciatica. In areas close to the sciatic nerve pathway—her low back or down her posterior thigh—Emily's perception of pressure and pain may be disrupted, resulting in her either feeling more pain or being unaware of pressure, and she may be unable to perform directed actions to their fullest range without eliciting acute pain.

Case #3

Suzanne, 57, has a chronic autoimmune disease—lupus. She takes multiple medications for her condition, including steroids and prescribed narcotics for pain. What steps will you take to ensure that your palpation of Suzanne's tissues is appropriate and takes into account the possible side effects of her medications that may interfere with her perception of touch?

■ **Discussion points:** the first recommended step is to obtain information about the dosages and specific side effects of Suzanne's medications, including their cumulative effects over time. Next, ask Suzanne how long she has been taking the medications at their current dosage, and whether she is aware of any increase in side effects. Long-term steroid use may degrade soft tissues in the body and destabilize joints, and narcotics interfere with the client's ability to perceive pressure, temperature, and pain appropriately. Palpation pressure should be very light and movement of her joints through their range of motion should be minimal, with the massage therapist being sure to fully support the joints during the movement.

CHAPTER 6 CASE PROFILES

Case #1

Phil is a 38-year-old mechanic who complains of pain and stiffness in his right shoulder that sometimes radiates all the way down his arm, into his hand. What target structures would you palpate on this client? What positions would you place this client in for palpation? Describe the structures you would locate and the procedure for locating them.

- **Discussion points:** the structures in the upper-right quadrant and surrounding Phil's right shoulder are targets for palpation, including the glenohumeral joint, the cervical and upper thoracic vertebrae, the muscles of the rotator cuff, and Trapezius, Levator scapulae, and the Rhomboids. Many of the structures are most easily palpated with the client in side-lying position. Refer to Chapter 7, Palpating Bony Landmarks and Fascial Structures and Chapter 8, Palpating Superficial Muscles of the Axial Skeleton, for information on locating and palpating these structures.

Case #2

Amy is a 45-year-old dancer who has pain and stiffness in her right hip and the lateral side of her right thigh when she walks or climbs stairs. What target structures would you palpate on this client? What positions would you place this client in for palpation? Describe the structures you would locate, the muscle actions you would direct, and your process for adding resistance to movement.

- **Discussion points:** target structures for palpation on Amy may include the iliac crest, the greater trochanter, and the ITB, plus Tensor fasciae latae, the Gluteals, and Quadratus lumborum. Having the client in side-lying position is recommended for directing actions and adding resistance during adduction, extension, and medial and lateral rotation of the thigh at the acetabulofemoral joint. Prone position is a secondary positioning recommendation.

Case #3

Carl is a 56-year-old writer who is quite sedentary and overweight. He has come to a massage therapist because of persistent pain across his upper back. What target structures would you palpate on this client? What positions would you place this client in for palpation? Describe the structures you would locate, the muscle actions you would direct, and your process for adding resistance to movement. What palpation skills will help you meet the challenge of this client's body structure?

- **Discussion points:** Carl's target structures for palpation may include those involved in a head-forward and rounded shoulders posture, such as the cervical and thoracic spinal curves of the spine and the position of each shoulder. Muscles and muscle-group targets may include Trapezius, the Rhomboids, Levator scapulae, Splenius capitis, the rotator cuff muscles, SCM, the Scalenes, plus Pectoralis major and minor. Palpation may be best accomplished in seated and side-lying positions. Muscle actions to be directed and resisted may include flexion, lateral flexion, and extension of the head at the spinal joints and medial and lateral rotation of the arm at the glenohumeral joints. Carl's excessive weight and sedentary lifestyle may present the palpation challenges of tender tissues and limited range of motion.

CHAPTER 7 CASE PROFILES

Case #1

Sandra, 45, drives a delivery truck all day, five days a week. She has pain in her right axilla (armpit) that has been evaluated by her primary care physician, who found no pathology or disease process that would cause the pain, which is worse toward the end of the day and the end of the week. Sandra thinks her work has something to do with the pain. What bony structures would you palpate first in evaluating Sandra's presenting problem? What client positions would you use for these palpations?

- **Discussion points:** target bony structures for palpation may include all the landmarks on the posterior and anterior scapula, the spinous processes of cervical and upper thoracic vertebrae, and the glenohumeral joint. Palpating spinous processes and the posterior scapula are easily palpated with the client prone.

Case #2

Marie is a 71-year-old woman who recently retired from her work as a ski instructor. After decades on the slops, Marie has ongoing pain, stiffness, and poor mobility in her hips and knees. What bony and fascial structures would you palpate first in evaluating Marie's hips and knees? What changes in position and pressure might be indicated for Marie because of her age and frailty?

- **Discussion points:** target bony and fascial structures for palpation include the iliac crest, the greater trochanter, the ITB, the patella and the patellar ligament, and the pes anserine tendon. Although side-lying is recommended for palpating many of these structures, Marie's age, pain, and stiffness may put too much pressure on the greater trochanter while she is side-lying if she does not have significant padding beneath her hip. Palpation pressure may need to be kept very light, and adding resistance to movement may be contraindicated for Marie.

Case #3

Tom is a 39-year-old entrepreneur who runs his Internet dating service business from his home, using his laptop as he reclines in his easy chair. He has come for a massage because of persistent headaches and neck pain. When you ask Tom to duplicate his position at his "workstation," you see that he semi-reclines and slumps his head forward. What bony and fascial structures would you palpate first in evaluating Tom's presenting complaints? What positions would you place Tom in for palpation?

- **Discussion points:** bony landmarks and fascial structures for palpation may include the cervical and thoracic spinous processes, the nuchal ligament, the posterior scapula, and the glenohumeral joint structures. You may decide to palpate Tom in seated, prone, and side-lying positions to palpate these structures comfortably.

CHAPTER 8 CASE PROFILES

Case #1

Maria, 49, was involved in a minor car accident two weeks ago when her car was hit from behind in a parking lot. She felt okay at first, but now is experiencing some dizziness and headaches, plus pain on the right side of her neck. What muscles will you target for palpation? What other assessments will you perform? Describe any cautions, positioning, or draping considerations for the palpations you plan to perform.

- **Discussion points:** it sounds as if Maria has suffered a whiplash-type injury. Target muscles for palpation may include the upper fibers of Trapezius, Splenius capitis, Levator scapulae, SCM, the Scalenes, and Longus colli. Additional assessment may include assessment of the position of the mandible, palpation of Temporalis and Masseter, and ROM at the cervical spinal joints. Cautions may include accommodating Maria's sensitivity to pressure, limited ROM, and discomfort in certain positions. Seated palpation may be a viable option, if Maria is comfortable supporting the weight of her head unassisted.

Case #2

Eddie, 27, is a house painter. He works long hours holding a paint sprayer, which is connected to a hose, in his right hand, sweeping it back and forth to apply the paint evenly. After four years at this job, Eddie is experiencing shooting pains and sometimes numbness and tingling down his right arm. By the end of the day, his right arm is so weak that he has to support his right elbow with his left hand. The symptoms are sometimes worst in the morning, after he has slept on his right shoulder. What muscles will you target for palpation? What other assessments will you perform? Describe any cautions, positioning, or draping considerations for the palpations you plan to perform.

- **Discussion points:** target muscles for palpation may include Trapezius, Levator scapulae, the Rhomboids, Serratus anterior, Pectoralis major and minor, the rotator cuff muscles, Deltoid, Biceps brachii, and Brachialis, plus forearm flexors and extensors. Other assessments may include observation of Eddie's standing posture, noting his head position and symmetry of his shoulders; ROM at the neck, shoulder, elbow, and wrist; and comparison of hand strength in each hand. Cautions may include accommodating Eddie's discomfort level and awareness of his altered perception of pain and pressure in areas of numbness. Seated, standing, supine, side-lying, and prone positions are all indicated, as long as his joints are supported and no weight is placed in his affected shoulder.

Case #3

David, 60, is experiencing pain in his neck, mostly on the right side, that runs down from his jaw and up into his head. A lawyer for a telecom company, David has lots of stress in his job and admits he takes the stress home and sometimes wakes up at night in pain because he's clenching his teeth so hard. What muscles will you target for palpation? What other assessments will you perform? Describe any cautions, positioning, or draping considerations for the palpations you plan to perform.

■ **Discussion points:** it sounds as if David is experiencing symptoms of temporomandibular joint disorder. Palpation targets include simultaneous palpation of the mandible and palpation of Temporalis, the Masseter and the Pterygoids, plus SCM, upper Trapezius, and the Scalene group. Other assessments may include range of motion (ROM) at the temporomandibular joint in elevation, depression, and medial and lateral deviation. Cautions may include accommodating David's limited ROM at the jaw, and potentially in the cervical spinal joints. These palpations may be done with David seated or supine.

CHAPTER 9 CASE PROFILES

Case #1

Stephanie is a 22-year-old MFA student, majoring in dance. In addition to her dance classes and rehearsals, Stephanie teaches aerobics every weekend at a community center on a hard concrete floor, to help pay her tuition. Stephanie has pain in her right lateral knee and hip and experiences sharper pain in her left shin. What muscles or muscle groups will you target for palpation on Stephanie? What client positions and draping will you use for these palpations?

■ **Discussion points:** Stephanie describes the symptoms of shin splints on one side of her body and iliotibial band (ITB) syndrome on the other. Palpation targets include Stephanie's right ITB, TFL, and the Quadriceps group, as well as her left Tibialis anterior and posterior, Extensor digitorum, and Peroneal muscles. These palpations may be done with Stephanie seated or supine.

Case #2

Oscar, 45, plays soccer three evenings a week and coaches a soccer team on the weekends. He complains of burning pain down the back of his right thigh and high on the inside of his thigh. The pain down the back of his right thigh doesn't get better even when he works out harder before and after soccer. What muscles or muscle groups will you target for Oscar? What client positions and draping will you use for these palpations?

■ **Discussion points:** Oscar may be experiencing Hamstrings and/ or Adductor strain. Palpation targets include the muscles of both groups, along with the ITB, Sartorius, and Gracilis and the pes anserine tendon, which receives the distal tendons of three muscles in this palpation. Palpation positions for Oscar include supine, side-lying and prone, with specific attention to secure draping.

Case #3

Myla, 29, works as a sales consultant for an interior design firm. Myla carries a large, heavy portfolio of fabric samples with her to her sales calls, over her left shoulder. She also pitches with her right arm in a softball league on weekends. Myla has persistent pain and stiffness in both shoulders and pain in her upper-right back. What muscles or muscle groups will you target for palpation on Myla? What client positions and draping will you use for these palpations?

■ **Discussion points:** Myla may be straining both shoulders, her left by the weight of her heavy portfolio and the right by pitching. Because of the difference in root cause, the muscles strained in each shoulder and the postural compensations on each side of her body will probably differ. Palpation targets on Myla's left side may include Trapezius, Levator scapulae, SCM, and the Scalene group. On her right side, palpation targets may include the rotator cuff group, Deltoid, Serratus anterior, and the Rhomboids. Although the client in side-lying position may be recommended for these palpations, it will exert pressure on whichever shoulder is bearing the weight of her torso in side-lying. The resulting discomfort may make the side-lying position a contraindication and indicate that seated, supine, and prone positions as more appropriate.

CHAPTER 10 CASE PROFILES

Case #1

Jim, 24, lost 50 pounds in the last year and is training hard for his first marathon, after years without exercising. After the first few miles, Jim begins to suffer intense pain in his right buttock, which soon spreads to his groin. The pain worsens when he runs in the desert, where he has to make frequent, sudden turns to avoid low-lying cactus. Sometimes, the pain is accompanied by tingling and "pins and needles" down his right leg. What muscles or muscle groups will you target for palpation on Jim? What client positions and draping will you use for these palpations? Which antagonist muscles will you also palpate?

■ **Discussion points:** Jim may have strained his lateral rotators during one of his sudden turns. Palpation targets include Piriformis, Quadratus lumborum, the lumbar Erector spinae and Transversospinalis groups, the Gluteals, and Psoas major. Several of these muscles are antagonists to another muscle used in some of the movements Jim does as he runs. Additional antagonist muscles as palpation targets may include TFL, Rectus abdominis, and the External obliques. Palpation positions may include supine, semi-side-lying, and full side-lying, as well as prone.

Case #2

Andre, 32, is afraid he's developing heart disease: he has pain and tenderness in his upper chest and weakness in his left arm. His symptoms have developed since he was in a car accident six months ago, when he was hit from behind, and his stress level has been high ever since. He's not sleeping well and often wakes up at night with his left shoulder hurting and tingling. What muscles or muscle groups will you target for palpation on Andre? What client positions and draping will you use for these palpations? Which antagonist muscles will you also palpate? Will you refer Andre to his doctor for an evaluation, and if so, why?

- **Discussion points:** Andre should be referred to his primary health care provider for an evaluation of his symptoms before assessment by a massage therapist. Once he has received clearance from that provider to receive massage, the following muscles and muscle groups are palpation targets: Temporalis, Masseter, SCM and the Scalenes, Longus colli, Trapezius, Levator scapulae, and the Rhomboids, as well as the rotator cuff muscles as Serratus anterior. Many of the muscles listed are antagonists in the actions to be directed during palpation.

Case #3

Katie, 19, a student, has chronic pain and stiffness on the right side of her low back and hip. The pain is always worse after she walks several miles to campus each day carrying her two-year-old daughter to campus day care. Once in class, the pain can get even worse: at 6 feet tall (183 cm), Katie is uncomfortable in the cramped chairs in her crowded classroom. What muscles or muscle groups will you target for palpation on Katie? What client positions and draping will you use for these palpations? Which antagonist muscles will you also palpate?

- **Discussion points:** Katie may be chronically elevating one hip as she carries her toddler to school and then after her long trek, immobilizing her lower body at her cramped desk. Palpation target structures may include the lumbar spinous processes; the symmetry of her pelvis, the Erector spinae and Transversospinalis muscle groups; the Gluteals, TFL, and the ITB; Quadratus lumborum and Psoas major; and the Quadriceps, Adductor, and Hamstrings groups. Supine, prone, and side-lying positions may all be necessary for these palpations, with specific attention to secure draping. In addition to the muscles listed above that are antagonistic during actions you will direct during palpation, Rectus abdominis and the External obliques may be palpation targets.

INDEPENDENT STUDY ACTIVITIES

Included in this Appendix are five templates for deconstructing common complex movements, for readers who care to explore movement deconstruction on additional movements. Also included are additional touch sensitivity exercises that interested readers may practice independently.

COMMON COMPLEX MOVEMENTS TEMPLATES

Movement for deconstruction: _____

Initiation stage:

At the trunk:
- Joint actions at the spinal joints: _____
- Muscles acting on the trunk: _____
- Joint actions at cervical spinal joints: _____
- Muscles acting on the head: _____
- Joint actions at the lumbosacral joint: _____
- Muscles acting on the pelvis: _____

At the proximal joints:
- Joint actions at each acetabulofemoral joint: _____
- Muscles acting on each thigh: _____
- Joint actions at each glenohumeral joint: _____
- Muscles acting on each arm: _____
- Joint actions at each tibiofemoral joint: _____
- Muscles acting on each leg: _____
- Joint actions at each humeroulnar joint: _____
- Muscles acting on each forearm: _____

At the distal joints:
- Joint actions at each talocrural joint: _____
- Muscles acting on each foot: _____
- Joint actions at each radiocarpal joint: _____
- Muscles acting on each hand: _____
- Joint actions within the hands and feet: _____
- Muscles acting within the hands and feet: _____

Action stage:

At the trunk:
- Joint actions at the spinal joints: _____
- Muscles acting on the trunk: _____
- Joint actions at cervical spinal joints: _____
- Muscles acting on the head: _____
- Joint actions at the lumbosacral joint: _____
- Muscles acting on the pelvis: _____

At the proximal joints:
- Joint actions at each acetabulofemoral joint: _____
- Muscles acting on each thigh: _____

- Joint actions at each glenohumeral joint: _____
- Muscles acting on each arm: _____
- Joint actions at each tibiofemoral joint: _____
- Muscles acting on each leg: _____
- Joint actions at each humeroulnar joint: _____
- Muscles acting on each forearm: _____

At the distal joints:
- Joint actions at each talocrural joint: _____
- Muscles acting on each foot: _____
- Joint actions at each radiocarpal joint: _____
- Muscles acting on each hand: _____
- Joint actions within the hands and feet: _____
- Muscles acting within the hands and feet: _____

Transition stage:

At the trunk:
- Joint actions at the spinal joints: _____
- Muscles acting on the trunk: _____
- Joint actions at cervical spinal joints: _____
- Muscles acting on the head: _____
- Joint actions at the lumbosacral joint: _____
- Muscles acting on the pelvis: _____

At the proximal joints:
- Joint actions at each acetabulofemoral joint: _____
- Muscles acting on each thigh: _____
- Joint actions at each glenohumeral joint: _____
- Muscles acting on each arm: _____
- Joint actions at each tibiofemoral joint: _____
- Muscles acting on each leg: _____
- Joint actions at each humeroulnar joint: _____
- Muscles acting on each forearm: _____

At the distal joints:
- Joint actions at each talocrural joint: _____
- Muscles acting on each foot: _____
- Joint actions at each radiocarpal joint: _____
- Muscles acting on each hand: _____
- Joint actions within the hands and feet: _____
- Muscles acting within the hands and feet: _____

COMMON COMPLEX MOVEMENTS TEMPLATES

Movement for deconstruction: _____

Initiation stage:

At the trunk:
- Joint actions at the spinal joints: _____
- Muscles acting on the trunk: _____

- Joint actions at cervical spinal joints: _____
- Muscles acting on the head: _____
- Joint actions at the lumbosacral joint: _____
- Muscles acting on the pelvis: _____

At the proximal joints:

- Joint actions at each acetabulofemoral joint: _____
- Muscles acting on each thigh: _____
- Joint actions at each glenohumeral joint: _____
- Muscles acting on each arm: _____
- Joint actions at each tibiofemoral joint: _____
- Muscles acting on each leg: _____
- Joint actions at each humeroulnar joint: _____
- Muscles acting on each forearm: _____

At the distal joints:

- Joint actions at each talocrural joint: _____
- Muscles acting on each foot: _____
- Joint actions at each radiocarpal joint: _____
- Muscles acting on each hand: _____
- Joint actions within the hands and feet: _____
- Muscles acting within the hands and feet: _____

Action stage:

At the trunk:

- Joint actions at the spinal joints: _____
- Muscles acting on the trunk: _____
- Joint actions at cervical spinal joints: _____
- Muscles acting on the head: _____
- Joint actions at the lumbosacral joint: _____
- Muscles acting on the pelvis: _____

At the proximal joints:

- Joint actions at each acetabulofemoral joint: _____
- Muscles acting on each thigh: _____
- Joint actions at each glenohumeral joint: _____
- Muscles acting on each arm: _____
- Joint actions at each tibiofemoral joint: _____
- Muscles acting on each leg: _____
- Joint actions at each humeroulnar joint: _____
- Muscles acting on each forearm: _____

At the distal joints:

- Joint actions at each talocrural joint: _____
- Muscles acting on each foot: _____
- Joint actions at each radiocarpal joint: _____
- Muscles acting on each hand: _____
- Joint actions within the hands and feet: _____
- Muscles acting within the hands and feet: _____

Transition stage:

At the trunk:
- Joint actions at the spinal joints: _____
- Muscles acting on the trunk: _____
- Joint actions at cervical spinal joints: _____
- Muscles acting on the head: _____
- Joint actions at the lumbosacral joint: _____
- Muscles acting on the pelvis: _____

At the proximal joints:
- Joint actions at each acetabulofemoral joint: _____
- Muscles acting on each thigh: _____
- Joint actions at each glenohumeral joint: _____
- Muscles acting on each arm: _____
- Joint actions at each tibiofemoral joint: _____
- Muscles acting on each leg: _____
- Joint actions at each humeroulnar joint: _____
- Muscles acting on each forearm: _____

At the distal joints:
- Joint actions at each talocrural joint: _____
- Muscles acting on each foot: _____
- Joint actions at each radiocarpal joint: _____
- Muscles acting on each hand: _____
- Joint actions within the hands and feet: _____
- Muscles acting within the hands and feet: _____

COMMON COMPLEX MOVEMENTS TEMPLATES

Movement for deconstruction: _____

Initiation stage:

At the trunk:
- Joint actions at the spinal joints: _____
- Muscles acting on the trunk: _____
- Joint actions at cervical spinal joints: _____
- Muscles acting on the head: _____
- Joint actions at the lumbosacral joint: _____
- Muscles acting on the pelvis: _____

At the proximal joints:
- Joint actions at each acetabulofemoral joint: _____
- Muscles acting on each thigh: _____
- Joint actions at each glenohumeral joint: _____
- Muscles acting on each arm: _____
- Joint actions at each tibiofemoral joint: _____
- Muscles acting on each leg: _____
- Joint actions at each humeroulnar joint: _____
- Muscles acting on each forearm: _____

At the distal joints:

- Joint actions at each talocrural joint: _____
- Muscles acting on each foot: _____
- Joint actions at each radiocarpal joint: _____
- Muscles acting on each hand: _____
- Joint actions within the hands and feet: _____
- Muscles acting within the hands and feet: _____

Action stage:

At the trunk:

- Joint actions at the spinal joints: _____
- Muscles acting on the trunk: _____
- Joint actions at cervical spinal joints: _____
- Muscles acting on the head: _____
- Joint actions at the lumbosacral joint: _____
- Muscles acting on the pelvis: _____

At the proximal joints:

- Joint actions at each acetabulofemoral joint: _____
- Muscles acting on each thigh: _____
- Joint actions at each glenohumeral joint: _____
- Muscles acting on each arm: _____
- Joint actions at each tibiofemoral joint: _____
- Muscles acting on each leg: _____
- Joint actions at each humeroulnar joint: _____
- Muscles acting on each forearm: _____

At the distal joints:

- Joint actions at each talocrural joint: _____
- Muscles acting on each foot: _____
- Joint actions at each radiocarpal joint: _____
- Muscles acting on each hand: _____
- Joint actions within the hands and feet: _____
- Muscles acting within the hands and feet: _____

Transition stage:

At the trunk:

- Joint actions at the spinal joints: _____
- Muscles acting on the trunk: _____
- Joint actions at cervical spinal joints: _____
- Muscles acting on the head: _____
- Joint actions at the lumbosacral joint: _____
- Muscles acting on the pelvis: _____

At the proximal joints:

- Joint actions at each acetabulofemoral joint: _____
- Muscles acting on each thigh: _____
- Joint actions at each glenohumeral joint: _____
- Muscles acting on each arm: _____
- Joint actions at each tibiofemoral joint: _____

- Muscles acting on each leg: _____
- Joint actions at each humeroulnar joint: _____
- Muscles acting on each forearm: _____

At the distal joints:
- Joint actions at each talocrural joint: _____
- Muscles acting on each foot: _____
- Joint actions at each radiocarpal joint: _____
- Muscles acting on each hand: _____
- Joint actions within the hands and feet: _____
- Muscles acting within the hands and feet: _____

COMMON COMPLEX MOVEMENTS TEMPLATES

Movement for deconstruction: _____

Initiation stage:

At the trunk:
- Joint actions at the spinal joints: _____
- Muscles acting on the trunk: _____
- Joint actions at cervical spinal joints: _____
- Muscles acting on the head: _____
- Joint actions at the lumbosacral joint: _____
- Muscles acting on the pelvis: _____

At the proximal joints:
- Joint actions at each acetabulofemoral joint: _____
- Muscles acting on each thigh: _____
- Joint actions at each glenohumeral joint: _____
- Muscles acting on each arm: _____
- Joint actions at each tibiofemoral joint: _____
- Muscles acting on each leg: _____
- Joint actions at each humeroulnar joint: _____
- Muscles acting on each forearm: _____

At the distal joints:
- Joint actions at each talocrural joint: _____
- Muscles acting on each foot: _____
- Joint actions at each radiocarpal joint: _____
- Muscles acting on each hand: _____
- Joint actions within the hands and feet: _____
- Muscles acting within the hands and feet: _____

Action stage:

At the trunk:
- Joint actions at the spinal joints: _____
- Muscles acting on the trunk: _____
- Joint actions at cervical spinal joints: _____

- Muscles acting on the head: _____
- Joint actions at the lumbosacral joint: _____
- Muscles acting on the pelvis: _____

At the proximal joints:
- Joint actions at each acetabulofemoral joint: _____
- Muscles acting on each thigh: _____
- Joint actions at each glenohumeral joint: _____
- Muscles acting on each arm: _____
- Joint actions at each tibiofemoral joint: _____
- Muscles acting on each leg: _____
- Joint actions at each humeroulnar joint: _____
- Muscles acting on each forearm: _____

At the distal joints:
- Joint actions at each talocrural joint: _____
- Muscles acting on each foot: _____
- Joint actions at each radiocarpal joint: _____
- Muscles acting on each hand: _____
- Joint actions within the hands and feet: _____
- Muscles acting within the hands and feet: _____

Transition stage:

At the trunk:
- Joint actions at the spinal joints: _____
- Muscles acting on the trunk: _____
- Joint actions at cervical spinal joints: _____
- Muscles acting on the head: _____
- Joint actions at the lumbosacral joint: _____
- Muscles acting on the pelvis: _____

At the proximal joints:
- Joint actions at each acetabulofemoral joint: _____
- Muscles acting on each thigh: _____
- Joint actions at each glenohumeral joint: _____
- Muscles acting on each arm: _____
- Joint actions at each tibiofemoral joint: _____
- Muscles acting on each leg: _____
- Joint actions at each humeroulnar joint: _____
- Muscles acting on each forearm: _____

At the distal joints:
- Joint actions at each talocrural joint: _____
- Muscles acting on each foot: _____
- Joint actions at each radiocarpal joint: _____
- Muscles acting on each hand: _____
- Joint actions within the hands and feet: _____
- Muscles acting within the hands and feet: _____

COMMON COMPLEX MOVEMENTS TEMPLATES

Movement for deconstruction: _____

Initiation stage:

At the trunk:
- Joint actions at the spinal joints: _____
- Muscles acting on the trunk: _____
- Joint actions at cervical spinal joints: _____
- Muscles acting on the head: _____
- Joint actions at the lumbosacral joint: _____
- Muscles acting on the pelvis: _____

At the proximal joints:
- Joint actions at each acetabulofemoral joint: _____
- Muscles acting on each thigh: _____
- Joint actions at each glenohumeral joint: _____
- Muscles acting on each arm: _____
- Joint actions at each tibiofemoral joint: _____
- Muscles acting on each leg: _____
- Joint actions at each humeroulnar joint: _____
- Muscles acting on each forearm: _____

At the distal joints:
- Joint actions at each talocrural joint: _____
- Muscles acting on each foot: _____
- Joint actions at each radiocarpal joint: _____
- Muscles acting on each hand: _____
- Joint actions within the hands and feet: _____
- Muscles acting within the hands and feet: _____

Action stage:

At the trunk:
- Joint actions at the spinal joints: _____
- Muscles acting on the trunk: _____
- Joint actions at cervical spinal joints: _____
- Muscles acting on the head: _____
- Joint actions at the lumbosacral joint: _____
- Muscles acting on the pelvis: _____

At the proximal joints:
- Joint actions at each acetabulofemoral joint: _____
- Muscles acting on each thigh: _____
- Joint actions at each glenohumeral joint: _____
- Muscles acting on each arm: _____
- Joint actions at each tibiofemoral joint: _____
- Muscles acting on each leg: _____
- Joint actions at each humeroulnar joint: _____
- Muscles acting on each forearm: _____

At the distal joints:

- Joint actions at each talocrural joint: _____
- Muscles acting on each foot: _____
- Joint actions at each radiocarpal joint: _____
- Muscles acting on each hand: _____
- Joint actions within the hands and feet: _____
- Muscles acting within the hands and feet: _____

Transition stage:

At the trunk:

- Joint actions at the spinal joints: _____
- Muscles acting on the trunk: _____
- Joint actions at cervical spinal joints: _____
- Muscles acting on the head: _____
- Joint actions at the lumbosacral joint: _____
- Muscles acting on the pelvis: _____

At the proximal joints:

- Joint actions at each acetabulofemoral joint: _____
- Muscles acting on each thigh: _____
- Joint actions at each glenohumeral joint: _____
- Muscles acting on each arm: _____
- Joint actions at each tibiofemoral joint: _____
- Muscles acting on each leg: _____
- Joint actions at each humeroulnar joint: _____
- Muscles acting on each forearm: _____

At the distal joints:

- Joint actions at each talocrural joint: _____
- Muscles acting on each foot: _____
- Joint actions at each radiocarpal joint: _____
- Muscles acting on each hand: _____
- Joint actions within the hands and feet: _____
- Muscles acting within the hands and feet: _____

TOUCH SENSITIVITY EXERCISES

The following exercises are described to include a partner or an observer, but they can also be performed solo.

Exercise #1

Materials needed: a table or desk that has clear access to its underside surface and a very heavy, dense object such as a pile of thick books, a heavy briefcase, a large bucket filled with water, etc., to place atop the surface.

   Strategy: a blindfolded massage therapist must correctly identify the placement site of a heavy object on a surface by palpating the underside of that surface with his hands to sense the density of energy that may be felt beneath where the object is placed.

Exercise:
1. Working blindfolded, preferably seated in a rolling chair for ease of movement and with an observer, place both your hands on the underside of the table or desk.
2. Slowly palpate, exploring the underside surface completely, to assess the placement of the heavy object. *Hint: there will be a "density" of energy where the object lies.* Tell your observer what your conclusion is.
3. Move the object to a different site on the same surface and repeat the exercise. Assess your results, gauging how successfully you sensed the presence of the heavy object through your fingertips.

Exercise #2

Materials needed: a thick telephone book or another book that has very thin paper, a spool of heavy-duty thread, and a spool of super-fine thread or a human hair.

Strategy: a blindfolded massage therapist must locate a length of heavy thread, followed by a length of fine thread or hair, placed within the pages of a telephone book. A partner will place the thread to be palpated approximately 30 pages into the telephone book, centered on the page vertically, horizontally, or at an angle, visible to others. The therapist will locate the thread by palpating from a depth of 30 pages, then 20 pages, then 10 pages and so on, if need be, to assess fine touch and texture sensitivity.

Exercise:
1. Working blindfolded and with a partner: gently palpate the pages of the open telephone book with your dominant hand, with sequentially fewer pages over the thread, until you can locate it by your touch.
2. Repeat the palpation with your non-dominant hand.
3. Assess the results with your partner: what was the difference between your fine touch sensitivity of your dominant and non-dominant hands?

A

Abduction: movement of a limb or a structure away from the midline of the body.

Acetylcholine (ACh): a neurotransmitter that triggers mechanisms at the neuromuscular junction that change the electrical charge inside the myofiber.

Acetylcholinesterase (AChE): an enzyme that inactivates acetylcholine (ACh), at the neuromuscular junction, ensuring a single and complete filament slide before another can be triggered by the presence of ACh.

Actin: a contractile protein within a myofiber that forms micro and thin filaments.

Action stage: the stage of complex movement during which multiple joints and muscles in the axial and appendicular skeleton are engaged; the action stage includes the aspects of movement that occur immediately after initiation.

Active movement: the client makes a muscle action unassisted by the massage therapist.

Acute pain: pain of less than six months' duration.

Adaptation: the decrease, over time, in the perception of a sensation, even though the stimulus remains.

Adduction: movement of a limb or a structure toward the midline of the body.

Agonist: the prime skeletal mover in a muscle action.

Allodynia: pain in response to a usually non-painful stimulus.

Alzheimer's disease: one form of dementia in which plaques, sticky deposits of a protein called beta amyloid, accumulate in the brain and result in the death of brain cells.

Ambidextrous: having equal facility with either hand.

Amyotrophic lateral sclerosis (ALS): a progressive neurological disease characterized by the degeneration of motor neurons and progressive atrophy of voluntary muscles.

Anatomical position: the position in which body is erect, the head faces forward, the palms of the hands face forward, and the feet are flat and face forward.

Angular: joint actions that result in an increase or a decrease in the angle between the articulating bones.

Ankylosing spondylitis: an inflammatory condition, usually inherited, in which bony overgrowths on the anterior of vertebral bodies join and eventually fuses the vertebrae.

Antagonist: a skeletal muscle that allows and limits the movement of an agonist in a muscle action.

Aponeurosis: a broad, flat layer of fascia that extends to connect muscles or other tendons.

Appendicular skeleton: portion of the skeleton that includes the clavicle, the scapula, and the upper extremity and the pelvis and the lower extremity.

AROM: active range of motion; the client demonstrates the range of motion at a joint, unassisted.

Arthrosis: another term for a joint.

Articulation: the joint itself or where the bones in a joint connect.

Asymmetry: an imbalance in the body's structure from one side of the body to the other; marked differences in the size or shape of contralateral structures.

Axial skeleton: portion of the skeleton that includes the skull, the hyoid bone, the thorax, the spine, and the sacrum.

Axis: a stationary pivot around which another structure may rotate.

B

Ball-and-socket joint: a joint in which a ball-shaped bone end fits into the deep socket of another bone, such as at the shoulder and the hip.

Bow legs: see *Genu varum*.

Breakthrough pain: pain that occurs when chronic pain no longer is controlled by medication.

Bruxism: grinding of the teeth often associated with temporomandibular joint dysfunction.

Bunion: see *Hallux valgus*.

Bursa: a sac filled with synovial fluid that reduces friction and cushion joint parts.

C

Cadence: the speed of one's gait.

Carpal tunnel syndrome: compression of the median nerve caused by swelling and irritation of the tissues that travel through the carpal tunnel or by misalignment of one or more of the carpal bones.

Carpal tunnel: a narrow passageway through the wrist formed by the Flexor retinaculum on the anterior and the carpal bones at its posterior.

Carpal tunnel syndrome: pain, tingling, or numbness caused by compression or entrapment of the median nerve as it travels beneath the transverse carpal ligament, the flexor retinaculum, of the wrist.

Caution: a client's local or systemic conditions that indicate extra care should be taken by the massage therapist before proceeding with palpation or massage treatment.

Chronic pain: pain of more than six months' duration.

Circumduction: circular movement of the distal part of a limb as the proximal part of the limb remains stationary.

Claw toe: when the foot is chronically everted, the resulting contraction of the distal tendons of extensor muscles toes may buckle the toes upward, giving them a claw-like appearance.

Compensation: the reactive accommodation by body structures to dysfunction that allows the body to maintain equilibrium.

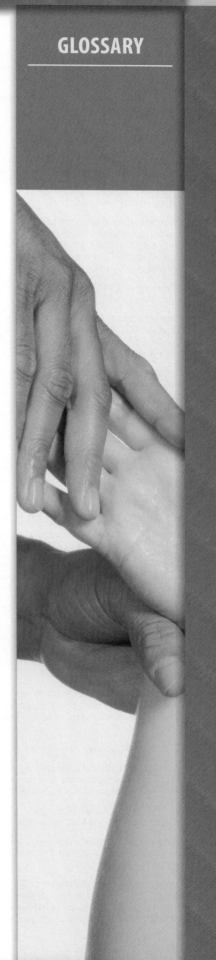

Complex movement: movement that involves multiple joint and muscle actions in both the axial and appendicular skeleton.

Concentric contraction: contraction that shortens a skeletal muscle.

Condyle: a large, round protuberance at the end of a long bone.

Condyloid joint: a joint in which an oval-shaped condyle of a bone fits into a basin-shaped bone.

Congenital: present at birth.

Contraindication: a condition that renders massage treatment, including palpation, potentially harmful. Contraindications may be local, confined to the area affected, or systemic, bodywide.

Convergent muscle: a muscle with an origin that is wider than its insertion.

Chronic obstructive pulmonary disease (COPD): a chronic, progressive lung condition that includes chronic bronchitis and emphysema.

Crest: a prominent ridge or an elongated projection on a bone.

Crude touch: the type of touch that detects that something has touched the skin; it does not perceive the exact location of the touch, nor the exact size, shape, or texture of the stimulus.

Cutaneous pain: pain that is detected by nociceptors in the epidermis.

D

Deep fascia: a type of dense connective tissue that lines the walls of the body and holds muscle groups together.

Dementia: a group of chronic, progressive neurological conditions that affect memory and cognitive function.

Depression: movement of a body part downward, away from the head.

Dermatomes: areas on the skin that provide sensory input to the central nervous system via specific spinal nerves and correspond to the sensory nerve pathway.

Deviation: a term for certain movements of structures away from anatomical position; a variation from the standard or normal expectation.

Diarthrotic: a freely moving joint.

Dominance (hand): the preference for using one hand over the other for reaching, grasping, holding, and manipulating objects.

Dorsiflexion: flexion of the dorsal aspect of the foot, pointing the toes toward the head.

Double support: the amount of time during gait when both limbs are touching the ground at the same time.

Dupuytren's contracture: a condition in which the fascia in the palm of the hand, either the palmar aponeurosis itself or one of the tendons deep to it, contracts, puckering the palm of the hand and maintaining one or more fingers in a flexed position.

Dynamic equilibrium: the type of equilibrium that maintains the position of your head in response to movement to keep you upright and balanced.

Dystonia: a neurological disorder that affects the ability of the brain to process certain neurotransmitters. The resulting bursts of stimulation to certain skeletal muscles cause involuntary movements, muscle strain, and contractures that disrupt gait.

E

Eccentric contraction: contraction that slackens or lengthens a skeletal muscle.

Elevation: movement of a body part upward, toward the head.

End feel: the palpation feedback during passive range of motion movements that indicates the limits of a joint's range of motion.

Endangerment site: a discrete, specific area on the body that indicates potential injury to the client because of its location near or over major nerves, blood vessels, or vital organs and that is vulnerable to injury from direct or significant pressure.

Endomysium: the inner layer of connective tissue that extends into the fascicles of a skeletal muscle to surround and separate individual muscle fibers.

Epicondyle: a small condyle; a rounded projection found above a condyle.

Epimysium: an extension of deep fascia that surrounds an entire skeletal muscle.

Equilibrium: the state of balance that maintains uprightness of posture.

Eversion: movement of the sole of the foot outward, away from the midline of the body.

Extension: an increase in the angle between articulating bones.

F

Facet: a flat, smooth articular surface.

Fascia: connective tissue that surrounds, supports, and separates structures.

Fascicle: a bundle of muscle fibers.

Fast pain: pain that occurs in response to a stimulus in about one-tenth of a second.

Fibromyalgia: a syndrome characterized by pain, fatigue, and stiffness in the connective tissue of the muscles, tendons, and ligaments.

Fine touch: touch that provides the detailed information lacking in crude touch: the exact location, size, shape, and texture of the stimulating source.

Flat feet: when the foot is chronically everted, transferring the weight of the body unequally onto the medial aspect of the plantar foot, flattening the medial longitudinal arch.

Flexion: a decrease in the angle between articulating bones.

Flexor retinaculum: also called the transverse carpal ligament, a strong fascial band around the anterior aspect of the carpals.

Foot drop: weak dorsiflexors cause the toes to fail to clear the ground during the swing phase of gait.

Foot flat: also called the loading response stage of the stance phase, when the foot is flat on the ground.

Foot slap: weak dorsiflexor muscles fail to keep the foot from slapping the ground during the stance phase of gait.

Fossa: a shallow depression in a bone.

Frontal plane: a plane that divides the body into anterior and posterior.

Fusiform muscle: a spindle-shaped skeletal muscle, with a belly that is wider than either the origin or the insertion.

G

Gait cycle: the stance and swing phases together. The gait cycle is equivalent to one stride or stride length.

Gait: an individual's style or manner of walking.

Genu recurvatum: the knee is hyperextended. The shaft of the femur angles toward the posterior, while the tibia and fibula angle toward the anterior.

Genu valgum: also called knock knees. The shaft of the femur angles toward the midline, while the tibia and fibula angle away from the midline.

Genu varum: also called bow legs. The shaft of the femur angles away from the midline, while the tibia and fibula angle toward the midline.

Gliding: a joint action during which relatively flat bones move back and forth and side to side over one another, with no significant change in the relative angle between the bones.

Goniometer: a device for measuring range of joint movement.

H

Hallux valgus: also called bunion; a bony prominence that develops at the first metatarsophalangeal joint, pushing the big toe (the hallux) toward and sometimes over the second toe.

Hammertoe: when the foot is chronically everted, the resulting contraction of the distal tendons of flexor muscles in the toes may buckle the toes upward, giving them a hammer-like appearance.

Heel-bone spurs: overgrowths of bone, also called osteophytes, that may develop on the plantar surface of the calcaneus; painful, heel-bone spurs affect posture and gait.

Heel off: stage four of the stance phase, also called terminal stance. The weight of the body, which shifted entirely onto this limb during midstance, now begins to transfer again as the foot prepares to leave the ground. Included in this stage is the preparatory push off, during which the body is propelled forward.

Heel strike: also called initial contact, heel strike occurs as the heel first makes contact with the ground. Heel strike is the beginning of the stance phase of gait.

Herniated disc: a condition in which disc material protrudes from between the bodies of adjacent vertebrae.

Hinge joint: a joint in which a convex bone end fits into a concave bone end.

Horizontal abduction: movement of a flexed limb away from the midline of the body, in the horizontal or transverse plane.

Horizontal adduction: movement of a flexed limb toward the midline of the body, in the horizontal or transverse plane.

Hyperesthesia: increased sensitivity to touch, often involving dysfunction of touch or pain receptors in the skin.

Hyperextension: extension of a body part beyond anatomical position.

Hyperkyphosis: another term for kyphosis, an exaggeration of the posterior thoracic curve of the spine.

Hyperlordosis: another term for lordosis, an exaggeration of the anterior lumbar curve of the spine.

Hypermobility: an excess of range of motion at a joint, sometimes the result of loose or stretched ligaments that fail to provide adequate support to the articulation.

Hypertonic: an excess of tone in a skeletal muscle.

Hypodermis: the layer of superficial fascia that separates skin from muscles.

Hypotonic: a lack of functional tone in a skeletal muscle.

I

Iliopsoas syndrome: also called iliopsoas tendonitis; an inflammation of the distal fibers of Iliopsoas, aggravated by forceful or repeated thigh flexion.

Iliotibial syndrome: strain along the iliotibial band in the lateral leg that may refer pain into the knee.

Initial contact: another term for heel strike, as the heel first makes contact with the ground. Heel strike is the beginning of the stance phase of gait.

Initiation stage: the first stage of a complex movement, when joints and muscles within the trunk and at the shoulder and hip are being arranged to carry out the active stages of movement; initiation includes the beginning posture from which action occurs.

Insertion: the skeletal muscle attachment on the bone that is usually mobile during contraction.

Inversion: movement of the sole of the foot inward, toward the midline of the body.

Isometric contraction: a skeletal muscle contraction that does not change the length of the muscle.

Isotonic contraction: a skeletal muscle contraction that changes the length of the muscle.

Itching: a local inflammatory response, often to chemical irritation.

J

Joint fit: the overall structure of an articulation, including its bony parts, ligaments, and other accessory structures.

K

Kinesiology: the study of the anatomy and mechanics of human movements, large and small.

Knock knees: see *Genu valgum*.

Kyphosis: an exaggeration of the posterior thoracic curve of the spine.

L

Laminectomy: a surgical procedure in which the laminae of adjoining vertebrae may be trimmed or removed to relieve pressure on the spinal cord by enlarging the spinal canal or the vertebrae themselves may be fused during the procedure.

Lateral epicondylitis: also called tennis elbow, a condition including pain, inflammation, and tenderness to touch at or near the lateral epicondyle of the humerus; often follows intensive lifting or gripping.

Lateral flexion: bending of the head or the trunk to one side.

Lateral rotation: the anterior surface of a long bone rotates away from the midline of the body, sometimes called external rotation.

Lateralization: a phenomenon of the brain; the left side of the brain sends messages to and controls the right side of the body and vice versa.

Ligament: a band of dense, fibrous connective tissue that connects bone to bone.

Line of pull: an imaginary line drawn on a muscle from its origin to its insertion that indicates the direction in which it will act on the joint it crosses.

Lines of cleavage: the linear clefts in the skin that indicate the direction of its fibers.

Loading response: another term for the foot-flat stage of the stance phase that follows the heel strike, when the foot is flat on the ground.

Lordosis: an exaggeration of the anterior lumbar curve of the spine.

M

Mechanoreceptor: a sensory receptor that detects mechanical pressure and senses touch, pressure, vibration, proprioception, and hearing and equilibrium.

Medial epicondylitis: also called golfer's elbow, a condition including pain, inflammation, and tenderness to touch at or near the medial epicondyle of the humerus; common in golfers.

Medial rotation: the anterior surface of a long bone rotates toward the midline of the body, sometimes called internal rotation.

Meniscus: a plate of cartilage found at synovial joints that allows bones of different shapes to articulate and stabilizes them during movement.

Midstance: in this stage of the stance phase, the weight of the body has entirely shifted onto the limb that has been mobile and is now in stance. The body can now balance completely on that limb.

Mother hand: the non-palpating hand, which is used to stabilize the client's body, to provide secure touch and to balance the massage therapist's body position.

Motor-unit recruitment: the process that ensures safe, smooth, muscle contraction and delays muscle fatigue; it allows some motor units to relieve strain on other motor units by alternating contraction.

Motor unit: a motor neuron and all the myofibers it stimulates.

Multipennate muscle: a skeletal muscle with fibers arranged diagonally in multiple rows. A central tendon may itself branch into other tendons.

Multiple sclerosis: the progressive destruction of myelin, the protective covering around sensory and motor neurons in the central nervous system. Symptoms include the progressive loss of motor control and perception of sensations, including touch, pressure, and pain.

Myasthenia gravis: an autoimmune disease in which neurotransmitter receptor sites at the neuromuscular junction degenerate or are destroyed, interfering with muscle contraction and progressively weakening muscles.

Myofiber: a muscle cell.

Myosin: a contractile protein within a myofiber that forms thick filaments.

N

Nerve entrapment: pain, tingling, numbness, weakness, and possible loss of function caused by compression of a nerve by nearby tissues.

Neuromuscular junction: the functional junction between the nervous and muscular systems.

Neuron: a nerve cell.

Neuropathic pain: pain that results from damage to nervous system structures.

Neuropathy: pain, numbness, or tingling caused by damage to peripheral nerves (those outside the central nervous system).

Neurotransmitter: a chemical messenger from the nervous system that assists a nerve impulse across the synaptic gaps along its route.

Nociceptive pain: pain that results from damage to tissues.

Nociceptors: sensory receptors that detect physical or chemical damage to tissues (pain).

Non-support: the period of time when both feet are off the ground, usually only during a running gait.

O

Oblique plane: a plane that divides the body or a section of the body at an angle.

Opposition: a diagonal movement of the thumb across the hand, making contact with the other digits.

Origin: the skeletal muscle attachment on the bone that usually remains fixed during contraction.

Orthotics: inserts that fit into one or both shoes, designed to compensate for unequal leg length and dysfunctions in the arches and other aspects of the foot.

Osteoarthritis: degeneration of the articular cartilage around synovial joints, due to age-related wear and tear on the joints.

Osteoporosis: a chronic, progressive condition that is the result of calcium being "pulled off" the bones.

P

Palpation feedback: the characteristics of the palpated tissue experienced by the palpating massage therapist.

Palpation: the application of purposeful focused touch for therapeutic assessment of somatic structures.

Parallel muscle: a skeletal muscle with fibers that run parallel to each other; sometimes called a strap muscle.

Paresthesia: tingling, pricking, or burning, usually not painful, in one area.

Parkinson's disease: a neurological disorder in which neurons in the substantia nigra area of the brain that produces dopamine degenerate and eventually die. Dopamine is the neurotransmitter that produces smooth muscle movement by balancing the contractions of agonists and antagonists.

Passive movement: the therapist moves the structure during an action; the client does not participate.

Pectoralis minor syndrome: one type of thoracic outlet syndrome in which Pectoralis minor entraps nearby structures: the shoulders are rounded to the anterior when protraction of the scapula is sustained by a tight Pectoralis minor and is not counterbalanced due to weakness in Serratus anterior.

Pennate muscle: a skeletal muscle with many fibers per motor unit. A pennate muscle is strong, but tires easily.

Perception: the conscious awareness and interpretation of sensations.

Perimysium: the intermediate layer of connective tissue within a skeletal muscle; surrounds groups of muscle fibers into fascicles.

Phantom pain: pain that persists in a body limb that has been amputated.

Phasic muscle: a skeletal muscle that is a mover of the skeleton, used for quick, powerful movement.

Piriformis syndrome: the Piriformis muscle of the deep lateral rotators of the thigh creates pressure or irritation on the sciatic nerve as it travels between Piriformis and Superior gemellus, causing pain, numbness, or tingling in the gluteal region or referring symptoms down the posterior leg and even into the groin. The pain from piriformis syndrome is deep and made worse by walking, stepping up stairs, or squatting.

Pivot joint: at a pivot joint, a bony process rotates around an axis.

Planar joint: at a planar joint, flat or slightly curved bones glide against one another.

Plantar fasciitis: a painful condition that impacts standing posture and gait, often the result of irritation or inflammation of the plantar aponeurosis.

Plantarflexion: flexion of the plantar aspect of the foot, pointing the toes away from the head.

Posterior axillary fold: a mass of tissue created by the junction of Latissimus dorsi and Teres major and a pad of adipose tissue.

Postural muscle: a skeletal muscle that stabilizes and supports the posture of the body.

Posture: the arrangement of your body and limbs while standing, sitting, or reclining.

Pressure: touch that displaces tissue.

Preswing: also called toe off; the last stage of the stance phase, representing the snippet of time before and during which the toes leave the ground.

Process: a projection on a bone that serves as attachment sites for ligaments and tendons.

PROM: passive range of motion; a therapist moves a client's joint through its range of motion without the client's participation.

Pronation: rotation of the radius around the ulna to turn the palm of the hand downward.

Proprioception: internal perception of the position of one's body parts without looking at them.

Protraction: movement of the shoulder or the jaw forward, toward the anterior.

Push off: during stage four of the stance phase is the preparatory push off, during which the body is propelled forward—the point of walking—by the muscles that strongly plantarflex the foot.

R

Radial deviation: abduction of the hand at the wrist, moving it away from the midline of the body.

Range of motion: the degree of movement, measured in a circle, allowed at a synovial joint.

Referred pain: pain that is felt on or just deep to the skin, but which does not arise from the site where the pain sensation is perceived.

Resistance to movement: the application of gentle pressure on a body structure to elicit stronger muscle contraction during palpation.

Resisted movement: muscle action by the client while the massage therapist provides resistance against the movement.

Resting length: the normal length of the non-contracting muscle, maintained by its tone.

Retraction: movement of the shoulder or the jaw backward, toward the posterior.

Retinaculum: a fibrous, transverse band of deep fascia that holds body structures in place.

Reverse action: an action in which the structure that is usually mobile is fixed, while the structure that is usually fixed is mobile.

Rheumatoid arthritis: a progressive autoimmune disease in which the body's immune system attacks the synovial membranes of multiple joints.

Rocking-horse gait: a type of gait that occurs when a weak Gluteus maximus leaves the thigh in continuing extension during the stance phase; as the trunk shifts toward the posterior to compensate, gait takes on a forward-to-backward shifting motion, like a rocking horse.

Rotation: revolution of a bone around a single longitudinal axis.

Rounded shoulders: one result of a kyphotic thoracic curve; the scapulae are moved laterally, altering the position of the glenohumeral joint and bringing the head of the humerus down and toward the anterior.

S

Saddle joint: a joint in which the shape of one bone's articular surface looks like a saddle, while its joint partner is shaped to sit in it, as a rider would sit in a saddle.

Sagittal plane: a plane that divides the body into left and right halves.

Sciatica: pain, tingling, or numbness in the hip or groin caused by compression of the sciatic nerve root, usually by a disc herniation in the lumbar region.

Scoliosis: a spinal curvature that is laterally S-shaped or C-shaped, usually in the thoracic and lumbar regions. The vertebrae are not stacked squarely over one another at the midline.

Secondary gain: the experience of reaping benefit from a usually negative experience, such as when a client gains physical or emotional benefit from maintaining the status quo of an injury or chronic condition.

Sensation: the awareness of change in a condition.

Sensory receptor: a specialized neuron in the peripheral nervous system that converts a stimulus into an electrical signal strong enough to produce nerve impulses.

Shin splints: pain along the tibia caused by stress on the connective tissue that attaches Tibialis anterior to the bone.

Short-leg syndrome: a discrepancy in leg length that may be structural, in which one leg is truly anatomically shorter than the other, or functional, perhaps as a compensation for scoliosis.

Single support: the stage during the stance phase of gait when the entire weight of the body is on the limb that is in contact with the ground.

Slow pain: pain that develops about a second or so after the stimulating event and gradually increases in intensity.

Somatic pain: pain that arises from a body structure.

Somatic sensory receptors: sensory receptors that detect stimuli arising from body structures.

Spine: a long, raised ridge on a bone.

Spinous process: a sharp, slender projection on a bone.

Stabilizer: a skeletal muscle that fixes proximal joints in place during an action, so that distal limbs can bear weight more effectively, unhindered by unnecessary movements.

Stance phase: the period of time during which one or both limbs are in contact with the ground; the weight-bearing phase of the gait cycle.

Static equilibrium: the maintenance of the position of your body in relation to your environment, or the force of gravity.

Stenosing tenosynovitis: another term for trigger finger, when one or more fingers or the thumb is chronically flexed, or extends only with difficulty in a snap-like movement similar to pulling a trigger, caused by a narrowing of the sheath surrounding the tendon of either Flexor digitorum superficialis or Flexor digitorum profundus as it travels to the distal phalanx.

Step length: the distance between the heel strikes of the left and right feet.

Step width: the usual distance between the feet during the stance phase of gait.

Stimulus: a change in the environment that produces a physiological response.

Strap muscle: another name for a parallel muscle.

Striated: the appearance of skeletal or cardiac muscle tissue that when viewed under a microscope has alternating light and dark bands.

Stride or stride length: the distance between one heel strike and the subsequent heel strike of the same foot.

Stroke: also called a CVA, or cerebrovascular accident. When a stroke occurs, an area of the brain is deprived of oxygen, either because a blood clot has blocked an artery, called an ischemic stroke, or because there has been bleeding in the brain, called a hemorrhagic stroke.

Styloid process: a sharp, pointed projection on a bone.

Superficial fascia: connective tissue that separates the skin from the muscles beneath it; sometimes called the hypodermis.

Supination: rotation of the radius around the ulna to turn the palm of the hand upward.

Supraspinatus tendonitis: pain, tenderness to touch, swelling, and local inflammation caused by a strain, tearing, or rupture of the supraspinatus tendon.

Swing phase: the period of time during which one limb is off the ground and swinging forward during the gait cycle.

Synergist: an adjacent skeletal muscle that assists the agonist or antagonist in an action.

Synovial joint: joint structure characterized by a surrounding fibrous capsule and an inner membrane-lined cavity filled with fluid; a freely moveable joint.

T

Tactile receptor: sensory receptor that detects touch and pressure.

Tactile sensation: sensation that results from touch, including fine and crude touch, pressure, vibration, itching, and tickling.

Target structure: the bony landmark, soft tissue structure, or muscle that is selected as a primary palpation site.

Temporomandibular joint disorder (TMJD): a condition characterized by headaches or dizziness, clicking or popping in the temporomandibular joint, pain, tinnitus, loss of full range of motion, or even locking in the joint. One cause of TMJD may be bruxism; other causes include osteoarthritis or an injury to the jaw, such as dislocation.

Tendon sheath: a tube-like bursa that wraps around tendons traveling through areas of great friction, such as at the wrist and the ankle.

Tendon: a cord of fascial connective tissue that attaches muscles to bone.

Terminal stance: another term for the heel-off stage of the stance phase of gait. The weight of the body, which shifted entirely onto this limb during midstance, now begins to

transfer weight again as the foot prepares to leave the ground. Included in this stage is the preparatory push off, during which the body is propelled forward.

Texture: the palpatory feel of the "grain" of muscle fibers.

Thermal sensations: sensations that result from warmth or coolness.

Thermoreceptor: sensory receptor that detects absolutes of and changes in temperature.

Thermoregulation: the adjusting of body temperature to within normal range.

Thixotropy: the property of fascia that allows it to melt and turn from gel-like to more liquid when a form of energy is applied, such as the heat and mechanical energy of massage.

Thoracic outlet syndrome: compression or entrapment of nerves in the brachial plexus and/or blood vessels that supply the arm, causing shooting pains, numbness and weakness, and possibly discoloration in the affected arm due to inadequate circulation.

Tickling: a sensory receptor response stimulated usually only by the touch of another person or by an object, such as a feather.

Tilt: the slight movement of one aspect of a structure away from anatomical position.

Tinnitus: persistent ringing or noise in the ears that is internally generated.

Tissue barrier: a pre-existing limitation on the manipulation of a tissue.

Toe off: The last stage of the stance phase, sometimes called preswing, representing the snippet of time before and during which the toes leave the ground.

Tone: the small amount of contraction remaining in the skeletal muscles of the trunk even during relaxation that helps to maintain posture.

Torticollis: also called wry neck; a condition in which the neck is kept in a twisted position by hypertonic muscles and/or postural compensation patterns.

Touch sensitivity: the ability of a massage therapist to place his or her hand on a client's body and accurately perceive and characterize the temperature, tone, texture, health, and energy of the tissue layers.

Transition stage: the stage of a complex movement during which the movement is concluding or has ended.

Transverse plane: a plane that divides the body into upper and lower (superior and inferior) sections.

Trendelenberg gait: a type of gait that results when a weak Gluteus medius on one side of the hip causes the opposite hip to drop during the swing phase of gait, shifting the trunk toward the weakened Gluteus medius during the stance phase in compensation.

Triangular muscle: another name for a convergent muscle.

Trigger finger: another term for *Stenosing tenosynovitis*.

Trigger point: an extremely irritable nodule in muscle tissue—usually near a tendinous attachment—that elicits acute pain at the site or refers pain elsewhere when palpated directly.

Trochanter: a very large, protruding projection on a bone.

Tropomyosin: a regulatory protein within a myofiber that allows or prohibits the slide of filaments to create skeletal muscle contraction by regulating the action of troponin.

Troponin: a regulatory protein within a myofiber whose action, governed by tropomyosin, allows or prohibits the slide of filaments to create skeletal muscle contraction.

Tubercle: a small, rounded projection on a bone.

Tuberosity: a large, usually roughened projection on a bone.

U

Ulnar deviation: adduction of the hand at the wrist, moving it toward the midline of the body.

Unipennate muscle: a skeletal muscle with fibers arranged to insert diagonally into a tendon, which creates great strength.

V

Vibration: sensations that result from tactile receptor signals that are both rapid and repetitive.

Visceral pain: pain that arises from a body organ.

W

Whiplash: a sudden, forceful flexion followed by extension, or vice versa, of the cervical spine, such as that experienced when struck on the head or hit from behind in a rear-end collision.

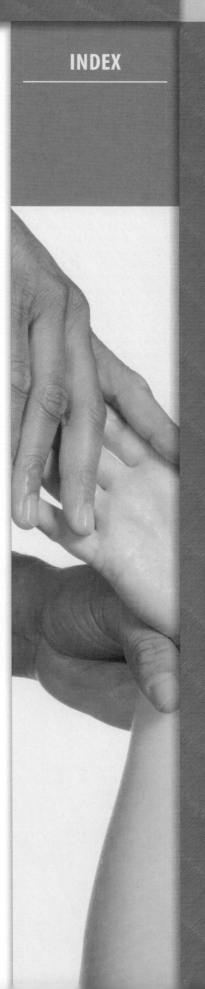

Note: Bold page numbers refer to figures (f) or tables (t)